PRINCIPLES OF DIABETES MELLITUS

PRINCIPLES OF DIABETES MELLITUS

7/3/02
To Eve Bloomgarden,
With best wishes and
great confidence in her
bright future.
good luck! Len Poretsky

edited by

Leonid Poretsky, M.D.
Beth Israel Medical Center, U.S.A.

KLUWER ACADEMIC PUBLISHERS
Boston / Dordrecht / London

Distributors for North, Central and South America:
Kluwer Academic Publishers
101 Philip Drive
Assinippi Park
Norwell, Massachusetts 02061 USA
Telephone (781) 871-6600
Fax (781) 681-9045
E-Mail: kluwer@wkap.com

Distributors for all other countries:
Kluwer Academic Publishers Group
Post Office Box 322
3300 AH Dordrecht, THE NETHERLANDS
Telephone 31 786 576 000
Fax 31 786 576 474
E-Mail: services@wkap.nl

 Electronic Services < http://www.wkap.nl >

Library of Congress Cataloging-in-Publication Data

A C.I.P. Catalogue record for this book is available
from the Library of Congress.

ISBN# 1-4020-7114-0

Printed on acid-free paper.

Printed in the United States of America.

The Publisher offers discounts on this book for course use and bulk purchases.
For further information, send email to melissa.ramondetta@wkap.com.

Contents

List of Contributors

Gerald B. Appel, M.D.
Director of Clinical Nephrology,
The Presbyterian Division of
New York Presbyterian Hospital,
Professor of Clinical Medicine,
Columbia University
College of Physicians and
Surgeons,
New York, New York.

Hisham Alrefai, M.D.
Research Fellow,
Division of Endocrinology,
Department of Internal Medicine,
Wayne State University,
Detroit, Michigan.

Mary Beyreuther, R.N., C.D.E.
Diabetes Nurse Educator,
Division of Endocrinology and
Metabolism,
Beth Israel Medical Center,
New York, New York.

Rajiv Bhambri, M.D.
Fellow in Endocrinology,
Robert Wood Johnson
University Medical School,
New Brunswick, New Jersey.

Zachary Bloomgarden, M.D.
Associate Clinical Professor of
Medicine,
Mount Sinai School of Medicine,
New York, New York.

Barry Brass, M.D., Ph.D.
Director, Diabetes Center,
Division of Endocrinology and
Metabolism,
Beth Israel Medical Center,
New York, New York.

David J. Brillon, M.D.
Director, Diabetes Care Center,
Associate Professor of Clinical
Medicine,
Weill Medical College of Cornell
University,
New York, New York.

Rochelle L. Chaiken, M.D.
Medical Director,
Diabetes Worldwide Team,
Pfizer, Inc.,
Associate Professor of Medicine,
State University of New York,
Downstate Medical Center,
Brooklyn, New York.

Russell L. Chin, M.D.
Fellow in Electromyography and
Clinical Neurophysiology,
Hospital for Special Surgery and
New York Presbyterian Hospital,
Weill Medical College of Cornell
University,
New York, New York.

Ken C. Chiu, M.D.
Assistant Professor of Medicine,
Division of Endocrinology,
Diabetes and Hypertension,
University of California at Los
Angeles Medical Center,
Los Angeles, California.

Theodore P. Ciaraldi, Ph.D.
Project Endocrinologist,
Division of Endocrinology,
Department of Medicine,
University of California at San
Diego,
La Jolla, California.

Richard Devereux, M.D.
Professor of Medicine,
Director, Laboratory of
Echocardiography,
New York Presbyterian Hospital,
Weill Medical College of Cornell
University,
New York, New York.

Daniel S. Donovan, Jr., M.D.
Assistant Clinical Professor of
Medicine,
Columbia University
College of Physician and
Surgeons,
New York, New York.

Andrew Drexler, M.D.
Director, The Mount Sinai
Diabetes Center,
Clinical Associate Professor of
Medicine,
Mount Sinai School of Medicine,
New York, New York.

Amal F. Farag, M.D.
Associate Professor of Medicine,
Director of Endocrinology,
Veteran's Affairs Medical Center,
State University of New York,
Brooklyn, New York.

Adrienne M. Fleckman, M.D.
Associate Chairperson of
Medicine,
Beth Israel Medical Center,
Professor of Clinical Medicine,
Albert Einstein College of
Medicine,
New York, New York.

Christine L. Frissora, M.D.
Assistant Professor of Medicine,
Division of Gastroenterology and
Hepatology,
The Weill Medical College of
Cornell University,
New York, New York.

Asha Thomas-Geevarghese, M.D.
Clinical Fellow,
Division of Endocrinology,
Department of Medicine,
Columbia University College of
Physicians
and Surgeons,
New York, New York.

John E. Gerich, M.D.
Director of the General Clinical
Research Center,
Head of Diabetes Research
Laboratory,
Professor of Medicine,
University of Rochester School of
Medicine,
Rochester, New York.

10

Ira J. Goldberg, M.D.
Chief, Division of Preventive
Medicine,
Professor of Medicine,
Columbia University College of
Physicians
and Surgeons,
New York, New York.

Alina Gouller, M.D.
Director, Endocrine Clinic,
Division of Endocrinology and
Metabolism,
Beth Israel Medical Center,
New York, New York.

George Grunberger, M.D.
Director, Diabetes Program,
Detroit Medical Center,
Professor, Department of Internal
Medicine,
Professor, Center for Molecular
Medicine and Genetics,
Wayne State University,
Detroit, Michigan.

Martin Haluzik, M.D., PhD.
Research Fellow,
Diabetes Branch,
National Institute of Diabetes and
Digestive and Kidney Diseases,
National Institutes of Health,
Bethesda, Maryland.

Kevan C. Herold, M.D.
Associate Professor of Clinical
Medicine,
Columbia University College of
Physicians and Surgeons,
New York, New York.

William C. Hsu, M.D.
Joslin Diabetes Center,
Instructor in Medicine,
Harvard Medical School,
Boston, Massachusetts.

Alan M. Jacobson, M.D.
Senior Vice President,
Joslin Diabetes Center,
Professor of Psychiatry,
Harvard Medical School,
Boston, Massachusetts.

Ira M. Jacobson, M.D.
Chief, Division of
Gastroenterology and Hepatology,
Vincent Astor Professor of
Clinical Medicine,
New York Presbyterian Hospital,
Weill Medical College of Cornell
University,
New York, New York.

Yolanta Kruszynska, M.D., Ph.D.
Associate Adjunct Professor of
Medicine,
Division of Endocrinology,
Department of Medicine,
University of California,
San Diego, California.

Albert C. Leung, M.D.
Resident,
Department of Urology,
Montefiore Medical Center,
Albert Einstein College of
Medicine,
Bronx, New York.

Jennifer Liu, M.D.
Assistant Professor of Medicine,
Weill Medical College of Cornell
University,
New York, New York.

Christos Mantzoros, M.D., D.Sc.
Associate Program Director in
Endocrinology and Diabetes,
Beth Israel Deaconess Medical
Center,
Assistant Professor of Medicine,
Harvard Medical School,
Boston, Massachusetts.

Dorothy S. Martinez, M.D.
Fellow,
Division of Endocrinology,
Diabetes and Hypertension,
Department of Medicine,
University of California at Los
Angeles
School of Medicine,
Los Angeles, California.

Ellen S. Marmur, M.D.
Resident,
Department of Dermatology,
New York Presbyterian Hospital,
New York, New York.

Samy McFarlane, M.D.
Assistant Professor of Medicine,
Program Director, Division of
Endocrinology,
Diabetes and Hypertension,
State University of New York,
Downstate Medical Center,
Brooklyn, New York.

Maria A. Mendoza, R.N.
Nurse Practitioner, Coordinator
of Diabetes Education,
Jacobi Medical Center,
Assistant Professor of Nursing,
City University of New York,
New York, New York.

Arnold Melman, M.D.
Professor and Chairman,
Department of Urology,
Albert Einstein College of
Medicine,
Montefiore Medical Center,
Bronx, New York.

Christian Meyer, M.D.
Fellow in Endocrinology,
Department of Medicine,
University of Rochester School of
Medicine,
Rochester, New York.

Joseph A. Murphy, M.D.
Instructor in Ophthalmology,
Weill Medical College of Cornell
University,
New York Presbyterian Hospital,
New York, New York.

Jocelyn Myers, M.D.
Fellow, Division of
Endocrinology,
Department of Medicine,
Albert Einstein College of
Medicine,
Bronx, New York.

Fiona R. Pasternack, B.A.
Thomas Jefferson University
Hospital,
Jefferson Medical College,
Philadelphia, Pennsylvania.

Leonid Poretsky, M.D.
Chief, Division of Endocrinology,
Beth Israel Medical Center,
Professor of Medicine,
Albert Einstein College of
Medicine,
New York, New York.

Firas Rahhal, M.D.
Assistant Clinical Professor of
Ophthalmology,
Retinal Surgery Division,
University of California at Los
Angeles
School of Medicine,
San Luis Obispo, California.

Elliot J. Rayfield, M.D.
Clinical Professor of Medicine,
Mount Sinai School of Medicine,
New York, New York.

Eileen Reilly, R.N., F.N.P., C.D.E.
Diabetes Nurse Educator/Nurse
Practitioner,
Division of Endocrinology and
Metabolism,
Beth Israel Medical Center,
New York, New York.

Marc L. Reitman, M.D., Ph.D.
Chief, Molecular Biology and
Gene Regulation Section,
Diabetes Branch, National
Institute of Diabetes and
Digestive and Kidney Diseases,
National Institutes of Health,
Bethesda, Maryland.

Marian Rewers, M.D., Ph.D.
Clinical Director,
Barbara Davis Center for
Childhood Diabetes,
Professor of Pediatrics and
Preventive Medicine,
University of Colorado Health
Sciences Center,
Denver, Colorado.

Carolyn Robertson, APRN, MSN
Associate Director,
The Mount Sinai Diabetes Center,
The Mount Sinai Medical Center,
New York, New York.

Laura Ronen, R.D., C.D.E.
Staff Nutritionist,
Division of Endocrinology and
Metabolism,
Beth Israel Medical Center,
New York, New York.

Jordan L. Rosenstock, M.D.
Fellow in Nephrology
Division of Nephrology,
Department of Medicine
Columbia University College of
Physicians and Surgeons,
Presbyterian Division of the New
York Presbyterian Hospital,
New York, New York.

Michael Rubin, M.D.
Chief, Neuromuscular Service,
Director, Electromyography
Laboratory,
New York Presbyterian Hospital,
Professor of Clinical Neurology,
Weill Medical College of Cornell
University,
New York, New York.

Tamer N. Sargios, M.D.
Fellow,
Division of Gastroenterology and
Hepatology,
Department of Medicine,
Beth Israel Medical Center,
New York, New York.

Adina E. Schneider, M.D.
Clinical Fellow in Endocrinology
and Metabolism,
Mount Sinai School of Medicine,
Division of Endocrinology and
Metabolism,
New York, New York.

Stephen H. Schneider, M.D.
Director, Diabetes Center,
Professor of Medicine,
Robert Wood Johnson
University Medical School,
New Brunswick, New Jersey.

Dennis Shavelson, D.P.M.
Faculty Podiatrist,
Beth Israel Medical Center and
Weill Medical College of Cornell
University,
New York, New York.

Anil Shrestha, M.D.
Fellow,
Division of Endocrinology and
Metabolism,
Beth Israel Medical Center,
New York, New York.

James R. Sowers, M.D.
Chief, Division of Endocrinology,
Professor of Medicine,
State University of New York,
Downstate Medical Center,
Brooklyn, New York.

Gladys Witt Strain, Ph.D., R.D.
Associate Clinical Professor of
Medicine,
Mount Sinai School of Medicine,
New York, New York.

Markus Stoffel, M.D.
Professor,
Director, Laboratory of Metabolic
Diseases,
The Rockefeller University,
New York, New York.

Jennifer K. Svahn, M.D.
Attending Surgeon,
Department of Surgery,
Division of Vascular Surgery,
Beth Israel Medical Center,
New York, New York.

Marsha C. Tolentino, M.D.
Fellow,
Division of Endocrinology and
Metabolism,
Beth Israel Medical Center,
New York, New York.

Matthew C. Varghese, M.D., M.P.H.
Associate Professor of Clinical
Dermatology,
Department of Dermatology,
New York Presbyterian Hospital,
Weill Medical College of Cornell
University,
New York, New York.

Elizabeth Walker, D.N.Sc., R.N.
Associate Professor of Medicine,
Director, Prevention and Control
Component,
The Diabetes Research and
Training Center,
Albert Einstein College of
Medicine,
Bronx, New York.

Katie Weinger, Ed.D.
Instructor in Psychiatry,
Joslin Diabetes Center,
Harvard Medical School,
Boston, Massachusetts.

Garry W. Welch, Ph.D.
Assistant Professor of Psychiatry,
Joslin Diabetes Center,
Harvard Medical School,
Boston, Massachusetts.

Steven D. Wittlin, M.D.
Associate Professor of Medicine,
University of Rochester School of
Medicine,
Rochester, New York.

Vincent Yen, M.D.
Assistant Attending Physician,
St. Vincent's Medical Center,
Assistant Professor of Medicine,
New York Medical College,
New York, New York.

Jacek Zajac, M.D.
Fellow,
Division of Endocrinology and
Metabolism,
Beth Israel Medical Center,
New York, New York.

Joel Zonszein, M.D.
Director, Clinical Diabetes
Center, Montefiore Medical
Center,
Professor of Clinical Medicine,
Albert Einstein College of
Medicine,
New York, New York.

Susan B. Zweig, M.D.
Fellow,
Division of Endocrinology and
Metabolism,
Beth Israel Medical Center,
New York, New York.

Preface

Diabetes mellitus is a very common disease. Described initially in the Egyptian papyrus *Ebers* in 1500 BC and now affecting approximately 150,000,000 people worldwide, with its prevalence rising rapidly, diabetes continues to mystify and fascinate both practitioners and investigators by its elusive causes and multitude of manifestations.

A neurosurgeon operating on a patient with a life-threatening brain tumor, an obstetrician delivering a baby, a psychiatrist trying to penetrate deep into a patient's emotional life – all will encounter diabetes from their very early days of medical practice. This disease will significantly affect the choice of therapeutic approaches throughout their careers, regardless of their specialty. Hence, there is need for every student of medicine, whatever his or her ultimate career goals, to understand and learn to manage diabetes.

Many excellent diabetes textbooks exist. Most of them, however, are written for endocrinologists. This textbook is written not only for endocrinologists, but also for other specialists, primary care physicians, housestaff, and particularly for medical students.

The needs of the latter group are well understood by the authors of this text, most of whom have been medical students and all of whom continue to teach medical students on a regular basis. The main challenge for a medical student is to "digest" a large amount of complicated, rapidly changing information under heavy time pressure. Therefore, a book written for medical students must not only be up-to-date and cover all aspects of the disease, from its pathogenesis on the molecular and cellular levels to its most modern therapy, but must also be concise, clear, and easy to use. To achieve these goals, we have made liberal use of illustrations and tables, provided a summary after each chapter, and added website addresses where additional information can be found to the lists of references. Each chapter is written to stand on its own, and readers who wish to explore a particular subject should not have to search through many chapters. This may have resulted in redundancies noticeable to readers of the entire text, but the pages where the most detailed discussion of a given topic can be found are highlighted in the index in bold print.

We hope that these features will make **Principles of Diabetes Mellitus** user-friendly. We also hope that readers will find this volume useful for studies of diabetes throughout their professional lives: first in medical school, then during the years of residency, and, finally, as they enter their chosen specialty.

The authors would like to dedicate this book to those from whom we learned and continue to learn about diabetes: our teachers, who inspired us to undertake studies of the challenging diabetes problems and then supported us throughout these studies; our students, who lead us to ponder new questions; and finally, our patients, who live with the disease every moment of every day and in some ways know more about it than we do.

We thank Jill Gregory for her expert help with illustrations and Anthony J. DiCarlo for help with computer programming. We also gratefully acknowledge the efforts of Marilyn Small Jefferson, who helped coordinate the work of sixty nine writers, and without whose patience, diligence, and dedication this book would not have been possible.

The authors.

I. The Main Events in the History of Diabetes Mellitus[*]

Jacek Zajac, Anil Shrestha and Leonid Poretsky

IN ANTIQUITY

A medical condition producing excessive thirst, continuous urination and severe weight loss has interested medical authors for over three millennia. Unfortunately, until the early part of 20th century the prognosis for a patient with this condition was no better than it was over 3000 years ago. Since the ancient physicians described almost exclusively cases of what is today known as type 1 diabetes mellitus, the outcome was invariably fatal.

Ebers Papyrus, which was written around 1500 BC, excavated in 1862 AD from an ancient grave in Thebes, Egypt, and published by egyptologist Georg Ebers in 1874, describes, among various other ailments and their remedies, a condition of "too great emptying of the urine"– perhaps, the reference to diabetes mellitus. For the treatment of this condition ancient Egyptian physicians were advocating the use of wheat grains, fruit and sweet beer.[1, 2]

Physicians in India at around the same time developed what can be described as the first clinical test for diabetes. They observed that the urine from people with diabetes attracted ants and flies. They named the condition "madhumeha" or "honey urine". Indian physicians also noted that patients with "madhumeha" suffered from extreme thirst and foul breath (probably, from ketosis). Although the polyuria associated with diabetes was well recognized, ancient clinicians could not distinguish between the polyuria due to what we now call diabetes mellitus from polyuria due to other conditions.[3]

Around 230 BC Apollonius of Mephis for the first time used the term "diabetes", which in Greek means "to pass through" (dia–through, betes–to go). He and his contemporaries considered diabetes a disease of the kidneys and recommended, among other ineffective treatments, such measures as bloodletting and dehydration.[4]

---

[*] Although the term "diabetes mellitus" was not firmly established until the nineteenth century, we will refer to this disease using its modern name throughout this chapter, even for the earlier periods.

The first complete clinical description of diabetes appears to have been made by Aulus Cornelius Celsus (30 BC–50 AD). Often called "Cicero medicorum" for his elegant Latin, Celsus included the description of diabetes in his monumental eight-volume work entitled "De medicina".[5, 6]

Aretaeus of Cappadocia, a Greek physician who practiced in Rome and Alexandria in the second century AD, was the first to distinguish between what we now call diabetes mellitus and diabetes insipidus. In his work "On the Causes and Indications of Acute and Chronic Diseases" he gave detailed account of diabetes mellitus and made several astute observations, noting, for example, that the onset of diabetes commonly follows acute illness, injury or emotional stress. Aretaeus wrote:

"Diabetes is a dreadful affliction, not very frequent among men, being a melting down of the flesh and limbs into urine. The patients never stop making water and the flow is incessant, like the opening of the aqueducts. Life is short, unpleasant and painful, thirst unquenchable, drinking excessive and disproportionate to the large quantity of urine, for yet more urine is passed....If for a while they abstain from drinking, their mouths become parched and their bodies dry; the viscera seem scorched up, the patients are affected by nausea, restlessness and a burning thirst, and within a short time they expire.[4, 5]

Both Aretaeus and the renowned Roman physician Galen observed that diabetes was a rare disease. In fact, Galen mentioned that he encountered only two such cases in his entire career.[4] Galen attributed the development of diabetes to weakness of the kidney and gave it a name "diarrhea of the urine" (diarrhoea urinosa).[5]

In the 5th century AD Susruta and Charaka, two Indian physicians, were the first to differentiate between the two types of diabetes mellitus, observing that thin diabetics developed diabetes at a younger age in contrast to heavier diabetics, who had a later onset and lived longer. In 7th century AD in China, Li Hsuan noted that the diabetics were prone to boils and lung infections. He prescribed avoidance of sex and wine as treatments for diabetes. Avicenna, or Ibn-Sina (980–1037 AD), a court physician to Caliphs of Baghdad, compiled an exhaustive medical text ("Canon Avicennae"), which included a detailed description of diabetes. Its clinical features, such as sweet urine and increased appetite, and complications, such as diabetic gangrene and sexual dysfunction, were described by Avicenna in detail.[7]

RENAISSANCE AND AFTER

The origin of current understanding of some aspects of diabetes can be traced to discoveries made in Europe between 16th and 18th centuries. Aureolus Theophrastus Bombastus von Hohenheim, a Swiss physician better known as Paracelsus (1494–1541), allowed the urine of diabetics to evaporate and observed a white residue. He incorrectly thought that this residue consisted of salt and proceeded to attribute excessive thirst and urination in diabetics to salt deposition in the kidneys.[8] In 1670 Thomas Willis in Oxford noticed the sweet taste of urine of patients with diabetes. Thomas Cawley, in 1788, was the first to suggest the link between the pancreas and diabetes after he observed that people with pancreatic injury developed diabetes.[8]

In 1776, British physiologist Matthew Dobson (1713–1784) in his "Experiments and observations on the urine in diabetics" was the first to show that the sweet tasting substance in the urine of diabetics was sugar. He also noted the sweet taste of serum of diabetics and therefore discovered hyperglycemia. Dobson put forward the theory that the diabetes was systemic disease, rather than one of the kidneys.[9]

THE NINETEENTH AND EARLY TWENTIETH CENTURY; DISCOVERY OF INSULIN

The important elements of current understanding of diabetes mellitus can be traced to 19th century, when modern scientific disciplines, including biochemistry and experimental physiology, acquired prominence in biological studies.

In 1815 Eugene Chevreul in Paris proved that the sugar in urine of diabetics was glucose. Von Fehling developed quantitative test for glucose in urine in 1848.[9] Thus, in the nineteenth century glucosuria became an accepted diagnostic criterion for diabetes.

Claude Bernard (1813–1878), professor of physiology at Sorbonne University, was one of the most prominent and prolific experimental physiologists in nineteenth century Europe. Because of the scope of Bernard's interests, Louis Pasteur referred to him as "Physiology itself".[10] In the course of his work on the physiology of gastrointestinal tract Bernard developed an experimental operation during which the pancreatic ducts were ligated. Degeneration of the pancreas followed. This technique proved invaluable for later experiments searching for pancreatic substance which controlled glucose level. In addition to developing the technique for pancreatic duct ligation, Bernard also discovered that the liver stored glycogen and secreted sugary substance into the blood. He assumed that it was an excess of this secretion that caused diabetes. Bernard's theory of sugar over-secretion leading to diabetes received wide acceptance.[11]

At the same time as researchers were looking for the cause of diabetes, clinicians were further advancing the understanding of diabetes mellitus as a systemic disease with various manifestations and complications. William Prout (1785–1850) was the first to describe diabetic coma and Wilhelm Petters in 1857 demonstrated the presence of acetone in the urine of diabetics. Adolf Kussmaul (1822–1902) proposed that acetonemia was the cause of diabetic coma. Henry Noyes in 1869 described retinopathy in a person with advanced diabetes. M. Troiser in 1871 observed diabetes in patients with hemochromatosis, naming it "bronze diabetes". [12]

John Rollo, Surgeon General to the British Army, added the term "mellitus" (derived from the Greek word for honey) to "diabetes" in order to distinguish it from diabetes insipidus. In 1897 Rollo developed a high protein, low carbohydrate diet and prescribed anorexic agents, such as antimony, digitalis and opium to suppress appetite in patients with diabetes.[4]

During the years prior to insulin discovery diabetes treatment mostly consisted of starvation diets. Frederick Allen, a leading American diabetologist of the time, believed that, since diabetics could not utilize the food efficiently, limiting the amount of food would improve the disease. The dietary restriction treatment was harsh and death from starvation was not uncommon in patients with type 1 diabetes on this therapy. On the other hand, it is easy to understand why outcomes of low calorie diets were often quite good in patients with type 2 diabetes.[12, 13]

Discovery of insulin by Frederick Banting and Charles Best was the final step in identifying the substance whose deficiency had been postulated to be responsible for development of diabetes. This milestone, however, was preceded by a number of earlier significant advances.

Oscar Minkowski (1858–1931) and Joseph von Mering (1849–1908), working in Strasbourg in 1889, observed that the dogs whose pancreas was removed developed severe thirst, excessive urination and weight loss with increased appetite. Minkowski, suspecting that such symptoms were caused by diabetes, tested the urine of these dogs and found glucose. Since Minkowski was working in the laboratory of Bernard Naunyn (1839–1925), who was interested in carbohydrate metabolism and was a leading authority on diabetes at the time, Minkowski's research received enthusiastic endorsement by Naunyn. Work on pancreatic extraction ensued, but the investigators were not able to obtain presumed anti-diabetic substance. They suspected that digestive juices produced by pancreas might have interfered with their ability to purify this substance. To prove that the absence of exocrine pancreatic secretion was not related to the development of diabetes, they ligated dog's pancreatic duct. This procedure led to the development of digestive problems but not the diabetes.[12, 14]

In 1893 a very important contribution was made by French investigator Edouard Hedon (1863–1933) in Montpellier, who showed that the total pancreatectomy was necessary for the development of diabetes. After removing the pancreas, he grafted a small piece of it under the skin. No evidence of diabetes in experimental animals was present at this stage. However, removal of the graft caused the symptoms of diabetes to develop immediately. Similar results were independently obtained by Minkowski. It was becoming clear that the internal secretion of the pancreas was pivotal to the pathogenesis of diabetes mellitus.[14]

In 1893 French scientist Gustave–Edouard Laguesse (1861–1927) suggested that tiny islands of pancreatic tissue described in 1869 by Paul Langerhans might be the source of the substance involved in blood glucose control. Paul Langerhans (1847–1888), distinguished German pathologist, was a student of Rudolf Virchow. In his doctoral thesis, at the age of 22, he described small groupings of pancreatic cells that were not drained by pancreatic ducts. In 1909, the Belgian physician Jean de Mayer named the presumed substance produced by the islets of Langerhans "Insulin". [15]

A number of researchers worked on the isolating of active component of internal pancreatic secretion. In 1902, John Rennie and Thomas Fraser in Aberdeen, Scotland, extracted a substance from the endocrine pancreas of codfish (Gadus callurious) whose endocrine and exocrine pancreata are anatomically separate. They injected the extract into the dog who soon died, presumably from severe hypoglycemia. In 1907 Georg Ludwig Zuelzer (1870–1949), a German physician, removed pancreas from the dog and then injected the dog with pancreatic extract. His experiments resulted in lowered amount of glucosuria and raised blood pH. Zuelzer patented the extract in the USA under the name Acomatol. In 1908, he used it successfully to rescue a comatose diabetic patient, but, owing to likely contamination of the extract by other substances, the treatment produced severe complications and led to withdrawal of further funding of Zuelzer's work by Schering. Zuelzer continued his investigations, however, and developed a new extract for Hoffman–La Roche. The new extract, extraction method for which he never published, produced convulsive reaction, most likely caused by hypoglycemia. [12,14] Nicolas Constantin Paulesco (1869–1931), professor of physiology at Bucharest University in Romania, was also involved in research on pancreatic extracts. In 1916 in the course of his first experiment, he injected the diabetic dog with the pancreatic extract. The injection resulted in the death of the animal with symptoms of hypoglycemia. During the experiment dog's blood glucose fell from 140 mg% to 26 mg%. Because of World War I Paulesco did not publish the report of his experiments until 1921. [12]

Frederick Grant Banting (1891–1941) was a young (and not very successful) orthopedic surgeon when he developed interest in diabetes. A war veteran, wounded in France in 1918, he was decorated with Military Cross for heroism. After returning from Europe, he briefly practiced orthopedic surgery and then took the position as a demonstrator in physiology at the University of Western Ontario, Canada. [16] On October 31, 1920 Banting wrote in his notebook:

"Diabetus (sic!). Ligate pancreatic ducts of the dog. Keep dog alive till acini degenerate leaving Islets. Try to isolate the internal secretion of these to relieve glycosurea". [16]

The technique of pancreatic duct ligation, leading to pancreatic degeneration, was developed and used for pancreatic function studies by

Claude Bernard, as discussed earlier. Banting approached John J.R. MacLeod, professor of physiology at the University of Toronto, who agreed to provide Banting with limited space in his laboratory for the eight-week summer period in 1921. McLeod assigned a physiology student Charles Best (1899–1978) to assist Banting with the experiments (Best apparently won the opportunity to work alongside Banting on the toss of coin with another student).[16]

In July 1921, after initial delays caused by insufficient ligature of the pancreatic ducts, Banting and Best were able to harvest atrophied pancreatic glands from the dogs, chop them up, grind the tissue in the mortar, strain the solution and inject the extract into the vein of pancreatectomized (diabetic) dog. When it was clear that the dog's condition improved, they proceeded to repeat the experiments with other diabetic dogs, with similar dramatic results. They also experimented with fresh pancreata, fetal calf pancreata and different routes of administration (rectal, subcutaneous, and intravenous).

At the end of 1921, biochemist James Collip joined the team of Banting and Best and was instrumental in developing better extraction and purification techniques.[12] First report of successful animal experiments with Banting's pancreatic extracts was presented at Physiological Journal Club of Toronto on November 14th, 1921 and American Physiological Society later that year.[17]

On January 11, 1922 Banting and Best injected with their extract Leonard Thompson, a 14-year old boy being treated for diabetes at Toronto General Hospital. At the time Thompson's weight was only 64 lb. After having 15 cc of "thick brown" substance injected into the buttocks, Thompson became acutely ill upon developing abscesses at the injection sites. Second injection, using a much improved preparation made with Collip's method, followed on January 23. This time the patient's blood glucose fell from 520 to 120 mg/dl within about 24 hours, urinary ketones disappeared, and Thompson quickly began to gain weight. He received ongoing therapy and lived for another 13 years, but died of pneumonia at the age 27.[16, 18]

On May 3, 1922 McLeod presented results of Toronto group's research to the Association of American Physicians and received standing ovation.[18] Banting and Best were not present at the meeting. In 1923, the Nobel Prize was awarded for discovery of insulin, but only to Banting and MacLeod, who shared their portions of the prize with Best and Collip, respectively.[12] The new proposed antidiabetic substance was named by Banting "Isletin". The name was later changed by MacLeod to Insulin, who did not know that this name had already been coined by de Mayer in 1909. Later on Banting and Best fully acknowledged this fact.[18]

In April 1922 Banting and Best accepted the offer by Eli Lilly Company to work on purification and large-scale commercial production of insulin. The Board of Governors of the University of Toronto and Eli Lilly signed the agreement, providing that Lilly would pay royalties to the

University of Toronto to support research in exchange for manufacturing rights for North and South America.[19]

The announcement of insulin discovery was greeted with tremendous enthusiasm around the world. Press was bringing numerous reports of miraculous cures. The following two examples are transcribed newspaper articles from Banting family scrapbook. The sources of the articles are not known: [20]

Insulin as a Life Saver
No deaths From Diabetes in Three Months in London

London, Ont., Oct. 2 – According to medical records made public to-day, for the first time in the history of the city of London, a three month period has elapsed without a death from diabetes. It is explained, however, that there have been several deaths in which diabetes existed with other complications, but no patient suffering alone from diabetes has succumbed. The Banting insulin treatment is the cause of happy change.

Edmonton Cure for Diabetic Coma Predates that in New York

Edmonton, Dec. 7 – A child in a state of diabetic coma, practically at death's door, is reported to have been brought back to life at the University of Alberta. This wonderful recovery was made possible through the use of insulin serum, manufactured in the University of Alberta laboratory by Dr. J.E.Collip, professor of biochemistry at the institution. Some two weeks ago a girl, eight-year old, was brought to the university hospital from her home near Vulcan, in southern Alberta. When he arrived, the child was in the state of diabetic coma, a condition, from which, as far as have been known, there had never been a recovery. This information was secured from Dr. E.H. Tory, president of the university, following the receipt of the dispatch from New York, which reported what was believed to be the first case of diabetic coma to be successfully treated in the annals of medicine in that city. The Edmonton cure apparently pre-dates that recorded in the dispatch from New York City.

Previously doomed patients were getting the new lease on life. Indeed, Ted Ryder, one of the first four children to receive insulin in 1922 in Toronto, died at the age of 76 in 1993.

Over the years insulin purification methods improved and new insulin formulations were developed. Protamine–zinc insulin, a long acting insulin, was introduced in 1930s; Neutral Hagedorn (NPH) was introduced in 1940s; and Lente series of insulin in 1950s.[19]

Among the people who first witnessed the introduction of insulin into the clinical use was a Portuguese physician named Ernesto Roma who was visiting Boston shortly after insulin became available. Upon returning to Portugal he founded the world's first organization for diabetics – the

Portuguese Association for Protection of Poor Diabetics. The association provided insulin free of charge to the poor. Founding of British Diabetic Association by Robin Lawrence, a physician with diabetes whose life was saved by insulin, and the writer H.G. Wells, who was also a diabetic, followed shortly in 1934.[21]

In 1922, August Krogh of Denmark, winner of the Nobel Prize for his studies of capillaries, was lecturing in the USA, accompanied by his wife Marie, who had recently been diagnosed with diabetes. Krogh and his wife were informed by famous diabetologist of the time Eliot P. Joslin about new diabetes treatment developed in Toronto by Banting's group. Marie and August Krogh decided, therefore, to visit Toronto and stayed as John McLeod's guests. After return to Denmark, Krogh, with H.C. Hagedorn, founded Nordisk Insulin Company, a not-for-profit concern that, together with Novo Company, was responsible for making Denmark the main insulin producing country outside of the USA.[22]

ORAL AGENTS IN DIABETES

Oral hypoglycemic agents were discovered following the fortuitous observations of hypoglycemia as a side effect of various investigative substances. In 1918, while investigating biological effects of guanidine, C.K. Watanabe noted that guanidine, under certain condition, can cause hypoglycemia. Watanabe injected guanidine subcutaneously into rabbits, initially causing hyperglycemia followed by hypoglycemia within several hours. Inspired by these findings, E. Frank, M. Nothmann and A. Wagner tried to modify the guanidine molecule. Several guanidine derivatives were studied, including monoguanidines and biguanidines. The biguanidines were found to have greatest hypoglycemic effect. The first commercially available guanidine derivative, dekamethyl–diguanidine, was introduced in 1928 and marketed in Europe under the name Synthalin. In USA phenylethyl–biguanidine was introduced for treatment of diabetes in 1957 and was available for clinical use in 1959 under the name Phenformin. Synthalin was discontinued from the use because of liver and kidney toxicity.[23]

Celestino Ruiz and L.L. Silva of Argentina noted the hypoglycemic properties of certain sulphonamide derivatives in 1939. In 1942 in occupied France professor of pharmacology at Montpellier University M.J. Janbon discovered that the sulphonylurea agent tested for the treatment of typhoid fever produced bizzare toxic side effects. Janbon correctly attributed these effects, which included confusion, cramps and coma, to hypoglycemia.[4, 23] This compound was then administered to diabetic patients, lowering their blood glucose. The researchers explored the potential mechanism of action of the substance and found that it became ineffective if experimental animal had been pancreatectomized. After well publicized research by German investigators Hans Franke and Joachim Fuchs, sulphonylureas were studied extensively. Franke and Fuchs discovered hypoglycemic actions of sulphonylureas during testing of the new long acting sulphonamide antibiotic. Chemists at Hoechst manufactured a compound D 860, which was marketed in the USA as tolbutamide in 1956. This compound became the first commercially available sulphonylurea agent.[23]

Many chemical substances have been studied for their hypoglycemic effect but extremely few have made it to the market. As an example, from 1962 to 1977 Boehringer–Mannheim and Hoechst studied eight thousand different chemicals for hypoglycemic properties, of which six thousand produced hypoglycemia in laboratory animals. Out of these only five made it as far as clinical tests and ultimately just one, HB 419 (glybenclamide/glyburide), was marketed. [23]

In addition to biguanides and sulphonylureas a number of other classes of oral hypoglycemic agents were ultimately discovered and are currently in clinical use. These are discussed in detail in chapter VIII.6.

USE OF RADIOIMMUNOASSAY FOR MEASUREMENT OF CIRCULATING INSULIN LEVEL

One of the most important milestones in the understanding of pathophysiology of diabetes was the development of radioimmunoassay (RIA) by Rosalyn Sussman Yalow (b.1921) and Salomon A. Berson (1919–1972).

During her graduate studies at the University of Chicago, Yalow, a nuclear physicist, worked on the development of the device to measure radioactive substances. In 1947 she became a consultant in nuclear physics at Veteran Administration Hospital in the Bronx, New York. She became a full time faculty member at the Bronx VA Hospital in 1950. Here Yalow worked with Salomon A. Berson investigating the use of radioactive isotopes in physiologic systems. Yalow and Berson developed the technique called radioimmunoassay (RIA), which allowed quantification of very small amounts of biological substances. The first report of the new technique in 1959 was largely ignored. [24]

The RIA is based on a principle of competition between the radio labeled compound of interest with unlabeled compound in the patient's serum for limited number of binding sites on the antibody against this compound. After the incubation period, which allows for equilibrium to develop, the antibody–antigen complexes are precipitated and the amount of radioactive label attached to the antibody is measured. Because of the competition for binding sites on the antibody, the higher the concentration of unlabeled compound in the patient's serum, the smaller amount of labeled compound will bind to the precipitated antibody. [25]

In 1959, using their method, Yalow and Berson demonstrated that diabetics did not always suffer from deficiency of insulin in their blood. Thus, insulin was the first hormone measured with the new technique. [24]

For this groundbreaking work Rosalyn Yalow was awarded many honors, including Nobel Prize in 1977, which she accepted on behalf of herself and Berson, who had died five years earlier. The Nobel Prize Committee called the RIA the most valuable advance in basic clinical research in the previous two decades. [24]

Yalow and Berson never patented the RIA technique, instead sparing no effort to make it more popular and accessible for the use by both the clinicians and investigators.

RECOMBINANT DNA TECHNOLOGY IN THE SYNTHESIS OF HUMAN INSULIN

The groundwork for the production of large quantities of human insulin was laid by Frederick Sanger (b. 1918), who published the structural formula of bovine insulin in 1955 while working at Cambridge University. He received Nobel Prize for this work in 1958.[23] Dorothy Hodgkin (1910–1994) described the three-dimensional structure of porcine insulin in 1969 at Oxford using X-ray crystallography.[26]

Prior to the development of recombinant DNA technology diabetics mostly received bovine or porcine insulin. Although bovine insulin differs from human insulin only by three amino acids and porcine only by one amino acid, these differences are sufficient for human immune system to produce antibodies against insulin, neutralizing its action and causing local inflammatory reactions. The pharmacokinetics of insulin are altered by its binding to antibodies, resulting in increased half-life of the circulating insulin and prolongation of its action. These considerations and growing demand for insulin, coupled with the difficulties in animal insulin production (it is estimated that 8000 lbs. of animal pancreatic tissue is needed to produce 1 lb. of insulin) prompted work on developing alternative sources of insulin. [27]

The gene coding for human insulin is located on the short arm of chromosome 11. Once incorporated in the bacterial plasmid of *E.coli* the human insulin gene became active resulting in the production of alpha and beta chains of insulin, which then were combined to construct complete insulin molecule. [28]

In 1978 Genentech, Inc. and City of Hope National Medical Center, a private research institution in Duarte, California announced the successful laboratory production of human insulin using recombinant DNA technology. This was achieved by team of scientists led by Robert Crea and David Goeddel. Insulin thus became the first genetically manufactured drug to be approved by the FDA. [27]

In July 1996, the FDA approved the first recombinant DNA human insulin analog, the insulin lispro. At present more than 300 human insulin molecule analogs have been identified, including about 70 animal insulins, 80 chemically modified insulins and 150 biosynthetic insulins.

LANDMARK CLINICAL TRIALS IN DIABETES

One of the major questions in diabetes therapy, which had remained unresolved until recently, was that of the relationship between glycemic control and the development of the complications of diabetes. The evidence supporting the role of metabolic abnormalities in the development of diabetic complications had long been known. It was not clear, however, if meticulous glycemic control could prevent the development of these complications.

Two very important studies were conducted to answer this question. Diabetes Control and Complications Trial (DCCT) was a large multi-center diabetes study conducted by NIH from 1983 to 1993. The study was designed to evaluate whether tight glucose control can prevent or reduce the rate of progression of long-term complications of diabetes. DCCT involved 1441 volunteers 13 to 39 years of age in 29 centers in the USA. They all had type 1 diabetes for at least one year but no longer than 15 years. The subjects were divided into 2 groups. The Primary Prevention group consisted of patients with type 1 diabetes of one to five years duration and no complications of diabetes. The subjects in the Secondary Intervention group had type 1 diabetes for 1 to 15 years. They also had mild diabetic nephropathy and retinopathy. Patients in both groups were randomized to receive either intensive or conventional therapy. The goal of intensive therapy was to keep pre-meal blood glucose between 70–120 mg/dl and post–meal glucose less than 180 mg/dl. In the conventional therapy group the aim was to keep the patients free of diabetic symptoms. [29]

At the conclusion, the study showed that the hemoglobin A1C (a measure of glycemic control within previous 3-months) in the intensively treated patients was almost 2% lower than in those treated conventionally. The average blood glucose level in the intensive therapy group was 155 mg/dl, as compared to average blood glucose of 231 mg/dl in the conventional therapy group. Intensive therapy resulted in 76% reduction in retinopathy, 34% reduction in the development of early nephropathy and 69% reduction in the development of neuropathy. In the Secondary Intervention group intensive therapy resulted in 54% reduction in progression of established eye disease. The risk of hypoglycemia, however, was increased three times in those receiving intensive therapy; this group also experienced weight gain 1.6 times more frequently. [29]

The United Kingdom Prospective Diabetes Study (UKPDS), completed in 1998, was the largest study of patients with type 2 diabetes mellitus. The study was designed to observe the effects of glycemic control on long-term complications of diabetes. Researchers enrolled 5102 patients with newly diagnosed type 2 diabetes and followed them for a median of 11 years. Intensive treatment (insulin or oral agents or both) was compared to conventional therapy (diet and, if necessary, pharmacological therapy).

Median level of HbA1C in intensively treated group was 7.0%; it was 7.9% in conventionally treated group. Intensively treated group had significantly decreased (by 12%) risk of aggregated diabetes related endpoints (sudden death, death from hyperglycemia or hypoglycemia, fatal or non-fatal myocardial infarction, angina, heart failure, stroke, renal failure, amputation, vitreous hemorrhage, retinal photocoagulation, blindness or cataract extraction). Risk reduction for progression of retinopathy was 17%, and for appearance of microalbuminuria 30%. Cardiovascular events were not decreased significantly, however. Tight blood pressure control (mean blood pressure 144/82 mmHg) compared to less tight control (mean blood pressure 154/87 mmHg) significantly decreased the risk of microvascular complications. Adding metformin in the diet treated, overweight patients, reduced the risk of any diabetes-related endpoints, diabetes related death, and all-cause mortality and did not induce weight gain. [30]

Collectively DCCT and UKPDS, along with other studies (discussed in detail in chapters VII.1 and VII.7), established that improvement in the control of metabolic abnormalities of diabetes decreases the risk of the development of dreaded complications responsible for severe and chronic disabilities associated with the disease, such as blindness and renal failure.

ATTEMPTS TO CURE DIABETES; WHOLE PANCREAS AND PANCREATIC ISLET CELL TRANSPLANTION

Majority of the treatment methods available for the management of diabetes offer means of controlling the disease. The ultimate goal of the physicians treating patients with diabetes is to achieve cure. There have been many attempts to develop the safe and effective methods of curing diabetes. Although very intensive research is done in this field, current protocols still have limited applications.

In 1966, University of Minnesota surgeons performed the first cadaver pancreas transplant. The first living donor transplant was performed in 1978.[31] Because of the need for ongoing immunosuppression after the transplant, pancreatic transplants are usually done at the time of kidney transplant in patients with renal failure. Overall, one-year patient survival rate is about 90% and about 60 % of the grafts are functioning after one year. Although the risk of the procedure and the rates of the graft failure have declined, the complications associated with prolonged immunosuppression limit the use of this procedure to a small number of patients with type 1 diabetes.

In 1972, Paul Lacy and coworkers published the paper on methods of isolation of intact pancreatic islet cells.[32] First attempts at islet cell transplants were performed in animals with experimental diabetes and resulted in the reversal of hyperglycemia.

First autologus islet cell transplant was performed by surgeons at the University of Minnesota in 1977.[31] Autologus islet cell transplants are reported to have 75% long-term success rate. Autologus transplants are usually used in the setting of chronic pancreatitis requiring removal of pancreas, which renders the patient diabetic.

Success with autologus cell transplants has foreshadowed the recent very promising developments in the field of allogenic islet cell transplants. Early experience with human allogenic transplants was not promising. It is thought that the poor success rate with the early allogenic transplants was related to the use of immunosuppressants like prednisone, which is diabetogenic. That may have been compounded by insufficient number of islets used for transplantation.

In 1999 a group of researchers from Edmonton in Alberta, Canada, reported in The New England Journal of Medicine their experience with seven patients with type 1 diabetes mellitus who had a history of severe, recurrent hypoglycemia and poor metabolic control. These patients received islet cell transplants from non-HLA (human leukocyte antigen) matched cadaveric pancreata, with the use of glucocorticoid-free immunosuppressive regimen. The regimen consisted of sirolimus, tacrolimus and daclizumab. All seven patients quickly attained insulin independence. Each recipient required islets from two donors and one required a third transplant for sustained insulin independence. The mean glycosylated hemoglobin values were normal after transplantation in all recipients. There were no further episodes of hypoglycemic coma. During the mean follow-up of 11 months patients continued to maintain insulin independence. Half the patients went home or back to work within 12 to 24 hours after the procedure.[33]

The most serious limitation to the use of donor islet cells is the shortage of available donors. This limitation has led to a search for alternative islet cell sources. Porcine cells have been suggested as a potential source of islet cells for the transplant. The development of transgenic pigs (expressing human genes to diminish immunological reaction) might decrease the need for immunosupression after the transplant procedure. The disadvantage of using cells from transgenic pigs involves the risk of cross-species infection with porcine retroviruses, which can adapt to human hosts. These concerns have led the FDA to halt trials of porcine xenografts until those patients who have already received grafts are assessed for possible infections.[34]

Other possible sources of islet cells under investigation are human pancreatic duct cells, fetal pancreatic stem cells and embryonic stem cells.[34]

DIABETES PREVENTION

It is proper at the present time to devote not alone to treatment but still more to prevention of diabetes. The results may not be as striking or immediate, but they are sure to come and to be important."

Elliot P. Joslin, 1921

Studies have clearly demonstrated that diet and exercise improve glycemic control and some patients with diabetes treated with diet and exercise alone enter a sustained remission state lasting up to five years.

Since 1991 the number of obese Americans has grown by nearly 60%. Thirty percent of adults age 20–70 are overweight.[35] More than 84% of Americans eat too much fat and only about 30% comply with the daily recommended five servings of fruit and vegetables. [36]

The Physician Health Study has demonstrated inverse relationship between physical activity and a rate of development of diabetes.[37] Similar results were reported from Nurses Health Study.[38] National Health Interview Survey, completed in 1990, has shown that diabetic individuals were less likely to participate in regular physical exercise than were people without the diabetes.[39]

Several clinical studies present the evidence, suggesting that diet and exercise can reduce the incidence of type 2 diabetes. Tuomilehto and coworkers demonstrated that the individuals on a consistent diet and exercise program had 10% incidence of diabetes during 4 years of follow-up compared to 22% for patients in the control group, who met only once a year with the dietician and the physician.[40] A six-year randomized trial conducted by Pan and colleagues demonstrated that exercise resulted in 46% reduction in the incidence of diabetes in patients with impaired glucose tolerance.[41] Helmrich and coworkers administered questionnaires evaluating the pattern of physical activity to 5990 male alumni of University of Pennsylvania. The researchers found that the leisure time activity (like walking, stair climbing and participation in sports) during 14-year of follow-up was inversely related to the risk of development of type 2 diabetes. The protective effect was strongest among the people at the highest risk for diabetes.[42] Study by Manson and coworkers followed 87,253 women (age 34–59) free of diabetes, cardiovascular disease or cancer for 8 years. Women who engaged in vigorous exercise at least once per week, after adjusting for age, family history, body mass index and other factors, had 46% relative risk reduction for development of diabetes. [38]

In 1993, National Institute of Diabetes and Digestive and Kidney Diseases initiated a multi-center study with the objective of developing methods to prevent new cases of type 2 diabetes in adults. The study was named Diabetes Prevention Program (DPP). DPP was a 27-center randomized clinical trial designed to evaluate the safety and efficacy of interventions that may delay or prevent development of diabetes in people with the increased risk. 3234 obese patients with impaired glucose tolerance and fasting plasma glucose of 5.3-6.9 mmol/l were randomized into three groups: intensive lifestyle modification, standard care plus metformin or standard care plus placebo. Trial was terminated one year prematurely because the data had clearly addressed main research objectives. Results of DPP were reported in 2001. About 29% of DPP control subjects developed diabetes during the average follow-up period of three years. In contrast, 14 % of the diet and exercise subgroup, and 22% in metformin arm developed diabetes. Volunteers in the diet and exercise arm achieved average weight loss of about 5% during the duration of the study. [43]

Efforts are also underway to determine if it is possible to prevent or delay the development of type 1 diabetes. Diabetes Prevention Trial (DPT-1) is a nationwide, randomized, controlled clinical study designed to answer this question. This multi-center study is sponsored by the National Institute of Diabetes and Digestive and Kidney Diseases in cooperation with the National Center for Research Resources, the Juvenile Diabetes Foundation International, and the American Diabetes Association. DPT-1 started in 1994. During the study subjects at more than 50% risk for developing type 1 diabetes within 5 years are given insulin injections or placebo. Subjects with the risk between 25–50% are placed on oral insulin or placebo. Both groups of patients are evaluated to establish if insulin administration can delay the development of type 1 diabetes. Since only 3% of all relatives of individuals with type 1 diabetes are at risk for developing diabetes, it is estimated that at least 60, 000 people will need to be screened to complete the trial. [43]

SUMMARY

Diabetes mellitus has been observed and reported throughout written history since at least 1500 BC. It is only relatively recently that the perception of this disease has changed. Type 1 diabetes no longer carries the stigma of inevitably fast progressing and deadly disease. Intensive scientific research worldwide has brought new insight into this disease with modern management methods. Yet, much remains to be done and the cure has remained elusive. With improving standard of living and affluence the western world is now witnessing the rising epidemic of obesity predisposing to type 2 diabetes. As the disease itself and its complications impose great social and economical burdens, attention of medical professionals should increasingly be directed towards raising awareness of diabetes and promoting healthy lifestyle to prevent the development of this disease. Ultimately, with effective strategies for prevention and cure of diabetes, this disease will be eliminated.

DIABETES TIMELINE

CIRCA 1500 BC, EBERS PAPYRUS	First written reference to diabetes by ancient Egyptian physicians.
230 BC, APOLLONIUS OF MEMPHIS	The name diabetes (from Greek "to pass through") given to the disease.
FIRST CENTURY AD, AULUS CORNELIUS CELSUS	First clinical description of diabetes.
5TH CENTURY AD, SUSRUTA AND CHARAKA, INDIA	First distinction between type 1 and type 2 diabetes mellitus.
1776, MATHEW DOBSON, ENGLAND	Determined that the sweet tasting substance in the urine of diabetics is sugar.
1788, THOMAS COWLEY, ENGLAND	First link between diabetes and pancreas.
1869, PAUL LANGERHANS, GERMANY	Discovery of small cell clusters in the pancreas, not drained by the pancreatic ducts. These cell clusters later named "Islets of Langerhans".
1889, OSCAR MINKOWSKI, JOSEPH VON MEHRING, GERMANY	Removal of the pancreas in the dogs causing immediate development of diabetes.
1893, EDOUARD LAGUESSE, FRANCE	Islets of Langerhans might be the source of anti-diabetic substance.
1907, GEORG ZUELZER, GERMANY	Pancreatic extract "Acomatol", produced by Zuelzer, decreased glucosuria and raised blood pH in diabetic dogs.
1921-1922, FREDERICK BANTING, CHARLES BEST, JAMES COLLIP AND JOHN.J.R. MACLEOD, CANADA	Dog's pancreatic extracts shown to decrease glucosuria. First successful clinical use of refined pancreatic extract for diabetic patient. Eli Lilly Company begins the work on the commercial development of insulin.
1928, GERMANY	Synthalin–a guanidine derivative introduced for treatment of diabetes.
1939, C. RUIZ, L.L. SILVA, ARGENTINA	Hypoglycemic properties of sulphonamide antibiotics observed for the first time.
1958, FREDERIC SANGER, GREAT BRITAIN	Nobel prize for the structural formula of bovine insulin.
1959, ROSALYN YALOW AND SALOMON BERSON, USA	Development of radioimmunoassay. Rosalyn Yalow received Nobel Prize for RIA in 1977.
1966, UNIVERSITY OF MINNESOTA, USA	First transplant of the pancreas performed.
1969, DOROTHY HODGKIN, GREAT BRITAIN	Description of the three-dimensional structure of porcine insulin using X-ray crystallography.

1978, ROBERT CREA, DAVID GOEDDEL, USA	Human insulin production using recombinant DNA technology.
1993, DIABETES CONTROL AND COMPLICATIONS TRIAL, USA	Relation of the metabolic control of type 1 diabetes to the development of diabetic complications.
1998, UNITED KINGDOM PROSPECTIVE DIABETES STUDY, GREAT BRITAIN	Relation of the metabolic control of type 2 diabetes to the development of diabetic complications
2001, DIABETES PREVENTION PROGRAM, USA	Relation of diet and exercise to the rate of development of type 2 diabetes in high risk population

REFERENCES

1. Papaspyros NS. The history of diabetes. In: The history of diabetes mellitus. Thieme, Stuttgart, p. 4, 1964.
2. www.crystalinks.com/egyptmedicine.html–ancient Egyptian medicine, Ebers papyrus.
3. Papaspyros NS. The history of diabetes. In: The history of diabetes mellitus. Thieme, Stuttgart, p. 4-5, 1964.
4. www.diabetesmanager.com–history of diabetes from ancient times till twentieth century.
5. Medvei VC. The Greco – Roman period. In: The history of clinical endocrinology: a comprehensive account of endocrinology from earliest times to the present day. Parthenon Publishing, New York, p.34, 37, 1993.
6. Southgate TM. De medicina. JAMA 10:921, 1999.
7. Medvei VC. Mediaeval scene. In: The history of clinical endocrinology: a comprehensive account of endocrinology from earliest times to the present day. Parthenon Publishing, New York, p. 46, 49, 1993.
8. Medvei VC. The 16th century and the Renaissance. In: The history of clinical endocrinology: a comprehensive account of endocrinology from earliest times to the present day. Parthenon Publishing, New York, p. 55-56, 1993.
9. Medvei VC. The 18th century and the beginning of the 19th century. In: The history of clinical endocrinology: a comprehensive account of endocrinology from earliest times to the present day. Parthenon Publishing, New York, p. 97, 1993.
10. www.uic.edu–Claude Bernard.
11. www.britannica.com–Claude Bernard
12. Medvei VC. Story of Insulin. In: The history of clinical endocrinology: a comprehensive account of endocrinology from earliest times to the present day. Parthenon Publishing, New York, p.249-251, 253-256, 1993.

13. Bliss M. A long prelude. In: The discovery of insulin. The University of Chicago Press, Chicago, p. 33-39, 1982.

14. Minkowski O. Introduction and translation by R. Levine. Historical development of the theory of pancreatic diabetes. Diabetes 38 :1-6, 1989.

15. Medvei VC. The birth of endocrinology. In: The history of clinical endocrinology: a comprehensive account of endocrinology from earliest times to the present day. Parthenon Publishing, New York, p. 151, 1993.

16. Bliss M. Banting's idea. In: The discovery of insulin. University of Chicago Press, Chicago, p. 45-58, 1990.

17. Bliss M. A mysterious something. In: The discovery of insulin. University of Chicago Press, Chicago, p. 90, 1990.

18. Bliss M. Triumph. In: The discovery of insulin. University of Chicago Press, Chicago, p. 112-113, 120-121, 127, 1990.

19. MacCracken J. From ants to analogues. Puzzles and promises in diabetes management. Postgraduate Medicine 4:138-150, 1997.

20. www.discoveryofinsulin.com

21. Pratt P. History of insulin. Hutchinson family encyclopedia, online edition. Helicon Publishing Ltd., 2000.

22. www.nobel.se–August Krogh

23. Medvei VC. Present trends and outlook for the future – Part III. In: The history of clinical endocrinology: a comprehensive account of endocrinology from earliest times to the present day. Parthenon Publishing, New York, p. 380-383, 1993.

24. www.netsrq.com–Rosalyn Yalow, Salomon Berson, RIA.

25. Segre GV, Brown EN. Measurement of hormones. In: Williams textbook of endocrinology. Wilson JD, Foster DW, Kronenberg HM, Larsen PR. Editors. 9th Edition. WB Saunders, Philadelphia, p. 44-45, 1998.

26. Medvei VC. Chronological tables. In: The history of clinical endocrinology: a comprehensive account of endocrinology from earliest times to the present day. Parthenon Publishing, New York, p. 495, 1993.

27. www.gene.com–recombinant DNA technology in insulin production.

28. Galloway J, deShazo R. Insulin chemistry and pharmacology: insulin allergy, resistance, and lipodystrophy. In: Diabetes mellitus. Theory and practice. Rifkin H, Porte D, Jr. Editors. Fourth edition. Elsevier, New York, p. 498, 1990.

29. Diabetes Control and Complications Trial Research Group. The effect of intensive treatment of diabetes on the development and progression of long-term complications in insulin-dependent diabetes mellitus. N Engl J Med 329:997-86, 1993.

30. UK Prospective Diabetes Study Group. Intensive blood-glucose control with sulphonylures or insulin compared with conventional treatment and risk of complications in patients with type 2 diabetes (UKPDS 33). Lancet 352:837-53, 1998.

31. www.fairviewtransplant.org–pancreatic transplant.

32. Lacy PE, Kostianovsky M. Methods for the isolation of intact islets of Langerhans from rat pancreas. Diabetes 16:35-9, 1967.

33. Shapiro JAM, Lakey JRT, Ryan EA, Korbutt GS, Toth E, L. Warnock GL, Kneteman NM, Rajotte RV. Islet transplantation in seven patients with type 1 diabetes mellitus using a glucocorticoid-free immunosuppressive regimen. N Engl J Med 343:230-23, 2000.

34. Serup P, Madsen DO, Mandrup–Poulsen T. Islet and stem cell transplantation for treating diabetes. Brit Med J 322:29-32, 2001.

35. National Heart, Lung and Blood Institute: Clinical guidelines on the identification, evaluation, and treatment of overweight and obesity in adults. Bethesda, MD, National Heart, Lung and Blood Institute, 1998.

36. Centers for Disease Control and Prevention: National diabetes fact sheet: national estimates and general information on diabetes in the United States. Revised edition. Atlanta, GA, US Department of Health and Human Services, Centers for Disease Control and Prevention, 1998.

37. Manson JE, Nathan DM, Krolewski AS, Stampfer MJ, Willett WC, Hennekens CH. A prospective study of exercise and incidence of diabetes among U.S. male physicians. JAMA 268:63-67, 1992.

38. Manson JE, Rimm EB, Stampfer MJ, Colditz GA, Willett WC, Hennekens CH, Speizer FE. A prospective study of physical activity and incidence of non insulin–dependent diabetes mellitus in women. Lancet 338:774-77, 1991.

39. U.S. Department of Health and Human Services: Healthy People 2000: Summary Report. Washington, D.C., U.S. Department of Health and Human Services (DHHS Publ. PHSSs 91-50213), p. 6-8, 55, 91-92, 1992.

40. Tuomilehto J, Lindstrom J, Eriksson JG, Valle TT, Hamalainen H, Ilanne–Parikka P, Keinanen–Kiukaanniemi S, Laakso M, Louheranta A, Rastas M, Salminen V, Uusitupa M. Finnish Diabetes Prevention Study Group. Prevention of type 2 diabetes mellitus by changes in lifestyle among subjects with impaired glucose tolerance. N Engl J Med 344(18):1343-50, 2001.

41. Pan XR, Li GW, Wang JX, Yang WY, An ZX, Lin J, Xiao JZ, Cao XB, Liu PA, Jiang XG, Jiang YY, Wang JP, Zheng H, Bennet PH, Howard BV. Effects of diet and exercise in preventing NIDDM in people with impaired glucose tolerance: the Da Qing IGT and Diabetes Study. Diabetes Care 20:537-544, 1997.

42. Helmrich SP, Ragland DR, Leung RW, Paffenbarger RS. Physical activity and reduced occurrence of non-insulin-dependent diabetes mellitus. N Engl J Med 325:147-152, 1991.

43. www.niddk.nih.gov–results of Diabetes Prevention Program, Diabetes Prevention Trial.

II. Physiology of Glucose Metabolism

Chapter 1. Normal Glucose Homeostasis

John E. Gerich, Steven D. Wittlin, and Christian Meyer

INTRODUCTION

Plasma glucose values are normally maintained within a relatively narrow range throughout the day (70-170 mg/dl) despite wide fluctuations in the delivery (e.g. meals) and removal (e.g. exercise) of glucose from the circulation. Teleologically, this is consistent with the fact that hyperglycemia is to be avoided because of its potential to cause macro- and microvascular complications.[1,2] Conversely, this is also consistent with the fact that hypoglycemia is to be avoided because it can injure the brain. Limitations in the availability of alternate fuels (e.g. ketone bodies) or in their transport across the blood brain barrier (e.g. free fatty acids [FFA]) make glucose the usual source of energy for the brain. After prolonged fasting, however, because of an increase in their circulating concentration, ketone bodies may be used by the brain.[3]

Since the brain cannot store or produce glucose, it depends on plasma glucose as its fuel source for its immediate survival. A decrement in plasma glucose levels as little as 20 mg/dl (i.e. from 90 mg/dl to 70) can decrease glucose uptake in certain areas of the brain (e.g. in the hypothalamus where glucose sensors are located) and trigger the release of counterregulatory hormones (glucagon, catecholamines, cortisol and growth hormone) to prevent a further decrease and restore normoglycemia. This decrease in plasma glucose also suppresses insulin release which also helps to prevent further decrements.[4] On the other hand, a 10 mg/dl increment in plasma glucose will stimulate insulin release and suppress glucagon secretion so as to prevent further increments and restore normoglycemia.

GENERAL CONSIDERATIONS

Importance of relative changes in glucose fluxes

Plasma glucose concentrations are determined by the relative rates at which glucose enters and leaves the circulation. Thus the plasma glucose concentration will increase only if the rate of glucose entry exceeds its rate of exit and, conversely, plasma glucose levels will decrease only if rates of exit exceed rates of entry. Both rates may simultaneously decrease, such as during prolonged fasting or development of hypoglycemia in insulinoma patients, but it is the relative change that determines the direction of change in plasma glucose. In the above examples, the decrease in glucose entry into the circulation exceeds the decrease in glucose exit from the circulation and therefore plasma glucose concentrations decrease. Changes in glucose clearance, an index of the efficiency of glucose removal from the circulation, by itself will not affect plasma glucose concentrations independent of changes in rates of glucose entry and exit.

Factors influencing glucose fluxes

Rates of glucose entry into and exit from plasma are regulated by several factors: for practical purposes, the most important on a moment to moment basis are hormones, substrate concentrations and sympathetic nervous system activity. On a prolonged time frame (hours/days), nutritional factors (e.g. diet composition, caloric balance), exercise/physical fitness, and concomitant changes in the sensitivity to hormones become important.

Fasting vs postprandial states

The sources for supplying glucose (as well as the mechanisms involved, i.e. glycogenolysis vs. gluconeogenesis) and the sites for glucose disposal will vary depending on duration of fasting since the last meal. Therefore the following description of normal glucose homeostasis will deal separately with the postabsorptive state (12-14 hr fast), prolonged fasting (>24 hours) and the immediate postprandial state (0-6 hrs after meal ingestion).

Actions of key regulatory factors

In order to understand the interactions of factors involved in maintenance of normal glucose homeostasis, it is necessary to know how they work (Table 1).

Table 1. Mechanism of Action of Key Metabolic Regulators

	Glucose Production	Glucose Utilization	Lipolysis
Insulin	↓	↑	↓
Glucagon	↑	-	-
Epinephrine	↑	↓	↑
Cortisol	↑	↓	↑
Growth Hormone	↑	↓	↑
FFA	↑	↓	-

Insulin

Insulin regulates glucose metabolism by direct and indirect actions. Binding of insulin to its receptors in liver, kidney, muscle and adipose tissue leads to activation of its signalling pathway which involves a complex cascade of protein kinases and regulatory proteins of which IRS-1 and IRS-2 are most important. This causes suppression of glucose release from liver and kidney,[5] translocation of glucose transporters in muscle and adipose tissue to increase their glucose uptake, and inhibition of release of FFA into the circulation due to suppression of the activity of hormone-sensitive lipase and a simultaneous increase in their clearance from the circulation. Although insulin does not increase glucose transport into liver, it promotes glycogen accumulation by inhibiting glucose-6-phosphatase and phosphorylase while stimulating glycogen synthase. The effects of insulin on circulating FFA levels indirectly reduce glucose release into the circulation and promote glucose removal since FFA stimulate gluconeogenesis and reduce glucose transport into cells.

The main regulator of insulin secretion is the plasma glucose concentration; increases in plasma glucose stimulate while decreases in plasma glucose inhibit insulin secretion. Thus the increase in plasma glucose after meal ingestion will result in a 3-4-fold increase in plasma insulin within 30-60 min whereas a decrease in plasma glucose below 50 mg/dl will result in a 80-90% reduction in plasma insulin levels. Acute increases in plasma amino acids and, to a lesser extent, FFA can also increase insulin secretion. After meal ingestion, intestinal factors called incretins (e.g. Gastrointestinal Peptide, Glucagon-like Peptide I) augment insulin secretion. This is why plasma insulin concentrations increase to a greater extent after oral glucose than after intravenous glucose despite identical plasma glucose concentrations.

Different metabolic processes vary in their sensitivity to insulin and in their dose-response characteristics. At basal levels observed in the postabsorptive state (~5-10 μU/ml), insulin is already inhibiting glucose and FFA release 30-50% (counteracting the effects of glucagon and the sympathetic nervous system) while having a trivial effect on tissue glucose uptake. Maximal suppression of glucose and FFA release normally is observed with plasma insulin concentrations seen postprandially (~40-50 μU/ml) whereas maximal stimulation of tissue glucose uptake requires plasma insulin concentrations greater than 300 μU/ml—levels not seen under normal physiological conditions except in extremely insulin resistant individuals in whom, of course, such levels would not produce a maximal effect.

Glucagon

Glucagon acts exclusively on the liver. Binding of glucagon to its hepatic receptors activates adenylate cyclase. The immediate response to the increase in intracellular C-AMP levels is an increase in glycogenolysis due to stimulation of phosphorylase.[6] This wanes and, after several hours, is followed by a later increase in gluconeogenesis due to a complex process involving both increased substrate uptake and enzyme activation. Thus the

41

main action of glucagon to increase plasma glucose levels is the stimulation of hepatic glycogenolysis.

Glucagon secretion is generally reciprocal to that of insulin being suppressed by increases in plasma glucose and stimulated by decreases in plasma glucose. Increases in plasma amino acid levels also are a potent stimulus for glucagon release so that after ingestion of a protein meal, plasma glucagon levels do not decrease despite increases in plasma glucose and insulin levels. Increases in plasma FFA and insulin levels suppress glucagon secretion. Glucagon secretion increases during stress and prolonged fasting; these effects are probably mediated by increases in sympathetic nervous system activity.

Catecholamines (epinephrine/norepinephrine)

Catecholamine release is mediated through changes in sympathetic nervous system, being increased during various stresses and hypoglycemia. Acting as both hormones (epinephrine) and neurotransmittors (norepinephrine), they are potent hyperglycemic factors whose actions, unlike those of glucagon, are sustained and affect both glucose release and glucose removal. Their metabolic actions are complex, being mediated for the most part via beta 2 adrenergic receptors: at the liver they directly increase glycogenolysis via C-AMP activation of phosphorylase and, to a lesser extent, augment gluconeogenesis indirectly through increasing gluconeogenic substrate availability and plasma FFA. At the kidney they are potent stimulators of gluconeogenesis both directly and indirectly as on the liver and are actually more potent stimulators of renal glucose release than hepatic glucose release.[7] In skeletal muscle, they reduce glucose uptake and stimulate glycogenolysis which results in an increase in release of lactate—the major gluconeogenic precursor. In adipose tissue, catecholamines stimulate lipolysis via activation of hormone-sensitive lipase which results in an increase in the release of FFA and glycerol, another key gluconeogenic precursor.

Growth hormone and cortisol

In contrast to glucagon and catecholamines which act almost immediately, the metabolic actions of growth hormone and cortisol generally take several hours to become evident. These can be summarized as being antagonistic to the actions of insulin, i.e. they reduce the ability of insulin to suppress glucose release, stimulate glucose uptake and inhibit lipolysis. Both hormones increase the synthesis of gluconeogenic enzymes and reduce glucose transport. In addition, cortisol can impair insulin secretion. Accordingly, the mechanism for deterioration in glucose tolerance during immunosuppressive glucocorticoid treatment involves induction of insulin resistance and prevention of an appropriate compensatory increase in insulin secretion.

Stress and hypoglycemia are the major factors stimulating secretion of these hormones due to hypothalamic release of growth hormone releasing

42

factor and corticotrophin releasing factor. Changes in plasma FFA levels are also involved in regulation of growth hormone secretion, increases suppressing and decreases stimulating its release.

It is important to note that since all of the counterregulatory hormones work via different intracellular mechanisms which reinforce/synergize with one another, simultaneous small increases in their plasma levels will have greater effects than large increases in the plasma level of only one hormone.[4]

Free fatty acids (FFA)

FFA are the major fuel used by most tissues of the body, the major exceptions being the brain, renal medulla and blood cells.[8,9] Increases in their circulating concentrations have many potentially important metabolic consequences:[10,11] stimulation of hepatic and renal gluconeogenesis; inhibition of muscle glucose transport and competition with glucose as an oxidative fuel. The major regulators of circulating FFA levels are the sympathetic nervous system and growth hormone (which increases plasma FFA levels), and insulin and hyperglycemia (which reduce plasma FFA levels by suppressing lipolysis and increasing FFA clearance). There is evidence for heterogeneity of adipose depots with visceral fat being more metabolically active.

THE POSTABSORPTIVE STATE

Glucose utilization (Table 2)

The period after a 14-16 hour overnight fast is commonly referred to as the postabsorptive state. In this time plasma glucose concentrations average about 90 mg/dl (range 70-110 mg/dl) and are relatively stable since rates of release of glucose into the circulation closely approximate rates of glucose exit from the circulation ($\sim$10 μg $\cdot$ kg^{-1} $\cdot$ min^{-1}). Although this situation is often considered to represent a steady-state, it is actually a pseudosteady state. Rates of glucose removal slightly, often undetectably, exceed rates of glucose release into the circulation so that if fasting is prolonged, plasma glucose levels gradually decrease: by 20-24 hours of fasting they may be 15-20% lower. However, even after 72 hours of fasting, they are usually maintained above 50 mg/dl.[12]

In the postabsorptive state, there is no net storage of glucose; consequently, glucose taken up by tissues is either completely oxidized to CO_2 or released back into the circulation as lactate, alanine, and glutamine[13] for reincorporation into glucose via gluconeogenesis (Table 2).

Most glucose used by the body can be accounted for by five tissues: the brain (45-60%), skeletal muscle (15-20%), kidney (10-15%), blood cells (5-10%), splanchnic organs (3-6%), and adipose tissue (2-4%).[14]

Table 2. Glucose Disposal in the Postabsorptive State

	Rate	% of Total
Overall	$10 \ \mu mol \cdot kg^{-1} \cdot min^{-1}$	100
Oxidation	$\sim 7 \ \mu mol \cdot kg^{-1} \cdot min^{-1}$	~70
Glycolysis	$\sim 3 \ \mu mol \cdot kg^{-1} \cdot min^{-1}$	~30
Tissues		
Brain	$5 \ \mu mol \cdot kg^{-1} \cdot min^{-1}$	~50
Skeletal Muscle	$2 \ \mu mol \cdot kg^{-1} \cdot min^{-1}$	~20
Splanchnic Organs	$1 \ \mu mol \cdot kg^{-1} \cdot min^{-1}$	~10
Kidney	$1 \ \mu mol \cdot kg^{-1} \cdot min^{-1}$	~10
Adipose Tissue	$0.5 \ \mu mol \cdot kg^{-1} \cdot min^{-1}$	~5
Blood Cells	$0.5 \ \mu mol \cdot kg^{-1} \cdot min^{-1}$	~5

All glucose taken up by brain is completely oxidized whereas that taken up in kidney, blood cells, splanchnic tissues and muscle mainly undergoes glycolysis. Recall that most of the body's energy requirements are met by oxidation of FFA which compete with glucose as the fuel of choice in certain organs (e.g. skeletal muscle, heart and possibly kidney).[10]

Glucose uptake by brain, blood cells, renal medulla, and splanchnic tissues occurs largely independent of insulin, and plasma insulin levels are low in the postabsorptive state (<10 μU/ml), Under these conditions, the amount of glucose removed from the circulation is determined almost exclusively by tissue demands, the mass action effects of the plasma glucose concentration per se, and the number and characteristics of the glucose transporters in specific tissues rather than by insulin. Insulin may be viewed as playing a permissive role; counterregulatory hormones that antagonize the actions of insulin (e.g. cortisol, growth hormone, epinephrine, and thyroid hormone) can be viewed as modulating the sensitivity of tissues to the effects of insulin on tissue glucose uptake and utilization.

Glucose production (Table 3)

Glucose release into the circulation, on the other hand, is under considerably more regulation by both hormonal and nonhormonal mechanisms. Until recently it was thought that the liver was the sole source of glucose entering the circulation except during acidosis and after prolonged fasting. However, recent studies now indicate that both liver and kidney release glucose in the postabsorptive state.[15] Although many tissues contain enzymes to break down glycogen to glucose-6-phosphate (glycogenolysis) or to synthesize glucose-6-phosphate from glycerol, lactate and amino acids (gluconeogenesis), only liver and kidney contain enough glucose-6-phosphatase to make significant amounts of free glucose available for release.

Table 3. Summary of Postabsorptive Glucose Release

	Rate $\mu mol \cdot kg^{-1} \cdot min^{-1}$	% of Total
I. Glucose Release	10.0	100
A. Hepatic	8.0	80
1. Glycogenolysis	5.0	50
2. Gluconeogenesis	3.0	30
Lactate	1.3	13
Alanine	0.8	8
Other amino acids	0.2	2
Glycerol	0.4	4
Glutamine	0.3	3
B. Renal	2.0	20
1. Glycogenolysis	0	0
2. Gluconeogenesis	2.0	20
Lactate	1.2	12
Glutamine	0.4	4
Glycerol	0.2	2
Other amino acids	0.1	1
Alanine	0.1	1

The liver is responsible for approximately 80% of the glucose released into the circulation in the postabsorptive state[15]. Under these conditions, ~50% of the glucose entering the circulation is due to glycogenolysis and the remainder (~5.0 $\mu mol \cdot kg^{-1} \cdot min^{-1}$) to gluconeogenesis.[16] The proportion owing to gluconeogenesis rapidly increases with the duration of fasting, as glycogen stores become depleted; by 24 hours from the last meal, gluconeogenesis accounts for about 70% of all glucose released into the circulation, and by 48 hours it accounts for over 90% of all the glucose released into the circulation.[12,16]

The kidney normally contains little glycogen, and renal cells that could make glycogen lack glucose-6-phosphatase. Consequently, virtually all the glucose released by the kidney is the result of gluconeogenesis[15]. Although the liver releases about four times as much glucose as the kidney under postabsorptive conditions, both organs release about the same amount (2.5-3.0 $\mu mol \cdot kg^{-1} \cdot min^{-1}$) from gluconeogenesis. The proportion of overall glucose release owing to renal gluconeogenesis increases with prolongation of the fast.[17]

The liver releases glucose both by glycogenolysis and gluconeogenesis and can be considered to be the sole source of glucose due to glycogenolysis. In overnight fasted people, the liver contains about 75 gm of glycogen. Thus if it releases glycogen at a rate of 63 mg/min (5 $\mu mol \cdot kg^{-1} \cdot min^{-1}$), glycogen stores would be totally depleted in about 20 hours.

Glucose release by liver and kidney are regulated differently. Insulin suppresses glucose release by both organs directly by affecting enzyme activation/deactivation and indirectly through such actions as limitation of gluconeogenic substrate availability and gluconeogenic activators (e.g. suppression of FFA and glucagon)[5]. However glucagon, which increases both glycogenolysis and gluconeogenesis in the liver, has no effect on the kidney.[18] Epinephrine, which can directly activate hepatic glycogenolysis, nevertheless appears to increase glucose release, predominantly by directly stimulating renal gluconeogenesis and, to a lesser extent, by increasing availability of gluconeogenic precursors/activators (e.g. glycerol and FFA).[7,19]

The major precursors for gluconeogenesis are lactate, glycerol, glutamine and alanine.[14] Most amino acids released from skeletal muscle protein are converted to alanine and glutamine for transport through plasma to liver and kidney. There is a slightly different pattern in the use of these substrates in liver and kidney: alanine being selectively used by liver, glutamine being preferentially used in kidney, while lactate and glycerol are used to a roughly comparable extent by both organs. In the resting postabsorptive state, lactate is the major gluconeogenic precursor, accounting for about half of all gluconeogenesis.

Insulin, glucagon and catecholamines (norepinephrine released postsynaptically in the abundantly innervated liver and kidney and epinephrine released from the adrenal medulla) are the most important acute glucoregulatory hormones. Physiologic changes in their circulating levels are able to change glucose release in a matter of minutes. Other important glucoregulatory factors such as growth hormone, cortisol, and thyroid hormone take hours for their effects to become evident. Their effects are mediated through affecting the sensitivity of kidney and liver to insulin, glucagon and catecholamines and by altering the amount of key enzymes, glycogen stores, and availability of circulating precursors/activators of gluconeogenesis. Increases in circulating FFA augment hepatic and renal gluconeogenesis by affecting the activity of key enzymes, providing the necessary adenosine triphosphate (ATP) and reducing equivalents.[10,20]

PROLONGED FASTING (TABLE 4)

With prolongation of fasting, plasma insulin levels decrease while those of glucagon, catecholamines, growth hormone and cortisol increase. Consequently, plasma FFA, glycerol and the products of FFA oxidation, the ketone bodies beta hydroxybutyrate and acetoacetate increase. Since hepatic glycogen stores become depleted by 60 hours, virtually all of glucose release at this time is due to gluconeogenesis. Initially, hepatic gluconeogenesis decreases while renal gluconeogenesis increases, with an overall result of a decrease in overall glucose release and a slight increase in gluconeogenesis. With more prolonged fasting there is a further decrease in glucose release as gluconeogenesis decreases. Although more glycerol is available for gluconeogenesis, less lactate is available due to less being produced by glycolysis, and less amino acids are available because muscle proteolysis decreases. These changes limit gluconeogenesis despite increases in plasma FFA and counterregulatory hormones which promote gluconeogenesis.

Table 4. Glucose Release and Disposal after Prolonged Fasting (~60 hr)

	Glucose Disposal*		Glucose Release*
Overall	6.0	Overall	6.0
Oxidation	4.8	Gluconeogenesis	5.5
Glycolysis	1.2	Glycogenolysis	0.5
Tissues		Tissues	
Brain	3.5	Liver	2.7
Skeletal Muscle	1.0	Kidney	2.8
Splanchnic Organs	0.5		
Kidney	0.4		
Adipose Tissue	0.2		
Blood Cells	0.4		

*$\mu mol \cdot kg^{-1} \cdot min^{-1}$

Initially during the course of the fast, decreases in glucose release are slightly greater than decreases in glucose uptake so that plasma glucose levels decrease. Eventually, however, the rates of release and uptake approximate one another so that a new pseudosteady state is established after 60-70 hours with plasma glucose levels usually averaging 55-65 mg/dl. This stabilization forms the basis for the 72 hr fast for the diagnosis of an insulinoma. In such patients insulin secretion is not appropriately reduced and this leads to the development of hypoglycemia (i.e. plasma glucose levels <45 mg/dl).

These changes during prolonged fasting are relevant to changes seen in chronically ill patients who often are anorexic, malnourished, and miss meals in hospital because of diagnostic or therapeutic procedures. Because of the limitations on gluconeogenesis, such patients, i.e. those with chronic renal failure, severe liver disease, heart failure, are prone to develop hypoglycemia during infections or other situations which increase the body's glucose utilization.

THE POSTPRANDIAL STATE

Complete assimilation of the constituents of a mixed meal containing fat, protein and carbohydrate and restoration of the postabsorptive state takes at least six hours.[21] Assimilation is generally complete within four-five hours after ingestion of a pure carbohydrate load. Despite these differences, there is little evidence that the fate of ingested carbohydrate differs markedly under the two conditions.[21] Clearly, therefore, with ingestion of three meals, most of the day is spent in the postprandial state.

Various factors can affect the extent of circulating glucose excursions after meal ingestion. These include the time and degree of physical activity since the last meal, the composition and form (liquid vs. solid), rate of gastric emptying, digestion within the lumen of the small intestine, absorption into the portal vein, extraction by the liver, suppression of endogenous glucose release, and finally the uptake, storage, oxidation and glycolysis of glucose in posthepatic tissues.[22]

From a practical point of view, however, the major factors influencing postprandial glucose homeostasis are those that affect suppression of endogenous glucose release and those that affect hepatic and posthepatic tissue glucose uptake. Recent studies have used dual isotope approaches to measure splanchnic sequestration (i.e. first-pass hepatic uptake), endogenous glucose release, and total glucose appearance into and disappearance from the systemic circulation. At the same time, investigators have measured net balance across limbs, splanchnic tissues, and the kidney as well as NMR-determined glycogen accumulation in liver and muscle[23,24]to gain insight into the fate of an ingested glucose load.[21,25,26] The dual isotope approach makes it possible to distinguish the amount of plasma glucose molecules originating from the ingestate from endogenous molecules.

Changes in plasma hormone and substrate concentrations

After ingestion of 75 gm glucose, plasma glucose levels increase to a peak in 60-90 minutes, usually not exceeding 160 mg/dl, and gradually return to or slightly below postabsorptive values by 3-4 hours. It is important to note that although plasma glucose levels have returned to postabsorptive levels, glucose fluxes and organ glucose exchange have not. Plasma insulin concentrations follow a similar profile and average only about four-fold basal values during this period. Plasma glucagon concentrations change reciprocally and are generally suppressed about 50% during the interval. Numerous studies have demonstrated a critical role of early insulin release (i.e. that occurring within the first 30-60 min) in maintaining normal postprandial glucose homeostasis.[22]

Plasma FFA and glycerol levels decrease due to inhibition of lipolysis while plasma lactate concentrations increase as a result of increased glycolysis in liver, muscle, adipose tissue and kidney. After ingestion of a mixed meal containing protein, the circulating concentrations of several amino acids increase.

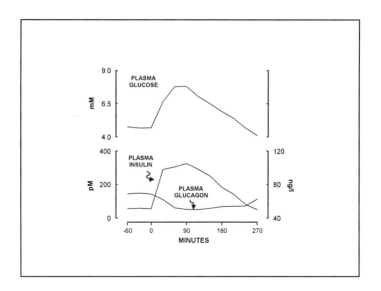

Figure 1. Changes in plasma glucose, insulin and glucagon after ingestion of a 75 gm oral glucose load in normal volunteers.

Changes in rates of glucose entry into and exit from plasma

Rates of glucose appearance in plasma represent the sum of glucose escaping first pass splanchnic (hepatic) extraction and the residual release of endogenous glucose by liver and kidney. Appearance of ingested glucose in the systemic circulation is detected as early as 15 minutes, reaches a peak at 80-120 minutes, and gradually decreases thereafter. On average during a 4-5 hr postprandial period about 75% of the glucose molecules in plasma represent those from the meal. Endogenous glucose release by the liver decreases rapidly and is suppressed nearly 80% during the 5 hour postprandial period. As a result, nearly 25 gm less glucose due to endogenous production reaches the systemic circulation during this interval. In contrast to the liver, recent studies indicate that endogenous renal glucose release is not suppressed and actually increases during this period so that it exceeds hepatic glucose release.[27] This increase in renal glucose release would permit more complete suppression of hepatic glucose release and facilitate more efficient glycogen replenishment.[27]

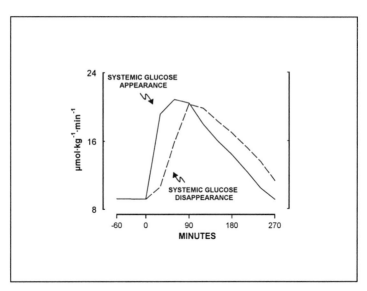

Figure 2. Changes in rates of glucose entry into and removal from plasma after ingestion of a 75 gm oral glucose load in normal volunteers.

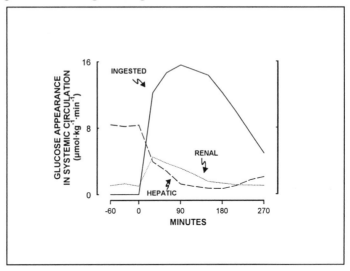

Figure 3. Changes in rates of entry of glucose into the circulation from ingested glucose, liver and kidney.

Tissues responsible for disposal of ingested glucose

Based on a survey of published studies, a consensus view of the disposal of a hypothetical meal containing 100 gm carbohydrate is depicted in Figure 4. About 30% of the ingested glucose (~33 gm) is initially extracted by splanchnic tissues.[21,25,26,28-32] Most is taken up by the liver and immediately incorporated into glycogen via the "direct pathway" to hepatic glycogen.[23,24] A significant portion of glucose taken up by the liver probably undergoes glycolysis and is released as lactate which is eventually taken up by the liver where it undergoes gluconeogenesis and is subsequently incorporated into glycogen via the "indirect pathway."[24,25,33,34] Inhibition of glucose-6-phosphatase causes the glucose-6-phosphate made from this lactate to enter glycogen rather than being released into the circulation as free glucose.

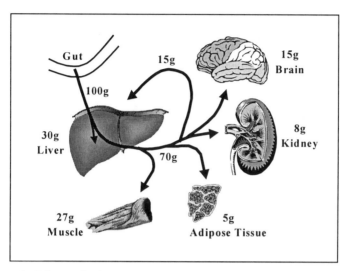

Figure 4. Disposal of a 100 gm oral glucose load.

Of the remaining 70 gm glucose, which enters the systemic circulation, 25-30 gm is taken up by skeletal muscle,[21,25,26,28,30-32,35] initially to be oxidized in place of FFA and later (after 2-3 hours) to be stored as glycogen.[36,37] Relatively little of the glucose taken up by muscle is released into the circulation as lactate and alanine.[25,38]

About 15 gm (~20% of the ingested glucose entering the circulation) is taken up by brain as a substitute for the endogenously produced glucose that it normally would have taken up during this period. Recall that endogenous release of glucose from the liver is markedly reduced postprandially.

Another 15 gm is extracted from the systemic circulation by the liver either as intact glucose (direct pathway) or as lactate, alanine and glutamine, whose carbon backbone originated from the ingested glucose, for further glycogen formation (indirect pathway).[33] Thus, ultimately splanchnic tissues dispose of nearly half of the ingested glucose.[39]

Recent studies[27] indicate that the kidney may take up as much as 8 gm (~10% of the ingested glucose entering the circulation). This would leave 5-10 gm (7-15% of the ingested glucose reaching the systemic circulation) to be taken up by adipose and other tissues.[37]

From the above description of postprandial events, it can be readily appreciated that three factors normally predominate in regulating postprandial glucose excursions: suppression of endogenous glucose release, initial hepatic glucose extraction, and subsequent uptake of glucose from the systemic circulation. Suppression of endogenous glucose release and initial hepatic glucose extraction depends largely on the coordinated reciprocal secretion of insulin and glucagon, in particular the early release of insulin.[32] Seventy to eighty percent of posthepatic glucose uptake occurs in insulin-sensitive tissues. Insulin plays a major role in this process via its action to increase glucose transport; for example, skeletal muscle glucose fractional extraction (an index of the efficiency of glucose uptake) increases about three-fold whereas glucose fractional extraction by brain, an insulin insensitive tissue, actually decreases.[27]

Another factor to be considered, which may represent an indirect effect of insulin, is the postprandial suppression of lipolysis with the consequent decrease in circulating FFA concentrations. This would decrease the availability of a promoter of hepatic glucose release and a competitor to glucose as a metabolic fuel. For example, recent studies using nuclear magnetic resonance to measure glycogen accumulation in skeletal muscle found that during the initial two hours after meal ingestion, when skeletal muscle glucose uptake is markedly increased, there is no net accumulation of glycogen in skeletal muscle.[36] This has been attributed to the use of the glucose taken up as an oxidative fuel in place of FFA. A similar phenomenon has been invoked to explain the postprandial increase in renal glucose uptake.[27] Finally, recent studies have found that infusion of a triglyceride emulsion to prevent the decrease in circulating FFA reduces suppression of endogenous glucose release.[40]

SUMMARY

For both the fasting and postprandial states, factors which affect the rate of entry of glucose into the circulation are more important for maintaining normal glucose homeostasis than those which affect the rate of removal of glucose from the circulation. In type 2 diabetes, for example, absolute rates of glucose disposal are generally normal whereas rates of glucose entry into the circulation in both the fasting and postprandial states are increased.[22] Although glucose disposal is relatively impaired, i.e. inappropriate for the prevailing plasma glucose and insulin concentrations, rates of glucose entry are increased in an absolute sense and are therefore the more important determinant of hyperglycemia.

The regulation of glucose entry into the circulation is complex, being influenced by hormones, the sympathetic nervous system and substrates (i.e. free fatty acid concentrations and availability of gluconeogenic precursors). Moreover, recent studies have provided evidence for hepatorenal reciprocity. According to this concept, when release of glucose by either liver or kidney is reduced, release of glucose by the other organ will increase in order to maintain appropriate release of glucose into the circulation. There are several examples of the possible operation of this reciprocity. During prolonged fasting (when liver decreases its release)[41] and in anhepatic patients undergoing liver transplantation (when liver glucose release is absent)[42] the kidney increases its release of glucose. Presumably, the reverse happens in patients with renal failure since hypoglycemia is uncommon in uncomplicated cases. As indicated earlier, postprandially hepatic glucose release decreases while renal glucose release increases, these reciprocal changes would permit more efficient repletion of hepatic glycogen stores. Another example of this concept is counterregulation of hypoglycemia in patients with type 2 diabetes; as a result of reduced glucagon responses and decreased liver glycogen stores, hepatic glucose release is decreased. However, there is a compensatory increase in renal glucose release. This is probably due to increased catecholamine responses and at least in part explains the reduced tendency for hypoglycemia in insulin-treated type 2 diabetic patients compared to type 1 diabetic patients. The latter, because of impaired glucagon and catecholamine responses, have reductions in both hepatic and renal glucose release during counterregulation of hypoglycemia and hepatorenal reciprocity is inoperative.[43]

REFERENCES

1. DCCT Research Group. The effect of intensive treatment of diabetes on the development and progression of long-term complications in insulin dependent diabetes mellitus. N Engl J Med 329:977-986, 1993.
2. UK Prospective Diabetes Study (UKPDS) Group. Intensive blood-glucose control with sulphonylureas or insulin compared with conventional treatment and risk of complications in patients with type 2 diabetes (UKPDS 33). Lancet 352:837-853, 1998.
3. Owen O, Morgan A, Kemp H, Sullivan J, Herrera M, Cahill G. Brain metabolism during fasting. J Clin Invest 46:1589-1595, 1967.
4. Gerich J. Glucose counterregulation and its impact on diabetes mellitus. Diabetes 37:1608-1617, 1988.
5. Meyer C, Dostou J, Nadkarni V, Gerich J. Effects of physiological hyperinsulinemia on systemic, renal and hepatic substrate metabolism. Am J Physiol 275:F915-F921, 1998.
6. Magnusson I, Rothman D, Gerard D, Katz L, Shulman G. Contribution of hepatic glycogenolysis to glucose production in humans in response to a physiological increase in plasma glucagon concentration. Diabetes 44:185-189, 1995.
7. Stumvoll M, Chintalapudi U, Perriello G, Welle S, Gutierrez O, Gerich J. Uptake and release of glucose by the human kidney: postabsorptive rates and responses to epinephrine. J Clin Invest 96:2528-2533, 1995.

8. Cahill G. Starvation in man. N Engl J Med 282:668-675, 1970.
9. Havel R. Caloric homeostasis and disorders of fuel transport. N Engl J Med 287:1186-1192, 1972.
10. Boden G. Role of fatty acids in the pathogenesis of insulin resistance and NIDDM. Diabetes 46:3-10, 1997.
11. McGarry J. Glucose-fatty acid interactions in health and disease. Am J Clin Nutr 67(3 Suppl):500S-504S, 1998.
12. Consoli A, Kennedy F, Miles J, Gerich J. Determination of Krebs cycle metabolic carbon exchange in vivo and its use to estimate the individual contributions of gluconeogenesis and glycogenolysis to overall glucose output in man. J Clin Invest 80:1303-1310, 1987.
13. Perriello G, Jorde R, Nurjhan N, Stumvoll M, Dailey G, Jenssen T, Bier D, Gerich J. Estimation of the glucose-alanine-lactate-glutamine cycles in postabsorptive man: role of the skeletal muscle. Am J Physiol 269:E443-E450, 1995.
14. Gerich J. Control of glycaemia. Bailliere's Clinical Endocrinology and Metabolism 7:551-586, 1993.
15. Stumvoll M, Meyer C, Mitrakou A, Nadkarni V, Gerich J. Renal glucose production and utilization: new aspects in humans. Diabetologia 40:749-757, 1997.
16. Landau B, Wahren J, Chandramouli V, Schuman W, Ekberg K, Kalhan S. Contributions of gluconeogenesis to glucose production in the fasted state. J Clin Invest 98:378-385, 1996.
17. Ekberg K, Landau B, Wajngot A, Chandramouli V, Efendic S, Brunengraber H, Wahren J. Contributions by kidney and liver to glucose production in the postabsorptive state and after 60 h of fasting. Diabetes 48:292-298, 1999.
18. Stumvoll M, Meyer C, Kreider M, Perriello G, Gerich J. Effects of glucagon on renal and hepatic glutamine gluconeogenesis in normal postabsorptive humans. Metabolism 47:1227-1232, 1998.
19. Stumvoll M, Meyer C, Perriello G, Kreider M, Welle S, Gerich J. Human kidney and liver gluconeogenesis: evidence for organ substrate selectivity. Am J Physiol 274:E817-E826, 1998.
20. Krebs H, Speake R, Hems R. Acceleration of renal gluconeogenesis by ketone bodies and fatty acids. Biochem J 94:712-720, 1965.
21. McMahon M, Marsh H, Rizza R. Comparison of the pattern of postprandial carbohydrate metabolism after ingestion of a glucose drink or a mixed meal. J Clin Endocrinol & Metab 68:647-653, 1989.
22. Dinneen S, Gerich J, Rizza R. Carbohydrate metabolism in noninsulin-dependent diabetes mellitus. N Engl J Med 327:707-713, 1992.
23. Beckmann N, Fried R, Turkalj I, Seelig J, Keller U, Stalder G. Noninvasive observation of hepatic glycogen formation in man by ^{13}C MRS after oral and intravenous glucose administration. Magn Reson Med 29:583-590, 1993.

24. Petersen K, Cline G, Gerard D, Magnusson I, Rothman D, Shulman G. Contribution of net hepatic glycogen synthesis to disposal of an oral glucose load in humans. Metabolism 50:598-601, 2001.

25. Kelley D, Mitrakou A, Marsh H, Schwenk F, Benn J, Sonnenberg G, Archangeli M, Aoki T, Sorensen J, Berger M, Sonksen P, Gerich J. Skeletal muscle glycolysis, oxidation, and storage of an oral glucose load. J Clin Invest 81:1563-1571, 1988.

26. Kelley D, Mokan M, Veneman T. Impaired postprandial glucose utilization in non-insulin-dependent diabetes mellitus. Metabolism 43:1549-1557, 1994.

27. Meyer C, Dostou J, Welle S, Gerich J. Role of liver, kidney and skeletal muscle in the disposition of an oral glucose load. Diabetes 48(Suppl 1):A289, 1999(Abstract).

28. Butler P, Kryshak E, Rizza R. Mechanism of growth hormone-induced postprandial carbohydrate intolerance in humans. Am J Physiol 260:E513-E520, 1991.

29. Ferrannini E, Bjorkman O, Reichard G, Pilo A, Olsson M, Wahren J, DeFronzo R. The disposal of an oral glucose load in healthy subjects: a quantitative study. Diabetes 34:580-588, 1985.

30. Jackson R, Roshania R, Hawa M, Sim B, DiSilvio L. Impact of glucose ingestion on hepatic and peripheral glucose metabolism in man: an analysis based on simultaneous use of the forearm and double isotope techniques. J Clin Endo & Metab 63:541-549, 1986.

31. McMahon M, Marsh H, Rizza R. Effects of basal insulin supplementation on disposition of a mixed meal in obese patients with NIDDM. Diabetes 38:291-303, 1989.

32. Mitrakou A, Kelley D, Mokan M, Veneman T, Pangburn T, Reilly J, Gerich J. Role of reduced suppression of glucose production and diminished early insulin release in impaired glucose tolerance. N Engl J Med 326:22-29, 1992.

33. Taylor R, Magnusson I, Rothman D. Direct assessment of liver glycogen storage by ^{13}C nuclear magnetic resonance spectroscopy and regulation of glucose homeostasis after a mixed meal in normal subjects. J Clin Invest 97:126-132, 1996.

34. Mitrakou A, Jones R, Okuda Y, Pena J, Nurjhan N, Field J, Gerich J. Pathway and carbon sources for hepatic glycogen repletion in the dog. Am J Physiol 260:E194-202, 1991.

35. Firth R, Bell P, Marsh H, Hansen I, Rizza R. Postprandial hyperglycemia in patients with noninsulin-dependent diabetes mellitus. Role of hepatic and extrahepatic tissues. J Clin Invest 77:1525-1532, 1986.

36. Taylor R, Price T, Katz L, Shulman R, Shulman G. Direct measurement of change in muscle glycogen concentration after a mixed meal in normal subjects. Am J Physiol 265:E224-E229, 1993.

37. Marin P, Hogh-Kristiansen I, Jansson S, Krotkiewski M, Holm G, Bjorntorp P. Uptake of glucose carbon in muscle glycogen and adipose tissue triglycerides in vivo in humans. Am J Physiol 263:E473-E480, 1992.

38. Radziuk J, Inculet R. The effects of ingested and intravenous glucose on forearm uptake of glucose and glucogenic substrate in normal man. Diabetes 32:977-981, 1983.

39. Ferrannini E, Wahren J, Felig P, DeFronzo R. The role of fractional glucose extraction in the regulation of splanchnic glucose metabolism in normal and diabetic man. Metabolism 29:28-35, 1980.

40. Kruszynska Y, Mulford M, Yu J, Armstrong D, Olefsky J. Effects of nonesterified fatty acids on glucose metabolism after glucose ingestion. Diabetes 46:1586-1593, 1997.

41. Owen O, Felig P, Morgan A, Wahren J, Cahill G. Liver and kidney metabolism during prolonged starvation. J Clin Invest 48:574-583, 1969.

42. Joseph S, Heaton N, Potter D, Pernet A, Umpleby M, Amiel S. Renal glucose production compensates for the liver during the anhepatic phase of liver transplantation. Diabetes 49:450-456, 2000.

43. Cersosimo E, Ferretti J, Sasvary D, Garlick P. Adrenergic stimulation of renal glucose release is impaired in type 1 diabetes. Diabetes 50(Suppl 2):A54, 2001.

Chapter 2. Endocrine pancreas: mechanisms of insulin secretion by the β-cells; interactions among insulin, glucagon and somatostatin

Barry J. Brass

INTRODUCTION

The endocrine pancreas is composed of the islets of Langerhans which comprise approximately two million clusters of cells dispersed within the acinar tissue of the exocrine pancreas. In the adult, the islets constitute between one and two percent of the pancreatic mass. The islets are composed of four endocrine cell types: α-cells which secrete glucagon, β-cells which secrete insulin, δ-cells which secrete somatostatin, and PP cells which secrete pancreatic polypeptide (Table 1).

Table 1. Islet Cell Types

Cell Type	Percentage of total	Hormone
Alpha (α)	15	Glucagon
Beta (ß)	60	Insulin
Delta (δ)	10	Somatostatin
PP	15	Pancreatic polypeptide

The principal role of the pancreatic hormones is to regulate the uptake and release of metabolic fuels from the hormone sensitive tissues, liver, muscle and fat. After meals, when nutrient levels in the blood are high, insulin secretion is stimulated, glucagon secretion is inhibited, and the high insulin to glucagon ratio promotes nutrient storage. At times of fasting, when stored fuel energy is needed, insulin secretion is inhibited, glucagon secretion is stimulated, and the low insulin to glucagon ratio promotes nutrient release from storage. Figure 1 shows the concentrations of insulin, C-peptide and glucose in the blood of normal and diabetic subjects over a 24-hour period.[1] The subjects were fed three standard meals totaling 30 kcal/kg body weight and composed of 50% carbohydrate, 15% protein and 35% fat. The meals were served at 9:00 a.m., 1:00 p.m. and 6:00 p.m. In the normal subjects, insulin and C-peptide concentrations rose to a sharp peak after meals and then rapidly declined. Glucose rose to approximately 50%

above basal levels and then returned to baseline within one to two hours. In the type 2 diabetic subjects, insulin and C-peptide peaked less sharply and rose to lower levels. Glucose levels were higher and their peaks were more prolonged.

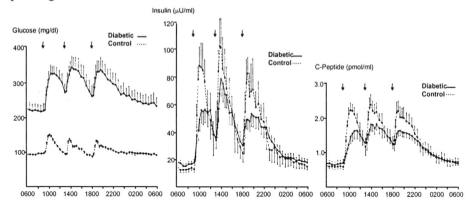

Figure 1. Blood glucose, insulin and C-peptide levels over a 24-hour period in normal subjects and type 2 diabetics. Post-prandial insulin and C-peptide levels are higher in normal subjects. Glucose levels are lower. (From: Polonsky KS et al. Abnormal patterns of insulin secretion in non-insulin-dependent diabetes mellitus. N Engl J Med 318:1231-9, 1988, with permission.)

The total amount of insulin secreted at any given time reflects the sum of the insulin secreted by individual islets. In type 2 diabetes an inadequate insulin secretory response reflects inadequate insulin secretion from the individual β-cells of the individual islets. This is referred to as beta cell dysfunction.

Figure 2 shows the concentrations of insulin, C-peptide and glucose in the blood of normal and obese subjects over a 24-hour period.[2] Note that the plasma glucose concentrations are similar, but the obese subjects require higher insulin and C-peptide levels to maintain the same glucose levels. This demonstrates the concept of insulin resistance, which is often present in obesity and is defined as impaired insulin-stimulated glucose disposal. The interpretation of this figure is that insulin resistance in obese subjects is compensated for by increased insulin secretion. Since there is no hyperglycemia relative to normal subjects, it can be inferred that there is no significant β-cell dysfunction. When both insulin resistance and beta cell dysfunction are present, the result is the sustained hyperglycemia of type 2 diabetes mellitus, as in Figure 1.

Islet hormones are secreted into the splenic vein and are carried directly to the hepatic portal system. In the liver, where a high insulin to glucagon ratio signals energy storage, glycogen synthesis is stimulated while glycogenolysis, gluconeogenesis, fatty acid oxidation and ketone production are inhibited. A low ratio signals energy utilization, and glycogenolysis, gluconeogenesis and fatty acid oxidation are increased. In adipose tissue, where a high ratio also favors energy storage, fatty acid and glucose uptake increase, and triglyceride formation is stimulated. A low ratio favors energy utilization, and fatty acids and glycerol are released into the circulation.

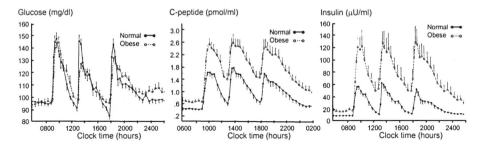

Figure 2. Blood glucose, insulin and C-peptide levels over a 24-hour period in normal and obese subjects. Insulin and C-peptide levels are higher in obese subjects. Glucose levels are similar. (From: Polonsky KS et al. Twenty-four-hour profiles and pulsatile patterns of insulin secretion in normal and obese subjects. J Clin Invest 81:422-8, 1988, with permission.)

Figure 3 shows the uptake of insulin and glucagon by the liver.[3] Greater than 50% of both insulin and glucagon bind to specific receptors on hepatocytes and are removed from the circulation. Since meal derived nutrients also enter the hepatic portal system, the first pass hepatic uptake of insulin and glucagon is a very efficient means of signalling hepatic processing of nutrients. With subcutaneously injected insulin, the first pass hepatic uptake of insulin is lost, and the uptake of meal related nutrients by the liver is not as efficient.

It is tempting to think that the amount of insulin secreted by islets is exclusively determined by the concentration of glucose in the blood. It must be emphasized that this is not the case. Just as insulin affects the uptake and storage of fatty acids and amino acids as well as glucose, so do fatty acids and amino acids exert an influence on beta cell insulin secretion. Consequently, islet hormones play a central role in maintaining total fuel energy homeostasis and not just carbohydrate homeostasis. Moreover, islet secretion is not solely determined by nutrients. Both extrapancreatic hormones and neural activity coordinate and magnify the effects of nutrients on pancreatic hormone secretion. Thus, there are four factors that are principally responsible for regulating insulin secretion: 1) the concentrations of nutrients bathing the islets including glucose, free fatty acids and amino acids; 2) the activity of the autonomic nerves innervating the islets; 3) blood borne hormonal inputs; and 4) interactions between the islet cells.

The architecture of the islets facilitates interactions that regulate hormone secretion. Insulin secreting cells are centrally located within the islets, and glucagon-secreting cells are located peripherally. Blood flow within the islets is from the center outward allowing β-cell secretion of insulin to exert a tonic inhibitory effect on α-cell secretion of glucagon. Small molecules and ions pass between islet cells through gap junctions allowing the islet to function as a coordinated secretory unit. The capillary network investing the islets brings gut derived hormones affecting islet hormone secretion, and the complex innervation of the islets plays a role in integrating the hormonal response. This chapter will discuss the mechanisms by which all of these factors acting together and separately affect insulin secretion.

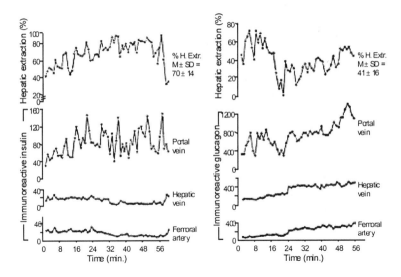

Figure 3. Uptake of insulin (left pane;) and glucagon (right panel) by the liver. (From: Jaspan et al. In vivo pulsatility of pancreatic islet peptides. Am J Physiol 14: E215-26, 1986, with permission.)

NUTRIENTS AND INSULIN SECRETION

Glucose and The Fuel Hypothesis of Insulin Secretion

Insulin is secreted at a rate that depends in part on the concentration of glucose in the blood. It was originally thought that islet cells possess glucose receptors, and it was theorized that increased blood concentrations of glucose leads to greater receptor occupancy which in turn leads to greater insulin secretion. This view was abandoned in light of a large body of evidence demonstrating that insulin secretion is proportional to the rate at which glucose is metabolized within the islet ß-cells (reviewed in ref. 4). This forms the basis of the well-accepted "fuel hypothesis" (Figure 4) which states that the intracellular glucose concentration determines the rate of glucose metabolism, and the rate of glucose metabolism determines the rate of insulin secretion.

Details of this mechanism have been well worked out. Metabolism of glucose increases the ratio of the concentrations of ATP to ADP. ATP interacts with ATP-dependent potassium channels closing the channels. Potassium channel closure depolarizes the plasma membrane potential which in turn opens L-type voltage gated calcium channels. The cytoplasmic calcium concentration, $[Ca^{++}]_c$, rises and calcium activates protein kinases and interacts with the cell's secretory machinery leading to exocytosis of insulin laden secretory vesicles, i.e. insulin secretion.

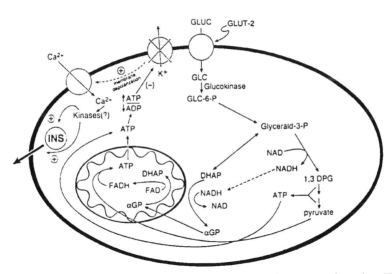

Figure 4. Schematic view of the fuel hypothesis (see text above). (From: Newgard, C.B. and McGarry, J.D. Metabolic coupling factors in pancreatic ß-cell signal transduction. Ann Rev Biochem 64:689-719, 1995, with permission.)

This cellular pathway explains the mechanism of action of sulfonylureas, the first class of drugs used to enhance insulin secretion in patients with type 2 diabetes mellitus. Sulfonylureas bind to the ATP-dependent potassium channel complex closing the channels. Subsequent membrane depolarization and calcium channel opening raises the intracellular calcium concentrations, and insulin secretion is increased.

Glucose enters the ß-cell through facilitated glucose transporters, GLUT-2, which are constitutively expressed in the plasma membrane of islet cells. The transporter has a Michaelis constant of approximately 15 to 20 mmol/L which is higher than the normal basal plasma glucose concentration of around 5.5 mmol/L. As a result changes in plasma glucose are reflected by changes in the free glucose concentration within islet cells. Glucose is trapped within the ß-cell by the first step in glycolysis, the phosphorylation of glucose to glucose-6-P. This reaction, catalyzed by glucokinase, is the rate-limiting step in glycolysis, and since insulin secretion is proportional to the rate of glucose metabolism, it can be said that the combined actions of GLUT-2 and glucokinase form a physiologic "glucose sensor".

The mechanism outlined above does not account for all of the insulin secretion stimulated by glucose. It has been shown that the mitochondrial metabolism of glycolytically derived pyruvate causes insulin secretion independently of increased $[Ca^{++}]_c$. The exact nature of the mitochondrial derived signals is unknown and is the subject of intensive investigation and very vigorous debate. There is strong evidence that mitochondrially derived glutamate provides the signal for insulin secretion in insulinoma cell lines[5]. However, several labs have shown that this does not appear to be the case in native islets. It is anticipated that further elucidation of the mechanism of insulin secretion will lead to new therapies.

The First and Second Phases of Insulin Secretion

Intravenously administered glucose elicits a biphasic insulin response (Figure 5). The first phase is rapid in onset, has a sharp peak and lasts for about 10 minutes. The second phase is a prolonged plateau that lasts for as long as the blood glucose remains elevated. As the figure shows, the first phase of secretion is lost in type 2 diabetics. However, in these same diabetic subjects the first phase response to intravenously administered arginine is intact demonstrating that the loss of the glucose stimulated first phase secretion is due to failure to transduce a glucose associated signal.

A plausible explanation for biphasic insulin secretion is that the first phase represents release of insulin from a population of secretory vesicles that are "docked " and "primed" at the β-cell membrane and awaiting a glucose dependent calcium signal for immediate release. The second phase represents replenishment of exocytosis-competent secretory vesicles.

Lipids and Insulin Secretion

Non-esterified fatty acids (NEFA), also known as free fatty acids (FFA), are an important energy source for many tissues of the body. In addition, they are metabolized in ß-cells where they also serve as important signalling molecules regulating ß-cell function. Acute exposure to free fatty acids increases both basal insulin secretion and glucose stimulated insulin secretion. Chronically elevated levels of free fatty acids such as that seen in patients with Type 2 Diabetes mellitus may have deleterious effects on ß-cell function, and may have an etiologic role in both the ß-cell dysfunction and insulin resistance of type 2 diabetes mellitus.[6]

The effect of free fatty acids on insulin secretion is illustrated in a study by Dobbins et al. (Ref. 7, Figures 6a and 6b). In this study, lean healthy subjects were fasted for 48 hours on three separate occasions prior to an experimental protocol in which circulating FFA levels were varied and glucose stimulated insulin secretion was measured. Fig. 6a, panel B, shows the striking effect of nicotinic acid in reducing circulating FFA. Panel B also shows that a glucose bolus at time 0 stimulated insulin secretion (panel C) which then led to a marked reduction in circulating FFA (panel B). Fig. 6a, panel A, and Fig. 6b, panel A, show that in all experiments blood glucose levels were equivalent, therefore differences in insulin secretion reflected the effects of circulating FFA and not glucose. Basal levels of insulin fell from 19.2 pmole/L in the saline experiment to 10.8 pmole/L in the nicotinic acid experiment. Insulin and C-peptide levels in response to glucose were lowest in the nicotinic acid experiment where FFA levels were lowest, and highest in the NA/intralipid/heparin experiment where FFA levels were highest (Fig. 6b, panels C and D). This experiment along with in vitro experiments on isolated islets established that acutely elevated levels of free fatty acids enhance both basal and glucose stimulated insulin secretion in normal subjects.

The cellular events leading to the fatty acid induced enhancement of glucose stimulated insulin secretion are illustrated in Figure 7. Glucose metabolism leads to increased mitochondrial citrate formation. Some of the citrate is oxidized in the Kreb's cycle producing ATP, and some is exported out of the mitochondria into the cytoplasm. Cytoplasmic citrate is converted to malonyl Co-A by the actions of the enzymes citrate lyase and acetyl-CoA carboxylase. Malonyl-CoA is a potent inhibitor of carnitine palmitoyltransferase 1 (CPT-1), the outer mitochondrial membrane ezyme that transports fatty acyl-CoA into the mitochondria. Inhibition of transport of fatty acyl Co-A into the mitochondria leads to an increase in cytoplasmic fatty acyl-CoA which then acts as a signalling molecule having several actions that increase insulin secretion. It increases the synthesis of diacylglycerol which activates protein kinase C, and as discussed below, protein kinase C enhances insulin secretion. Fatty acyl-CoA also increases insulin vesicle trafficking, alters ion channel activity, and promotes vesicle docking and fusion with the cell membrane.

The accumulation of lipids in muscle leads to insulin resistance.[10] Since fatty acids enhance insulin secretion, it may be that this enhancement arose as an adaptation to protect against the hyperglycemia that would otherwise have resulted from fatty acid mediated insulin resistance. The breakdown of this balance may occur in Type 2 diabetes mellitus. In early type 2 diabetes, the disease is characterized by prolonged elevation of FFA along with insulin resistance, basal hyperinsulinemia, and exagerated postprandial insulin secretion. It may be speculated that prolonged exposure to elevated fatty acids causes a decompensation in which ß-cell dysfunction cannot overcome the effects of insulin resistance.

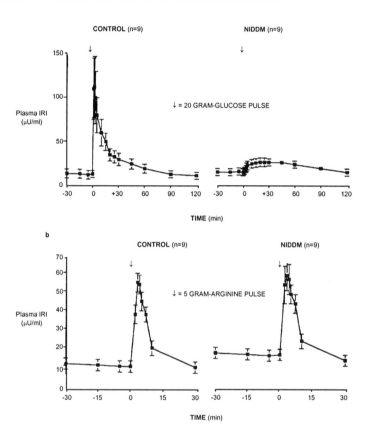

Figure 5. The top panel shows the first phase of insulin secretion in response to intravenous insulin in normal subjects (left plot) and the loss of the first phase in diabetic subjects (right plot). The bottom panel shows the intact insulin secretory response to intravenous arginine in normal subjects and diabetics. (From: Poitout V and Robertson RP. An integrated view of ß-cell dysfunction in type-II diabetes. Annu Rev Med 47:69-83, 1996, with permission.)

6a.   6b.

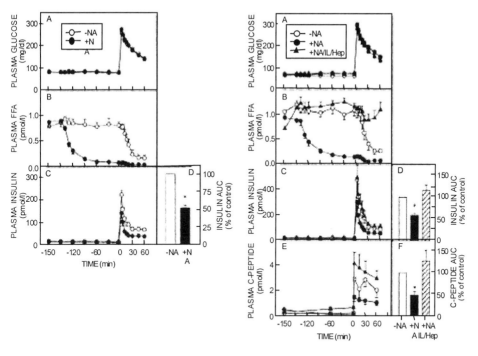

Figure 6. Higher circulating FFA (NA/IL/Hep) produce higher levels of insulin and C-peptide (see text). (From: Dobbins RL et al. Circulating fatty acids are essential for efficient glucose-stimulated insulin secretion after prolonged fasting in humans. Diabetes 47:1613-8, 1998, with permission.)

Experiments using animal models of diabetes support this view. In the male Zucker Diabetic Fatty rat there is a pronounced increase in plasma fatty acids, triglycerides, and islet triglycerides that occurs before hyperglycemia appears. Diet restriction as sole therapy reduces hyperlipidemia, islet hypertiglyceridemia and improves ß-cell function while preventing hyperglycemia. In another experiment using rats, circulating FFA was rapidly increased by infusing intralipid. It was found that elevated fatty acids enhanced glucose stimulated insulin secretion at three and six hours of exposure but suppressed it at 48 hours. Carpentier et al. 1999,[8] showed essentially the same results in healthy young men. Similar results have been obtained by several investigators using in vitro systems in which acute exposure of isolated islets to FFA enhanced insulin secretion while prolonged exposure suppressed it. Observations such as these raise the possibility that in diabetes prone individuals chronically elevated fatty acids play a role in the β-cell dysfunction of clinical diabetes.

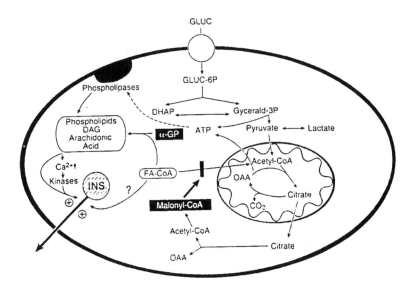

Figure 7. Glucose inhibits the oxidation of fatty acyl-CoA by increasing the productionn of malonyl-CoA which blocks transport of fatty acyl-CoA into the mitochondria. This ensures that cytoplasmic fatty acyl-CoA is available to enhance insulin secretion. (From: Newgard CB and McGarry JD. Metabolic coupling factors in pancreatic ß-cell signal transduction. Ann Rev Biochem 64:689-719, 1995, with permission.)

NEURAL REGULATION OF INSULIN SECRETION

The pancreatic islets are richly innervated by autonomic and sensory nerves (reviewed in ref. 9). Insulin secretion is enhanced by stimulation of parasympathetic nerves and inhibited by stimulation of sympatheitic nerves. Sensory pathways are for the most part inhibitory. Additional neural pathways mediate direct entero-pancreatic interactions.

The cephalic phase of insulin secretion refers to the first three to four minutes of insulin secretion triggered not by blood borne nutrients but by the sight, smell, and anticipation of food. The cephalic phase has been demonstrated in a number of ways: by imaginary feeding under hypnosis, by the ingestion of nonnutrient sweeteners, and by the rise in blood insulin levels prior to the rise in blood glucose after ingestion of a glucose load.

The neural effector pathways begin in the ventro-medial hypothalamus and dorsal motor nucleus of the vagus. The cephalic phase is abolished by vagotomy or by ganglionic blockade with muscarinic antagonists, demonstrating that it is mediated by cholinergic neurons of the parasympathetic nervous system. The question of the physiologic importance of the cephalic phase has been raised since it accounts for only 1% to 3% of the total insulin response to a meal. A possible role may be to maintain glucose tolerance defined as the ability of insulin to lower blood glucose in response to an ingested glucose load. Accordingly, it has been shown that insulin treatment of subjects with Type 2 diabetes in the first 15 minutes after food ingestion improves glucose tolerance.

The insulin output of an individual islet derives from the coordinated function of many ß-cells. Within islet cells oscillatory patterns can be seen in oxygen consumption, production of ATP, and concentrations of cytosolic calcium. Electrical coupling by gap junctions serves to help coordinate activity. In addition, insulin secretion from the pancreas as a whole is pulsatile suggesting synchronization between the islets as well. Blockade of pancreatic ganglia abolishes this synchronization. The clinical importance of oscillatory insulin secretion is suggested by its loss in patients with impaired glucose tolerance and type 2 diabetes.

Parasympathetic Nerves

The parasympathetic nerves innervating the islets originate in the dorsal motor nuclei of the vagus. Preganglionic fibers traverse the vagus as parts of the bulbar outflow tract and the hepatic and gastric branches of the vagus. They enter the pancreas and terminate in intrapancreatic ganglia from which postganglionic fibers emerge to innervate the islets. The postganglionic nerve terminals contain the classical neurotransmitter acetylcholine and the neuropeptides gastrin releasing peptide (GRP), vasoactive intestinal polypeptide (VIP) and pituitary adenylate cyclase activating polypeptide (PACAP).

Vagal activation stimulates insulin secretion. Stimulation of the postganglionic fibers releases acetylcholine which binds to m3 muscarinic receptors on islet cells. The hormones secreted by the other three islet cell types, glucagon, somatostatin, and pancreatic polypeptide are also stimulated by acetylcholine via m3 receptors. In ß-cells, binding of acetylcholine to its receptor stimulates phospholipase C (PLC) activation via a G protein coupled mechanism. This stimulates phosphoinositde hydrolysis to IP$_3$ and diacylglycerol (DAG). Phospholipase A$_2$ (PLA$_2$) is also activated producing arachadonic acid. Insulin secretion is stimulated by subsequent increased $[Ca^{++}]_c$ and protein phosphorylation. The mechanisms by which PLC and PLA$_2$ stimulate insulin secretion are discussed in the section on insulin secretion and second messengers. The intracellular pathways by which acetylcholine stimulates secretion of the other islet hormones have not been elucidated.

VIP, PACAP, and GRP stimulate insulin secretion upon binding to their respective G protein coupled receptors. VIP and PACAP exert their effects by stimulating adenylate cyclase and increasing levels of cAMP. GRP binding to its receptor activates PLC and phospholipase D (PLD). The mechanisms by which cAMP and PLD stimulate insulin secretion are discussed in the section on insulin secretion and second messengers.

Sympathetic Nerves

At times of physiologic stress such as prolonged fasting, excercise, hypoglycemia or hypovolemia maintaining blood glucose levels becomes vitally important. Glucose output by the liver plays the main role in this process stimulated in part by the counter regulatory hormones cortisol, epinephrine and growth hormone. In addition, activation of local sympathetic nerves stimulates glucagon secretion, while insulin secretion is concurrently inhibited. The decreased insulin to glucagon ratio provides the signal for hepatic glucose production and output.

The adrenergic nerves innervating the islets are postganglionic fibers whose cell bodies are located in the celiac ganglion and paravertebral sympathetic ganglia. The preganglionic nerves originate in the hypothalamus and leave the spinal cord at the level of C8 to L3 and traverse the lesser and greater splanchnic nerves to reach the postganglionic cell bodies. The postganglionic nerve terminals contain the classical sympathetic neurotransmitter, norepinephrine, along with the neuropeptides galanin and neuropeptide Y (NPY).

Norepinephrine inhibition of glucose stimulated insulin secretion is mediated by a2-adrenoreceptors. It is not known whether the inhibition of basal insulin secretion is also mediated by norepinephrine. Sympathetic activation also stimulates glucagon and pancreatic polypeptide secretion, while somatostatin secretion is inhibited.

The norepinephrine induced inhibition of insulin secretion is mediated by several signalling pathways: First, a2-adrenoreceptor activation leads to hyperpolarization of the ß-cell through opening of the ATP-dependent potassium channels. This prevents opening of the voltage-gated calcium channels thereby preventing increased $[Ca^{++}]_c$ and subsequent exocytosis of secretory granules. Second, the formation of cyclic AMP is inhibited, and, third, there is an inhibitory action on the distal exocytotic machinery.

The concept that sympathetic neuropeptides inhibit glucose stimulated insulin secretion derives from animal experiments in which sympathetic stimulation leads to inhibition of secretion under conditions in which a2-adrenoreceptors are blocked. The mediators of this inhibition are the neuropeptides galanin and NPY. Binding of these neuropeptides to their respective receptors activates pathways similar to those activated by norepinephrine.

Sensory and Other Nerves

The islets are extensively innervated with sensory afferents containing the neuropeptides calcitonin gene related peptide (CGRP) and substance P (SP). The afferent fibers leave the pancreas along with the sympathetic fibers of the splanchnic nerve and participate in reflexes whose effectors are the autonomic nerves. CGRP has an inhibitory effect on insulin secretion mediated by a decrease in islet cyclic AMP probably reflecting a2-adrenoreceptor activation. The CGRP neurons also stimulate glucagon secretion and thus likely participate in the islet's reflex response to hypoglycemia. The actions of SP neurons are less well characterized and both stimulatory and inhibitory effects have been demonstrated.

Other nerves that innervate the islets and affect insulin secretion include neurons that contain nitric oxide synthase (NOS) and cholecystokinin (CCK). The NOS neurons stimulate insulin secretion. The CCK neurons stimulate insulin secretion via mechanisms that involve PLC and PLA_2 pathways. In addition, nerves originating in the duodenal ganglia directly innervate islets suggesting the existence of direct entero-pancreatic neural mechanisms.

GLUCAGON AND GLUCAGON-LIKE PEPTIDES

Glucagon and the glucagon-like peptides, GLP-1 and GLP-2, are the products of a single gene and are derived from differential posttranslational processing of a single proglucagon protein. Glucagon is produced by the alpha cells of the pancreatic islets, and the GLP's are produced by enteroendocrine cells of the small and large intestine. Glucagon and GLP-1 have important roles in maintaining glucose homeostasis.

Glucagon

Glucagon plays a central role in the maintenance of basal blood glucose levels. Hypoglycemia stimulates and hyperglycemia suppresses glucagon secretion. Glucagon levels rise with fasting and rise further with excercise. During times of nutrient need, blood glucose levels are maintained by hepatic glucose production stimulated by low insulin-glucagon ratios. The binding of glucagon to its G-protein coupled receptor on hepatocytes increases intracellular levels of cAMP leading to activation of protein kinase A, phosphorylase kinase, and phosphorylase. Glycogen synthase is inactivated. The result is stimulation of gluconeogenesis and glycogenolysis and inhibition of glycolysis. Increased hepatic fatty acid oxidation and ketone body formation provide additional energy substrate. In adipocytes, glucagon acts via increased cAMP to stimulate lipolysis liberating fatty acids into the circulation. In addition, glucose uptake into adipocytes is inhibited thereby decreasing triglyceride synthesis.

Positive regulators of glucagon secretion include sympathetic nerve stimulation, epinephrine, CCK, PACAP, and GIP. Insulin released by ß-cells tonically suppresses glucagon secretion. Conversely, during hypoglycemia insulin levels are low releasing glucagon from tonic suppression. Additionally, glucose suppresses glucagon secretion by inducing ß-cell release of the inhibitory neurotransmitter GABA.

GLP-1

The majority of GLP-1 producing cells are in the terminal ileum and proximal colon. Proglucagon synthesis in the gut is stimulated by nutrient intake, and GLP-1 levels in the blood increase rapidly after a meal. The activity of GLP-1 is largely regulated by its rate of degradation with its half-life being very short, approximately one minute. GLP-1 binding to its G-protein coupled receptor on ß-cells increases glucose stimulated insulin secretion via both increased cyclic AMP and increased intracellular calcium.

GLP-1 infused into healthy subjects decreases gastric emptying, causes a sensation of satiety and decreases appetite. Thus, in addition to enhancing insulin secretion, GLP-1 has effects outside of the pancreas that serve to limit postprandial hyperglycemia. In rodents, intracerebroventricularly administered GLP-1 inhibits food intake demonstrating CNS actions. Infusion of the GLP-1 antagonist exendin into healthy subjects increases blood glucose and reduces glucose stimulated insulin secretion[14]. The multiple actions of GLP-1 in lowering blood glucose make the development of a GLP-1-like agent modified for a longer half-life an interesting approach to be used in the treatment diabetes mellitus.

SOMATOSTATIN

Somatostatin was originally identified in 1973 in hypothalamic extracts as a 14 amino acid peptide that inhibits the release of growth hormone from dispersed rat pituitary cells. Since then, somatostatin and its receptors have been found in all neuroendocrine tissues, as well as in the central and peripheral nervous systems. A single somatostatin gene codes for two biologically active peptides of 14 and 28 amino acids, named somatostatin-14 and somatostatin-28, respectively. In addition to acting as hormones transported in the blood, the peptides act as neurotransmitters, neuromodulators and local paracrine regulators. Their diverse physiologic actions include modulation of secretion, neurotransmission, smooth muscle contractility and cell proliferation.

There are five different somatostatin receptors designated sst1, sst2A, sst3, sst4 and sst5. All are members of the G protein-coupled receptor family, and all inhibit adenylate cyclase activity. Other effectors linked to the sst's via G proteins include voltage sensitive calcium channels, potassium channels, ser/thr phosphatases amd tyrosine phosphatases

Somatostatin is produced in neurons of the hypothalamic periventricular area that terminate near the pituitary portal capillaries. Release of somatostatin by these neurons inhibits growth hormone secretion by cells of the anterior pituitary. Elsewhere in the brain, somatostatin acts as a neurotransmitter or neuromodulator. It is stored in synaptic vesicles, released by a calcium dependent mechanism upon depolarization and produces post synaptic hyperpolarization upon its release.

In the gastrointestinal tract, somatostatin is found in the stomach, duodenum, submucosal neurons and myenteric plexis of the intestinal tract. It is produced both by gastrointestinal endocrine D cells and by visceral autonomic neurons. Thus it has paracrine and hormonal functions as well as acting as a neurotransmitter. It inhibits the secretion of a variety of hormones including insulin, VIP, GIP, gastrin, cholecystokinin, secretin, motilin and GLP-1, and reduces gastrintestinal motility, gallbladder contraction and blood flow. Its concentration in the blood increases after meals as a consequence of both gastrointestinal and pancreatic secretion.

Intravenous administration of somatostatin inhibits insulin secretion as well as exocrine pancreatic secretion. However, the precise role of somatostatin in islet function has not been determined. Sst2A receptors are present on islet β-cells and α-cells suggesting that somatostatin may have a direct role in regulating insulin and glucagon secretion.

ISLET AMYLOID POLYPEPTIDE (IAPP)

IAPP is a 37 amino acid protein that is the principal component of islet amyloid deposits. These deposits are formed in normal islets during aging but are more abundant in the islets of type 2 diabetics. The amino acid sequences of IAPP from normal and diabetic subjects are identical, and consequently the increased deposition of amyloid deposits in diabetics is not due to structural abnormalities in the amyloid protein.

IAPP is localized in the secretory vesicles of β-cells and is cosecreted with insulin. Levels of IAPP are in the range of 0.2% to 3.0% of that of insulin in islets, and the amount cosecreted with insulin in about 5.0%. Several hormonal effects of IAPP have been proposed, but the data in support of a precise physiologic role for IAPP is far from compelling. Studies showing that amidated-IAPP inhibits insulin-stimulated glucose disposal used nonphysiologically high concentrations of IAPP. Other studies showed IAPP having complementary action to insulin. Still other studies showed that extremely high concentrations of IAPP inhibit insulin secretion.

REGULATION OF INSULIN SYNTHESIS

The immediate translation product of proinsulin messenger mRNA is an 1150 dalton peptide, preproinsulin, synthesized on polysomes of the rough endoplasmic reticulum. Within minutes of preproinsulin synthesis an N-terminal 24 residue signal peptide is cleaved by microsomal proteases forming proinsulin. Proinsulin, the precursor of mature insulin, is a single ~9000 dalton peptide chain that includes the A and B chains of mature insulin plus the C-peptide. Following translocation and cleavage of the signal sequence, proinsulin folds and rapidly forms three disulfide bonds to assume its native three dimensional structure. Proinsulin is then transferred in small coated vesicles to the *cis* and then the *trans* Golgi where it is sorted into secretory vesicles (Figure 8).

Insulin is concentrated within secretory vesicles by a process of protein sorting by subtraction in which non-insulin peptides are removed from the maturing vesicle by the budding off of clatrin-coated microvesicles. The process begins in the trans-golgi network, and leaves behind increasingly concentrated insulin within a developing secretory vesicle. The insulin condenses into tightly packed aggregates as proinsulin is enzymatically processed to mature insulin, and proton pumps acidify the environment of the vesicle. The end result is a mature secretory vesicle that contains predominently highly condensed insulin plus soluble C-peptide.

Theoretically, there are several ways in which proinsulin may be secreted from the ß-cell, but none of them involve the regulated secretory pathway. The clathrin-coated microvesicles that bud from the maturing secretory vesicle contain a small fraction of the proinsulin synthesized. Some of these vesicles fuse with endosomes, and their contents are cycled to the cell membrane and released. This is referred to as the constitutive-like (CL) pathway. Other vesicles fuse directly with the cell membrane prior to vesicle maturation and release their contents. This is referred to as the constitutive pathway. Finally, proinsulin may be released from immature secretory vesicles that fuse prematurely with the plasma membrane. The process of secretory vesicle maturation is highly efficient and less than 15% of the total insulins are secreted as proinsulin. This figure is much higher in conditions in which insulin secretion is less well regulated as in patients with type 2 diabetes mellitus or with inulinomas.

Proinsulin is converted to insulin by the action of two prohormone convertases, designated PC2 and PC3, which become activated in the *trans* Golgi network. Thus mature insulin is produced only in membrane bound vesicles which participate in regulated secretion. The proinsulin chain is cleaved at positions 31,32 and 64,65 producing mature insulin composed of a 21 residue A chain connected to a 30 residue B chain by two disulfide bonds plus a free 24 residue C-peptide. Partially processed proinsulin, called des-31,32 proinsulin, is secreted to some extent in the process of exocytosis and makes up a large proportion of the circulating proinsulin. As proinsulin processing proceeds, the interior of the granules become acidic by the action of vesicular proton pumps creating condtions for the optimum crystallization of insulin within the granules.

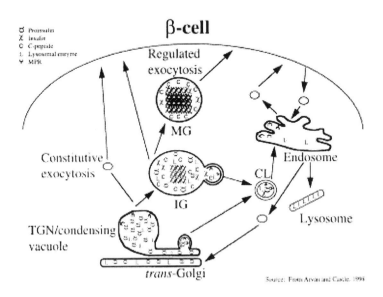

Figure 8. Cartoon illustrating the packageing of insulin into seretory vesicles. Mature insulin is secreted only by the regulated pathway. Proinsulin may be secreted by the constitutive or "constitutive-like" (CL) pathways. (From: Arvan P and Castle D. Sorting and storage during secretory granule biogenesis: looking backward and looking forward. Biochem J 332:513-610, 1998, with permission.)

C-peptide is secreted with insulin in equimolar amounts and serves as a useful marker of insulin secretion. It had been presumed that C-peptide had no biological activity, however in the last ten years reports have appeared describing biologic effects of C-peptide. Proposed effects include enhancement of glucose transport and utilization, improvements in microcirculation in muscle, skin, retina, and nerve, stimulation of renal tubular Na+,K+ ATPase, and stimulation of islet cell proliferation. However, C-peptide receptors have not been demonstrated, and physiologic actions of C-peptide would require novel interactions with membrane bilayers or other cellular constituents. The proposed actions of C-peptide raise the possibility that combined insulin and C-peptide therapy might be useful in the treatment of diabetics, and clinical trials are currently underway.

The regulation of insulin synthesis is an important aspect of ß-cell homeostasis. Secretion per se does not stimulate insulin synthesis. For example, insulin secretion stimulated by acute exposure to free fatty acids does not increase insulin synthesis. The major stimulators of insulin synthesis are glucose and cyclic AMP. Glucose stimulates insulin synthesis by increasing insulin mRNA translation via effects on both proinsulin chain initiation and elongation and by increasing the half-life of the mRNA. Hypoglycemia can lead to rapid declines in insulin mRNA, while prolonged glucose stimulation significantly increases insulin production. Additionally, transcription of insulin mRNA is upregulated by both glucose and cAMP resulting in part from phosphorylation of PDX1, a homeodomain protein that binds to regulatory regions of the insulin promotor.

The Insulin Gene and Insulinopathies

The human insulin gene is a single copy gene located on the short arm of chromosome 11 in band 15. Unlike other members of the insulin gene family which include IGF-1 and IGF-2 and which are synthesized by most tissues, insulin is produced only by islet β-cells. The selective expression of the insulin gene is brought about by the actions of transactivating factors that bind to specific DNA recognition sequences.

Six families have been identified in whom a structurally abnormal insulin is produced. The disorder is inherited in an autosomal fashion and presents with mild hyperinsulinemia and glucose intolerance. The hyperinsulinemia is likely due to impaired receptor binding leading to reduced insulin clearance. In all six cases, a single nucleotide substitution leads to a single amino acid replacement. In another type of variant, an amino acid substitution at the proconvertase cleavage site leads to increased proinsulin secretion via the constitutive secretory pathway.[15]

It is unlikely that variations in either coding or noncoding sequences of the insulin gene are associated with a significant number of cases of diabetes. However, it is possible that variants in promotor regions or defects in regulatory proteins may lead to decreased insulin gene expression and to diabetes of the MODY type (see Chapter V.3).

Insulin Release and Second Messenger Signal Transduction

Neurotransmitters and hormones bind to specific cell surface receptors activating second messenger systems that regulate insulin secretion (Fig. 9). Cyclic AMP generated by binding of GLP-1, VIP, PACAP and gastric inhibitory peptide to their respective stimulatory G protein coupled receptors magnifies glucose stimulated insulin secretion. Conversely, norepinephrine binding to its inhibitory G protein coupled receptor inhibits cyclic AMP formation and consequently inhibits insulin secretion.

Cyclic AMP increases $[Ca^{++}]_c$ both directly, by activating L-type calcium channels, and indirectly, by activating protein kinase A which phosphorylates and closes potassium channels depolarizing the plasma membrane potential. In addition, cyclic AMP sensitizes the insulin secretory machinery by shifting the dose-response curve of calcium-induced insulin secretion to lower calcium concentrations. Protein kinase A also rapidly phosphorylates a set of proteins that potentiate insulin secretion. Finally, cyclic AMP stimulates insulin gene transcription both directly, by binding to a cyclic AMP response element of the insulin promoter, and indirectly, by phosphorylating (via protein kinase A) a cyclic AMP response element binding protein.

Three phospholipases in β-cells, phospholipase A2, C, and D play a role in regulating insulin secretion. Binding of acetylcholine to its G protein coupled receptor activates phospholipase C which hydrolyzes membrane bound phospholipids to inositol triphosphate (IP3) and diacylglycerol (DAG). IP3 binds to specific receptors on intracellular membrane bound structures releasing calcium from inracellular stores and increasing the $[Ca^{++}]_c$. DAG activated protein kinase C phosphorylates proteins that elicit a variety of cellular responses amplifing glucose stimulated insulin. In addition, DAG stimulates insulin secretion by increasing the fusogenic potential of cell membranes and by activating DAG lipase which liberates arachadonic acid from phospholipids.

Arachadonic acid is a 20 carbon unsaturated fatty acid containing four double bonds that exists for the most part esterified in membrane phospholipids. It is released from the plasma membrane by the action of Phospholipase A2 upon binding of acetylcholine to its G protein coupled receptor. This is independent of its release by the action of DAG lipase. Aracadonic acid interacts with the voltage dependent calcium channels and amplifies insulin secretion by shifting the activation curve of the channels to more negative potentials. Arachadonic acid also activates protein kinase C and mobilizes calcium from intracellular stores.

Phosphatidic acid is released from membrane phospholipids upon binding of acetylcholine to its receptor with subsequent activation of phospholipase D. Increased phosphatidic acid levels stimulate insulin secretion by an as yet to be determined mechanism.

The resting membrane potential of ß-cells is determined primarily by potassium conductance through ATP dependent K^+-channels. When the cells are exposed to 3 mM glucose (below the threshhold for stimulated insulin secretion), the membrane potential is between -60 and -70 mV. As the glucose concentration is increased, the K^+-channels begin to close. This elicits an ocilatory pattern in which periods of more negative potentials are interspersed with plateaus of membrane depolarizaton upon which spikes of calcium dependent action potentials are superimposed. As the glucose concentration increases, the duration of the depolarized plateaus increase and the interplateau durations decrease until, at a concentration of 20 mM, the depolarization is continuous. Membrane depolarization opens voltage-gated calcium channels increasing $[Ca^{++}]_c$ and leading to insulin secretion. Two other potassium channels, the delayed rectifier K^+-channel and the Ca^{++}-dependent K^+ channel, function to repolarize the membrane potential. As mentioned above, sulfonylureas bind to and close the ATP dependent K^+-channels providing the mechanism by which these agents stimulate insulin secretion.

A second source of increased $[Ca^{++}]_c$ is release of calcium from intracellular stores. The endoplasmic reticulum contains a large number of low affinity calcium binding sites. Two specific receptors, the IP$_3$ receptor and the ryanodine receptor, serve as intracellular channels for mobilizing stored calcium. The IP$_3$ receptor can be phosphorylated by cyclic AMP-dependent protein kinase, protein kinase C and calcium calmodulin-dependent protein kinase II providing mechanisms by which several second messenger systems affect insulin secretion. Calcium itself activates the ryanodine receptor, and it has been proposed that this calcium induced calcium release may be important in the calcium oscillations observed in ß-cells.

CONCLUSIONS

The endocrine pancreas has a central role in maintaining energy homeostasis by regulating nutrient uptake and release by the hormone sensitive storage tissues, liver, fat and muscle. When the circulating levels of nutrient fuels, such as glucose and FFA, are high, energy metabolism within islet β-cells is increased, and intracellular signals are generated that increase insulin secretion. At the same time, glucagon secretion from islet α-cells is inhibited. Thus, a high insulin to glucagon ratio signals nutrient storage, and a low ratio signals nutrient release. The islet response is further regulated by autonomic and sensory nerves and by blood borne hormones produced at distant sites of the gastrointestinal tract.

Type 2 diabetes mellitus is a condition marked by both insulin resistance and β-cell dysfunction in which insulin secretion is inadequate to fully signal storage of circulating nutrient fuels. β-cell dysfunction is the descriptive term for the condition in which there is a breakdown in the intracellular chain of events that leads to insulin secretion. This is manifested by blunted peaks of insulin secretion in response to meals and by an inappropriately high concentration of circulating proinsulin. In addition, there is dysregulation involving the autonomic nervous system so that both interislet communication and intraislet stimulation of secretion are lost.

Both obesity and type 2 diabetes are characterized by insulin resistance. However, in non-diabetics insulin resistance is compensated for by increased insulin secretion. Only when β-cell dysfunction is also present does type 2 diabetes mellitus result.

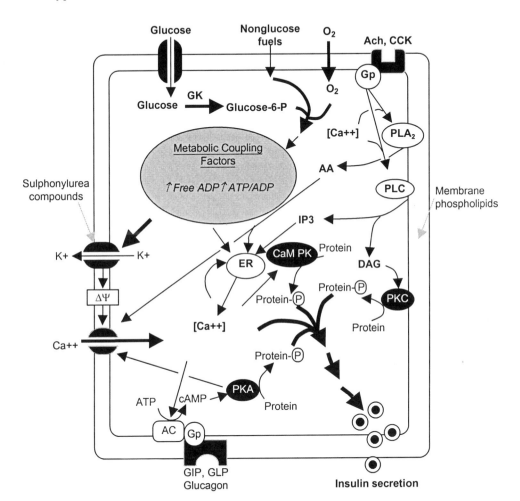

Figure 9. Intracellular pathways involved in insulin secretion (see text). Ach, acetylcholine; CCK, cholecystokinin; Gp, G-protein; GK, glucokinase; PLA2, phospholipase A2; AA, arachadonic acid; PLC, phospholipase C; CaM PK, calcium calmodulin dependent protein kinase; ER endoplasmic reticulum; P, phosphate; GIP, gastric inhibitory peptide; GLP, glucagon-like peptide. (From: Liang Y and Matschinsky FM. Mechanisms of action of nonglucose insulin secretagogues. Ann Rev Nutr 14:59-81,1994, with permission.)

REFERENCES

1. Polonsky KS, Given, BD, Hirsch LJ, et al. Abnormal patterns of insulin secretion in non-insulin-dependent diabetes mellitus. N Engl J Med 318:1231-1239, 1988.
2. Polonsky KS, Given BD, and Van Cauter E. Twenty-four hour profiles and pulsatile patterns of insulin secretion in normal and obese subjects. J Clin Invest 81:442-448, 1988.
3. Jaspan JB, Lever E, Polonsky KS, and Van Cauter E. In vivo pulsatility of pancreatic islet peptides. Am J Physiol 251:E215-226, 1986.
4. Newgard CB, and McGary JD. Metabolic coupling factors in pancreatic ß-cell signal transduction. Annu Rev Biochem 64:689-719, 1995.
5. Maechler P, and Wollheim, CB. Mitochondrial glutamate acts as a messenger in glucose-induced insulin exocytosis. Nature 402:685-689, 1999.
6. Bergman RN and Ader M. Free fatty acids and pathogenesis of type 2 diabetes mellitus. Trends Endocrinol Metab 11:351-356, 2000.
7. Dobbins RL, Chester MW, Daniels MB, et al. Circulating fatty acids are essential for efficient glucose-stimulated insulin secretion after prolonged fasting in humans. Diabetes 47:1613-1618, 1998.
8. Carpentier A, Mittelman SD, Lamarche B, et al. Acute enhancement of insulin secretion by FFA in humans is lost with prolonged FFA elevation. Am J Physiol 276:E1055-1066, 1999.
9. Ahren B. Autonomic regulation of islet hormone secretion - implications for health and disease. Diabetologia 43:393-410, 2000.
10. Schmitz-Peiffer C. Signaling aspects of insulin resistance in skeletal muscle: mechanisms induced by lipid oversupply. Cellular Signal 12:583-594, 2000.
11. Poitout V and Robertson RP. An integrated view of ß-cell dysfunction in type 2 diabetes. Annu Rev Med 47:69-83, 1996.
12. Arvan P, and Castle D. Sorting and storage during secretory granule biogenesis: looking backward and looking forward. Biochem J 332:593-610, 1998.
13. Liang Y, Matschinsky FM. Mechanisms of action of nonglucose insulin secretagogues. Annu Rev Nutr 14:59-81, 1994.
14. Edwards CM, Todd JF, and Mahmoudi M. Glucagon-like peptide 1 has a physiological role in the control of postprandial glucose in humans: studies with the antagonist exendin 9-39. Diabetes 48:86-93, 1999.
15. Carroll RJ, Hammer RE, Chan SJ, et al. A mutant human proinsulin is secreted from islets of Langerhans in increased amounts via an unregulated pathway. Proc Natl Acad Sci USA 85:8943-8947, 1988.

Chapter 3. Cellular Mechanisms of Insulin Action

Theodore P. Ciaraldi

INTRODUCTION

Insulin is a highly plieotrophic hormone, with predominantly anabolic actions in a variety of tissues. Selectivity of final responses to insulin arises both from cell specific expression of final effector proteins and by activation of different signaling pathways. We will consider first an overview of mechanisms of insulin action in normal human physiology, introducing the pathways, players and principles involved, before returning to consider how these elements are modulated in type 2 diabetes. While the critical initial studies in this area were performed in animal and cell systems and later confirmed in humans, for the consideration of pathophysiology we will concentrate on the literature concerning insulin action in humans.

Figure 1 presents a simplified schematic representation of the major pathways of insulin signaling. The organizing principles to note are that insulin signaling involves: 1) phosphorylation/dephosphorylation cascades, 2) phosphorylation of specific sites creates recognition domains that permit the formation of multi-molecular complexes, 3) complex formation involves scaffolding or adaptor proteins, and, 4) these multi-molecular complexes often target enzymes to specific intracellular locales where critical substrates reside.

NORMAL PHYSIOLOGY

The Insulin Receptor

The insulin receptor is a heterotetrameric protein consisting of two identical α subunits and two ß-subunits, linked by sulfhydryl bonds.[1] The alpha subunits are totally extracellular and contain the hormone recognition domain (Figure 2). The beta subunits are primarily intracellular. Most importantly, the ß-subunit contains an intrinsic tyrosine kinase activity, placing the insulin receptor in the large family of receptor tyrosine kinases. The vast majority of studies indicate that this tyrosine kinase activity is essential for the normal signaling function of the insulin receptor.[2]

Binding of insulin to the receptor generates a conformational change in the α-subunit that is transmitted to the ß-subunit, activating the intrinsic kinase activity. The next event is ordered *trans*-phosphorylation of three tyrosine residues in the kinase regulatory region on the adjacent ß-subunit (Y1146/Y1150/Y1151), further activating the kinase activity. Other tyrosines on the receptor are then phosphorylated, including Y960 in the juxtamembrane domain and Y1316/Y1322 in the C-terminus, creating recognition sites. These recognition sites permit high affinity association with other substrates, which are subsequently tyrosine phosphorylated, and then propagate the phosphorylation cascade.

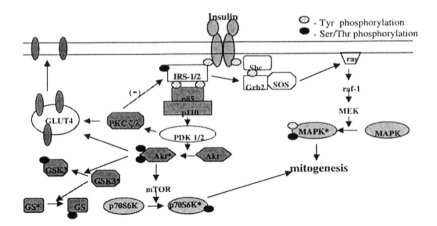

Figure 1. Pathways of insulin signaling. All events initiate from the insulin receptor after hormone binding. Phosphorylation of IRS-1/2 leads to control of both metabolism, represented by glucose uptake and glycogen synthase, and mitogenesis. The Shc/Grb2/ras/MAPK pathway regulates mitogenesis. Proteins are defined in the text. Activated forms of enzymes are indicated with*.

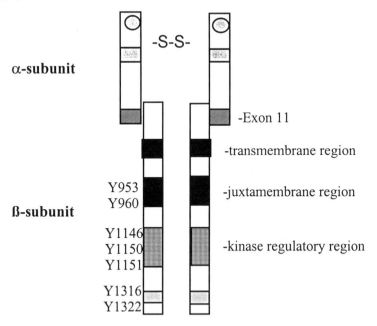

Figure 2. Insulin receptor structure. Regions of differing function are indicated by shading. Critical potential tyrosine phosphorylation sites are identified.

Insulin Receptor Substrates and the Importance of Recognition Domains

Insulin receptor substrates are, by definition, molecules phosphorylated by the insulin receptor kinase. They are most often adaptor or scaffolding proteins which have no catalytic activity but act rather, by means of multiple recognition domains, to form multimolecular complexes, bringing enzymes and substrates into proximity or to the proper intracellular localization. Best characterized, and most specific for insulin action are the insulin receptor substrates, IRSs. At least four different IRS molecules have been identified, of varying tissue distribution.[3] The common structural features of the IRS proteins are the presence of a pleckstrin homology (PH) domain, a phosphotyrosine binding (PTB) domain, and multiple tyrosines available for phosphorylation (Figure 3). IRS-1 and –2 each contain 21 tyrosine residues in their COOH-terminus that are potential phosphorylation sites. Another insulin receptor substrate, Shc, lacks the PH domain and has a single tyrosine phosphorylation site.

These varying domains provide the means by which insulin signaling is organized and specificity is provided for substrate recognition and complex formation. The PH domain binds specific lipid products with high affinity (Table 1), which would target the molecule to the inner surface of the plasma membrane, bringing it into close proximity to the insulin receptor. The PTB domain recognizes the phosphotyrosine residue present in an NPXpY sequence motif, such as that formed in the juxtamembrane region of

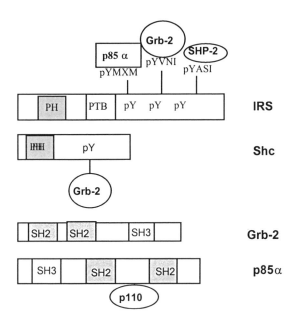

Figure 3. Representative examples of adaptor proteins and recognition domains involved in insulin signaling.

Table 1. Recognition domains important in insulin signaling

Domain	Recognition site
PH	Lipids: PIP3
PTB	Phosphotyrosine: NPXpY
SH2	Phosphotyrosine: ex, pYMXM
SH3	Proline-rich region: ex, PXXP

the receptor after phosphorylation of tyrosine 960 (Figure 2). Association of the protein with the insulin receptor through these interactions is transitory, during this association the substrate is phosphorylated, then released to propagate the signaling cascade. The next level of specificity is provided by src homology-2 (SH2) domains, which recognize specific amino acid motifs containing a phosphotyrosine. While there is some flexibility, the pY-SH2 association is of higher affinity that that involving the PTB domain. Beyond tyrosine phosphorylation, it is important to note that IRS-1 and IRS-2 have numerous potential serine/threonine phosphorylation sites. Serine phosphorylation of IRS-1 is stimulated by insulin[3], activators of PKA, classic PKC isoforms, and TNF-α.[4] In these instances serine phosphorylation reduces the ability of IRS-1 to transmit the insulin signal.[5]

Phosphatidylinositol 3-kinase

Key amongst the molecules that can associate with the IRS proteins is phosphatidylinositol 3'-kinase (PI 3-kinase). PI 3-kinase is a lipid kinase that phosphorylates the 3-position of the inositol ring in phosphatidylinositol. A major product is phosphatidylinositol-3',4'5'-trisphosphate (PIP3), an important lipid second messenger. PI 3-kinase consists of a regulatory subunit and a catalytic subunit. As many as 8 isoforms of the regulatory subunit, including alternative splicing forms, have been identified, that vary in their tissue distribution. The most ubiquitously expressed form is p85α (Figure 3). The regulatory subunit is not phosphorylated itself but associates with IRS proteins through it's SH2 domains after IRS-1/2 phosphorylation. The SH2 domains of p85 recognize phosphotyrosines in YMXM and YXXM motifs.[6] The p110 catalytic subunit is then recruited to p85 and activated. Complex formation and kinase activation has been disturbed by a number of complimentary approaches such as the use of chemical inhibitors of PI 3-kinase (e.g. wortmannin) , expression of dominant negative or interfering proteins, or reduction of the expression of endogenous proteins. The common result is that a number of insulin responses are reduced or eliminated; these include, stimulation of glucose transport, antilipolysis, activation of glycogen synthase, stimulation of protein and DNA synthesis, indicating that PI 3-kinase is essential for many of insulin's actions.[7]

A number of growth factors have been shown to stimulate PI 3-kinase activity yet do not generate the metabolic responses seen with insulin. For most growth factors, such as EGF, p85 can associate directly with the growth factor receptor, thus targeting PI 3-kinase to the proximity of the inner surface of the plasma membrane.[3] This association does not occur with the insulin receptor. Rather, IRS-1/2 is recruited from its primarily cytoplasmic distribution in resting cells to be phosphorylated by the insulin receptor. Binding to the receptor, mediated by the PTB domain, is weak and phosphorylated IRS-1/2 is released to intracellular membranous pools, where it complexes with the components of PI 3-kinase. In this manner insulin-stimulated PI 3-kinase is targeted to different sites than after stimulation by other growth factors, and PIP3 delivered to specific effectors.

Downstream Pathways

With regard to insulin action, the key effector or target of PIP3 generated by PI 3-kinase is 3'-phosphoinosotide-dependent kinase (PDK), a serine kinase that is activated by binding of PIP3 or PIP2 to it's C-terminal PTH domain.[8] Major substrates for PDK include the atypical forms of protein kinase C (PKC), PKC ζ and λ.[9] PDK mediated phosphorylation of atypical PKCs activates these enzymes. This activation is associated with insulin stimulation of glucose transport and GLUT4 translocation.[10] as well as stimulation of MAPK[11], implicating atypical PKCs as important elements in insulin signaling. Besides this positive intermediary role, atypical PKCs can also phosphorylate IRS-1, impairing stimulation of PI 3-kinase activity.[5] Thus PKC ζ/λ can participate in a negative feedback loop to limit insulin action. The classic, lipid dependent, PKC forms are also stimulated by insulin.[9] In this instance the result is negative, as classic PKCs also phosphorylate IRS-1, interfering with signaling.[12]

The other important substrate for PDK is yet another serine kinase, designated both Akt and protein kinase B (PKB). Akt contains an N-terminal PH domain.[13] Activation of Akt requires both binding of PIP3 (or PIP2) to the PH domain and phosphorylation by PDK.[13] A number of studies implicate Akt/PKB in stimulation of glucose transport[13], while others cast doubt on that role.[9,14] It is clear that glycogen synthase kinase 3 is a direct substrate for Akt[15], providing one pathway for insulin to stimulate glycogen synthesis (see below).

Also directly downstream of PI 3-kinase and Akt is the p70 ribosomal S6 kinase (Figure 1). Akt acts primarily on mammalian Target of Rapamycin (mTOR), which subsequently stimulates p70S6K to phosphorylate ribosomal protein S6 and accelerate translation of mRNA. P70S6K may also have some involvement in metabolic signaling, as blockade of p70S6K activation by rapamycin partially inhibits insulin action on glycogen synthesis.[16]

Protein Phosphatases

Dephosphorylation events also play an important role in insulin action, either to propagate or terminate the signal. Protein tyrosine phosphatases (PTPases) of interest can be placed in two categories: membrane-associated and cytoplasmic. The leukocyte antigen related phosphatase (LAR) is an example of the membrane associated PTPases.[17] LAR has been shown to associate with the phosphorylated insulin receptor and preferentially dephosphorylate a tyrosine in the kinase regulatory region (Y1150), reducing kinase activity.[18] Cytoplasmic phosphatases include PTP-1B and SH2-containing protein phosphatase-2 (designated as SH-PTP-2, SHP-2, or syp). PTP-1B has been shown to associate with the insulin receptor and dephosphorylate both the receptor and IRS-1, reducing association of the latter with p85 and stimulation of PI 3-kinase activity.[19]

SH-PTP-2 has been shown to associate with the insulin receptor, via phosphotyrosines in the C-terminal region[20] and dephosphorylate the receptor, though IRS-1 is the preferential substrate.[21] SH-PTP-2 can also associate with Shc.

Non- PI 3-kinase Pathways

While many of insulin's action occur through activation of PI 3-kinase, other pathways are also employed. The best characterized is one shared with other growth factors leading to activation of members of the mitogen activated protein kinase (MAPK) family of serine/threonine kinases. The prime mediator is Shc. Upon tyrosine phosphorylation by the insulin receptor, Shc is able to complex with another adaptor protein, Grb-2, through the SH2 domain on Grb-2 (Figure 3). Grb-2 exists in a constituative complex with the guanine nucleotide exchange factor son of sevenless (SOS). The Grb-2/SOS complex resides in the cytoplasm but upon binding to Shc associated with the insulin receptor, is recruited to the inner surface of the plasma membrane. There SOS is brought into proximity with the membrane localized small G-protein *ras*[22], activating *ras* and its associated phosphorylation cascade, leading to phosphorylation/activation of the p42/p44 forms of MAPK (Figure 1). The MAPK pathway represents the major, though not only[23], mechanism mediating nuclear effects of insulin on gene expression. The accumulation of evidence supports the conclusion that this pathway has no involvement in the acute metabolic responses to insulin.

Representative Final Responses

Glucose transport. Glucose entry into the primary insulin target tissues; skeletal muscle, heart, adipose tissue and liver, occurs by falicitated diffusion, mediated by a family of transport proteins. Up to 7 members of this family have been identified, designated GLUT1-7.[24] With regard to insulin action, the most important are GLUT1 and GLUT4. GLUT1 is near ubitquious in expression and resides primarily on the cell surface. GLUT4 is present in adipose tissue and cardiac and skeletal muscle and distributed mainly in a specific population of intracellular vesicles.[24] There is a constitutive recycling of GLUT4 between the plasma membrane and intracellular vesicles.[25] Insulin action on glucose uptake involves a multi-step process (Figure 1): translocation of GLUT4 containing vesicles to the plasma membrane, fusion of the vesicles with the membrane, insertion of GLUT4 into the membrane, and activation of the transporters. Similar events occur with GLUT1 and GLUT3, but to a lesser degree. Insulin primarily accelerates the rate of GLUT4 exocytosis, though transporter endocytosis is slowed as well. There appear to be multiple intracellular populations of GLUT4, subject to distinct control, as insulin stimulation and contraction of skeletal muscle cause loss of GLUT4 from distinct pools.[26] Considering the multiple steps involved in the glucose transport response, it is not surprising that multiple signaling pathways are also involved. That PI 3-kinase is necessary for the response is broadly accepted, but the relative importance of Akt/PKB and novel PKC isoforms is still under debate. Recent evidence also suggests that PI 3-kinase is not sufficient for the full transport response and there are PI 3-kinase-independent signaling pathways involved as well.

Glycogen synthesis. The ability of insulin to increase non-oxidative glucose utilization into muscle involves stimulation of glucose transport as well as activation of glycogen synthase (GS), the key enzyme catalyzing glycogen synthesis. Glycogen synthase activity is regulated by allosteric and covalent (phosphorylation/dephosphorylation) mechanisms.[27] While a number of kinases and phosphatases can act on GS , the most important enzymes with regard to insulin action are protein phosphatase-1 (PP1) and glycogen synthase kinase 3 (GSK3). PP1 activates GS while GSK3 deactivates. Insulin stimulates PP1 through a PI 3-kinase dependent mechanism.[28] The main target of insulin is the portion of PP1 activity that is localized with the glycogen particle. Insulin also removes a tonic inhibition of GS by suppressing GSK3 activity. Serine phosphorylation of GSK3 by Akt (Figure 1) reduces GSK3 activity, resulting in an augmentation of the effect on PP1. The relative importance of PP1 and GSK3 in mediating insulin action on GS may vary in a tissue specific manner.

Beyond these pathways, new work has revealed additional processes including; activation of heterotrimeric G proteins, the PI 3-kinase independent cbl-CAP pathway, and insulin activation of the stress-activated p38 MAP kinase. As these pathways have not yet been verified in humans, they have been omitted from the current presentation.

PATHOPHYSIOLOGY OF INSULIN ACTION IN DIABETES

Each of the elements involved in the pathways leading to insulin regulation of metabolism could represent a site of possible defects in insulin resistant states. Diabetes related differences could arise at several levels: the presence of mutations which influence protein turnover or activity, alterations in protein expression, or post-translational modifications which modify activity. Most of the work concerning this topic has been performed on type 2 diabetic subjects.

Insulin Receptor Regulation

Mutations of the insulin receptor that influence primarily intrinsic kinase activity are exceedingly rare and are usually associated with the syndromes of extreme insulin resistance discussed in chapter VI.6. In more typical cases of type 2 diabetes, a reduction in insulin receptor binding and receptor protein expression has been a common finding in skeletal muscle[29,30] and adipose tissue.[31] This downregulation of insulin receptors may be an acquired defect, resulting from hyperinsulinemia, as similar reductions were observed in obese, non-diabetic individuals.[31] More importantly, insulin receptor tyrosine kinase activity, especially toward the receptor itself, has been repeatedly shown to be impaired in tissues from diabetic subjects.[32,33] This defect in insulin-stimulated receptor autophosphorylation exists even when results are normalized to the amount of receptor protein. Thus the insulin-stimulated kinase activity of the receptor is impaired in diabetes. A possible cause for defects in receptor kinase activity could be augmented serine phosphorylation. However, in one report, phosphorylation of the serine and threonine residues most important for suppression of receptor kinase activity was normal in diabetic skeletal muscle.[34] Impaired receptor kinase activity may also be an acquired defect, as kinase activity in adipose tissue of obese diabetic subjects is improved by weight loss[35] or by normalization of glucose levels.[36] Under the usual conditions of hyperinsulinemia and hyperglycemia present in diabetes, it is clear that the initial events in insulin signaling, hormone recognition and receptor kinase activation, are impaired and can contribute to insulin resistance.

Insulin Receptor Substrates: acute and chronic regulation

A number of polymorphisms have been identified in the human IRS-1 gene[37] One of these, G972R, displays reduced functionality when expressed in cells[38] and is associated with obesity.[39] However, the allele frequency of each of these polymorphisms is similar in non-diabetic and diabetic populations.[37,39] A polymorphism has also been identified in the human IRS-2 gene, the frequency of this polymorphism, however, is also not associated with diabetes.[40,41]

Protein expression of IRS-1 has been reported to be reduced in adipose tissue of diabetic subjects, while that of IRS-2 was normal.[42] As a result, the relative importance of IRS-2 as a docking protein for PI 3-kinase was increased. Others have found IRS-1 expression to be normal in adipose tissue.[43] Skeletal muscle expression of IRS-1 has been reported as normal by several laboratories.[44] A common observation is that insulin stimulated tyrosine phosphorylation of IRS-1 is impaired in type 2 diabetes. This is true for both adipose tissue[45] and skeletal muscle[46,47] and the magnitude of the defect agrees with the extent of whole body insulin resistance. Thus, defects in IRS-1 phosphorylation and function (see below) appear to play an important role in insulin resistance. Weather augmented serine phosphorylation of IRS-1 is responsible for these defects has yet to be determined in human tissues.

Phosphatidylinositol 3-kinase

A single polymorphism has been identified in the p110ß catalytic subunit[48] that appears with the same frequency in non-diabetic and diabetic populations. A polymorphism resulting in a Met to Ile substitution at amino acid 326 in the p85α regulatory subunit has been reported by several groups.[49,50] In a population of Pima Indians the presence of this polymorphism is not associated with changes in insulin-stimulated glucose disposal, yet those expressing M326I have an impaired insulin response.[49] Individuals heterozygous for M326I appear with equal frequency in non-diabetic and diabetic populations, while those homozygous for the polymorphism do display glucose intolerance.[50]

While the importance of mutations in the components of PI 3-kinase to insulin resistance appears limited, post-translational regulatory mechanisms are critical. Insulin stimulated PI 3-kinase activity is reduced by ~50% in both skeletal muscle[44,46,47,51] and adipose tissue[45] from type 2 diabetic subjects. Impairments in PI 3-kinase activity are also seen in non-diabetic obese individuals[52], suggesting that dis-regulation of PI 3-kinase activity may appear early in the development of insulin resistance.

Downstream Pathways

There is, to date, a limited literature about the influence of diabetes on signaling events downstream of PI 3-kinase. Insulin-stimulated phosphorylation and activation of Akt/PKB is reduced in adipose tissue from type 2 diabetic subjects.[45] In skeletal muscle the story is mixed; two groups report that, at physiologic insulin levels, Akt/PKB activity is normal in diabetic subjects[46,47], even as PI 3-kinase activity is impaired. Such a discrepancy, together with defects in final insulin action, highlights the importance of regulation of PI 3-kinase. One of these groups did find Akt/PKB activity to be reduced at supraphysiologic insulin levels.[46] Activity of PKCθ was found to be elevated in skeletal muscle from diabetics.[53] Changes of this nature would be consistent with the postulate that classic PKC isoforms impede insulin action.

The only -PI 3-kinase independent pathway to be studied to date in diabetic individuals is activation of MAPK. Insulin stimulated phosphorylation and activation of MAPK in skeletal muscle was found to be normal in skeletal muscle .[51] Retention of normal mitogenic responses in the face of hyperinsulinemia could contribute to proliferative effects involved in the development of diabetic complications.

Protein Phosphatases

In adipose tissue PTP-1B protein expression is elevated, even as specific activity of the enzyme is reduced;[54] resulting in no net change in enzyme activity. Several groups have reported that basal PTPase activity in the particulate fraction, as well as protein expression is reduced in diabetic muscle[55,56,57], while others found activity to be elevated.[58] A common observation was that the insulin effect on PTPase activity was lost in diabetic muscle.[56,58] While augmented PTPase activity does not appear to be a major contributor to insulin resistance in diabetes, it is interesting to note that its regulation also displays insulin resistance.

Effectors

Glucose transporters. A number of polymorphisms have been identified in the GLUT4 gene. None of them have been linked to or found to be associated with type 2 diabetes in a variety of populations.[59,60] Interestingly, an association was found between a polymorphism in the human GLUT1 gene and type 2 diabetics[60] that was significant for obese women. Regulation of GLUT4 protein expression in diabetes occurs in a strongly tissue-specific manner. The total cellular complement of GLUT4 is reduced by 40-50% in subcutaneous adipocytes from diabetic subjects.[61] The magnitude of this impairment is sufficient to account for the reduction in maximal insulin-stimulated adipocyte glucose transport in the same subjects. A different situation exists in skeletal muscle, where the total cellular complement of GLUT4 is the same in non-diabetic and diabetic muscle.[62] Thus, in muscle, GLUT4 content is not the determinant of muscle glucose uptake. These differences in GLUT4 expression suggest tissue specific mechanisms for defective glucose uptake. In adipocytes it is the reduced intracellular GLUT4 pool that is responsible for impaired transport, while in skeletal muscle the problem lies at the level of late steps in signal transduction or GLUT4 translocation to the cell surface. A number of laboratories, using different and complimentary approaches, have verified that insulin-stimulated GLUT4 translocation is indeed impaired in diabetic muscle.[63,64] This resistance is specific to insulin signaling, for translocation in response to muscle contraction is intact in diabetes, as is the glucose transport response.[65]

Glycogen synthesis. Skeletal muscle glycogen synthesis is impaired in type 2 diabetes, in both the fasting state and in response to insulin. These defects are reflected at the level of glycogen synthase activity, which is also reduced.[66] Impairments in GS activity are not due to mutations in the GS gene.[67] Expression of immunoreactive GS protein is also normal in diabetic muscle[68], rather differences exist in the activation state of GS. While both the frequency of PPI polymorphisms and mRNA expression are normal in diabetes[69], glycogen synthase phosphatase activity has been reported to be lower in insulin resistant, though not necessarily diabetic, individuals.[70] On the other side of the equation, deactivation of GS, both the protein expression and total activity of GSK3 have been found to be elevated in diabetic skeletal muscle.[71] While GSK3 responds in a qualitatively normal manner to insulin with regard to both serine phosphorylation and a reduction in activity, there is still augmented activity compared to non-diabetic muscle. This diabetes-related qualitative overexpression of GSK3 could account for a large portion of the decrement in GS activity in diabetic muscle. Yet there is no apparent insulin resistance for regulation of GSK3 activity, which would be consistent with normal Ak/PKB activity in the same subjects.[47]

SUMMARY

A highly complex system has developed to transmit insulin signals from the cell surface to metabolic and mitogenic responses. Such a multiplicity of signaling pathways provides flexibility, redundancy and specificity. Tissue selectivity of insulin responsiveness is modulated, in large part, by the cell specific expression of different elements of the signaling pathways or of final effectors. Despite this complexity, there are several principles in the organization of insulin signaling: 1) phosphorylatio/dephosphorylation cascades initiated by the insulin receptor kinase, 2) formation of multimolecular complexes involving specific recognition domains on adapter proteins and, 3) targeting of signaling and effector molecules to appropriate intracellular locales. Impaired insulin action in type 2 diabetes most often involves defects in insulin receptor kinase and PI 3-kinase activation. It is unlikely that mutations in individual elements of insulin signaling are responsible for the majority of instances of insulin resistance. Such mutations, however, may represent susceptibility factors, reflecting the polygenic nature of diabetes.

REFERENCES:

1. Ottensmeyer FP, Beniac DR, Luo RZ, Yip CC. Mechanism of transmembrane signaling: insulin binding and the insulin receptor. Biochemistry 39:12103-12112, 2000.

2. Ellis L, Tavare JM, Levine BA. Insulin receptor tyrosine kinase structure and function. Biochem Soc Trans 43-426-432, 1991.
3. Myers MG, White MF. Insulin signal transduction and the IRS proteins. Annu Rev Pharmacol Toxicol 36:615-658, 1996.
4. Hotamisligil GS, Perald, P, Budavar, A, Ellis R, Whit, MF, Spiegelman BM. IRS-1-mediated inhibition of insulin receptor tyrosine kinase activity in TNF-alpha-and obesity-induced insulin resistance. Science 271:665-668, 1996.
5. Ravichandran LV, Esposito DL, Chen J, Quon MJ. Protein kinase C-zeta phosphorylates insulin receptor substrate-1 and impairs its ability to activate phosphatidylinositol 3-kinase in response to insulin. J Biol Chem 276:3543-3549, 2001.
6. Virkamaki A, Ueki K, Kahn CR. Protein-protein interaction in insulin signaling and the molecular mechanisms of insulin resistance. J Clin Invest 103:931-943, 1999.
7. Shepherd PR, Withers DJ, Siddle K. Phosphoinositide 3-kinase: the key switch mechanism in insulin signalling. Biochem J 333:471-490, 1998.
8. Alessi DR, Deak M, Casamayor A, et al. 3-Phosphoinositide-dependent protein kinase-1 (PDK1): structural and functional homology with the Drospohila DSTPK61 kinase. Current Biol 7:776-789, 1997.
9. Farese RV. Insulin-sensitive phospholipid signaling systems and glucose transport. Update II. Exp Biol Med 226:283-295, 2001.
10. Valverde AM, Lorenzo M, Navarro P, Mur C, Benito M. Okadiac acid inhibits insulin-induced glucose transport in fetal brown adipocytes in an Akt-independent and protein kinase C zeta-dependent manner. Febs Letts 472:153-158, 2000.
11. Sajan MP, Standaert ML, Bandyopadhyay G, Quon MJ, Burke TR, Farese RV. Protein kinase C-zeta and phosphoinositide-dependent protein kinase-1 are required for insulin induced activation of ERK in rat adipocytes. J Biol Chem 274:30495-30500, 1999.
12. Kellerer M, Mushack J, Seffe, E, Mischsak H, Ullrich A, Haring HU. Protein kinase C isoforms alpha, delta and theta require insulin receptor substrate-1 to inhibit the tyrosine kinase asctivty of the insulin receptor in human kidney embbyronic cells (HEK 293 cells). Diabetologia 41:833-838, 1998.
13. Downward J. Mechanisms and consequences of activation of protein kinase B/Akt. Curr Op Cell Biol 262-267, 1998.
14. Kitamura T, Ogawa W, Sakaue H, et al. Requirement for activation of the serine-threonine kinase Akt (protein kinase B) in insulin stimulation of protein synthesis but not of glucose transport. Mol Cell Biol 18:3708-3717, 1997.
15. Cross, BAE, Alessi DR, Cohen P, Andjelkovic, M, Hemmings BA. Inhibition of glycogen synthase kinase-3 by insulin mediated by protein kinase B. Nature 378:785-789, 1995.

16. Halse R, Rochford JJ, McCormack JG, Vandendeede JR, Hemmings BA, Yeaman SJ. Control of glycogen synthesis in cultured human muscle cells. J Biol Chem 274:776-780, 1999.
17. Elchebly M, Cheng A, Tremblay ML. Modulation of insulin signaling by protein tyrosine phosphatases. J Mol Med 78:473-482, 2000.
18. Hashimoto, N, Feener, EP, Zhang, W-R, Goldstein, BJ: Insulin receptor protein-tyrosine phosphatases. J Biol Chem 267:13811-13814, 1992.
19. Elchebly M, Payette P, Michaliszyn E, et al. Increased insulin sensitivity and obesity resistance in mice lacking the protein tyrosine phosphatase-1B gene. Science 282:1544-1548, 1999.
20. Rocchi S, Tartare-Decker, S, Sawka-Verhelle D, GamhaA, Van Obberghen E. Interaction of SH2-containing protein tyrosine phosphatase 2 with the insulin receptor and the insulin-like growth factor-I receptor: studies of the domains involved using the yeast two-hybrid system. Endocrinology 137:4944-4952, 1996.
21. Sugimoto S, Wandless TJ, Sholeson SE, Neel BG, Walsh CT. Activation of the SH2-containing protein tyrosine phosphatase, SH-PTP2, by phosphotyrosine-containing peptides derived from insulin receptor substrate-1. J Biol Chem 269:13614-13622, 1994.
22. Avruch J, Khokhlatchev A, Kyriakis JM, et al. Ras activation of the Raf kinaseL tyrosine kinase recruitment of the MAP kinase cascade. Rec Prog Horm Res 56:127-155, 2001.
23. Coffer PJ, van Puijenbroek A, Burgering BM, et al. Insulin activates Stat3 independently of p21ras-ERK and PI-3K signal transduction. Oncogene 15:2529-2539, 1997.
24. Mueckler M. Facilitative glucose transporters. Eur J Biochem 219:713-725, 1994.
25. Quon MJ. Advances in kinetic analysis of insulin-stimulated GLUT-4 translocation in adipose cells. Am J Physiol 266:E144-E150, 1994.
26. Goodyear LG, Kahn BB. Exercise, glucose transport and insulin sensitivity. Ann Rev Med 49:235-261, 1998.
27. Lawrence JC, Roach PJ. New insights into the role and mechanism of glycogen synthase activation by insulin. Diabetes 46:541-547, 1997.
28. Brady MJ, Saltiel AR. The role of protein phosphatase-1 in insulin action. Rec Prog Hormone Res 56:157-173, 2001.
29. Bak J, Jacobsen U, Jorgensen,F, Pedersen O. Insulin receptor function and glycogen sythase activity in skeletal muscle biopsies from the patients with insulin-dependent diabetes mellitus: Effects of physical training. J Clin Endocrinol Metab 69:158-164, 1989.
30. Handberg A, Vaag A, Vinte, J, Beck-Nielsen H. Decxreased tyrosine kinase activity in partially purified insulin receptors from muscle of young non-obese first degree relatives of patients with Type 2 (non-insulin-dependent) diabetes mellitus. Diabetologia 36:668-674, 1993.

31. Hunter SJ, Garvey WT. Insulin action and insulin resistance: diseases involving defects in insulin receptorss, signal transduction and the glucose transport effector system. Am J Med 105:331-345, 1998.

32. Obermaier-Kusser B, White MF, Pongrantz DE, et al. A defective intramolecular autoactivation cascade may cause the reduced kinase activity of skeletal muscle insulin receptor from patients with non-insulin-dependent diabetes mellitus. J Biol Chem 264:9497-9504, 1989.

33. Freidenberg GR, Henry RR, Klein HH, Reichart DR, Olefsky JM. Decreased kinase activity of insulin receptors from adipocytes of Non-insulin-dependent diabetic subjects. J Clin Invest 79:240-250, 1987.

34. Kellerer M, Coghlan M, Capp E, et al. Mechanism of insulin receptor kinase inhibition in non-insulin-dependent diabetes mellitus patients. J Clin Invest 96:6-11, 1995.

35. Freidenberg GR, Reichart D, Olefsky JM, Henry RR. Reversibility of defective adipocyte insulin receptor kinase activity in non-insulin-dependent diabetes mellitus. J Clin Invest 82:1398-1406, 1988.

36. Hajduch E, Hainault I, Meunier C, et al. Regulation of glucose transporters in cultured rat adipocytes: synergistic effect of insulin and dexamethasone on GLUT4 gene expression through promoter activation. Endocrinology 136:4782-4789, 1995.

37. Lei H-H, Coresh J, Shuldiner AR, Boerwinkle E, Brancati FL. Variants of the insulin receptor substrate-1 and fatty acid binding protein 2 genes and the risk of type 2 diabetes, obesity, and hyperinsulinemia in African Americans. Diabetes 48:1868-1872, 1999.

38. Yoshimura R, Araki E, Ura S, et al. Impact of IRS-1 mutations on insulin signals. Diabetes 46:929-936, 1997.

39. Ura S, Araki E, Kishikawa H, et al. Molecular scanning of the insulin receptor substrate-1 (IRS-1) gene in Japanese patients with NIDDM: identification of five novel polymorphisms. Diabetologia 39:600-608, 1996.

40. Bernal D, Almind K, Yenush L, et al. Insulin receptor substrate-2 amino acid polymorphisms are not associated with random type 2 diabetes among caucasians. Diabetes 47:976-979, 1998.

41. Bektas A, Warram JH, White MF, Krolewski AS, Doria A. Exclusion of insulin receptor substrate 2 (IRS-2) as a major locus for early-onset autosomal dominant type 2 diabetes. Diabetes 48:640-642, 1999.

42. Rondinone CM, Wang L-M, Lonnroth P, Wesslau C, Pierc, JH, Smith U. Insulin receptor substrate (IRS) 1 is reduced and IRS-2 is the main docking protein for phospahtidylinositol 3-kinase in adipocytes from subjects with non-insulin-dependent diabetes mellitus. Proc Natl Acad Sci USA 94:4171-4175, 1997.

43. Andreelli F, Laville M, Ducluzeau et al. Defective regulation of phosphatidylinositol-3-kinase gene expression in skeletal muscle and adipose tissue of non-insulin-dependent diabetes mellitus patients. Diabetologia 42:358-364, 1999.

44. Bjornholm M, Kawano Y, Lehtihet M, Zierath, JR. Insulin receptor substrate-1 phosphorylation and phosphatidylinositol 3-kinase activity in skeletal muscle from NIDDM subjects after in vivo insulin stimulation. Diabetes 46:524-527, 1997.

45. Smith U, Axelsen M, Carvalho E, Eliasson B, Jansson P. Insulin signaling and action in fat cells: associations with insulin resistance and type 2 diabetes. Ann NY Acad Sci 892:119-126, 1999.

46. Krook A, Roth RA, Jiang XJ, Zierat, JR, Wallberg-Henriksson H: Insulin-stimulated Akt kinase activity is reduced in skeletal muscle from NIDDM subjects. Diabetes 47:1281-1286, 1998.

47. Kim Y-B, Nikoulina SE, Ciaraldi TP, Henry RR, Kahn BB. Normal insulin-dependent activation of Akt/protein kinase B, with diminished activation of phosphoinositide 3-kinase, in muscle in type 2 diabetes. J Clin Invest 104:733-741, 1999.

48. Kossila M, Sinkovic M, Karkkaiinen P, et al. Gene coding for the catalytic subunit p110ß of human phosphatidylinositol 3-kinase. Cloniong, genomic structure, and screening for variant in patients with type 2 diabetes. Diabetes 49:1740-1743, 2000.

49. Baier,LJ, Wiedrich C, Hanson RL, Bogardus C: Variant in the regulatory subunit of phosphatidylinositol 3-kinase (p85alpha). Diabetes 47:973-975, 1998.

50. Hansen T, Andersen CB, Echwald SM, et al. Identification of a common amino acid polymorphism in the p85alpha regulatory subunit of phosphatidylinositol 3-kinase. Diabetes 46:494-501, 1997.

51. Cusi K, Maezono K, Osman A, et al. Insulin resistance differentially affects the PI 3-kinase- and MAP kinase-mediated signaling in human muscle. J Clin Invest 105:311-320, 2000.

52. Marsh BJ, Alm RA, McIntosh SR, James DE: Molecular regulation of GLUT-4 targeting in 3T3-L1 adipocytes. J Cell Biol 130:1081-1091, 1995.

53. Itani, SI, Pories WJ, Macdonald KG, Dohm GL. Increased protein kinase C theta in skeletal muscle of diabetic patients. Metabolism 50:553-557, 2001.

54. Cheung A, Kusari J, Jansen D, Bandyopadhyay D, Kusari A, Bryer-Ash M. Marked impairment of protein tyrosine phosphatase 1B activity in adipose tissue of obese subjects with and without type 2 diabetes mellitus. J Lab Clin Med 134:115-123, 1999.

55. Kusari J, Kenner KA, Suh K-L, Hill DE, Henry RR. Skeletal muscle protein tyrosine phosphatase activity and tyrosine phosphatase1B protein content are associated with insulin action and resistance. J Clin Invest 93:1156-1162, 1994.

56. Worm D, Vinten J, Staehr P, Henriksen JE, Handberg A, Beck-Nielsen H. Altered basal and insulin-stimulated phosphotyrosine phosphatase (PTPase) activity in skeletal muscle from NIDDM paitents compared with control subjects. Diabetologia 39:1208-1214, 1996.

57. Ahmad F, Azevedo JL, Cortright R, Dohm GL, Goldstein,BJ. Alterations in skeletal muscle protein-tyrosine phosphatase activity and expression in insulin-resistant human obesity and diabetes. J Clin Invest 100:449-458, 1997.

58. McGuire M, Fields R, Nyomba B, et al. Abnormal Regulation of Protein Tyrosine Phosphatase Activities in Skeletal Muscle of Insulin-Resistant Humans. Diabetes 40:939-942, 1991.

59. Lesage S, Zouali H, Vionnet N, et al. Genetic analyses of glucose transporter genes in French non-insulin-dependent diabetic families. Diabetes and Metabolism 23:137-142, 1997.

60. Pontiroli AE, Capra F, Vegila F, et al. Genetic contribution of polymorphism of the GLUT1 and GLUT4 genes to the susceptibility to type 2 (non-insulin-dependent) diabetes mellitus in different populations. Acta Diabetologia 33:193-197, 1996.

61. Garvey WT, Maianu L, Huecksteadt TP, Birnbaum MJ, Molina JM, Ciaraldi TP. Pretranslational suppression of GLUT4 glucose transporters causes insulin resistance in type II diabetes. J Clin Invest 87:1072-1081, 1991.

62. Garvey WT. Glucose transport and NIDDM. Diabetes Care 15:396-417, 1992.

63. Ryder JW, Yang, J, Galuska D, et al. Use of a novel impermeable biotinylated photolabeling reagent to assess insulin- and hypoxia-stimulated cell surface GLUT4 content in skeletal muscle from type 3 diabetic patients. Diabetes 49:647-654, 2000.

64. Garvey WT, Maianu L, Zhu J-H, Brechtel-Hook G, Wallace P, Baron AD. Evidence for defects in the trafficking and translocation of GLUT4 glucose transporters in skeletal muscle as a cause of human insulin resistance. J Clin Invest 101:2377-2386, 1998.

65. Kennedy JW, Hirshman MF, Gervino EV, et al. Acute exercise induces GLUT4 translocation in skeletal muscle of normal human subjects and subjects with type 2 diabetes. Diabetes 48:1192-1197, 1999.

66. Thornburn AW, Gumbiner B, Bulacan F, Wallace P, Henry RR. Intracellular glucose oxidation and glycogen synthase activity are reduced in non-insulin dependent (Type II) diabetes independent of impaired glucose uptake. J Clin Invest 85:522-529, 1990.

67. Bjorbaek C, Echwald SM, Hubrich, P, et al. Genetic varients in promoters and coding regions of the muscle glycogen synthase and the insulin responsive GLUT4 genes in NIDDM. Diabetes 43:976-983, 1994.

68. Vestergaard H, Lund S, Larsen FS, Bjerrum OJ, Pedersen O. Glycogen synthase and phosphofructokinase protein ans mRNA levels in skeletal msucle from insulin-resistant patients with non-insulin-dependent diabetes mellitus. J Clin Invest 91:2342-2350, 1993.

69. Bjorbaek C, Vik TA, Echwald SM, et al. Cloning of a human insulin-stimulated protein kinase (ISPK-1) gene and analysis of coding regions and mRNA levels of the ISPK-1 and protein phosphatase-1 genes in muscle from NIDDM patients. Diabetes 44:90-97, 1995.
70. Freymond D, Bogardus C, Okubo M, Stone K, Mott D. Impaired insulin-stimulated muscle glycogen synthase activation in vivo in man is related to low fasting glycogen synthase phosphatase activity. J Clin Invest 82:1503-1509, 1988.
71. Nikoulina SE, Ciaraldi TP, Mudaliar S, Mohideen P, Carter L, Henry RR. Role of glycogen synthase kinase 3 in skeletal muscle insulin resistance of Type 2 diabetes. Diabetes 49:263-271, 2000.

III. Diagnosis and Epidemiology of Diabetes

Chapter 1. Diagnostic Criteria and Classification of Diabetes

Jocelyn Myers and Joel Zonszein

DEFINITION AND DESCRIPTION OF DIABETES

Diabetes mellitus is a heterogeneous group of metabolic diseases characterized by hyperglycemia resulting from defects in insulin secretion, insulin action, or both. Chronic hyperglycemia is associated with pathognomonic changes and failure of various organs, especially the eyes, kidneys, and nerves. Individuals with hyperglycemia are also subject to the accelerated cardiovascular disease that causes premature morbidity and mortality. Pathogenic processes involved in the development of diabetes range from autoimmune destruction of the β-cells of the pancreas with consequent insulin deficiency, to abnormalities in insulin signaling that result in resistance to insulin action. The vast majority of cases of diabetes fall into two broad etiopathogenetic groups. In one group (type 1 diabetes), the cause is an absolute deficiency of insulin secretion. Individuals at increased risk of developing this type of diabetes can often be identified by serological evidence of an autoimmune process of the pancreatic islets and by genetic markers. In the second and more prevalent group (type 2 diabetes), the cause is a combination of resistance to insulin action with inadequate compensatory insulin secretory response.

DIAGNOSTIC CRITERIA

The current classification and diagnosis of diabetes used in the U.S., developed by the World Health Organization (WHO) and National Diabetes Data Group (NDDG) and published in 1979,[1] has been further modified by the International Expert Committee under the sponsorship of the American Diabetes Association.[2] The terms "insulin dependent diabetes mellitus" and "non-insulin dependent diabetes mellitus" and their acronyms, IDDM and NIDDM, are no longer valid. They have been eliminated, as they were confusing and based on treatment rather than etiology. The terms type 1 and type 2 diabetes, with Arabic numerals rather than roman numerals, are now used.

The diagnosis can be established by documentation of abnormal glycemic values. Blood glucose determinations can be made during a fasting (12-hours overnight fast) state, known as fasting plasma glucose (FPG) or at random. Timely determinations after a meal (post-meal), or after a 75g or 100g glucose challenge, known as oral glucose tolerance test (OGTT), can also be used. It is important to recognize the difference between a physiological post-meal glucose value, and a non-physiological glucose challenge of 75g to 100g, often used for research purposes. Glycemic values vary greatly, and the degree of hyperglycemia or glucose intolerance can be a moving target. Glycemic values can improve or worsen according to changes in body weight, food intake, physical activity, stress, pregnancy, corticosteroids, medications, etc. For instance an individual treated with corticosteroids can develop hyperglycemia consistent with the diagnosis of diabetes, but this condition can improve or even normalize after the discontinuation of corticosteroids.

Diagnosis of Diabetes Mellitus. While plasma glucose concentrations are distributed over a continuum, there is a threshold (FPG $\geq$ 126 mg/dl) where adverse outcomes related to microvascular complications start to occur. In the early stages, particularly in type 2 diabetes, the degree of hyperglycemia is sufficient to cause pathologic changes, but it is not enough to cause clinical symptoms. Thus, a silent phase of the disease can exist for prolonged periods of time before it is diagnosed. During this asymptomatic period, it is possible to demonstrate abnormal carbohydrate metabolism. Derangement of carbohydrate metabolism in the more common form of type 2 diabetes evolves from a pre-diabetic condition known as impaired glucose tolerance (IGT) to overt type 2 diabetes. The criteria for the diagnosis of diabetes and IGT are shown in **Table 1** and **Table 2** respectively.

Table 1. Criteria for the diagnosis of diabetes mellitus

- Symptoms of diabetes + random plasma glucose concentration $\geq$ 200 mg/dl (11.1 mmol/L)
- Fasting plasma glucose $\geq$ 126 mg/dl (7.0 mmol/L)
- Two hour plasma glucose $\geq$ 200 mg/dl (11.1 mmol/L) during an 75 grm Oral Glucose Tolerance Test

There are three possible ways to diagnose diabetes mellitus with the revised criteria shown in **Table 1**. To establish the diagnosis, each value must be confirmed on a subsequent day by any one of the three criteria given. For example, symptoms with a casual plasma glucose >200 mg/dl, needs to be confirmed *on a subsequent day* by either *1*) FPG ≥126 mg/dl, *2*) 2-h post-load (meal or OGTT) ≥ 200 mg/dl, or *3*) symptoms with random plasma glucose ≥ 200 mg/dl. Preferably, the diagnosis should be based on FPG ≥ 126 mg/dl, as it is an easier test. The OGTT is an acceptable diagnostic test, valuable for research, however it is impractical for clinical purposes as it is costly, needs to be done under controlled conditions and close supervision, and causes excessive demands on participants' time. Using the FPG test criteria results in a lower prevalence than using the WHO criteria (4.35% vs. 6.34%) in those individuals without a medical history of diabetes. However, a widespread adoption of the new criteria may have a large impact on the number of people actually diagnosed. This is important since presently, about 1/3 of adults with diabetes in the U.S. remain undiagnosed.[3]

Diagnosis of Impaired Glucose Tolerance (IGT) and Impaired Fasting Glucose (IFG). There is an intermediate group of subjects whose glucose levels do not meet the criteria for diabetes, but are too high to be considered normal (**Table 2.**)

Table 2. Criteria for the diagnosis of Glucose Intolerance

	Normal	Impaired Glucose Tolerance	Diabetes Mellitus
Fasting Plasma Glucose mg/dl	≤110	≥110 or ≤126	≥126
Mmol/l	≤6.1	≥6.1 or ≤ 7.0	≥7.0
2-hour post OGTT challenge mg/dl	≤140	≥140 or ≤ 200	≥200
mmol/l	≤7.8	≥7.8 or ≤11.1	≥11.1

OGTT= Oral Glucose Tolerance Test

To establish the diagnosis of IGT an OGTT needs to be performed. However, because of the cost and inconvenience, fasting plasma glucose (FPG) values alone are used in clinical practice as they correlate with those diagnosed as IGT. Individuals with FPG between 110 and 126 mg/dl are classified as having impaired fasting glucose (IFG).[4] While this is an arbitrary choice, individuals with IFG are at a threshold where the acute phase of insulin secretion is lost in response to intravenous administration of glucose,[5] and are at a greater risk of developing micro- and macrovascular complications;[6,7] they also often progress to type 2 diabetes. Individuals with IGT or IFG have other associated comorbidities and cardiovascular risk factors that include central obesity, dyslipidemia, hypertension, and abnormal hemostasis.[8] These individuals need to be properly screened, closely monitored and encouraged to make lifestyle changes in order to avoid conversion to type 2 diabetes and ameliorate the rate of cardiovascular events.

The use of HbA_{1c} for the diagnosis of diabetes is not currently recommended. Some studies however, have shown that the frequency distributions for HbA_{1c} are concordant with FPG and the 2-h PG determinations. These observations have led to the recommendation of HbA_{1c} measurement for diagnostic purposes,[9] but due to lack of uniformity in the assays, a nationwide standardization will be necessary prior to its approval for this use.[10,11] HbA_{1c} levels are closely correlated with macro- and or microvascular complications in diabetes and have become the gold standard test in monitoring the treatment of diabetes, utilizing it for decisions on when and how to implement therapy. It is also an excellent marker for cardiovascular mortality in diabetes, and in those prior to the development of the disease.[12] The 2-h PG determinations are also valuable for early diagnosis and detection of complications, however more information from clinical studies will be necessary in order to utilize this test.

Diagnosis of Gestational Diabetes. Gestational diabetes mellitus (GDM) is defined as any degree of glucose intolerance with onset or first recognition during pregnancy. (for more detail, please see the chapter on "Diabetes in pregnancy). The definition applies regardless of therapy or whether the condition persists after pregnancy.[13] A FPG level >126 mg/dl, or a casual plasma glucose >200 mg/dl, makes the diagnosis of diabetes, when confirmed on a subsequent day. In the absence of these criteria, evaluation for GDM should follow one of two approaches:

1) Perform a diagnostic OGTT without prior plasma or serum glucose screening. This one-step approach may be cost-effective in high-risk patients.
2) Perform an initial screening by measuring the plasma or serum glucose concentration 1 h after a 50g oral glucose load; if the glucose value is over >140 mg/dl, a diagnostic OGTT needs to be performed.

With the above tests, approximately 80% of women with GDM can be identified. The yield can further increase to 90% when using a cutoff of >130 mg/dl. With either approach, the diagnosis of GDM is based on an OGTT. Diagnostic criteria for the 100g OGTT is derived from the original work of O'Sullivan and Mahan, modified by Carpenter and Coustan, and is shown in the following table:

Table 3. Diagnosis of GDM with a 100-g or 75-g glucose challenge

	mg/dl	mmol/l
Fasting	95	5.3
1 hour	180	10
2 hour	155	8.6
3 hour	140	7.8

Test should be done in the morning after an overnight fast and at least three days of unrestricted diet, rich in carbohydrates. The subject should remain seated and not smoking throughout the test. Two or more values must be met or exceeded for a diagnosis.

The diagnosis of GDM should be entertained at the first prenatal visit, particularly in high risk populations (**Table 4**). If found not to have GDM at that initial screening, women should be retested between 24 and 28 weeks of gestation, as is the recommendation for women of average risk. It is good medical practice to restudy the patient six weeks or more after the termination of pregnancy with a glucose challenge, in order to reclassify them into one of the following categories: *1*) diabetes, *2*) IFG, *3*) IGT, or *4*) normoglycemia. In the majority, glucose regulation returns to normal after delivery.

Testing for diabetes in presumably healthy individuals. Undiagnosed type 2 diabetes is common in the U.S. Detection, and consequently early treatment, might well reduce the burden of type 2 diabetes and its complications. In order to increase the cost-effectiveness of diagnosing otherwise healthy individuals, testing should be considered in high-risk populations[14] (**Table 4**).

Table 4. Populations at high risk for diabetes

Age > 45 years old
Age < 45 with:
- Member of a minority population
- Obesity (> 120% desirable bodyweight or BMI > 27 kg/m^2
- First relative with diabetes
- Previous history of GDM or delivered a baby weighting > 9 lb
- Previous evidence of IGT or IFG
- Hypertension, dyslipidemia

Although the OGTT and FPG are both suitable tests, the FPG is strongly recommended in clinical settings as it easier and more acceptable to the patients.

DIABETES CLASSIFICATION

Diabetes is a complex and heterogeneous disorder with diverse etiopathogenetic mechanisms, thus any classification becomes arbitrary and simplistic. The generally accepted systematic categorization recognized two major forms of diabetes, type 1 and type 2 diabetes (1). This classification was modified by the Expert Committee Group (2) based on etiology rather than the pharmacology of treatment, which made it less confusing and more informative **(Table 5).** It is not within the scope of this chapter to review each of these forms, however a summary and highlights of several of these entities are briefly described.

Table 5. Etiologic classification of diabetes mellitus

I. Type 1 diabetes
    A. Autoimmune
    B. Idiopathic

II. Type 2 diabetes

III. Others
    A. Genetic defects of β-cell function
    B. Diseases of the exocrine pancreas
    C. Endocrinopathies
    D. Drug or chemical induced
    E. Infections
    F. Uncommon immune-mediated
    G. Other genetic syndromes associated with diabetes

IV. Gestational Diabetes

Type 1 diabetes (β-cell destruction, usually leading to absolute insulin deficiency) This form of diabetes accounts for 5-10% of all cases. It results from a progressive cellular-mediated autoimmune destruction of the β-cells of the pancreas.[15] Markers of the immune destruction of the β-cell include islet cell autoantibodies (ICAs), autoantibodies to insulin (IAAs), autoantibodies to glutamic acid decarboxylase (GAD_{65}), and autoantibodies to the tyrosine phosphatases IA-2 and IA-2$_\alpha$.[16-19] At least one or more of these autoantibodies are present in the majority (85 to 90%). The disease has also strong HLA associations, with linkage to the DQA and B genes, and influenced by the DRB genes.[20] Immune-mediated diabetes commonly occurs in childhood and adolescence, but it can occur at any age, even in the 8th and 9th decades of life. The pancreatic β-cells suffer a progressive and relentless attack that terminates in failure to produce insulin. The rate of β-cell destruction can be rapid, particularly in infants and children, but can be slow in others.[21] At a later stage of the disease, there is little or no insulin secretion that can be assessed by low levels of plasma C-peptide determinations. The typical patient with newly diagnosed Type 1 DM is young Caucasian, who often presents in diabetic ketoacidosis. Family history of type 1 diabetes is not a common feature, found only in 10%. In identical twins there is only 35-50% concordance. Thus, while there is a genetic predisposition, there clearly are other factors. Because of the autoimmune nature of type 1 DM, patients are at increased risk for developing other disorders such as autoimmune thyroid disease, rheumatoid arthritis, etc. Some individuals may retain residual β-cell function sufficient to prevent ketoacidosis for many years, but eventually become dependent on insulin. The total lack of insulin makes these patients more susceptible to ketosis, and makes treatment with exogenous insulin a necessity in order to survive. Therapy therefore, consists in mimicking the pancreatic physiologic insulin secretion patterns, through giving exogenous insulin, still an elusive goal. The adult form of this type of diabetes can account for up to > 30% of all cases in certain populations in Northern Europe. The defect of insulin secretion can be prolonged due to slower β-cell destruction. This type of diabetes is known as Latent Autoimmune Diabetes of the Adult (LADA). The diagnosis is often overlooked thus patients are improperly treated as type 2 diabetes during the early stages.[21]

Idiopathic diabetes. Some forms of type 1 diabetes are less well understood, and can present with a variety of β-cell dysfunction. Some have intermittent, moderate to severe forms of insulinopenia, and while they can present in ketoacidosis, there is often a partial recovery of the pancreatic β-cell. Thus, requirements for insulin replacement therapy may come and go[22]. This form of diabetes is inherited, lacks evidence for β-cell autoimmunity, and is not HLA associated. Only a minority of patients falls under this category, and most are from African-Caribbean origin.

Type 2 diabetes (ranging from predominantly insulin resistance to predominantly insulin secretory defect) This type of diabetes is a group of heterogeneous conditions responsible for nearly 90% of all individuals with diabetes. It is characterized by a dual defect of insulin resistance and β-cell dysfunction. Circulating insulin levels are higher early in the disease due to the insulin-resistance, but eventually insulin production becomes less sufficient. In the typical progression of the disease, impaired insulin mediated glucose utilization results first in postprandial hyperglycemia (or IGT). Fasting hyperglycemia ($\geq$126 mg/dl), the hallmark of type 2 diabetes, ensues at a later stage due to excessive hepatic glucose production. The presence of insulin in these patients is enough to prevent ketosis with the occasional exception of severe stressors (i.e. infection, trauma). The typical patient with type 2 diabetes is often obese, with associated comorbidities and cardiovascular risk factors, that result in a high and premature morbidity and mortality rate. Unfortunately, this disease is becoming more common in progressive societies and is afflicting younger individuals particularly among ethnic minorities.

Other specific types. These numerous conditions summarized in **Table 5** account for only a minor portion of all cases. Genetic defects of pancreatic β-cells are also referred as Maturity Onset Diabetes of the Young (MODY) a group of monogenetic disorders in which a genetic mutation causes hyperglycemia via a defect in glucose sensing or insulin secretion. Abnormalities at three genetic loci on different chromosomes have already been identified. The most common form is associated with mutations on chromosome 12 in a hepatic transcription factor (referred to as hepatocyte nuclear factor (HNF)-1α).[23] A second form has a mutation in the glucokinase gene on chromosome 7p,[24,25] and affects glucokinase ("glucose sensor"). A third form is associated with a mutation in the HNF-4α gene on chromosome 20q.[26] The typical MODY patient is less than 25 years old, non-obese, with a strong family history of diabetes. Hyperglycemia tends to be milder and may be accompanied with less sever chronic complications. Point mutations in mitochondrial DNA (most common at position 3243 in the tRNA leucine gene, leading to an A-to-G transition) are associated with an uncommon condition of diabetes mellitus and deafness.[27] Genetic defects causing an abnormal conversion of proinsulin to insulin,[28] and cases with production of insulin mutants with impaired insulin receptor binding[29] have been identified. Genetic defects in insulin action are more common, and can be associated with acanthosis nigricans and polycystic ovarian (PCO) syndrome. This is characterized clinically by the typical skin abnormalities (acanthosis nigricans), obesity, hyperandrogenism, and enlarged cystic ovaries.[30-32] The genetic defect in insulin action of this syndrome was named Type A insulin resistance.[31] Patients with PCO syndrome also have a premature and accelerated rate of arteriosclerosis, thus, need to be properly identified and treated early. Other causes of diabetes include abnormalities of the exocrine pancreas (pancreatitis, trauma, and cystic fibrosis), several endocrinopathies that cause increased demand in insulin secretion such as Cushing's syndrome or acromegaly. Hyperglycemia can also be induced or precipitated by a number of drugs such as thiazides, dilantin, α-interferon, diazoxide and glucocorticoids. Viral infections such as Hepatitis C, coxsackie virus B, cytomegalovirus, adenovirus, and mumps are also associated with β-cell dysfunction or destruction.[33-34]

Gestational Diabetes Mellitus (GDM), complicates ~4% of all pregnancies in the U.S. The prevalence may range from 1 to 14% of pregnancies, depending on the population studied and it represents nearly 90% of all pregnancies complicated by diabetes.[35] As aforementioned, early diagnosis is important as proper therapy can reduce perinatal morbidity and mortality.[36,37] These women are at higher risk of developing type 2 diabetes and need to be continuously monitored.

SUMMARY

Diabetes mellitus is a heterogeneous and multifactorial disorder. There is now a well-established and easier set of criteria to screen the high-risk population, allowing for an earlier diagnosis and a more focused treatment. The classification of the disease is now based on disease etiology rather than pharmacological treatment, making it more uniform, and reflecting the current knowledge of the disease.

REFERENCES:

1. National Diabetes Data Group. Classification and diagnosis of diabetes mellitus and other categories of glucose intolerance. Diabetes 28:1039–1057, 1979.
2. The Expert Committee on the Diagnosis and Classification of Diabetes Mellitus. Report of the Expert Committee on the diagnosis and classification of Diabetes Mellitus. Diabetes Care 24 (Suppl. 1): S5-S20, 2001.
3. Harris MI, Hadden WC, Knowler WC, Bennett PH. Prevalence of diabetes and impaired glucose tolerance and plasma glucose levels in the U.S. population aged 20–74 yr. Diabetes 36:523–534, 1987.
4. Charles MA, Fontboune A, Thibult N, Warnet JM, Rosselin GE, Eschwege E. Risk factors for NIDDM in white population: Paris Prospective Study. Diabetes 40:796–799, 1991.
5. Brunzell JD, Robertson RP, Lerner RL, Hazzard WR, Ensink JW, Bierman EL, Porte D Jr. Relationships between fasting plasma glucose levels and insulin secretion during intravenous glucose tolerance tests. J Clin Endocrinol Metab 42:222–229, 1976.
6. Klein, R, Comor EB, Blount BA, Wingard DL. Visual impairment and retinopathy in people with normal glucose tolerance, impaired glucose tolerance and newly diagnosed NIDDM. Diabetes Care 14:914– 918, 1991.

7. Fuller JH, Shipley MJ, Rose G, Jarrett RJ, Keen H. Coronary-heart disease risk and impaired glucose tolerance: the Whitehall Study. Lancet i:1373–1376, 1980.

8. Klein R. Hyperglycemia and microvascular and macrovascular disease in diabetes. Diabetes Care 18:258–268, 1995.

9. McCance DR, Hanson RL, Charles MA, Jacobsson LTH, Pettitt DJ, Bennett PH, Knowler WC. Comparison of tests for glycated haemoglobin and fasting and two hour plasma glucose concentrations as diagnostic methods for diabetes. Brit Med J 308:1323–1328, 1994.

10. American Diabetes Association. Tests of glycemia in diabetes (Position Statement). Diabetes Care 24 (Suppl. 1):S80–S82, 2001.

11. Engelgau MM, Thompson TJ, Herman WH, Boyle JP, Aubert RE, Kenny SJ, Badran A, Sous ES, Ali MA. Comparison of fasting and 2-hour glucose and HbA_{1c} levels for diagnosing diabetes: diagnostic criteria and performance revisited. Diabetes Care 20:785–791, 1997.

12. Barrett-Connor E, Wingard DL. HbA1c levels predict mortality across population ranges. Brit Med J 322:5-6, 2001.

13. Metzger BE. Organizing committee summary and recommendations of the Third International Workshop-Conference on gestational diabetes mellitus. Diabetes 40:197–201, 1991.

14. Harris MI, Hadden WC, Knowler WC, Bennett PH: Prevalence of diabetes and impaired glucose tolerance and plasma glucose levels in the U.S. population aged 20–74 yr. Diabetes 36:523–534, 1987.

15. Atkinson MA, Maclaren NK. The pathogenesis of insulin dependent diabetes. N Engl J Med 331:1428–1436, 1994.

16. Kaufman D, Erlander M, Clare-Salzler M, Atkinson M, Maclaren N, Tobin A. Autoimmunity to two forms of glutamate decarboxylase in insulin-dependent mellitus. J Clin Invest 89:283–292, 1992.

17. Myers MA, Rabin DU, Rowley MJ. Pancreatic islet cell cytoplasmic antibody in diabetes is represented by antibodies to islet cell antigen 512 and glutamic acid decarboxylase. Diabetes 44:1290–1295, 1995.

18. Lan MS, Wasserfall C, Maclaren NK, Notkins AL. IA-2, a transmembrane protein of the protein tyrosine phosphatase family, is a major autoantigen in insulin-dependent diabetes mellitus. Proc Natl Acad Sci USA 93:6367–6370, 1996.

19. Lu J, Li Q, Xie H, Chen Z, Borovitskaya AE, Maclaren NK, Notkins AL, Lan MS. Identification of a second transmembrane protein tyrosine phosphatase, IA-2_α, as an autoantigen in insulin-dependent diabetes mellitus: precursor of the 37-kDa tryptic fragment. Proc Natl Acad Sci USA 93: 2307–2311, 1996.

20. Huang W, Connor E, DelaRosa T, Muir A, Schatz D, Silverstein J, Crockett S, She JX, Maclaren NK. Although DR3-DQB1* may be associated with multiple component diseases of the autoimmune polyglandular syndromes, the human leukocyte antigen DR4-DQB1I0302 haplotype is implicated only in beta cell autoimmunity. J Clin Endocrinol Metab 81:1–5, 1996.

21. Zimmet PZ, Tuomi T, Mackay R, Rowley MJ, Knowles W, Cohen M, Lang DA. Latent autoimmune diabetes mellitus in adults (LADA): the role of antibodies to glutamic acid decarboxylase in diagnosis and prediction of insulin dependency. Diabet Med 11:299–303, 1994.

22. Banerji M, Lebovitz H. Insulin sensitive and insulin resistant variants in IDDM. Diabetes 38:784–792, 1989.

23. Yamagata K, Oda N, Kaisaki PJ, Menzel S, Furuta H, Vaxillaire M, Southam L, Cox RD, Lathrop GM, Boriraj VV, Chen X, Cox NJ, Oda Y, Yano H, Le Beau MM, Yamada S, Nishigori H, Takeda J, Fajans SS, Hattersley AT, Iwasaki N, Hansen T, Pedersen O, Polonsky KS, Bell GI. Mutations in the hepatocyte nuclear factor-1̄ gene in maturity-onset diabetes of the young (MODY 3). Nature 384:455–458, 1996.

24. Froguel P, Vaxillaire M, Sun F, Velho G, Zouali H, Butel MO, Lesage S, Vionnet N, Clement K, Fougerousse F, et al. Close linkage of glucokinase locus on chromosome 7p to early-onset non-insulin-dependent diabetes mellitus. Nature 356:162–164, 1992.

25. Vionnet N, Stoffel M, Takeda J, Yasuda K, Bell GI, Zouali H, Lesage S, Velho G, Iris F, Passa P, et al. Nonsense mutation in the glucokinase gene causes early-onset non-insulin-dependent diabetes mellitus. Nature 356:721–1488, 1992.

26. Yamagata K, Furuta H, Oda N, Kaisaki PJ, Menzel S, Cox NJ, Fajans SS, Signorini S, Stoffel M, Bell GI. Mutations in the hepatocyte factor-4_α gene in maturity-onset diabetes of the young (MODY 1). Nature 384:458–460, 1996.

27. Kadowaki T, Kadowaki H, Mori Y, Tobe K, Sakuta R, Suzuki Y, Tanabe Y, Sakura H, Awata T, Goto Y, et al. A subtype of diabetes mellitus associated with a mutation of mitochondrial DNA. N Engl J Med 330:962–968, 1994.

28. Gruppuso PA, Gorden P, Kahn CR, Cornblath M, Zeller WP, Schwartz R. Familial hyperproinsulinemia due to a proposed defect in conversion of proinsulin to insulin. N Engl J Med 311:629–634, 1984.

29. Given BD, Mako ME, Tager HS, Baldwin D, Markese J, Rubenstein AH, Olefsky J, Kobayashi M, Kolterman O, Poucher R. Diabetes due to secretion of an abnormal insulin. N Engl J Med 302:129–135, 1980.

30. Taylor SI. Lilly Lecture: molecular mechanisms of insulin resistance: lessons from patients with mutations in the insulin-receptor gene. Diabetes 41:1473–1490, 1992.

31. Kahn CR, Flier JS, Bar RS, Archer JA, Gorden P, Martin MM, Roth J. The syndromes of insulin resistance and acanthosis nigricans. N Engl J Med 294:739–745, 1976.

32. Dunaif A, Segal KR, Shelley DR, Green G, Dobrjansky A, Licholai T. Evidence for distinctive and intrinsic defects in insulin action in polycystic ovary syndrome. Diabetes 41:1257–1266, 1992.

33. Karjalainen J, Knip M, Hyoty H, Linikki P, Ilonen J, Kaar M-L, Akerblom HK. Relationship between serum insulin antibodies, islet cell antibodies and Coxsackie-B4 and mumps virus–specific antibodies at the clinical manifestation of type I (insulin-dependent) diabetes. Diabetologia 31:146–152, 1988.

34. Pak CY, Eun H, McArthur RG, Yoon J. Association of cytomegalovirus infection with autoimmune type 1 diabetes. Lancet ii:1–4, 1988.

35. Engelgau MM, Herman WH, Smith PJ, German RR, Aubert RE. The epidemiology of diabetes and pregnancy in the U.S., 1988. Diabetes Care 18:1029–1033, 1995.

36. Magee MS, Walden CE, Benedetti TJ. Influence of diagnostic criteria on the incidence of gestational diabetes and perinatal morbidity. JAMA 269:609–615, 1993.

37. Langer O, Rodriguez DA, Xenakis EMJ, McFarland MB, Berkus MD, Arrendondo F. Intensified versus conventional management of gestational diabetes. Am J Obstet Gynecol 170:1036–1047, 1994.

Chapter 2. Epidemiology of Diabetes and its Burden in the World and in the United States

Daniel S. Donovan, Jr.

INTRODUCTION

An epidemic is defined as an increase in the usual or expected number of cases of a disease in a population. The increase in the number of cases of diabetes that the world has experienced and continues to experience certainly qualifies as epidemic. Diabetes mellitus is a growing public health problem throughout the world and in the U. S.[1] The disease and its attendant morbidity and mortality exact huge personal, public and economic costs.[2] This chapter will review current knowledge regarding the distribution and determinants of diabetes throughout the world and the U.S. Two terms used and confused frequently in epidemiological discussions of disease are incidence and prevalence and a review of their definitions may be useful. Prevalence is defined as the number of affected persons present in the population at a specific time divided by the number of persons in the population at that time and is a measure of the burden of disease in a population. Incidence, on the other hand, is the number of *new* cases of disease that occur during a specified time in a population and represents the risk for developing the disease.

THE WORLDWIDE BURDEN OF DIABETES

There is a growing burden to society for diabetes. Type 2 diabetes accounts for an estimated 90 to 95% of the total cases of diagnosed diabetes worldwide, type 1 for 5-10%, and other forms for 2-3%.

In the U.S. diabetes is the leading cause of new cases of adult blindness, end stage renal disease and non-traumatic amputations.[3] Diabetes mellitus is reported to be among the five leading causes of death in most countries. It is estimated that 30 to 50 percent of diabetes cases remain undiagnosed. The burden of diabetes in the world presently and predicted for the future is astounding.[4] While in 1985 there were approximately 30 million people diagnosed worldwide with diabetes, by 1995 the prevalence of diagnosed diabetes had increased to an estimated 135 million people or 4% of adults older than 20 years of age. In the year 2000 the number increased again to 150 million and the projection for the number of cases of diabetes in the world in the year 2025 is even more frightening. It is estimated that the prevalence of diabetes will rise to 5.4% and there will be 300 million adults with diabetes[5,6] (Figure 1).

This will be a 35% increase in the world wide prevalence of diabetes while at the same time the world population size is predicted to remain relatively stable, with only an 11% increase from 1995 to 2025. The prevalence of diabetes is currently higher in developed nations than in developing nations, however, there will be a 170% increase in the number of individuals with diabetes in developing countries with a 42% increase in developed countries. This change is the result of increased westernization, urbanization, and obesity.[7,8] The 10 countries with the largest numbers of individuals with diabetes in 1995 and 2025 are depicted in Table 1.

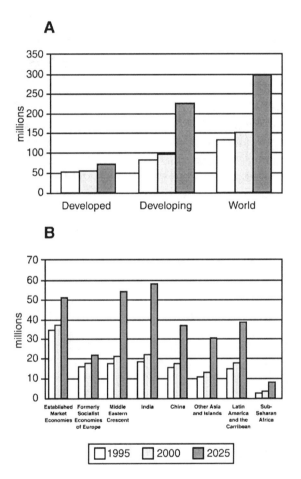

Figure 1. Number of people with diabetes in the adult population (aged≥20 years) by year and region. A: Developed and developing countries and world total. B: Major geographic areas. (From: King H, Aubert RE and Herman WH. Global burden of diabetes, 1995-2025: prevalence, numerical estimates, and projections. Diabetes Care 21(9): 1414-31,1998, with permission.[6])

In developed countries diabetes is most common in individuals who are 65 years of age or older. This is not true of developing countries, where individuals between 45 and 64 years of age make up the largest group.

In general there are more women than men with diabetes worldwide. This female preponderance is greatest in developed countries whereas the figures are more equal in developing countries. It is predicted that by the year 2025 there will be an excess of diabetes cases in urban areas compared with non-urban areas, more severe in developing countries.

Geographically, the Western Pacific Region has the highest number of individuals with diagnosed diabetes (approximately 44 million), but the prevalence of 3.6% is significantly lower than that of 7.8% seen in North America. The Eastern Mediterranean and Middle East regions have a similar prevalence of 7.7%.

Table 1. Top ten countries for estimated number of adults with diabetes, 1995 and 2025

	Country	1995 (millions)	Country	2025 (millions)
Rank				
1	India	19.4	India	57.2
2	China	16.0	China	37.6
3	U.S.	13.9	U.S.	21.9
4	Russian Federation	8.9	Pakistan	14.5
5	Japan	6.3	Indonesia	12.4
6	Brazil	4.9	Russian Federation	12.2
7	Indonesia	4.5	Mexico	11.7
8	Pakistan	4.3	Brazil	11.6
9	Mexico	3.8	Egypt	8.8
10	Ukraine	3.6	Japan	8.5
All other countries		49.7		103.6
Total		135.3		300.0

(From King H, Aubert RE, Herman WH. Global burden of diabetes. Diabetes Care 21:1414–1431, 1998, with permission.)

The increase in the prevalence of diabetes is alarming and projected to reach 300 million people worldwide by the year 2025, with developing countries suffering disproportionately. The urbanization, westernization and economic development in developing countries are likely contributors to substantial rise in diabetes.

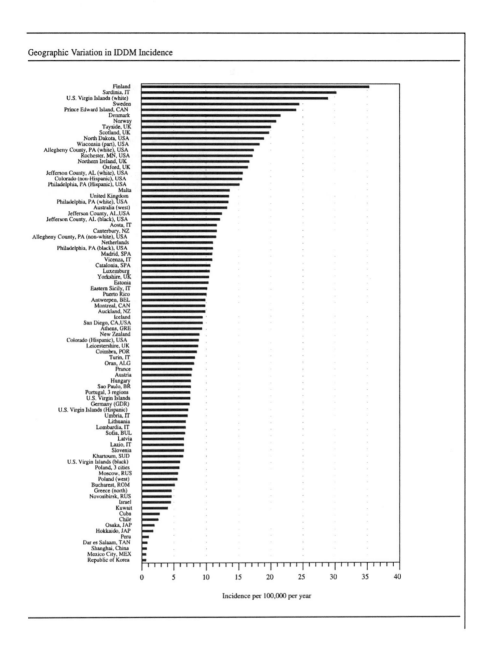

Figure 2. Geographic variation in IDDM incidence. Source : Diabetes in America, p. 41, 1995.[9]

While the majority of individuals with diagnosed diabetes have type 2 diabetes, it is estimated that approximately 4.9 million people (in all age groups) have type 1 diabetes, for a prevalence of 0.09%.[10,11] The variation is wide, with the European region having the highest estimated number of people with type 1 diabetes (1.27 million), followed by the North American

110

Region (1.04 million) and the South East Asian Region (0.91 million). The estimated prevalence of type 1 diabetes is highest in the North American Region (0.25%), followed by the European Region (0.19%) and lowest in Africa (0.02%) and the Western Pacific (0.03%).

The incidence of type 1 diabetes in people less than 15 years old varies widely across populations, as much as 60 fold between the highest and lowest rates. The highest reported incidence is in Finland, with 35 cases per annum per 100,000 population, and the lowest is in China and Peru, with approximately 0.5 cases per annum per 100,000 population.[3, 9, 12] (Figure 2)

Recent evidence indicates a global trend toward rising incidence rates, averaging approximately 2.5% per year. The incidence is higher in Caucasoid populations. Within ethnic groups, however, differences in incidence depend upon the racial admixture and possibly environmental exposures. Type 1 diabetes occurs at all ages and nearly 44 percent of all new cases of type 1 diabetes in Denmark are diagnosed after 30 years of age.[12]

THE BURDEN IN THE UNITED STATES OF AMERICA

The major sources of information regarding the prevalence and incidence of diabetes in the U.S. are from national surveys. The National Health and Information Survey (NHIS) and the Behavioral Risk Factor Surveillance System (BRFSS) assess diagnosed diabetes, and the third National Health and Nutrition Examination Survey (NHANES III) assess both diagnosed and undiagnosed diabetes.

TOTAL AND TYPE 2 DIABETES

NHANES III, 1988-1994 estimated the prevalence of both diagnosed and undiagnosed diabetes in adults ≥ 20 years old. When extrapolated to 1997 it was estimated that 15.7 million Americans or 5.9% of U.S. population had diabetes. Of these individuals 10.2 million were estimated to have been diagnosed with diabetes and 5.4 million had undiagnosed diabetes as assessed by glucose challenge. The prevalence of diagnosed diabetes increases with age. While 0.8% of the individuals less than 45 years of age had diagnosed diabetes, 11.7 percent of those age 65 to 74 years and 10.9 percent of those older than 75 years of age had diagnosed diabetes. The prevalence of diagnosed diabetes is similar for men and women, however, 45% of diagnosed individuals are males and 55 percent are females. It is estimated that 90-95% of individuals with diabetes have type 2 diabetes.[13]

There are marked racial and ethnic differences in the prevalence of diagnosed diabetes. The prevalence of diabetes is higher by 1.6 fold in African-Americans compared with whites at all ages. Individuals of

Mexican and Puerto Rican descent have an approximately 1.9 fold higher prevalence of diabetes compared with non-Hispanic whites.[9, 14, 15]

Although prevalence data are limited, Asians and Pacific Islanders also have a higher prevalence of diabetes than whites.[8, 16] The prevalence of diabetes is very high in Native American populations and varies by tribal groups. The highest prevalence of diabetes in the world is found in the Pima Indians of Arizona where 65 percent of those aged 45 to 74 years old have type 2 diabetes[17, 18] (Figure 3).

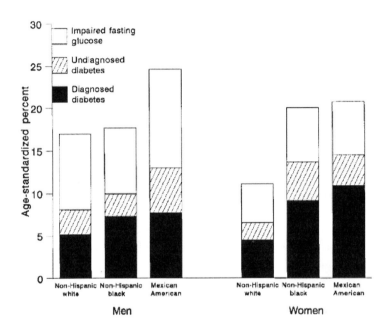

Figure 3. Age-standardized prevalence of diagnosed and undiagnosed diabetes and impaired fasting glucose in the U.S. population ≥ 20 years of age, presented according to sex and racial or ethnic group, based on NHANES III. Diagnosed diabetes was defined by medical history; undiagnosed diabetes by fasting plasma glucose ≥ 126 mg/dl, and impaired fasting glucose by fasting plasma glucose 110-125 mg/dl. (From Harris M I et al. Diabetes Care 21(4):518-24, 1998, with permission).

There has been a steady increase in the prevalence of diabetes in recent years with an 18% increase in the prevalence of diagnosed diabetes noted between NHIS evaluations conducted during 1979 to 1981 (2.5%) and 1995 to 1997 (3.0%). The BRFSS found a 33% increase in the prevalence of diagnosed diabetes from 1990 (4.9%) to 1998 (6.5%). The increase in prevalence by age group is shown in Table 2.[19] The BRFSS also reported a 6% increase in the prevalence of diagnosed diabetes during only the one year between 1998 and 1999 when the prevalence rose from 6.5% to 6.9%. Average weight increased during this period as well from 76.2 kg to 76.7 kg.

This trend continued into the following year 2000 when the prevalence had increased to 7.3%.[20]

Table 2. Increase in prevalence of diagnosed diabetes 1990 to 1998 (by age group).

Age (yr)	% Increase
30–39	70
40–49	40
50–59	31

Source: Diabetes Care 23(9): 1278-83.[19]

Figure 4 graphically demonstrates the increasing prevalence trends in the US.

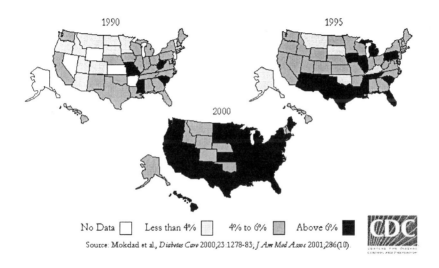

Figure 4. Diabetes and gestational diabetes trends among adults in the U.S., BRFSS 1990, 1995 and 2000. Source: www.cdc.gov

A number of factors have been implicated in the rising prevalence of diagnosed diabetes. These include the aging of the U.S. population, a reduction in mortality of people with diabetes, an increase in higher risk ethnic minorities, the improved detection of diabetes, and the lowering of the diagnostic threshold from 140 mg per deciliter to 126 mg per deciliter in 1996.[16] Obesity and overweight, especially upper body or abdominal adiposity, are strongly associated with development of type 2 diabetes. The BRFSS estimated there to be 9% increase in prevalence of diabetes for every 1 kg increase in weight. More than 70% of individuals with type 2 diabetes are overweight.[21] Sedentary lifestyle and physical inactivity have been implicated as risk factors as well. Evidence suggests that physical activity can decrease risk of diabetes.[22] Diet may also play a role. High calorie diets, including those high in fat, and especially saturated fat, have been implicated in the development of type 2 diabetes.[24-26] Family history is a very strong risk factor for type 2 diabetes. A strong genetic component is suggested by the 58-75% concordance rates for type 2 diabetes observed in identical twins (Table 3).[3]

Table 3. Estimated risk of developing type 2 diabetes by family history

One parent with type 2 diabetes	
Diagnosed before age 50	14% chance of type 2 diabetes
Diagnosed after age 50	7-8% chance of type 2 diabetes
Both parents with type 2 diabetes	
Both diagnosed before age 50	25% chance of type 2 diabetes before age 50
Both diagnosed after age 50	15% chance of type 2 diabetes after age 50
Overall risk	45% chance of type 2 diabetes by age 65
Sibling with type 2 diabetes	
Diagnosed before age 50	14% chance of type 2 diabetes
Diagnosed after age 50	7-8% chance of type 2 diabetes
Identical twin with type 2 diabetes	58-75% change of type 2 diabetes

Source: Diabetes 2001 Vital Statistics.[3]

NHANES II found that from 1976 to 1980 the prevalence of undiagnosed type 2 diabetes was equal to the prevalence of diagnosed diabetes or, alternatively, that 50% of diabetes cases were undiagnosed. In the follow up survey, NHANES III, the prevalence of diagnosed and undiagnosed diabetes was now 5.3% and 2.8% respectively, suggesting that there had been a reduction in the proportion of undiagnosed individuals with diabetes to approximately 35%. This was perhaps due, in part, to the change in fasting plasma glucose diagnostic criteria from 140 mg/dL to 126 mg/dL. The prevalence of both diagnosed and undiagnosed diabetes is higher in African-Americans and Mexican-Americans than in whites.[13]

Until recently, immune mediated type 1 diabetes was the only type of diabetes considered prevalent among children with only one to 2 percent of children considered to have type 2 diabetes or other rare forms of diabetes. Recent reports indicate that between 8-45% of children with newly diagnosed diabetes do not have immune mediated diabetes. Most children with type 2 diabetes present with glycosuria without ketonuria, absent or mild polyuria and polydipsia and little or no weight loss. However, up to 33 percent may have ketonuria at diagnosis. Eighty-five percent of affected children are either overweight or obese at diagnosis. A family history of diabetes is usually present: 74-100% of patients have a first or second degree relative with type 2 diabetes. Acanthosis nigricans is present in as many as 90 percent of children with type 2 diabetes. In the Pima Indians the prevalence of type 2 diabetes in children has been reported to be 22.3 per 1000 in the 10 to 14 year-old age group and 50.9 per 1000 in the 15 to 19 year-old age group. Type 2 diabetes constitutes an increasing percentage of the incident pediatric cases of diagnosed diabetes.[27-30]

Table 4: Risk Factors for Type 2 Diabetes

Older Age
Ethnic minority (African American, Hispanic, Native American, Asian American)
Family history
Obesity –Total body
        Upper body or central
Lifestyle factors : Physical inactivity
            Diet: high caloric intake, high fat, saturated fat
            Alcohol intake
            Cigarette smoking
            Acculturation
            Urbanization
Socioeconomic status
Impaired glucose tolerance or impaired fasting glucose
Gestational diabetes
Hypertension
Dyslipidemia

Source: Diabetes 2001 Vital Statistics, Diabetes in America.[3,9]

INCIDENCE

The incidence of diabetes was assessed during the NHIS from 1995 to 1997 and demonstrated that approximately 780,000 people in the U.S. are diagnosed with diabetes each year or about 2,200 people per day. Of these cases 42 percent occur in persons between the ages of 45 and 64 years. Women accounted for 57% of new cases with men accounting for 43%. Incidence rates for diagnosed diabetes have increased by 18% during the years 1980 to 1994. As is the case for prevalence, incidence of diabetes is higher in African Americans, Hispanics, and Native Americans than in white Americans.[8,31,32]

TYPE 1 DIABETES

PREVALENCE

The incidence and prevalence discussed above refer predominately to type 2 diabetes. The patterns and risk factors for type 1 diabetes are quite different. One problem in obtaining accurate prevalence and incidence data for type 1 diabetes is classification. The use of insulin and age of the individual are not reliable ways to classify the type of diabetes. Most information for type 1 diabetes comes from patients under the age of 20 years. The prevalence of type 1 diabetes varies from population to population across the United States but averages approximate 1.7 cases per 1000 people younger than the age of 20. Total prevalence has been estimated to be 0.25%. The prevalence of type 1 diabetes is lower among African-Americans, Hispanics, and Asian-Americans compared to whites and is rare in Native Americans.

INCIDENCE

There are approximately 13,200 new cases of type 1 diabetes diagnosed each year in children less than 20 years of age or 18 new cases per 100,000. The risk of developing type 1 diabetes before the age of 20 is approximately 0.5%. Estimate of the annual incidence of type 1 diabetes in U.S. adults older than 20 years of age is approximately nine per 100,000 or 16,500 cases. It is believed that 5-10% of adults initially diagnosed with type 2 diabetes actually have type 1 diabetes and these individuals are usually not overweight. Approximately 29,700 Americans develop type 1 diabetes each year. The incidence of type 1 diabetes increases with age until puberty, with a peak incidence at 10 to 12 years in girls and 12 to 14 years in boys. There is no clear sex difference in the risk of developing type 1 diabetes.[3,12]

The incidence of type 1 diabetes varies by season with a decline in cases seen during the summer months and a peak during the late winter and early spring in temperate climates. The seasonal variation and spiking patterns of incidence suggest that in addition to genetic influences environmental factors may play an important role. A marked rise in type 1 diabetes incidence occurred in Birmingham, Alabama, in 1983 coinciding with a Coxsackie virus epidemic highlighting the potential effect of environmental influences.[3]

RISK FACTORS

Race/ethnicity is an important risk factor for the development of type 1 diabetes. As noted earlier the incidence is highest in Scandinavian countries. White populations are at higher risk than ethnic minorities .

Sex and age play a role. A small peak in the incidence of type 1 diabetes is seen around the age of five in males and a larger peak near puberty for both sexes.

Family history is associated with increased risk. There is a 1 to 6% risk of developing type 1 diabetes before the age of 30 in North American whites with first-degree relatives with type 1 diabetes. This risk is less than 1% in families without a member with type 1 diabetes. If a child with type 1 diabetes has a parent with type 1 diabetes, that parent is more likely to be the father.

Table 5. Estimated risk of developing type 1 diabetes by family history

No diabetes in family	11% chance of type 2 diabetes by age 70
	1% chance of type 1 diabetes by age 50
One parent with type 1	Risk is 2 times higher if parent was
diabetes	diagnosed before age 11
Father	6% chance of type 1 diabetes
Mother who was	
<25 yr old at child's birth	4% chance of type 1 diabetes
≥25 yr old at child's birth	1% chance of type 1 diabetes
Sibling with type 1 diabetes	10% chance of type 1 diabetes by age 50
Identical twin with type 1	25-50% chance of type 1 diabetes
diabetes	

Source: Diabetes 2001 Vital Statistics, Diabetes in America.[3, 9]

Genetic factors may account for approximately 50 percent of the total risk for type 1 diabetes. There is an increased susceptibility conferred by genes located in the major histocompatibility complex or HLA region (primarily HLA -DQ and HLA-DR).

Environment influences such as early exposure to cow's milk have been cited as potential risk factors for the development of type 1 diabetes. Breast feeding through at least the first three months of an infant's life is protective, since there is an inverse association with type 1 diabetes. Bovine serum albumin has been proposed as a potential trigger for an immune reaction leading to the destruction of pancreatic beta cells although other components may play a role.

Viruses may play a role. A number of viral infections, such as Coxsackie B virus, cytomegalovirus, rubella, measles, and mumps have been associated with the subsequent development of type 1 diabetes.

GESTATIONAL DIABETES MELLITUS (GDM)

GDM occurs in about 7 percent of pregnant women and the abnormal glucose tolerance returns to normal in 81 to 94% of women after delivery. However, 30 to 40 percent of these women will later develop type 2 diabetes or impaired glucose tolerance. The risk factors for gestational diabetes are the same as those for type 2 diabetes, including older maternal age, a family history of diabetes, and obesity. The racial and ethnic distribution in gestational diabetes mellitus is similar to that found in type 2 diabetes. Thirty to forty percent of women with gestational diabetes who are obese will develop type 2 diabetes within four years after pregnancy.[3, 9, 33]

OTHER TYPES OF DIABETES

Approximately 1-2% of diabetes occurs secondary to other conditions such as pancreatic disease, endocrine disorders, drugs, malnutrition, and rare genetic disorders.[8, 31]

IMPAIRED FASTING GLUCOSE/IMPAIRED GLUCOSE TOLERANCE

The prevalence of impaired fasting glucose (IFG) was estimated to be 9.7 % and impaired glucose tolerance (IGT) 15.8% among adults 48 to 74 in NHANES III. Non-Hispanic blacks and Mexican-Americans had a higher prevalence of both when compared with Non-Hispanic whites.[13] These individuals are at high risk for subsequent development of diabetes. An estimated 1-5% of individuals with IGT will develop diabetes if no lifestyle changes are made.[3]

SUMMARY

The burden of diabetes in the world and in the US is epidemic and appears to be worsening. The rising prevalence and increasing incidence of diabetes are alarming. Current projections estimate that by the year 2025 there will be 300 million people with diabetes. Developing nations will experience a disproportionate increase in the number of cases of diabetes as well as the attendant morbidity, mortality, and economic costs associated with the disease. The U.S. faces an increase in the burden of diabetes as the population ages, the number of high risk ethnic minorities grow, and the prevalence of obesity/overweight, and sedentary lifestyles increases. It is likely that the prevalence of type 2 diabetes in children will continue to rise. An enormous public health challenge looms for the world and the U.S. Considerable resources will need to be expended to modify risk factors in order to prevent the disease. Diabetes epidemiology may be a useful tool in aiding research and improving the care of individuals with diabetes.[34]

REFERENCES

1. Vinicor F. Is diabetes a public-health disorder? Diabetes Care 17 (Suppl 1):22-27, 1994.
2. Venkat-Narayan KM, Gregg EW, Fagot-Campagna A, et al. Diabetes--a common, growing, serious, costly, and potentially preventable public health problem. Diabetes Research and Clinical Practice 50 (Suppl 2):S77-84, 2000.
3. American Diabetes Association. Diabetes 2001 Vital Statistics. Alexandria, Va, 2001.
4. Clark CM, Jr. How should we respond to the worldwide diabetes epidemic? Diabetes Care 21:475-476, 1998.
5. Amos AF, McCarty DJ, Zimmet P. The rising global burden of diabetes and its complications: estimates and projections to the year 2010. Diabetic Medicine 14:S1-85, 1997.
6. King H, Aubert RE, Herman WH. Global burden of diabetes, 1995-2025: prevalence, numerical estimates, and projections. Diabetes Care 21:1414-1431, 1998.
7. Narayan KM, Gregg EW, Fagot-Campagna A, et al. Diabetes--a common, growing, serious, costly, and potentially preventable public health problem. Diabetes Research & Clinical Practice - Supplement 50:S77-84, 2000.
8. HHS Fact Sheet: HHS targets efforts on diabetes. U.S. Department of Health and Human Services. August 8, 2001. (Accessed December 21, 2001, at http://www.hhs.gov/news/press/2001pres/01fsdiabetes.html.)
9. Diabetes in America. Bethesda, Md.: National Institutes of Health National Institute of Diabetes and Digestive and Kidney Diseases. p. 782, 1995.
10. DIABETES MELLITUS: Fact Sheet #138. WHO Information. November 1999. (Accessed December 21, 2001, at http://www.who.int/inf-fs/en/fact138.html.)

11. Internation Diabetes Federation. Diabetes Atlas 2000: Executive Summary. International Diabetes Federation, 2001. (Accessed December 21, 2001, at http://www.idf.org/media/buefx/filelib/DiabAtlas Summary.pdf.)

12. Onkamo P, Vaananen S, Karvonen M, et al. Worldwide increase in incidence of Type I diabetes--the analysis of the data on published incidence trends. Diabetologia 42:1395-1403, 1999.

13. Harris MI, Flegal KM, Cowie CC, et al. Prevalence of diabetes, impaired fasting glucose, and impaired glucose tolerance in U.S. adults. The Third National Health and Nutrition Examination Survey, 1988-1994. Diabetes Care 21:518-524, 1998.

14. Flegal KM, Ezzati TM, Harris MI, et al. Prevalence of diabetes in Mexican Americans, Cubans, and Puerto Ricans from the Hispanic Health and Nutrition Examination Survey, 1982-1984. Diabetes Care 14:628-638, 1991.

15. Self-reported prevalence of diabetes among Hispanics--United States, 1994-1997. MMWR Morb Mortal Wkly Rep 48:8-12, 1999.

16. United States. Dept. of Health and Human Services. Healthy people 2010. Washington DC, 2000.

17. Burrows NR, Geiss LS, Engelgau MM, et al. Prevalence of diabetes among Native Americans and Alaska Natives, 1990-1997: an increasing burden. Diabetes Care 23:1786-1790, 2000.

18. Prevalence of selected risk factors for chronic disease and injury among American Indians and Alaska Natives--United States, 1995-1998. MMWR Morb Mortal Wkly Rep 49:79-82, 91, 2000.

19. Mokdad AH, Ford ES, Bowman BA, et al. Diabetes trends in the U.S.: 1990-1998. Diabetes Care 23:1278-1283, 2000.

20. Mokdad AH, Ford ES, Bowman BA, et al. The continuing increase of diabetes in the US. Diabetes Care 24:412, 2001.

21. Mokdad AH, Bowman BA, Ford ES, et al. The continuing epidemics of obesity and diabetes in the United States. JAMA 286:1195-1200, 2001.

22. Wei M, Gibbons LW, Mitchell TL, et al. The association between cardiorespiratory fitness and impaired fasting glucose and type 2 diabetes mellitus in men. Ann Intern Med 130:89-96, 1999.

23. Diet and exercise dramatically delay type 2 diabetes. Press Release of the U.S. Department of Health and Human Services. August 6, 2001. (Accessed December 21, 2001, at http://www.nih.gov/news/pr/ aug2001/niddk-08.htm.)

24. Hu FB, Manson JE, Stampfer MJ, et al. Diet, lifestyle, and the risk of type 2 diabetes mellitus in women. New Engl J Med 345:790-797, 2001.

25. Tuomilehto J, Lindstrom J, Eriksson JG, et al. Prevention of type 2 diabetes mellitus by changes in lifestyle among subjects with impaired glucose tolerance. N Engl J Med 344:1343-1350, 2001.

26. Pan XR, Li GW, Hu YH, et al. Effects of diet and exercise in preventing NIDDM in people with impaired glucose tolerance. The Da Qing IGT and Diabetes Study. Diabetes Care 20:537-544, 1997.
27. Fagot-Campagna A, Pettitt DJ, Engelgau MM, et al. Type 2 diabetes among North American children and adolescents: an epidemiologic review and a public health perspective. J Pediatr 136:664-672, 2000.
28. Fagot-Campagna A, Burrows NR, Williamson DF. The public health epidemiology of type 2 diabetes in children and adolescents: a case study of American Indian adolescents in the Southwestern United States. Clin Chim Acta 286:81-95, 1999.
29. Rosenbloom AL, Joe JR, Young RS, et al. Emerging epidemic of type 2 diabetes in youth. Diabetes Care 22:345-354, 1999.
30. Type 2 diabetes in children and adolescents. American Diabetes Association. Diabetes Care 23:381-389, 2000.
31. Diabetes Statistics. NIDDK National Diabetes Information Clearinghouse. September 1999. (Accessed December 21, 2001, at http://www.niddk.nih.gov/health/diabetes/pubs/dmstats/dmstats.htm.)
32. National Diabetes Fact Sheet: National estimates and general information on diabetes in the United States. Atlanta, GA: U.S. Department of Health and Human Services, Centers for Disease Control and Prevention, 1998.
33. King H. Epidemiology of glucose intolerance and gestational diabetes in women of childbearing age. Diabetes Care 21 Suppl 2:B9-13, 1998.
34. Zimmet PZ. Diabetes epidemiology as a tool to trigger diabetes research and care. Diabetologia 42:499-518, 1999.

Internet Sites:

American Diabetes Association
www.diabetes.org
Centers for Disease Control and Prevention
www.cdc.gov/diabetes>
www.cdc.gov/nchswww>
Juvenile Diabetes Foundation International
www.jdfcure.org>
International Diabetes Federation
www.idf.org
National Diabetes Education Program
ndep.nih.gov>
www.cdc.gov/diabetes>
National Institute of Diabetes and Digestive and Kidney Diseases of the National Institutes of Health
www.niddk.nih.gov>
U.S. Department of Health and Human Services Office of Minority Health
www.omhrc.gov>

IV. Genes and diabetes

Chapter 1. DIABETES GENES
Human Genome Project and Diabetes Mellitus

Ken C. Chiu and Dorothy S. Martinez

INTRODUCTION

In contrast to primary beta cell failure mediated by autoimmunity in type 1 diabetes, type 2 diabetes is generally recognized as an imbalance between insulin sensitivity and beta cell function. Although most epidemiological studies have demonstrated the role of insulin resistance in the pathogenesis of type 2 diabetes, it is now well-accepted that failure of beta cells to compensate for prevailing insulin resistance is required for the development of overt diabetes. Since type 1 diabetes is an autoimmune disease, the term "diabetes genes" is generally applied to the genes involved in the pathogenesis of type 2 diabetes. This chapter will focus on the impact of human genome project on the genetic studies of diabetes with a brief discussion of the diabetes genes known to play a role in type 2 diabetes.

The Human Genome Project facilitates the discovery of linkage and identification of mutations in various Mendelian diseases that are related to diabetes. These diseases are maturity onset diabetes of the young (MODY), persistent hyperinsulinemic hypoglycemia of infancy (PHHI), and Wolfram syndrome (diabetes insipidus, diabetes mellitus, optic atrophy, and deafness). The Human Genome Project opens a new era of the "sequence-based" biology. Although substantial progress has been made in diabetes-related monogenic diseases, human genetics is now at a critical stage. The available strategies and molecular biology techniques used to identify the genes underlying rare Mendelian diseases are not very rewarding in identifying the genes causing the more common, familial, non-Mendelian diseases, such as diabetes. In the era of post-Human Genome Project, dissecting the genetics of diabetes remains one of the great challenges in human genetics.

Diabetes is a result of complex interactions between genetic and non-genetic (including environmental) factors. Although diabetes and its related traits have been shown to cluster within families, their transmission does not follow a Mendelian fashion, except for some rare syndromes such as MODY. Diabetes could be the result of few common variants with a relatively large effect, such as HLA alleles at the MHC locus and VNTR minisatellites of the insulin gene with type 1 diabetes. It could also be the result of a pool of alleles with low population frequency and a relative large effect, such as mutations of various genes in MODY. However, the majority of the common forms of type 2 diabetes is most likely a result of accumulating numerous polymorphisms (sequence variations within a species with an allelic frequency of the common allele less than 95%). Predisposing alleles of varying population frequencies could be found both in the same gene (allelic heterogeneity: various mutations which occur within one gene cause the same phenotype) and in different genes (locus heterogeneity: various loci cause the same phenotype) and act either independently or epistatically to influence disease outcome. With their interactions with environmental and other factors, a wide spectrum of clinical manifestations is observed in patients with diabetes (clinical heterogeneity).

GENETIC METHODS

Although not all the efforts have been successful in identifying the genes in diabetes, a variety of methods have been proven to be triumphant on various occasions.

Functional cloning

It is also known as candidate gene approach. By choosing a proper candidate gene within a known metabolic pathway, the gene of interest can be scrutinized in various ways: linkage analysis, association study, and molecular scanning. Glucokinase is a successful pay-off of functional cloning. It was chosen for its role as glucose sensor in both hepatocytes and pancreatic beta cells. The gene was first cloned to facilitate the genetic studies. Identification of two simple sequence repeat polymorphisms[1] allowed linkage analysis in the MODY pedigrees[2] and led to identification of mutated glucokinase. Its role in MODY is confirmed by functional analysis of mutated glucokinase and by the studies of transgenic mice.[3] The search for peroxidase proliferator-activated receptor γ (PPARγ) is a successful example of diabetes gene hunting by functional cloning (discussed later in this chapter). However, most of the candidate gene searches were not rewarding.

Positional cloning

This is performed without relying on prior knowledge of the underlying pathogenesis. The chromosomal region shared by the affected subjects can be identified by genotyping anonymous markers throughout the genome in multiple affected pedigrees or affected sib pairs (ASP), such as in the search of the gene for Wolfram syndrome. By recombination mapping, the disease locus can be further narrowed down to a small region; the region of interest can be constructed by using STS (sequence tag site); and eventually the disease gene (Wolfrin) can be identified by examining the genes located within the region of interest[4]. Positional cloning has been reasonably successful in the identification of a diabetes gene – Calpain 10 (discussed later in this chapter). Since Calpain 10 is not involved in any known pathway of diabetes, future study of this gene is highly likely to unfold a new pathway in diabetes and also to identify a new treatment for diabetes.

Positional candidate gene approach

This is an approach that takes advantage of the Human Genome Project. It places the various expressed sequence tags (ESTs) throughout the human genome. It saves tremendous effort in constructing the fine map of the region of interest and identifying all the genes located within that region. For example, the disease locus was first localized by genotyping anonymous markers throughout the genome in the search of the gene for PHHI.[5] After narrowing down by recombination mapping, the disease genes (SUR1 and Kir6.2) were identified by examining the known genes (or ESTs) within the region.[6] Fatty acid binding protein 2 is a successful testimonial of this approach (discussed later in this chapter).

Linkage disequilibrium mapping

Positional cloning relies on the analysis of chromosome sharing within biologically related diseased relatives, who are more difficult to recruit than unrelated diseased subjects. Although positional cloning has an excellent power to detect a genetic defect with a relatively large biological effect, it becomes less useful and less practical in detecting those with modest effects as in most complex diseases. With the availability of a dense genome-wide map of single nucleotide polymorphisms (or simple nucleotide polymorphisms, SNPs), linkage disequilibrium (LD) mapping, also known as genome-wide association study, has been developed theoretically.[7] This approach is particularly useful in the genetically isolated populations, for example, the Finnish population. Regions of chromosome shared by the affected subjects can be identified by comparing two groups of subjects with difference only in the disease status. Although there is no successful example available to date, it has been shown that LD in a United States population of north-European descent typically extends 60 kb from common alleles[8]. This implies that LD mapping is likely to be a practical approach in this population.

However, association studies are viewed as problematic and plagued by irreproducibility. Many associations have been reported for type 2 diabetes, but substantial associations have failed to be confirmed in multiple samples and with comprehensive controls. The selection of an appropriate control population is essential for this type of study.

GENETIC INFLUENCE: TYPE 1 VS. TYPE 2 DIABETES

The most widely used strategy to map the genes in a complex disease is the affected sib pair (ASP) method. The model independent nature of ASP becomes an advantage in the studies of diseases with an unknown mode of transmission, such as type 2 diabetes. By including only affected subjects in the study, the ASP method excludes the possibility of false-negative cases, such as those frequently seen in diseases like type 2 diabetes that have a variable and late onset of age. Furthermore, the ASP method

Table 1. Relative risk of diabetes from twin studies

	Population	Monozygotic twins	Dizygotic twins	Relative risk	First author
Type 1 diabetes					
	Finnish	0.23	0.05	4.79	Kaprio
	Danish	0.56	0.11	5.07	Kyvik
	Overall			4.93	
Type 2 diabetes					
	US male	0.58	0.17	3.35	Newman
	Finnish	0.34	0.16	2.10	Kaprio
	Japanese	0.83	0.40	2.08	Japanese
	German	0.69	0.24	1.63	Then
	Danish	0.50	0.37	1.35	Poulsen
	Overall			2.10	

eliminates the need to recruit parents of index cases who are often not available for the late-onset diseases. Although the ASP method has been successful in mapping the susceptible loci for type 1 diabetes, much less progress has been made in type 2 diabetes for the extent of genetic influence.

Genetic influence can be estimated by the relative risk of the disease between different types of twins. By comparing the concordance rate between monozygotic and dizygotic twins, the relative risk of genetic influence can be estimated for both type 1 and type 2 diabetes mellitus. Although a much higher concordance rate in monozygotic twins with type 2 diabetes has been reported, especially when the duration of follow-up increases, the relative risk is reduced by a high prevalence of type 2 diabetes that results in a high disease rate in dizygotic twins (Table 1).

Another way to estimate the genetic influence of a disease is to estimate the degree of familial clustering (λ_s). λ_s is estimated from the ratio of the risk for siblings of patients and the risk for population (prevalence). MODY accounts for no more than 5% of type 2 diabetes with an estimated population prevalence of 0.25%. As MODY is an autosomal dominant disorder, 50% of siblings will be affected. Thus, λ_s for MODY is 200 (50%/0.25%). In contrast to type 1 diabetes (λ_s being 6%/0.4% or about 15), λ_s of type 2 diabetes is much smaller due to a higher population prevalence of 5%. Based on the estimation of large-scale epidemiological surveys, λ_s of type 2 diabetes is about 2.5 - 3.5. Therefore, as compared to MODY and type 1 diabetes, hunting of the genes involved in type 2 diabetes is a much more difficult task.

Type 1 diabetes has a much greater genetic influence than type 2 diabetes, but there is a substantial controversy in the genetic studies using the ASP method. The initial positional cloning in type 1 diabetes not only confirms the known loci (MHC and insulin) but also identifies numerous new loci.[9] However, two attempts of replication by genotyping almost identical sample set of more than 1,000 sib pairs of patients with type 1 diabetes yielded contradictory results. The British group not only confirmed their original report but also identified some new loci.[10] The American group confirmed only the MHC locus and rejected other loci.[11] These discrepancies could have resulted from an imperfect nature of analytical methods, sample stratification, type 1 error, and intrinsic complexity of the disease.

MAGNITUDE OF GENETIC INFLUENCE IN DIABETES TRAITS

Table 2. Estimated genetic influence of insulin sensitivity and beta cell function

Population	Pedigree	Trait	Estimated genetic influence	First author
I. Insulin senstivity				
American Caucasians	20	Fasting insulin	33%	Schumacher
American Caucasians	26	S_I	33%	Elbein
Americans	33	S_I	20%	Martin
Pima Indians	45	M_{high}	34%	Lillioja
Pima Indians	45	M_{low}	15%	Lillioja
Pima Indians	153	M_{high}	49%	Sakul
Pima Indians	153	M_{low}	38%	Sakul
Mexican Americans	27	2-h insulin	31%	Mitchell
Dannish Twins	303	Fasting insulin	19%	Poulsen
Finnish Caucasians	184	S_I	28%	Watanabe
Amish	45	Fasting insulin	11%	Hsueh
Amish	45	2-h insulin	24%	Hsueh
II. Beta cell function				
American Caucasians	26	$AIR_{glucose}$	29%	Elbein
Dannish Twins	303	30-min insulin	47%	Poulsen
Finnish Caucasians	184	$AIR_{glucose}$	35%	Watanabe

S_I: insulin sensitivity by frequently sampled intravenous glucose tolerance test

$AIR_{glucose}$: acute insulin response to glucose by frequently sampled intravenous glucose tolerance test

M_{low}: insulin sensitivity by euglycemic clamp with an insulin concentration at ~130 μU/ml

M_{high}: insulin sensitivity by euglycemic clamp with an insulin concentration at ~2000 μU/ml

Although environmental factors are usually required for the development of overt type 2 diabetes, genetic influence is clearly supported by three types of data: twin studies, familial aggregation of the disease

127

evidenced by a very high positive rate of family history of diabetes, and drastically different prevalence in various ethnic groups. Therefore, there is no doubt that type 2 diabetes is a disease with a strong genetic influence. However, the prediction of the relative contribution of genetic influence and number of genes involved in the pathogenesis of the disease has changed in the past few years. Initially, enthusiastic searches of diabetes genes were generated by the euphoric propositions of monogenic (single gene) or oligogenic (few genes) hypotheses of type 2 diabetes or its traits from earlier studies. However, a polygenic nature appears more likely in most of the studies.

Heritability of various diabetes-related traits (how much of the phenotype is determined by genes) has been studied in different populations (Table 2). Since insulin sensitivity and beta cell function are the key determinants for the development of type 2 diabetes, the discussion here will be limited to these two traits. As shown in Table 2, no more than 50% of the variations in a given trait is affected by genetic factors. Furthermore, it is quite consistent throughout almost all studies that less than 40% of insulin sensitivity, measured by various methods, is under genetic influence. Similarly, less than 50% of the variation in beta cell function (AIR$_{glucose}$, 30-minute insulin) is controlled by genetic factors. That more than 50% of the trait variation is not controlled by genetic factors is consistently observed in all the populations studied. If type 2 diabetes is truly a polygenic disorder, each genetic factor (genetic variant) will have only a very modest impact (few percent) on the trait of interest. The past experience indicates that common genetic risk factors are not strong and strong genetic factors are not common. Therefore, it will be almost impossible to identify most of diabetes genes by using the ASP strategy, which is based on an assumption that type 2 diabetes is an oligogenic disorder.

PATHOETIOLOGY OF TYPE 2 DIABETES

As type 2 diabetes is a complex disease, genetic predisposition is only part of the story. The importance of nongenetic (environmental) factors cannot be overemphasized. Accordingly, two hypotheses have been proposed in the pursuit of the pathoetiology of type 2 diabetes by underscoring the relative importance of nature vs. nurture.

'Thrifty genotype' hypothesis

In search for the cause of rising prevalence of diabetes, a 'thrifty genotype' hypothesis was proposed.[12] It is suggested that the accumulation of diabetes gene(s) is a result of natural selection, which favors survival in famine of those individuals who store energy efficiently by secreting a higher insulin level when food supply is plentiful. To persist through centuries of evolution, the diabetes gene(s) must have had some survival advantage. This advantage could be the ability to respond with rapid insulin production so that energy could be stored more efficiently. Therefore, at the early stage of human evolution, a gene (or genes) for energy conservation is an asset to survive in the 'hunter-gathering' era (when food supply was erratic and obesity was rare). As a result, when food is available, extra energy is stored away enabling the individual to survive famine. Furthermore, during famine insulin resistance along with a lower insulin level will result in shunting of the fuel to vital organs for survival rather than facing fuel shortage. However, in the modern era (developed regions) when food supply is constant, diabetes gene(s) becomes a liability since it constantly stores extra energy away. This energy is rarely needed (as famine is extremely rare in the developed regions) resulting in obesity and insulin resistance.

In 'thrifty genotype' hypothesis, insulin resistance is the primary event. Insulin resistance is partly inherited (thrifty genotype) and partly acquired from such features of modernization as hypercaloric diet and lack of exercise. Those selected by evolution for efficient energy storage through insulin resistance secrete more insulin and develop hyperinsulinemia. Glucose intolerance and/or diabetes develop when the beta cells are exhausted.

'Thrifty phenotype' hypothesis

In contrast to 'thrifty genotype' hypothesis, a 'thrifty phenotype' hypothesis has been proposed.[13] Thrifty phenotype explains the role of nutrition in changes seen in fetal and infant growth. These changes in early life compromise the development of pancreatic beta cells, which becomes detrimental when nutrition becomes abundant in the adult life. As insulin resistance supervenes, the increased demand for insulin exceeds the capacity of the compromised beta cells, resulting in impaired glucose tolerance and overt diabetes. Subsequently, 'thrifty phenotype' is also implied to lead to insulin resistance and insulin resistance syndrome.

Since birth record and weight at one year were available for those born in Hertfordshire from 1911 onward, the initial study showed that the retardation of growth during fetal life and infancy was associated with increased death rates from cardiovascular disease in adult life. Since diabetes is a major risk factor for this disease, it is also noted that the prevalence of glucose intolerance increases as birth weight and weight at one year decrease. Subsequently, the association between poor early growth and glucose intolerance and/or insulin resistance syndrome was also reported in Pima Indians, Mexican Americans and non-Hispanic whites, Swedish men, schoolchildren in Jamaica, health professionals in US, and twins in Denmark. These observations underline two premises: i) growth retardation in early life (intrauterine and at the first year) has a nutritional basis, and the resulting altered fetal environment permanently alters the development and metabolic functions of organs and; ii) these phenomena are beneficial to survival in a poor nutritional environment during fetal and infant periods, but may lead to glucose intolerance and insulin resistance syndrome, when nutrition is abundant in adult life.

Since "thrifty phenotype" hypothesis is associated with glucose intolerance and insulin resistance syndrome, its relationship with insulin resistance has been examined. In 103 non-diabetic subjects, thinness at birth, as measured by a low ponderal index (birth weight/length^3) is associated with insulin resistance, which was measured by an insulin tolerance test, independent of duration of gestation, adult body mass index and waist-hip ratio, and social class at birth or currently. Furthermore, fasting insulin level in adult life (~50 years old), as an indicator of insulin resistance, was inversely correlated with abdominal circumference at birth in 216 subjects. Because abdominal circumference at birth is an indicator of the growth of the liver in fetal life, this association suggests that the sensitivity of the liver to insulin is permanently reduced if the intrauterine development of this organ is impaired. Interestingly, glucokinase and the VNTR of insulin gene have been shown to affect birth weight. Fetal insulin secretion in response to maternal glycemia plays a key role in fetal growth. Maternal insulin secretion is primarily dependent upon the state of glucose tolerance in the mother. A defect in sensing glucose (mutated glucokinase) or in insulin production (the VNTR of the insulin gene) in mother could reduce fetal growth and birth weight. These results indicate that the genetic factors also play a role in 'thrifty phenotype' hypothesis.

In laboratory rats, partial protein deprivation during pregnancy and lactation leads to a 50% decrease in glucokinase activity and 100% increase in phosphoenolpyruvate carboxykinase (PEPCK) in liver. It is associated with increased hepatic lobular volume and reduced perivenous concentration of glucokinase, leading to diminished glucose uptake in the distal perivenous region. As a result, there is a net increase in glucose production through decreased glucose uptake by glucokinase and gluconeogenesis via PEPCK in the isolated liver. Since insulin stimulates glucokinase and inhibits PEPCK in the liver, much more insulin is required to suppress the net increased glucose production by the liver (insulin resistance in the liver). Indeed, hyperinsulinemia is observed in these rats. These observations confirm that an unfavorable perinatal environment alters hepatic structure, affects enzyme activity, and leads to hepatic insulin resistance with compensatory hyperinsulinemia. In addition to insulin resistance, maternal protein deprivation also causes altered islet structure. The neonates had reduced pancreatic beta cell proliferation, islet size, and vascularization. Subsequently, it was shown that these offsprings had reduced insulin secretion and reduced glucose tolerance.

DIABETES GENES

The following examples are the diabetes genes, which affect at least 10% of type 2 diabetes. Their roles in the pathogenesis are reasonably well established, although some controversy might still exist.

Calpain 10 (CAPN10)

The first positional cloning study in type 2 diabetes was conducted on 170 Mexican-American families and found linkage near the terminus of chromosome 2q37 with a LOD (logarithm of odds) score of 3.2, designated NIDDM1.[14] This susceptibility locus originally encompassed about 10–20 cM, but was subsequently narrowed to 7 cM and shown to depend for its effect on the genotype at an unlinked locus, encompassing the CYP19 gene on chromosome 15.[15] Graeme Bell's group followed up on the NIDDM1 and identified the first positionally cloned gene for a complex disease with both polygenic and multifactorial natures.[16] The identification of the calpain 10 gene (CAPN10) as a diabetes gene suggests a new biochemical pathway involved in the regulation of blood glucose levels. However, the putative functioning polymorphism (UCSNP-43) was located within intron 3 of the CAPN10 gene with a G-to-A substitution. An increase in the frequency of the common G allele in diabetic patients was found compared with controls with evidence for linkage. Since the original population was ascertained by diabetes phenotype with very limited clinical phenotype, the functional study of UCSNP-43 was conducted in Pima Indians.[17] The G/G genotype was associated with small but significant differences in fasting glucose, 2-hour insulin, endogenous glucose output, glucose disposal, and carbohydrate oxidation, relative to those individuals with the G/A or A/A genotypes. Data from respiratory chamber studies revealed lower metabolic rates, higher lipid oxidation, and lower protein oxidation in the Pima Indians with the G/G genotype. In times of abundant food supply, the G/G phenotype might favor enhanced carbohydrate stores and secondary insulin resistance. In times of prolonged fasting, this phenotype could preserve skeletal muscle protein and glycogen, which might favor survival. These studies clearly show that the CAPN10 G/G genotype is associated with metabolic consequences in Pima Indians. However, they do not explain the genetic variation in the CAPN10 gene that causes these metabolic differences. The connection with glucose metabolism is still far from clear.

Fatty acid binding protein 2 (FABP2)

Pima Indians have one of the highest known prevalence of type 2 diabetes. The disease shows strong familial aggregation. In this group, insulin resistance is a major risk factor for the development of the disease. Maximal insulin action (i.e. glucose disposal rate at pharmacological insulin levels) was found to be determined by a codominantly inherited autosomal gene. Initially, the researchers observed an association and linkage between insulin resistance and red cell antigens on chromosome 4q, which were the only genetic markers available at that time. With additional families and additional genetic markers, a significant linkage was identified between the FABP2 and ANX5 loci with insulin resistance in non-diabetic Pima Indians.[18] Furthermore, the linkage of the FABP2 locus with insulin resistance (2-hour postchallenged insulin concentration) was also found in the Mexican-American population, which is genetically related to the Pima Indians.[19] However, no linkage was found between the FABP2 locus and diabetes, lipodystrophic diabetes, or obesity. The population association studies of the FABP2 locus with diabetes/impaired glucose tolerance were also negative in the UK, Finish, Welsh, and Japanese populations.

Subsequently, the A54T polymorphism was identified and it was found to be associated with increased fatty acid binding protein, increased fat oxidation and increased insulin resistance in the Pima Indians.[20] However, the population association studies of the A54T polymorphism with NIDDM, coronary artery disease, obesity, and hypertension were also essentially negative. Positive associations were mostly seen in the quantitative association studies. There are positive associations found between the A54T polymorphism with fasting plasma insulin concentration, fasting fat oxidation, glucose uptake, indices of insulin sensitivity, obesity indices, 2-hour post-challenged insulin, and various lipid metabolism parameters. However, numerous negative studies were also noted.

Clearly there is substantial controversy surrounding this locus and the A54T polymorphism in the pathogenesis of insulin resistance and type 2 diabetes as described above. Disagreement also occurred in the original Pima Indian study. Although significant linkages were identified at the FABP2 locus with fasting insulin concentration (p=0.0004) and with glucose uptake (p=0.0008) in the Pima Indians,[18] the differences regarding the A54T polymorphism with fasting insulin concentrations (p<0.04) and glucose uptake (p<0.04) were only marginally significant in the same population.[20] The significant linkage in the original sib-pair study could be the combined results of a highly polymorphic marker of the FABP2 locus (5 alleles vs. 2 alleles for the A54T polymorphism) and less intrafamilial difference in insulin sensitivity as the result of familial clustering of insulin sensitivity. In contrast, the marginal difference reflected a very modest influence on insulin sensitivity of the A54T polymorphism in the Pima Indian population, which is consistent with our observation that this polymorphism only accounted for 4-6% of the variation in insulin sensitivity in a Caucasian population.[21]

Furthermore, since 1) insulin resistance is neither necessary nor sufficient for the development of type 2 diabetes, 2) this polymorphism has only a very modest influence on insulin sensitivity, and 3) beta cell dysfunction, on which this polymorphism has no influence, plays a key role in the development of overt diabetes, the population association studies and linkage studies are not able to detect the interaction between this polymorphism and the overt diabetes phenotype. In contrast, quantitative studies of the diabetes-related (mainly insulin resistance-related) phenotypes become more rewarding in detecting a polymorphism of a very modest effect. The negative quantitative study could result from other confounding factors, such as inclusion of diabetic, impaired glucose tolerant or hypertensive subjects in the study.

The most convincing evidence supporting the A54T polymorphism as a caustic mutation is from a functional study of mutated FABP2. FABP2 plays a role in the absorption and intracellular transportation of dietary long-chain fatty acids. Thr54-containing FABP2 has a twofold greater affinity for the long-chain fatty acids than the Ala54-containing FABP2. As predicted by "Randle's cycle", an increased concentration of fatty acid inhibits glucose uptake in muscle and results in insulin resistance. Furthermore, two interventional studies showed that this A54T polymorphism affected lipid metabolism during the interventions.

Peroxidase proliferator-activated receptor γ (PPARγ)
Identification of a new class of antidiabetic drugs, thiazolidinediones (TZD), has brought back the interest in adipose tissue as a key player in the pathogenesis of type 2 diabetes. As TZD improve insulin sensitivity by activation of PPARγ, the role of PPARγ was examined in the patients with type 2 diabetes. A Pro12Ala substitution in PPARγ was associated with decreased receptor activity, lower body mass index, and improved insulin sensitivity.[22] Various studies also demonstrated the association of this SNP with obesity and type 2 diabetes.

The role of the Pro12Ala polymorphism in PPARγ in type 2 diabetes was confirmed in a large study using the family-based association study, in which population stratification is not required and a control population is not needed. By analyzing over 3,000 individuals, a modest (0.75-fold) but significant (P=0.002) decrease in diabetes risk is associated with the alanine allele (15% frequency). Meta-analysis of the published data confirmed the protective effect of the alanine allele for type 2 diabetes.[23] The data implicate an inherited variation in PPARγ in the pathogenesis of type 2 diabetes. Because the risk allele occurs at such high frequency, its modest effect translates into a large population attributable risk—influencing as much as 25% of type 2 diabetes in the general population. Moreover, the extrapolated analysis suggested that the contribution of this SNP would be impossible to discover by linkage analysis, which requires a genome scan of about 3 million sib pairs to obtain a LOD score of 3. It will be too costly to perform this type of analysis.

IMPACT OF HUMAN GENOME PROJECT ON DIABETES

Sequence-based biology will lead to several theoretical applications. Understanding the genetic basis of the disease will provide a better insight of the underlying pathophysiology of the disease with a potential of identifying a *de novo* pathway for the disease process. In turn, a new therapeutic approach and a better treatment strategy can be developed. It will also allow a more precise risk assessment. Application of preventive measurement and early intervention to high risk subjects will prevent or delay the development of overt diabetes and in turn will prevent the complications of diabetes, such as blindness and end-stage renal disease.

As it is generally believed that the functional SNPs play a major role in complex diseases such as diabetes, substantial work has been accomplished and confirmed that most SNPs carry at most a very modest impact on the traits of interest. We have demonstrated the 4-12% impact of the SNPs in the FABP2, hepatocyte nuclear factor 1α, liver glucokinase promoter, and vitamin D receptor on insulin sensitivity.[21;24] As compared to the effect of moderate physical activity that improves insulin sensitivity by 50% and insulin sensitizers, such metformin and TZD, that improve insulin sensitivity by 25-35%, the impact of each functional SNP is relatively small (4-12%). Furthermore, the frequencies of these SNPs are very high, reaching up to 50-60% or more in the population. Because of SNPs' high frequencies in the general population, relatively modest impact of each SNP, and relatively large number of SNPs, it will be more cost-effective to apply a public health approach to prevent type 2 diabetes by diet and exercise than application of genetic testing to identify the subjects at risk. For the same reasons, gene therapy will become a less practical approach for the treatment of type 2 diabetes.

Genetic differences among ethnic groups usually reflect differences in the phenotypic traits as a result of the distribution of polymorphisms, which occur at different frequencies in different populations. However, the differences could also be due to a trait unique to a particular ethnic group. The difference in the frequency of polymorphisms could in turn affect the prevalence of a disease. On the other hand, the underlying genetic determinants of the response (efficacy or adverse effect) to a drug are beginning to be unraveled. This appears to be based on the varying distributions of polymorphisms in the disease pathway or the pathway of drug metabolism/action. Therefore, for complex diseases such as type 2 diabetes, the Human Genome Project will facilitate the identification of new treatment (pharmacogenomics) and will also help physicians to choose the proper and specific medications while avoiding adverse effect of medications by performing a genetic profile on diabetic patients (pharmacogenetics). Furthermore, identification of genetic determinants of diabetic patients will better define the targets of current and future therapies, and will lead to therapies that are more specific for their genetic constitutes.

SUMMARY

With the advancement of the Human Genome Project, we enter the era of a sequence-based biology. Some progress has been made in the identification of genetic basis of the common form of type 2 diabetes, which mainly affects the susceptibility of the disease but is neither necessary nor sufficient to cause overt diabetes. Experience has taught us that common polymorphisms almost never have strong effect, and that strong genetic risk factors are rarely common. Thus, the common form of type 2 diabetes is most likely a combined result of multiple polymorphisms, each of which has a modest effect, with the influence of various non-genetic factors. As type 2 diabetes is a polygenic and multifactorial disease, each diabetes gene most likely accounts for a very modest influence on either insulin sensitivity or beta cell function. Evidence suggests that in addition to linkage analysis, which has rather limited power to detect the genes with a very modest effect, the successful hunting of diabetes genes will come from a carefully planned association study. To date only few diabetes genes have been reported and they are most likely the low laying fruits. A highly challenging work is ahead. The Human Genome Project will accelerate this process by stimulating the development of new genetic methods and analytical approaches, providing various maps (such as SNP, EST, and STS maps), and identifying unknown genes within human genome.

In the era of the post-Human Genome Project, the major utilization of the genetics of type 2 diabetes will focus in two areas: pharmacogenomics and pharmacogenetics. Pharmacogenomics will identify new pathways for the disease process through the study of the genetics of diabetes. New treatments and medications will be developed accordingly. Pharmacogenetics will prompt the individualized therapy for each diabetic patient based on her/his genetic profile to select the most effective medication(s) and to minimize the unwanted adverse effects of therapy.

REFERENCES

1. Tanizawa Y, Matsutani A, Chiu KC, Permutt MA. Human glucokinase gene: isolation, structural characterization, and identification of a microsatellite repeat polymorphism.   Mol Endocrinol 6:1070-1081, 1992.
2. Hattersley AT, Turner RC, Permutt MA, Patel P, Tanizawa Y, Chiu KC, O'Rahilly S, Watkins PJ, Wainscoat JS. Linkage of type 2 diabetes to the glucokinase gene. Lancet 339:1307-1310, 1992.
3. Matschinsky F, Liang Y, Kesavan P, Wang L, Froguel P, Velho G, Cohen D, Permutt MA, Tanizawa Y, Jetton TL. Glucokinase as pancreatic beta cell glucose sensor and diabetes gene. J Clin Invest 92:2092-2098, 1993.
4. Inoue H, Tanizawa Y, Wasson J, Behn P, Kalidas K, Bernal-Mizrachi E, Mueckler M, Marshall H, Donis-Keller H, Crock P, et al. A gene encoding a transmembrane protein is mutated in patients with diabetes mellitus and optic atrophy (Wolfram syndrome). Nat Genet 20:143-148, 1998.
5. Glaser B, Chiu KC, Anker R, Nestorowicz A, Landau H, Ben-Bassat H, Shlomai Z, Kaiser N, Thornton PS, Stanley CA. Familial hyperinsulinism maps to chromosome 11p14-15.1, 30 cM centromeric to the insulin gene. Nat Genet 7:185-188, 1994.

6. Nestorowicz A, Glaser B, Wilson BA, Shyng SL, Nichols CG, Stanley CA, Thornton PS, Permutt MA. Genetic heterogeneity in familial hyperinsulinism. Hum Mol Genet 7:1119-1128, 1998.

7. Risch NJ. Searching for genetic determinants in the new millennium. Nature 405:847-856, 2000.

8. Reich DE, Cargill M, Bolk S, Ireland J, Sabeti PC, Richter DJ, Lavery T, Kouyoumjian R, Farhadian SF, Ward R, et al. Linkage disequilibrium in the human genome. Nature 411:199-204, 2001.

9. Davies JL, Kawaguchi Y, Bennett ST, Copeman JB, Cordell HJ, Pritchard LE, Reed PW, Gough SC, Jenkins SC, Palmer SM. A genome-wide search for human type 1 diabetes susceptibility genes. Nature 371:130-136, 1994.

10. Mein CA, Esposito L, Dunn MG, Johnson GC, Timms AE, Goy JV, Smith AN, Sebag-Montefiore L, Merriman ME, Wilson AJ, et al. A search for type 1 diabetes susceptibility genes in families from the United Kingdom. Nat Genet 19:297-300, 1998.

11. Concannon P, Gogolin-Ewens KJ, Hinds DA, Wapelhorst B, Morrison VA, Stirling B, Mitra M, Farmer J, Williams SR, Cox NJ, et al. A second-generation screen of the human genome for susceptibility to insulin-dependent diabetes mellitus. Nat Genet 19:292-296, 1998.

12. Neel JV. Diabetes mellitus: a "thrifty" genotype rendered detrimental by "progress"? Am J Hum Genet 14:353-362, 1962.

13. Hales CN, Barker DJ: Type 2 (non-insulin-dependent) diabetes mellitus: the thrifty phenotype hypothesis. Diabetologia 35:595-601, 1992.

14. Hanis CL, Boerwinkle E, Chakraborty R, Ellsworth DL, Concannon P, Stirling B, Morrison VA, Wapelhorst B, Spielman RS, Gogolin-Ewens KJ, et al. A genome-wide search for human non-insulin-dependent (type 2) diabetes genes reveals a major susceptibility locus on chromosome 2. Nat Genet 13:161-166, 1996.

15. Cox NJ, Frigge M, Nicolae DL, Concannon P, Hanis CL, Bell GI, Kong A. Loci on chromosomes 2 NIDDM1 and 15 interact to increase susceptibility to diabetes in Mexican Americans. Nat Genet 21:213-215, 1999.

16. Horikawa Y, Oda N, Cox NJ, Li X, Orho-Melander M, Hara M, Hinokio Y, Lindner TH, Mashima H, Schwarz PE, et al. Genetic variation in the gene encoding calpain-10 is associated with type 2 diabetes mellitus. Nat Genet 26:163-175, 2000.

17. Baier LJ, Permana PA, Yang X, Pratley RE, Hanson RL, Shen GQ, Mott D, Knowler WC, Cox NJ, Horikawa Y, et al. A calpain-10 gene polymorphism is associated with reduced muscle mRNA levels and insulin resistance. J Clin Invest 106:R69-R73, 2000.

18. Prochazka M, Lillioja S, Tait JF, Knowler WC, Mott DM, Spraul M, Bennett PH, Bogardus C. Linkage of chromosomal markers on 4q with a putative gene determining maximal insulin action in Pima Indians. Diabetes 42:514-519, 1993.

19. Mitchell BD, Kammerer CM, O'Connell P, Harrison CR, Manire M, Shipman P, Moyer MP, Stern MP, Frazier ML. Evidence for linkage of postchallenge insulin levels with intestinal fatty acid-binding protein (FABP2) in Mexican-Americans. Diabetes 44:1046-1053, 1995.

20. Baier LJ, Sacchettini JC, Knowler WC, Eads J, Paolisso G, Tataranni PA, Mochizuki H, Bennett PH, Bogardus C, Prochazka M. An amino acid substitution in the human intestinal fatty acid binding protein is associated with increased fatty acid binding, increased fat oxidation, and insulin resistance. J Clin Invest 95:1281-1287, 1995.

21. Chiu KC, Chuang LM, Chu A, Yoon C. Fatty acid binding protein 2 and insulin resistance. Eur J Clin Invest 31:521-527, 2001.

22. Deeb SS, Fajas L, Nemoto M, Pihlajameaki J, Mykkeanen L, Kuusisto J, Laakso M, Fujimoto W, Auwerx J. A Pro12Ala substitution in PPARgamma2 associated with decreased receptor activity, lower body mass index and improved insulin sensitivity. Nat Genet 20:284-287, 1998.

23. Altshuler D, Hirschhorn JN, Klannemark M, Lindgren CM, Vohl MC, Nemesh J, Lane CR, Schaffner SF, Bolk S, Brewer C, et al. The common PPAR gamma Pro12Ala polymorphism is associated with decreased risk of type 2 diabetes. Nat Genet 26:76-80, 2000.

24. Chiu KC, Chuang LM, Ryu JM, Tsai GP, Saad MF. The I27L amino acid polymorphism of hepatic nuclear factor-1alpha is associated with insulin resistance. J Clin Endocrinol Metab 85:2178-2183, 2000.

USEFUL WEBSITES:

1. National Center for Biotechnology Information (NCBI)
http://www.ncbi.nlm.nih.gov
2. Online Mendelian Inheritance in Man (OMIM). This database is a catalog of human genes and genetic disorders authored and edited by Dr. Victor A. McKusick and his colleagues at Johns Hopkins and elsewhere. The database contains textual information and references.http://www.ncbi.nlm.nih.gov/entrez/ query.fcgi?db=OMIM.
3. Kyoto Encyclopedia of Genes and Genomes (KEGG)
This site attempts to computerize current knowledge of molecular and cellular biology in terms of information pathways consisting of interacting molecules or genes, and also provides links to gene catalogs produced by genome sequencing projects. http://www.gename.ad.jp/ kegg.

Chapter 2. Animal Models of Diabetes

Martin Haluzik and Marc L. Reitman

INTRODUCTION

General considerations

Animal models have had a major role in shaping our current understanding of diabetes, and should become even more important in the future. Two major purposes of animal models are to improve understanding the physiology of diabetes and promote development of new therapeutic compounds. Important contributions have come from both classical laboratory animal models and new ones made using advanced methods of genetic manipulation. This chapter reviews the different types of animal models, with emphasis on the more commonly used and informative animals. Models of type 1 diabetes, type 2 diabetes, and obesity are considered. For further information, the reader is referred to the more detailed reviews listed at the end of this chapter.[1,2]

The ideal animal model is simple to describe. It should be easy to produce, maintain, and study while accurately reproducing the human phenotype. One problem is immediately obvious. Humans develop diabetes in middle age or older. Must one study an animal that also develops diabetes later in its life span? The logistical advantages of studying an animal model with early onset of type 2 diabetes are obvious, assuming one can be assured that the information gathered is truly relevant. For example, imagine the difference in studying mouse genetics when the trait is scored at reproductive age (2 months) as compared to an aged animal (1 year).

In reality, the choice of animal model depends on the particular experimental question under investigation. For example, to study the complications of diabetes, streptozotocin can be used to induce diabetes at a known time, with disease onset shortly after treatment. Alternatively, one can use an autoimmune model, but then one must wait months to learn if the particular mouse will actually get diabetes, and wait longer for the complications to develop.

Why use animal models to study diabetes?

Diabetes mellitus is a systemic disease affecting many tissues. Some features of diabetes pathophysiology, such as insulin signaling, can easily be studied using cultured cells. However, other aspects of the disease cannot yet be studied except in whole animal models.

Classically, animal models have been used for identification of regulatory and metabolic pathways, for genetic studies of candidate genes for obesity, diabetes, and insulin resistance and for discovery of new drugs and subsequent testing of their efficacy and safety. The importance of animal models has been increased by the introduction of advanced methods for genetic manipulation, such as tissue-specific transgene expression and targeted gene inactivation. Using animal models for the study of diabetes is safe, relatively inexpensive and practical. Of course, known differences between the physiology of the model animal and human must be taken into account when interpreting the results. Moreover, unanticipated differences between the model and humans can always exist, so crucial conclusions should always be validated in human studies.

Species Considerations

The vast majority of animals used for diabetes research are rodents, usually rats or mice. Rats, being ~10-fold larger than mice, are typically the rodent of choice for physiology experiments. However, sophisticated techniques such as the hyperinsulinemic euglycemic clamp, have now been adapted to mice. In addition, the relative ease of genetic manipulation in mice and the more advanced state of the mouse genome project, have fostered the increasing use of mice.

The use of larger animals, such as dogs and primates will be mentioned only briefly. Experiments using these animals are expensive and require specialized expertise and facilities. However, the larger body size allows very sophisticated physiology experiments, such as those requiring frequent blood sampling, longitudinal tissue sampling, and use of multiple chronically indwelling catheters. Non-human primate experimentation is heavily regulated but has the major advantage that the biology and physiology are the most similar to humans. Thus, primate experiments are often performed prior to a human drug trial.

Sex, Genetics, and Age

Sex-related effects must always be considered in the choice of animal model. Typically male rodents have more severe diabetes (higher prevalence and/or higher mortality) than do females. These effects are thought to be mediated by the sex steroid hormones. However, not all models have more severe diabetes in males. In NOD mice, which get autoimmune diabetes, females have a higher prevalence.

The effects of background genotype are discussed in detail below. But it is worth emphasizing that background genotype effects are very significant and must be considered in every animal experiment. Ideally, background genotype should be controlled for by using littermates, by using genetically identical animals, and/or by using animals in which the phenotype or genes have been backcrossed onto a particular background for at least 10 generations.

GENETIC MODELS OF DIABETES

Classically, genetic models of diabetes and obesity have been produced in two ways. One is serendipitous observation of a spontaneously arising extreme phenotype, followed by selective breeding to fix the trait. The resulting model will often be monogenic, i.e. due to a single mutation. The other approach is by repeated selective breeding of initially normal-appearing members of a genetically diverse (outbred) population that are at one end of the distribution for the trait of interest. After multiple generations of selection, a polygenic model is produced. Thus the classical genetic models will, by definition, have the desired phenotype, although determining the underlying mutations is a major undertaking.

Recently, genetic models have been generated by different means and with a different purpose. Genetic engineering techniques are used to produce animals (predominantly mice) in which the mutations have been designed by the investigator. This 'reverse genetics' approach allows testing the hypothesis that a specific mutation, such as inactivation of a gene, causes diabetes. It is humbling that the results of these experiments often do not match the *a priori* predictions. Additionally, targeted genetic models can serendipitously reveal diabetes-related roles of genes not previously suspected of having such a function.

Types of Models

Table 1 lists a number of rodent models of diabetes. Diabetes can have environmental (islet-injuring drugs or a particular diet) and/or genetic (monogenic or polygenic) causes. We have grouped the models by cause and type of diabetes. While this grouping is reasonable and instructive, it can over-emphasize distinctions. For example, it is believed that beta cell failure (and/or poor islet regeneration) contributes to type 2 diabetes, but in their pure, severe form these processes cause type 1 diabetes.

MODELS OF INSULIN-DEFICIENT DIABETES

Human type 1 diabetes mellitus results from an autoimmune inflammatory response that destroys the insulin-producing pancreatic β-cells (referred to as insulitis). Inadequate β-cell regeneration may also contribute to the disease. The deficiency of β-cells leads to insulin deficiency, which in turn causes hyperglycemia, ketosis, and the rest of the symptoms of diabetes.

Common animal models of type 1 diabetes include those with selective destruction of pancreatic β-cells by chemicals (streptozotocin, alloxan) and animals that spontaneously develop autoimmune destruction of their islets (NOD mice, BB rats). The latter models resemble human type 1 diabetes closely both in the mechanism of induction and the pathophysiological consequences. They can therefore be used to study disease prevention, early markers of diabetes, and therapeutic approaches.

Pharmacologically induced insulin-deficient diabetes has virtually the same consequences as type 1 diabetes in humans but the mechanism of pancreatic β-cell damage is different. These models are used to study the long-term treatment of diabetes and the prevention and treatment of the complications of diabetes. Recently, transgenic mice with an insulin-deficiency phenotype have also been produced.

Animal models with spontaneous autoimmune insulin-dependent diabetes development

The discovery of animal models with spontaneous autoimmune diabetes has contributed significantly to the acceptance of an autoimmune etiology for human type 1 diabetes. A number of independently developed models exist.[3,4,5] The NOD (non-obese diabetic) mouse was discovered in 1974 at the Shionogi Research Laboratories in Osaka, Japan as a result of a selective breeding program searching for a new animal model of diabetes.[6] BB rats were first observed in a colony of Wistar rats at BioBreeding laboratories in Ottawa, Canada showing increased mortality due to a diabetic phenotype. The LETL (Long-Evans Tokushima Lean) rat and its subline, the KDP (Komeda Diabetes Prone) rat were developed in Japan. In addition to these parental strains, a number of genetically modified (congenic, etc) strains exist.

Much information about the development of autoimmune diabetes has been obtained using one or more of these animal models. For example, in the NOD mouse, lymphocytic infiltration of the islets and insulitis is seen as early as at 2 weeks of age, much before the onset of overt diabetes: At 30 weeks of age the incidence of diabetes reaches 80% in female and 20% in male mice. T-cell mediated immune responses to the islet β-cell occur, possibly due to both positive and negative mechanisms. Cell types implicated in development of insulitis include CD4+ and CD8+ T-cells, dendritic cells, and monocyte/macrophages. The ability of passively transferred lymphocytes to induce insulitis and diabetes in the recipients is convincing evidence of the role of these cells and also a powerful tool for dissecting out the detailed mechanisms underlying the autoimmunity.

Evidence to date demonstrates that the MHC class II genes are major contributors to the autoimmunity, and having the diabetogenic MHC class II genes is a necessary, but not sufficient, condition for development of the phenotype. Identification of the non-MHC genes that contribute is underway. For example, a genome-wide scan of the NOD mouse suggests that there are more than 10 loci contributing to the diabetes in this mouse strain, and that these loci are widely distributed in the genome. Due to the independent origins of the different autoimmune models, it is likely that some of the contributing genes will vary between the models.

Table 1. Rodent Models of Diabetes

GENETIC MODELS
Predisposition to immune-mediated β-cell injury (type 1)
- NOD mouse

BB rat
KDP rat
Genetic defects affecting insulin production
- Abnormal pancreas/islet development/function (*Ipf1*+/- mice)
- Abnormal coupling of glucose sensing to insulin secretion (β-cell glucokinase knockout)
- C57BL/6-*Ins2*$^{Akita/+}$ mouse
Classic monogenic obesity/diabetes (type 2)
- *ob/ob* mouse
- *db/db* mouse and Zucker *fa/fa* rat
- A^y mouse
Genetically engineered Transgenic, including polygenic
- IR/IRS1
- GLUT-4, GLUT-2
Classic polygenic
- OLETF rat
- GK rat
- SHR rat
- NZO mouse
- NON mouse
Susceptible genetic background
- C57BLKS/J mouse
- C57BL/6J mouse
- Spiny mouse
Lipoatrophic Diabetes Mellitus
- aP2/DTA mouse
- SREBP-1c overexpressing mouse
- A-ZIP/F-1 mouse
ENVIRONMENTAL MODELS
Pharmacologically induced β-cell injury
- Streptozotocin induced
- Alloxan induced
Surgical
Pancreatectomy
Diet-induced insulin resistance (type 2)
- high fat diet
- high available energy diet
- high fructose diet
- palatable ("cafeteria") diet

It is hard to underestimate the importance of rodent models to our knowledge of type 1 diabetes. Future research goals include understanding of the mechanisms of immune tolerance and devising strategies for preventing the development of human type 1 diabetes.

Pharmacologically induced insulin-dependent diabetes

The most frequently used β-cell injuring chemicals are streptozotocin and alloxan.[2] Alloxan is a pyrimidine that is given as a single dose. It is rapidly taken up by β-cells, causes the production of hydroxyl radicals, and produces irreversible β-cell damage within minutes to hours. The permanent insulinopenia with hyperglycemia and ketoacidosis typically starts after 12 hours and insulin therapy is required to keep the animals alive. The severity and lack of titratability of alloxan make it less frequently used than streptozotocin.

Streptozotocin is a fungal fermentation product that selectively damages pancreatic β-cells, possibly via oxidant damage. In many species, a single injection of a large dose of streptozotocin is sufficient to cause insulin-deficient diabetes. A regimen using multiple injections of a low dose of streptozotocin has also been devised. The multiple dose technique more consistently produces animals with sufficient β-cell loss to cause diabetes, while at the same time leaving enough residual insulin secretory capacity to avoid ketoacidosis and the need for treatment with insulin. This is a major practical advantage.

Surgical pancreatectomy to produce insulin-dependent diabetes

Surgical removal of the pancreas is of major historical interest. In 1889, Minkowsky and von Mering showed that pancreatectomy causes diabetes and in 1921-2 Banting, Best, Collip, and Macleod used pancreatectomized dogs to discover and purify insulin. Today, surgical pancreatectomy, whether complete or partial, is not a commonly used model.

Genetic defects in insulin production

Recently, great progress has been made in identifying the transcription factors controlling pancreas and islet organogenesis and β-cell physiology (some transcription factors: IPF1/PDX1, Isl1, NeuroD/β2, Pax4, Pax6, Nkx2.2, HNF-1α, HNF-1β, HNF-4α). Genetic ablation and targeted overexpression of these genes in mice are used to study their function. For mutations in some of these genes, the human and mouse phenotypes are similar, however other phenotypes are very different, a reminder to use caution in extrapolating between species.

A mouse severely deficient in insulin production, but with enough residual insulin to allow the animal to live, might substitute for some of the current uses of streptozotocin mice. Such a mouse was discovered at the Akita (Japan) University School of Medicine. The C57BL/6-*Ins2*[Akita/+]

mouse has small islets and greatly reduced insulin production. The *Akita* mutation is a cysteine to tyrosine change at position 7 of the A chain of the *Ins2* gene. Since mice have two insulin loci, the phenotype of heterozygous mice might have been predicted to be an asymptomatic ~25% reduction in insulin levels. However, the Akita insulin molecule has severe folding problems, causing toxicity to the β-cells making the protein, a dominant phenotype, and the reduction in β-cell mass.

RODENT MODELS OF TYPE 2 DIABETES MELLITUS

The correlation between obesity and insulin resistance/diabetes mellitus is well established in both humans and rodents. However, the mechanisms by which obesity causes insulin resistance are only partially understood. Diabetes and obesity in both animals and humans result from the combination of environmental and genetic factors. The genetic component of obesity and diabetes can be either monogenic or polygenic. Monogenic inheritance is caused by mutation of a single gene. There are some well-defined monogenic rodent models. In humans, monogenic obesity and diabetes exist as well, but are extremely rare.

Polygenic inheritance is the result of multiple contributing genes and is the predominant mode of inheritance in human type 2 diabetes. Multiple polygenic animal models are also available. However, even in monogenic animal models, genetic background plays an important influence. For example, mice carrying a specific mutation can be normoglycemic on one genetic background yet frankly diabetic on another (see *db* mutation, discussed below).

Monogenic rodent models of type 2 diabetes mellitus and obesity caused by spontaneous mutations

Leptin deficiency: ob/ob mouse
Leptin is a protein hormone produced by adipocytes in proportion to triglyceride content. Thus, the circulating leptin level signals body fat mass and a low leptin level is a signal for the body to adapt to starvation.[7] The *ob* mutation (now officially *Lep^ob^*) is a nonsense mutation and effectively a null allele that arose spontaneously at the Jackson laboratory. Features of *ob/ob* phenotype on the C57BL/6J genetic background (the most frequently studied) are severe, early onset obesity, hyperphagia, insulin resistance, and modest hyperglycemia. Other changes, all characteristic of the starving state, are decreased energy expenditure, hypercorticosteronism, central down regulation of the thyroid and reproductive axes. Chronically elevated corticosteroids contribute to the diabetic phenotype and adrenalectomy decreases glucose and insulin levels in *ob/ob* mice and blunts the obesity as well.

Leptin receptor deficiency: db/db mouse and fa/fa rat

Leptin signals through a single dimeric receptor that exists in multiple protein isoforms due to alternate mRNA splicing. The long leptin receptor isoform is essential for hypothalamic leptin signaling via the JAK/STAT signal transduction cascade. Leptin receptor mutations are known in the mouse as *db* (now officially *Lepr*^{db}) and the rat as *fa* (*fatty*, officially *Lepr*^{fa}). Both the *db* and *fa* mutations have arisen multiple independent times.

The *db/db* mouse is a classic example of the effect of genetic background in a monogenic disease. The *db* mutation arose on the C57BL/KsJ (now C57BLKS/J) genetic background, with a phenotype of hyperphagia, hyperinsulinemia, and hyperglycemia within the first month of age. By about four to five months of age the insulin production falls off, leading to insulin deficiency and death by 10 months of age from uncontrolled hyperglycemia. However, when the *db* mutation was moved onto the C57BL/6J genetic background, the homozygous phenotype was indistinguishable from that of *ob/ob* on this background, with severe obesity but much milder diabetes. Presumably the C57BL/6J strain has alleles that allow better β-cell survival and/or regeneration than does the C57BLKS/J genetic background. At present, little is known about the identity of the responsible modifier genes.

The original *fa* mutation arose spontaneously over forty years ago in an outbred stock of rats in the Zucker laboratory at Stow, Massachusetts. The phenotype of *fa/fa* rats is very similar to that of *db/db* mice including hyperphagia, hyperinsulinemia, insulin resistance, and infertility. Genetic background also plays an important role in determining the detailed phenotype of the *fa/fa* rats. The blood glucose levels of *fa/fa* rats on different genetic background can vary from mild hyperglycemia to severe hyperglycemia with subsequent β-cell failure.

Melanocortin pathway mutations: A^y and related mice

The yellow mouse models of obesity have been very useful and informative in our understanding of the hypothalamic regulation of energy metabolism. The mutations, such as A^y (*lethal yellow*) are autosomal dominant and cause a yellow coat color, obesity, insulin resistance, increased somatic growth, and a tendency to develop tumors. Each of the yellow mutations causes ectopic overexpression of the agouti protein, which is normally produced in the hair follicle and acts as a paracrine antagonist of melanocortin receptor signaling.[8] In A^y/a mice, the yellow coat color is due to heightened inhibition of α-melanocyte stimulating hormone (αMSH) action on the hair follicle type 1 melanocortin receptors (MC1R). The increased food intake, obesity, and insulin resistance are due to antagonism of αMSH on hypothalamic MC4R, and to a lesser extent, MC3R. However, in normal mice, agouti protein does not reach the hypothalamus, and the endogenous hypothalamic ligand is Agrp, Agouti-related protein. Our current understanding of hypothalamic physiology is that leptin stimulates αMSH and inhibits Agrp signaling, leading to increased MC4R/MC3R signaling and decreased food intake, increased energy expenditure, and increased insulin sensitivity.

Genetically modified mice have been used to elucidate and test this pathway. Thus some or all of the obesity/insulin resistance phenotype of the A^y/a (and other yellow allele) mice is found in mice null for MC4R, MC3R, or proopiomelanocortin (the precursor to αMSH) and in mice overexpressing Agrp or syndecan (a cell-surface heparan sulfate proteoglycan that potentiates Agrp action).

Genetically engineered monogenic rodent models of type 2 diabetes mellitus and obesity

The identification of a number of spontaneous gene mutations causing obesity and diabetes significantly augmented our understanding of this disease. The reverse approach is also used: the function and the importance of particular genes is directly tested by creation of the genetically modified mice with targeted gene knockouts or overexpression.[9,10] Conditional (tissue specific or inducible) knockouts can also be used to increase the specificity and selectivity of the changes. The number of genetically engineered models is growing rapidly, only a few are mentioned below.

Transgenic mice lacking the insulin receptor (IR) have severe diabetes with ketoacidosis, markedly increased plasma free fatty acids, triglycerides, and reduced hepatic glycogen content.[11] The phenotype is more severe than in humans lacking IR and the mice die by a week after birth. Mice lacking IR in muscle display severely reduced insulin-stimulated muscle glucose uptake and elevated fat mass, but their insulin and glucose levels are normal. In contrast, β-cell-specific IR ablated mice exhibit a selective loss of insulin secretion in response to glucose with progressively impaired glucose tolerance indicating an important functional role of IR in glucose sensing by the β-cells.

Mice lacking proteins downstream of the IR have also been studied. Insulin receptor substrate-1 (IRS-1) null mice have normal glucose levels, but develop an insulin resistance with compensatory hyperinsulinemia and other features resembling those of patients with type 2 diabetes mellitus.[12] IRS-2 knockout animals have reduced β-cell mass and a limited ability of compensatory increase of insulin secretion resulting in progressive glucose intolerance.[13] It is suggested that IRS-1 deficiency causes predominantly peripheral (muscle) insulin resistance with retained ability of compensatory insulin hypersecretion, while IRS-2 deficiency leads to milder peripheral insulin resistance with impaired liver response and β-cell compensatory function.

The ability of muscle and adipose tissue to take up glucose in response to insulin depends largely on glucose transporter-4 (GLUT4). Whole body GLUT4 null mice are insulin resistant, but euglycemic with a reduced amount of white adipose tissue and cardiac hypertrophy.[14] Selective muscle GLUT4 knockout results not only in severely decreased muscle insulin sensitivity, but also liver and white adipose tissue insulin resistance. Similarly, selective targeting of adipose tissue GLUT4 causes insulin resistance in the adipose tissue and probably secondary insulin resistance in muscle and liver.

Polygenic rodent models of type 2 diabetes mellitus and obesity

The phenotype of the polygenic obesity and type 2 diabetes mellitus is the result of multiple interacting genes.[15,16,17] The polygenic rodent models allow the discovery of diabetes/obesity genes. The contributing genes will sometimes be different and sometimes be the same between genetic models and between species. However, it is likely that the biological pathways using the identified gene will be important in all species, even if mutations in the particular gene identified in one model are not a cause of diabetes/obesity in another system.

Otsuka Long Evans Tokushima (OLETF) rat

One of the widely used selectively inbred type 2 diabetes mellitus rodent models is the OLETF rat, originally derived from spontaneously diabetic Long-Evans rats. OLETF rats manifest a spontaneous glucose intolerance, mild obesity, hyperglycemia, hyperinsulinemia, and insulin resistance at about 18 weeks of age. With aging, the severity of diabetes typically progresses to include late β-cell failure. OLETF rats thus represent a type 2 diabetes model with brittle pancreas.

Goto-Kakizaki (GK) rat

GK rats have been bred from an original Wistar population for more than 35 generations in Japan using relative intolerance to a glucose load as a selection criterion. The typical features of GK phenotype include glucose intolerance, hyperglycemia, and impaired glucose-stimulated insulin secretion without significant islet β-cell hyperplasia or obesity. Hyperglycemia, reduced β-cell number, and circulating insulin levels are present as early as in GK rat fetuses, indicating that those defects are the earliest steps in diabetes development in this strain.

Spontaneously Hypertensive Rat (SHR)

SHR were originally selected for hypertension from Wistar-Kyoto rat strain. The SHR males are hypertensive, hyperlipidemic, hyperinsulinemic, obese, and commonly exhibit non-fasting hyperglycemia. The SHR females, in contrast, are smaller and usually do not exhibit non-fasting hyperglycemia.

New Zealand obese (NZO) mice

The NZO strain was developed by selective inbreeding for obesity with mild hyperglycemia and marked hyperinsulinemia. NZO mice have severe, early onset obesity reaching comparable level of adiposity as the *ob/ob* or *db/db* mice. Insulin resistance is present in all of the NZO mice but only in some does it progress to frank type 2 diabetes mellitus.

Nonobese Nondiabetic (NON) mice

NON mice were inbred in Japan as a control line for the NOD mice (above). Male NON mice exhibit impaired glucose tolerance and mild visceral obesity at 9 weeks of age. Both insulin levels and insulin mRNA pancreatic islet content are decreased in NON mice, however the capacity for pancreatic islet hyperplasia is retained. The selective defect in insulin synthesis and/or secretion is suggested to be the reason of increased glucose levels in NON mice.

Diet-induced obesity, insulin resistance, and diabetes

Many animals will develop some degree of obesity and/or insulin resistance when fed a suitable diet. Most of the diets result in increased caloric intake. Specific diets include high fat diets, diets with varied, palatable foods (cafeteria diet), and diets with high available energy density (sucrose or fructose rich diets). Whether insulin resistance develops in response to diet can differ greatly between strains (for example, C57BL/6J mice are susceptible) and species (sand rats and spiny mice are susceptible). The causative genetic differences have not yet been identified. Although it is not known if the susceptibility genes involved in rodents' dietary obesity and diabetes are the same as those in human population, it is likely that the underlying biology is similar enough to make the use of animal models valid.

Lipoatrophic diabetes mellitus

While obesity is clearly a cause of insulin resistance and diabetes, paradoxically, rare patients with severe deficiency of adipose tissue are also at high risk of developing diabetes. Most studies of lipoatrophic (or lipodystrophic) diabetes have used one of three lines of transgenic mice.[18] Each line was produced by selective expression of a transgene in adipose tissue. The aP2-DTA mice were produced by expression of an attenuated diphtheria toxin. Animals expressing high levels of transgene developed a chylous ascites and died within a day of birth, precluding generation of lines. Mice expressing less transgene protein initially appeared normal, but lost almost all visible adipose tissue by ~10 months of age. The aP2-SREBP-1c mice express a constitutively active form of the SREBP-1c (sterol regulatory element binding protein-1c) transcription factor. For unclear reasons, this causes a marked reduction in white adipose tissue (35% of control at 12 weeks). The brown adipose tissue is increased in weight and resembles immature white adipose tissue in appearance. aP2-driven expression of a dominant negative to bZIP transcription factors produced the A-ZIP/F-1 line, which has the most complete deficiency of adipose tissue of the viable lipoatrophy models. These mice have virtually no visible white adipose tissue. Their brown adipose tissue appears normal at birth, but undergoes accelerated involution with aging, becoming metabolically inactive.

While differing in severity, the mouse models replicate the phenotype of the lipoatrophic patients, including severe insulin-resistant diabetes without ketoacidosis, decreased leptin levels, increased food intake, hepatomegaly, and increased triglyceride deposition in liver and muscle. Surgical transplantation of adipose tissue into lipoatrophic mice reduces the metabolic abnormalities associated with lipoatrophy. Leptin treatment also has a major effect, suggesting that much of the phenotype is due to leptin deficiency. The contribution of other adipocyte hormones and the role of adipose tissue as a sink for the storage of triglyceride to the pathophysiology of lipoatrophy are not yet resolved.

SUMMARY

Animal models of diabetes are important and powerful tools for unraveling the pathophysiological mechanisms of this disease, identifying candidate diabetic genes, and discovering and testing new therapeutic agents. The classical rodent models of diabetes allow unbiased discovery, while the new models made by genetic manipulation allow testing of the role of specific genes and tissues. Experimental animal models are an irreplaceable resource for diabetes research and are hastening the progress towards the goals of better treatment, prevention, and cure.

REFERENCES:

1. McNeill JH. Experimental models of diabetes. CRC Press, Boca Raton, Florida, pp. 418, 1999.
2. Shafrir E. Diabetes in animals. In *Diabetes Mellitus*. D Porte Jr. and RS Sherwin, Eds., Appleton & Lange, Stamford, CT, pp. 301-348, 1997.
3. Bone AJ and Gwilliam DJ. Animal models of insulin-dependent diabetes mellitus. In *Textbook of Diabetes*. JC Pickup and G Williams Eds., Blackwell Science, Cambridge, Mass, pp. 16.1-16.16, 1997.
4. Mathews CE, Leiter EH. Rodent models for the study of diabetes. In *Joslin's Diabetes Mellitus,* CR Kahn et al. Eds., in press, 2002.

5. Mordes JP, Greiner DL, Rossini AA. Animal models of autoimmune Diabetes mellitus. In *Diabetes mellitus: a fundamental and clinical text.* D LeRoith, SI Taylor and JM Olefsky, Eds. Lippincott Williams & Wilkins, Philadelphia, pp. 430-441, 2000.

6. Yoshida K, Kikutani H. Genetic and immunological basis of autoimmune diabetes in the NOD mouse. Rev Immunogenet 2(1):140-6, 2000.

7. Halaas JL, Gajiwala KS, Maffei M et al. Weight-reducing effects of the plasma protein encoded by the obese gene. Science 269(5223):543-546, 1995.

8. Ollmann, MM, Lamoreux, ML, Wilson, BD et al. Interaction of Agouti protein with the melanocortin 1 receptor in vitro and in vivo. Genes Dev 12(3):316-30, 1998.

9. Saltiel AR. New perspectives into the molecular pathogenesis and treatment of type 2 diabetes. Cell 104(4):517-29, 2001.

10. Kay TWH, and Harrison LC. Insights from transgenic and gene targeting strategies in type 1 diabetes mellitus. In *Diabetes mellitus: A fundamental and clinical text.* D LeRoith, SI Taylor, and JM Olefsky, Eds., Lippincott Williams & Wilkins, Philadelphia, pp. 441-454, 2000.

11. Accili D, Drago J, Lee EJ et al. Early neonatal death in mice homozygous for a null allele of the insulin receptor gene. Nat Genet 12(1):106-9, 1996.

12. Tamemoto H, Kadowaki T, Tobe K, et al. Insulin resistance and growth retardation in mice lacking insulin receptor substrate-1. Nature 372(6502):182-6, 1994.

13. Withers DJ, Gutierrez JS, Towery H, et al. Disruption of IRS-2 causes type 2 diabetes in mice. Nature 391:900-4, 1998.

14. Katz EB, Stenbit AE, Hatton K, et al. Cardiac and adipose tissue abnormalities but not diabetes in mice deficient in GLUT4. Nature 377(6545):151-5, 1995.

15. Bailey CJ and Flatt PR. Animal syndromes of non-insulin-dependent diabetes mellitus. In *Textbook of Diabetes.* JC Pickup, and G Williams, Eds., Blackwell Science, Cambridge, Mass, pp. 23.1-23.25, 1997.

16. Hansen BC. Primate animal models of type 2 diabetes mellitus. In *Diabetes mellitus: A fundamental and clinical text.* D LeRoith, SI Taylor, and JM Olefsky Eds., Lippincott Williams & Wilkins, Philadelphia, pp. 734-743, 2000.

17. Reitman ML. Rodent genetic models of obesity and type 2 diabetes mellitus, in: *Diabetes mellitus: A fundamental and clinical text.* D LeRoith, SI Taylor, and JM Olefsky, Eds., Lippincott Williams & Wilkins, Philadelphia, PA, pp. 723-734, 2000.

18. Reitman ML, Arioglu E, Gavrilova O et al. Lipoatrophy revisited. Trends Endocrinol Metab 11(10):410-6, 2000.

V. Diabetes Syndromes

Chapter 1. Type 1 Diabetes Mellitus: Epidemiology, Genetics, Pathogenesis And Clinical Manifestations

Marian Rewers

TYPE 1 DIABETES

Type 1 diabetes is caused by pancreatic β-cell destruction that leads to loss of insulin secretion and absolute insulin deficiency. Type 1 diabetes accounts for about 10% of all diabetes, affecting approximately 1.4 million people in the U.S., and 10-20 million globally.[1] Diabetes is one of the most common severe chronic diseases of childhood affecting 1 in 300 children and as many as 1 in 100 adults during the life span.[2]

The current classification of diabetes mellitus[3] distinguishes type 1a (autoimmune)[4] and type 1b (not immune-mediated) forms, the latter remaining poorly defined.[5] Type 1a is the most common form of diabetes among children and adolescents of European origin, usually characterized by acute onset and dependence on exogenous insulin for survival. In adults, the disease is nearly as frequent as in children, but often with less dramatic onset leading to misclassification as type 2 diabetes and a delayed insulin treatment. About 60% of persons with type 1 diabetes are diagnosed as adults.

NATURAL HISTORY OF TYPE 1a DIABETES

The natural history of type 1a diabetes (Figure 1) includes four distinct stages: 1) pre-clinical β-cell autoimmunity with progressive defect of insulin secretion; 2) onset of clinical diabetes; 3) transient remission; and 4) established diabetes associated with acute and chronic complications and premature death.

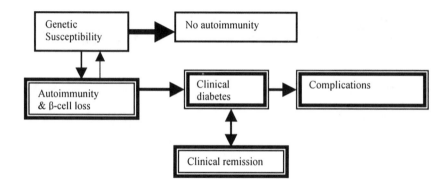

Figure 1. Natural history of type 1a diabetes.

B-cell autoimmunity

In most patients, the etiology of the autoimmune process and β-cell destruction is not known. The process is mediated by macrophages and T lymphocytes with detectable autoantibodies to various β-cell antigens. Currently, autoimmunity is defined by the presence of autoantibodies,[4] because their measurement is reliable and standardized across laboratories, in contrast to the cellular markers. The initial islet cell antibody (ICA) assay, using immunofluorescence and pancreatic tissue[6] has been notoriously difficult to standardize and has been replaced by a combination of specific β-cell autoantibodies to insulin (IAA),[7] glutamic acid decarboxylase (GAD),[8] and tyrosine phosphatase ICA512 (IA-2).[9] These tests have been shown to be quite sensitive and predictive in relatives of type 1 diabetes patients[10] and in the general population.[11]

Progression from β-cell autoimmunity to clinical diabetes

The duration of pre-clinical β-cell autoimmunity is variable and precedes the diagnosis of diabetes by up to 13 years.[12] In persons with persistent autoantibodies, there is an early loss of spontaneous pulsatile insulin secretion, progressive reduction in the acute insulin response to intravenous glucose load, followed by decreased response to other β-cell secretagogues, impaired oral glucose tolerance and fasting hyperglycemia.[13] However, a non-progressive β-cell defect has been shown to exist for many years in monozygotic twins and other relatives of type 1 diabetes persons.

Studies in the first-degree relatives of type 1 diabetes patients[14] and in school children with no family history of type 1 diabetes[15] have reported ICA "remission" rates between 10-78%. Newer data suggest that while individual islet-specific autoantibodies may fluctuate in titers, it is very unusual to observe remission after two or more of such autoantibodies were present for even a few months[16]. Some people may loose β-cell autoantibodies or remain positive for these antibodies but do not progress to diabetes due to incomplete penetrance of susceptibility genes or insufficient exposure to the causative environmental agent(s). It is possible that β-cell autoimmunity remits spontaneously in genetically resistant persons or when the offending factor is removed, similar to celiac disease. Age also plays a role: children younger than 10 years have a 3-fold increased risk of progressing from autoimmunity to type 1 diabetes, compared to older relatives.

B-cell autoimmunity may remit and reappear in the course of viral infections or variable exposure to dietary causal factors. The cumulative β-cell damage and increases in insulin resistance with obesity and physical inactivity may eventually cause diabetes at a later age. Those people in whom the disease process is slow may present with type 1 diabetes as adults, develop diabetes that does not require insulin treatment, or may even escape diabetes altogether. Markers of autoimmunity can be detected in 14-33% of diabetes patients classified on clinical grounds as "Type 2"[17] and are associated with early failure of oral hypoglycemic drug therapy and insulin dependence in these patients. A term "latent autoimmune diabetes of adults" (LADA)[18] has been coined for this slowly progressing form of type 1 diabetes.

Pathological lesions in the pancreas.

The β-cell destruction in the pancreas is though to involve apoptosis. The inflammatory pancreatic lesion, termed insulitis, is characterized by the mononuclear cell infiltration of the islets and the reduction of the β-cell mass. The cells involved in the insulitis include T and B lymphocytes and macrophages. Insulitis was initially described in necropsy specimens. Samples obtained during pancreatic biopsies in patients with a recent onset of type 1 diabetes uniformly show various degrees of reduction in the β-cell volume, but insulitis appears to be present only in half of these biopsies. Thus, further studies of the role of insulitis in β-cell destruction are needed.[19]

CLINICAL ONSET OF TYPE 1 DIABETES

In industrialized countries, 20-40% of type 1 diabetes patients younger than 20 years presents in diabetic ketoacidosis (DKA).[20] Younger age, female gender, HLA-DR4 allele,[21] lower socioeconomical status and lack of family history of diabetes have been associated with more severe presentation. Younger children present with more severe symptoms at diagnosis, because children younger than 7 have lost on average 80% of the islets, compared to 60% in those 7-14 year old and 40% in those older than 14.[22] Case fatality in industrialized countries ranges between 0.4-0.9%.[23] While brain edema is believed to be the major cause of death, the risk factors are poorly understood and heterogeneous.

Both DKA and onset deaths are largely preventable, because most of the patients have typical symptoms of polyuria, polydipsia, and weight loss for 2-4 weeks prior to diagnosis. The diagnosis is straightforward in almost all cases, based on the symptoms, random blood glucose over 200 mg/dl and/or HbA$_{1c}$ >7%. Oral glucose tolerance test (OGTT) is rarely needed for diagnosis. In questionable cases, negative OGTT allows to rule out current diabetes and, in combination with negative β-cell autoantibodies, offers reassurance that diabetes is not around the corner. Traditionally, nearly all children with newly diagnosed type 1 diabetes were hospitalized. More recently, an increasing proportion of these children have been managed on an outpatient basis, especially in urban centers with specialized diabetes education and treatment facilities. In Colorado, USA, the proportion of children receiving only outpatient care at onset increased from 6% in 1978 to 35% in 1988[24] and 75% in 2000. Hospitalization at onset does not improve short-term outcomes such as readmission for DKA or severe hypoglycemia,[25] if adequate family education and follow-up is available on outpatient basis. Onset hospitalizations and subsequent acute complications have similar predictors: biological (younger age, lower endogenous insulin secretion) and psychosocial (lower socioeconomic status, limited access to health care, dysfunctional family).

Incidence of type 1 diabetes

Geographic location One of the most striking characteristics of type 1 diabetes is the large geographic variability in the incidence[26] (Fig. 2).

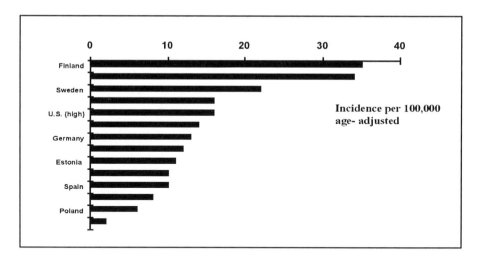

Figure 2. Incidence of type 1 diabetes, by age, in Hispanic and non-Hispanic white children living in the same geographic area. (Adapted from Kostraba JN, Gay EC, Cai Y, Cruickshanks KJ, Rewers MJ, Klingensmith GJ, Chase HP, Hamman RF. Incidence of insulin-dependent diabetes mellitus in Colorado. Epidemiology 3:232-238, 1992, with permission).

Scandinavia and the Mediterranean island of Sardinia have the highest incidence rates in the world while Oriental populations have the lowest rates. A child in Finland is 400 times more likely to develop diabetes than one in China. While there is a strong south-north gradient in the incidence, 'hot-spots' in warm climates have been reported (Sardinia, Puerto Rico, Kuwait). The geographic and ethnic variations in type 1 diabetes reflect the prevalence of susceptibility genes or that of causal environmental factors, or both.

In the general population, the prevalence of β-cell autoimmunity appears to be roughly proportional to the incidence of type 1 diabetes in the populations.[27] In contrast, the prevalence of β-cell autoimmunity in first-degree relatives of type 1 diabetic persons does not differ dramatically between high and low risk countries. The incidence of β-cell autoimmunity is higher in relatives younger than 5 years (3.7%/yr), compared to those 5-9 yr old (0.5%/yr)[28]. During 5 years of follow-up, none of the relatives older than 10 years has developed β-cell autoimmunity,[28] suggesting that β-cell autoimmunity develops primarily before the age of 5 and that it may remit in many cases.[15]

The clinical picture of the disease is similar in low- and high-risk areas,[29] making it unlikely that the inter-populations differences are due to misclassification of different types of diabetes. However, in many populations[30] type 2 diabetes is an increasing or already the predominant form of diabetes in children[31] making correct diagnosis and treatment increasingly difficult.

Age Type 1 diabetes incidence peaks at the ages of 2, 4-6 and 10-14 years, perhaps due to alterations in the pattern of infections or increases in insulin resistance. The age distribution of type 1 diabetes onset is similar across geographic areas and ethnic groups[29] (Figure 3). The incidence decreases in the third decade of life,[32] only to increase again in the fifth to seventh decades of life.[33] The prevalence of ICA decreased with age in first degree relatives participating in Diabetes Prevention Trial (DPT-1 screening. It is not known whether the etiology differs between childhood- and adult-onset type 1diabetes, but it was not apparent among adult participants in the United Kingdom Prospective Diabetes Study (UKPDS). Over 30% of those 25-34 years of age were positive for ICA and/or GAD autoantibodies, but the prevalence decreased with age, to less than 10% in those aged 55-65 years of age[34]. The presence of the autoantibodies and age of presentation of diabetes were strongly associated with the presence of the HLA-DRB1*03/DRB1*04-DQB1*0302 genotype.[35]

Race and ethnicity. There are striking racial differences in type 1 diabetes risk in multiracial populations, although not of the same magnitude as the geographic differences. In the U.S., non-Hispanic whites are about one and a half times as likely to develop type 1 diabetes as African Americans[36] or Hispanics[37] (Figure 3). This is similar to the differences reported from Montreal, where children of British descent had about one and a half the risk of type 1 diabetes in children of French descent.[38]

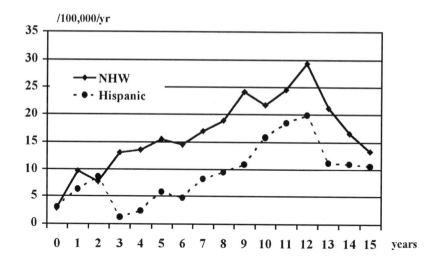

Figure 3 . Incidence of non-hispanic whites (NHW) type 1 diabetes mellitus in Colorado, 1978-88. (Adapted from Kostraba JN, Gay EC, Cai Y, Cruickshanks KJ, Rewers MJ, Klingensmith GJ, Chase HP, Hamman RF. Incidence of insulin-dependent diabetes mellitus in Colorado. Epidemiology 3:232-238, 1992, with permission.)

Little data concerning β-cell autoimmunity is available for non-Caucasian populations. Among 86,000 relatives of type 1 diabetic patients screened for the DPT-1 trail, lower prevalence of ICA was observed in Asian Americans (2.6%) and in Hispanics (2.7%), compared to African Americans (3.3%) or non-Hispanic whites (3.9%) (DPT-1, unpublished data 2001). Lower prevalence of GAD antibodies has also been reported in Oriental compared to Caucasian type 1 diabetes patients.[39]

Gender In general, males and females have similar risk of type 1 diabetes,[40] with the pubertal peak of incidence in females preceding that in males by 1-2 years. In lower-risk populations, such as Japan or U.S. blacks, there is a female preponderance, while in high-risk groups, there is a slight male excess.[41] Type 1 diabetes diagnosed in adulthood is associated with male excess[42] DPT-1 screening data (not adjusted for age, relation to proband of ethnicity) have suggested higher prevalence of ICA in male first-degree relatives (4.3%) than in females (3.3%).

Time The incidence of type 1 diabetes varies markedly over time, both seasonally and annually. In the Northern Hemisphere, the incidence declines during the warm summer months; similarly in the Southern Hemisphere, the seasonal pattern exhibits a decline during the warm months of December and January, implicating a climatic factor.[43] This seasonal pattern appears to occur only in older children[44] suggesting that factors triggering diabetes may be related to school attendance. The observed seasonality does not appear to be an artifact of health care seeking or access, but the seasonal patterns differ by the HLA-DR genotype.[45]

Most population-based registries have shown an increase in type 1 diabetes incidence over time.[46,47] Periodic outbreaks, sometimes of pandemic proportion, e.g., during 1984-86[46] appear to be superimposed on a steady secular increase in incidence. Figure 4 displays an example of parallel temporal incidence changes in populations that differ vastly in geographic location and the background risk of type 1 diabetes[29] (Allegheny Co., USA, and Wielkopolska, Poland). While the increase in type 1 diabetes incidence has affected all age groups, several studies reported particular increase among the youngest children[48]. No reliable information is available concerning potential seasonal or annual variation in the incidence of β-cell autoimmunity.

Genetic models are unable to explain the apparent temporal changes in the incidence.[49] The polio model, where autoimmune diabetes results from delayed exposure to infection that is benign when encountered in early childhood, could explain the recent increase in the incidence, but not the shift in diagnosis to earlier ages. Alternative explanation invokes the congenital rubella model where increased hygiene has led to a decline in herd immunity to common infections among women in child-bearing age. These women are more likely to develop viremia during pregnancy resulting in congenital persistent infection of β-cells and early onset type 1 diabetes in the offspring. This model could explain both the increasing incidence of diabetes and the decreasing age of disease onset.

Genetic factors

Family history of type 1 diabetes. In moderate type 1 diabetes risk areas, such as the United States, the risk of type 1 diabetes by the age of 20 years is approximately 1:300 (Table 1). The risk is increased to about 1:50 in offspring of type 1 diabetes mothers and 1:15 in offspring of type 1 diabetes fathers (the reason for this parental gender difference is not known). The risk to siblings of type 1 diabetes probands ranges from 1:12 to 1:35[50] and is further increased in HLA-identical siblings. It is estimated that by the age of 60 years approximately 10% of the first degree relatives develop type 1 diabetes.[51] Family history of type 1 diabetes is a surrogate measure of the combination of type 1 diabetes genes and environmental exposures shared by family members.

The risk of β-cell autoimmunity is higher, because not all autoantibody positive children develop diabetes by the age of 20. Prevalence estimates from cross-sectional studies shown in Table 1 are obviously less precise than cumulative incidence rates available for clinical diabetes.

159

Table 1. Risk, by the age of 20 years, of type 1 diabetes and beta-cell autoimmunity in the general population and family members of type 1 diabetic patients.

Risk Group	Type 1 Diabetes	Pre-Diabetic Autoimmunity
General Population		
All HLA genotypes	1:300	1:30-1:100
HLA-DR3/4,DQB1*0302	1:15	1:10(?)
Family Members		
Maternal offspring	1:50	1:15
Paternal offspring	1:15	1:5
Siblings (all)	1:12 - 1:35	1:5
Monozygotic twins	1:3	1:1(?)
HLA-identical siblings	1:4	1:2(?)

'Familial' cases represent about 10% of type 1 diabetes and do not appear to be etiologically different from 'sporadic' cases in terms of the HLA-DR,DQ gene frequencies, seasonality of onset, prevalence of islet autoantibodies.[52] 'Familial' cases tend to have lower HbA1c and higher C-peptide levels than 'sporadic' cases, because relatives recognize diabetes symptoms earlier, however, these differences disappear soon after diagnosis.

Candidate genes. The primary loci of genetic susceptibility to type 1 diabetes have been mapped to the HLA-DR and DQ regions[53] While 50 percent of non-Hispanic whites in the United States have HLA-DR3 or DR4 allele, at least one of these alleles is present in 95 percent of patients with type 1 diabetes. The estimated risk for general population children who have the HLA-DR3/4,DQB1*0302 genotype is approximately 1:15.[54] Only 2.4% of the general population carries this genotype, compared to 30-40% of type 1 diabetes patients.

No particular HLA type seems to be associated with β-cell autoimmunity, although inconsistent associations between insulin or GAD autoantibodies and HLA-DR, DQ phenotypes have been reported. The HLA-DR2,DQB1*0602 haplotype, which almost completely protects from type 1 diabetes[53], is found in about 15% of GAD and IAA positive young relatives of type 1 diabetes patients.[55] However, 90% of the first-degree relatives[56] and general population children who stay persistently autoantibody positive[57] express the HLA-DRB1*04,DQB1*0302. This may suggest that HLA genes are not involved in the initiation of β-cell autoimmunity, but rather determine progression to diabetes.

Candidate genes outside the HLA region are being identified[58] (see chapter "Diabetes Genes"). More subjects with β-cell autoimmunity need to be genotyped to precisely determine the role of HLA and additional type 1 diabetes candidate genes in the initiation of autoimmunity and progression to diabetes.

Environmental factors

Twin[59] and family studies indicate that genetic factors alone cannot explain the etiology of type 1 diabetes. Seasonality, increasing incidence and epidemics of type 1 diabetes as well as numerous ecological, cross-sectional and retrospective studies suggest that certain viruses and components of early childhood diet may cause type 1 diabetes.

Viruses. Herpesviruses,[60] mumps,[61] rubella,[62] retroviruses,[63] and rotavirus[64] have been implicated. Viral infections appear to initiate autoimmunity rather than precipitate diabetes in subjects with autoimmunity. Two or more infections with similar viruses may be needed: mice persistently expressing a viral protein in the β-cells do not develop β-cell autoimmunity unless exposed to the same virus later in life.[65] ICA or IAA has been detected after mumps,[66] rubella, measles, chickenpox[67], Coxsackie,[68] and rotavirus[64] infections. Newborns and infants are particularly likely to develop a persistent infection and among patients with congenital rubella syndrome, 70% have ICA.[62]

An increased incidence of type 1 diabetes in patients with congenital rubella syndrome (CRS) is particularly interesting. While CRS is responsible for a minute proportion of type 1 diabetes and there is little evidence that postnatal rubella exposure to the wild strain[67] or to the MMR vaccine[69] causes type 1 diabetes, CRS provides an example of viral persistence leading to type 1 diabetes. The incubation period of type 1 diabetes in CRS patients is 5-20 years[70] and persistent rubella virus infection of the pancreas has been demonstrated in some cases. While CRS is not associated with particular HLA-DR alleles, the distribution of the HLA-DR3 and 4 alleles among patients with CRS and diabetes resembles that in non-CRS type 1 diabetes patients.[62] Finally, a molecular mimicry has been reported between a rubella virus protein and a 52 kD β-cell autoantigen.[71]

The evidence is strongest for picornaviruses, which include human (enteroviruses and rhinoviruses) and animal pathogens (e.g., mouse EMC virus and Theiler's virus). Enteroviruses have been most strongly linked to human type 1 diabetes, but convincing proof of causality remains elusive (for review see[72,73]). Case and autopsy reports,[74] epidemics of type 1 diabetes associated with concurrent epidemics of enteroviruses[75] and multiple cross-sectional seroepidemiological studies have been suggestive, but not entirely convincing. At least 90% of type 1 diabetes patients demonstrate prolonged period of β-cell autoimmunity that is hardly compatible with an acute cytolytic enteroviral infection being a major cause. Enteroviral infection could, however, initiate β-cell autoimmunity through molecular mimicry between CBV P2-C protein and GAD[76] or a persistent β-cell infection with impairment of insulin secretion and expression of self-antigens.

Cross-sectional studies of anti-Coxsackie antibodies in β-cell autoimmunity have been week and inconclusive[77] and have been recently replaced by studies based on detection of picornaviral RNA in bodily fluids using polymerase chain reaction (PCR). Prospective studies of non-diabetic relatives and general population children found a strong relation between enteroviral infections, defined by PCR, and development of islet autoantibodies in Finland[78] but not in the U.S (P. Graves, unpublished data 2000). Studies from Finland[79] and Sweden[80] have suggested that *in utero* enteroviral infections can lead to type 1 diabetes in a significant proportion of the cases. Additional perinatal factors[81] and season of birth[82] have been associated with type 1 diabetes.

Possible protective effect of infections. In animal models, viral infection may protect the host from developing type 1 diabetes[83]. Evidence for such a protective effect in humans is speculative, at best.[84,85]

Routine childhood immunization. None of the routine childhood immunization have been shown to increase the risk of diabetes[85] or pre-diabetic autoimmunity.[86]

Dietary factors. Cow's milk or wheat introduced at weaning trigger insulitis and diabetes in animal models[87] perhaps through a molecular mimicry.[88] Human data are conflicting, but predominantly negative.[89] An ecological study suggested an association between decrease in breast-feeding and increase in type 1 diabetes incidence between 1940 and 1980.[90] Subsequent case-control studies have shown a negative,[91] positive[92] or no association.[93] Certain studies[94] but not others[93] suggested a dose-response relationship between the duration of breast-feeding and protection from type 1 diabetes. A meta-analysis found a 50% increase in type 1 diabetes risk associated with a breast-feeding duration of less than 3 months, and exposure to breast-milk substitutes prior to 3 months of age,[95] but a subsequent meta-analysis reported much lower risk estimates.[96] Breast-feeding may be viewed as a surrogate for the delay in the introduction of diabetogenic substances present in formula or early childhood diet. The reports that newly diagnosed diabetic children, compared with age-matched controls, have higher levels of serum antibodies against cow's milk and beta-lactoglobulin[97] as well as against bovine serum albumin[98] have been difficult to reproduce.[87] More recent cohort studies failed to find an association between infant diet exposures and beta-cell autoimmunity.[99] Interestingly, a study from Finland suggested that current cow's milk consumption was more closely linked to pre-diabetic autoimmunity and diabetes than infant exposure[100]. To resolve this controversy, a dietary intervention trial to prevent type diabetes by a short-term elimination of cow's milk from infant diet (TRIGR) is underway.[101]

Chemical compounds. Streptozotocin[102] or dietary nitrates and nitrozamines[103] induce β-cell autoimmunity in animal models. Circumstantial evidence suggests a connection between type 1 diabetes and consumption of foods and water containing nitrates, nitrites or nitrosamines.[104] Multiple hits of dietary β-cell toxins may render genetically resistant individuals susceptible to diabetogenic viruses leading to type 1 diabetes.[105]

Gene-environment interactions

Type 1 diabetes is likely caused by an interactive effect of genetic and environmental factors within a limited age-window. While both the susceptibility genes and the candidate environmental exposures appear to be quite common, the disease is still uncommon, raising a possibility of low penetrance.[106]

In mice, the host's genes restrict the diabetogenic effect of picornaviruses in a manner compatible with a recessive trait not related to the MHC. In humans, on the other hand, susceptibility to diabetogenic enteroviruses appears to be genetically restricted by HLA-DR and DQ alleles. However, the allelic specificity is controversial[107] and may depend on the viral type and epidemicity. In general, the HLA-DR3 allele, present in most patients with type 1 diabetes, is associated with viral persistence.

Very few studies have examined a possibility of an interaction between the HLA genes and dietary exposured[108,100]. The epidemiological data are limited, but suggest that an early exposure to cow's milk in relatives with HLA-DR3/4,DQB1*0302, DR3/3 or DRx/4,DQB1*0302 is not associated with development of β-cell autoantibodies[109]. It is unclear whether other genes are involved.

REMISSION ("HONEYMOON PERIOD")

Shortly after clinical onset, most of the patients experience a transient fall in insulin requirements due to improving β-cell function. Total and partial remissions have been reported in, respectively, 2-12% and 18-62% of young type 1 diabetes patients[25] age and less severe initial presentation of diabetes[110] and low or absent ICA[110] or IA-2 have been consistently associated with deeper and longer remission. Evidence relating GAD autoantibodies,[110] non-Caucasian origin, HLA-DR3 allele, female gender and family history of type 1 diabetes to a less severe presentation, greater frequency of remission and slower deterioration of insulin secretion is inconclusive. Most studies,[111] but not all[112] agree that preserved β-cell function is associated with better glycemic control (lower HbA_{1c}) and preserved α-cell glucagon response to hypoglycemia.[113] The prevalence of ICA (but not GAA) decreases from 87% at the time of type 1 diabetes diagnosis to 38-62% 2-3 years later,[114] faster in young boys, subjects lacking HLA-DR3 and 4, and those diagnosed between July and December.[115]

The natural remission is always temporary, ending with a gradual or abrupt increase in exogenous insulin requirements. Destruction of β-cells is complete within 3 years of diagnosis in most young children, especially those with the HLA DR3/4 phenotype.[116] It is much slower and often only partial in older patients[117], 15% of whom have still some β-cell function preserved 10 years after diagnosis.[118]

ESTABLISHED DIABETES

Complications. Acute complications of type 1 diabetes, such as DKA, and hypoglycemia and infections, are described in detail in other chapters. The risk of hospital admission for acute complication is 30/100 patient-years (p-yrs) in the first year of the disease and 20/100 p-yrs in the subsequent 3 years.[25] An estimated 26% of the patients have at least one episode of severe hypoglycemia within the initial 4 years of diagnosis, with little relation to the demographic or socioeconomical factors. The incidence of severe hypoglycemic episodes varies between 6 and 20 per 100 person-years, depending on age, geographic location, and intensity of insulin treatment.[25]

Type 1 diabetes is the leading cause of end-stage renal disease, blindness and amputation and a major cause of cardiovascular disease and premature death in the general population.[119] The disease results in over $5 billion in medical care expenditures per year, with costs for patients over 10 times that for non-diabetics.[120] These aspects of type 1 diabetes are highlighted in other chapters of this book.

Mortality. Insulin treatment dramatically prolongs survival but it does not cure diabetes. Although the absolute mortality at onset and within the first 20 years of type 1 diabetes is low (3-6%), it is 5 times higher for diabetic males and 12 times higher for diabetic females, compared to the general population.[121] This excess mortality is lowest in Scandinavia, intermediate in the U.S. and highest in countries where type 1 diabetes is rare, e.g. Japan,[122,123] probably due to a combination of the quality of care and access. Even in Finland, at least a half of the death is due to currently preventable causes such as acute complications, infections and suicide.[124] On the other hand, 40% of the patients survive over 40 years and a half of these have no major complications. Survival and avoidance of complications has been related to better metabolic control,[125] however, genetic factors also appear to be involved. Inconsistent associations have been reported between diabetic nephropathy and HLA-DR4[126] and several genes involved in blood pressure regulation.[127] Polymorphisms of paraoxonase[128] and A-IV[129] appear to play an important role in development of coronary artery disease in type 2 diabetes patients, but have not been extensively studied in persons with type 1 diabetes.

PREVENTION

The high incidence, associated severe morbidity, mortality, and enormous health care expenditures make type 1 diabetes a prime target for prevention. Unfortunately, many attempts to modify the natural history of events leading to clinical diabetes (primary prevention) have been unsuccessful, so far. More invasive interventions in persons with newly diagnosed diabetes, to induce deep and lasting remission (secondary prevention) have also been largely futile. At the time this book is written, new generation of preventive efforts is being launched through the NIH-funded TrialNet, Immunotolerance Network, Trial to Reduce Insulin-Dependent Diabetes in the Genetically at Risk (TRIGR), and other initiatives.

Primary prevention of β-cell autoimmunity

Prevention of diabetogenic viral infection. In mice, it is possible to prevent encephalomyocarditis virus-induced diabetes by immunization with a nondiabetogenic variant of the virus.[130] The interactions between HLA, antigen and T-cell receptor as well as the genetic determinants of viral diabetogenecity are being disentangled. It may become possible to design recombinant vaccines that would provide optimal antigenic stimulus in the context of the host's HLA leading to a long-term protection against diabetogenic strains. Approaches alternative to vaccination include antiviral agents.[131]

Dietary factors If early exposure to cow's milk triggers β-cell autoimmunity in humans, a logical primary prevention would include avoidance of cow's milk, especially in those with type 1 diabetes associated HLA alleles. Such an intervention has been piloted in newborn relatives of type 1 diabetes patients[101] and a large multiceneter trial (TRIGR) is underway.

Primary prevention of type 1 diabetes in persons with β-cell autoimmunity

ICA positive relatives of type 1 diabetes patients have become the primary target of clinical trials to prevent type 1 diabetes.[132] The effectiveness of oral nicotinamide[133] is being tested in the European Nicotinamide Diabetes Intervention Tiral Group (ENDIT) study[134] (results expected in 2002), but smaller studies[135] have not been promising. Preliminary results of a pilot trial with parenteral insulin[136] gave impetus to a large randomized unmasked trial of low-dose subcutaenous or intravenous insulin in relatives with confirmed ICA positivity and low acute insulin response to intravenous glucose (Diabetes Prevention Trial-1). The results of this trial were announced in 2000, but unfortunately showed no efficacy of insulin injections in preventing or delaying diabetes onset. The oral insulin arm of the DPT-1 is in progress, but results of smaller studies in newly diagnosed patients have not been encouraging.[137] Studies involving induction of tolerance to insulin or GAD using altered peptide ligands are at the stage of in phase II clinical trails.

Secondary prevention in new onset type 1 diabetes patients

A number of placebo controlled randomized trials using azathioprine, cyclosporin A, nicotinamide, prednisone and other immunosupressive agents have attempted to increase the rate and the duration of type 1 diabetes remission. Some of these interventions were associated with significant adverse effects [138]. Only cyclosporin A has been shown to be partially effective, inducing total remission in 25-40% and sustaining it for one year in 18-24% of newly diagnosed patients, compared to 0-10% in the placebo group.[139] However, the drug is nephrotoxic, of little value in children, and effective for only as long as it is administered,[140] rendering this approach to secondary prevention of type 1 diabetes unacceptable. Trials using intensive insulin treatment,[141] oral insulin,[137] or immunomodulation[142] have been even less successful than cyclosporine A trails. Recent ideas to be tested trough the TrialNet include humanized anti-CD3 antibodies,[143] mycophenolate mofetil,[144] and daclizumab.[145]

SUMMARY

Type 1 diabetes can be diagnosed at any age, but clinical course, genetic, and environmental determinants appear to be heterogenous by age. The common pathway begins with pre-clinical β-cell autoimmunity with progressive defect of insulin secretion, followed by onset of hyperglycemia, transient and usually partial remission, and finally complete insulinopenia associated with acute and chronic complications and premature death. Current research effort is focused on identification of the genetic and environmental determinants of this process and the ways they interact. Numerous attempts at prevention of type 1 diabetes have failed, but new promising approaches are under evaluation.

REFERENCES

1. Rewers M. The changing face of the epidemiology of insulin-dependent diabetes mellitus (IDDM): Research designs and models of disease causation. Ann Med 23:419-426, 1991.
2. Rewers M, LaPorte RE, King H, Tuomilehto J. Trends in the prevalence and incidence of diabetes: insulin-dependent diabetes mellitus in childhood. World Health Stat Q 41:179- 189, 1988.
3. American Diabetes Association. Report of the Expert Committee on the Diagnosis and Classification of Diabetes Mellitus. Diabetes Care 20:1183-1197, 1997.
4. Atkinson MAEisenbarth GS. Type 1 Diabetes: New Perspectives on Disease Pathogenesis and Treatment. Lancet 2000.

5. Imagawa A, Hanafusa T, Miyagawa J, Matsuzawa Y. A novel subtype of type 1 diabetes mellitus characterized by a rapid onset and an absence of diabetes-related antibodies. Osaka IDDM Study Group. New Engl J Med 342:301-307, 2000.

6. Bottazzo GF, Florin-Christensen A, Doniach D. Islet-cell antibodies in diabetes mellitus with autoimmune polyendocrine deficiencies. Lancet 2:1279-1283, 1974.

7. Williams AJK, Bingley PJ, Bonifacio E, Palmer JP, Gale EAM. A novel micro-assay for insulin autoantibodies. J Autoimmun 10:473-478, 1997.

8. Baekkeskov S, Aanstoot H-J, Christgau S, Reetz A, Solimena M, Cascalho M, Folli F, Richter-Olesen H, DeCamilli P. Identification of the 64K autoantigen in insulin-dependent diabetes as the GABA-synthesizing enzyme glutamic acid decarboxylase [published erratum appears in Nature 1990 Oct 25;347(6295):782]. Nature 347:151-156, 1990.

9. Rabin DU, Pleasic SM, Shapiro JA, Yoo-Warren H, Oles J, Hicks JM, Goldstein DE, Rae PM. Islet cell antigen 512 is a diabetes-specific islet autoantigen related to protein tyrosine phosphatases. J Immunol 152:3183-3188, 1994.

10. Verge CF, Gianani R, Kawasaki E, Yu L, Pietropaolo M, Jackson RA, Chase HP, Eisenbarth GS. Prediction of type I diabetes in first-degree relatives using a combination of insulin, GAD, and ICA512bdc/IA-2 autoantibodies. Diabetes 45:926- 933, 1996.

11. Bingley PJ, Bonifacio E, Williams AJ, Genovese S, Bottazzo GF, Gale, EA. Prediction of IDDM in the general population: strategies based on combinations of autoantibody markers. Diabetes 46:1701-1710, 1997.

12. Bonifacio E, Bingley PJ, Shattock M, Dean BM , Dunger D, Gale EAM, Bottazzo GF. Quantification of islet-cell antibodies and prediction of insulin-dependent diabetes. Lancet 335:147-149, 1990.

13. McCulloch DKPalmer JP. The appropriate use of B-cell function testing in the preclinical period of Type 1 diabetes. Diabetic Med 8:800-804, 1991.

14. Johnston C, Millward BA, Hoskins P, Leslie RD, Bottazzo GF, Pyke DA. Islet-cell antibodies as predictors of the later development of type 1 (insulin-dependent) diabetes. A study in identical twins. Diabetologia 32:382-386, 1989.

15. Yu J, Yu L, Bugawan TL, Erlich HA, Barriga K, Hoffman M, Rewers M, Eisenbarth GS. Transient anti-islet autoantibodies: infrequent occurrence and lack of association with genetic risk factors. J Clin Endocrinol Metab 85:2421-2428, 2000.

16. Yu J, Yu L, Bugawan TL, Erlich HA, Barriga K, Hoffman M, Rewers M, Eisenbarth GS. Transient anti-islet autoantibodies: infrequent occurrence and lack of association with genetic risk factors. J Clin Endocrinol Metab 85:2421-2428, 2000.

17. Tuomi T, Groop LC, Zimmet PZ, Rowley MJ, Knowles W, Mackay IR. Antibodies to glutamic acid decarboxylase reveal latent autoimmune diabetes mellitus in adults with a non-insulin- dependent onset of disease. Diabetes 42:359-362, 1993.

18. Zimmet PZ, Tuomi T, Mackay IR, Rowley MJ, Knowles W, Cohen M, Lang DA. Latent autoimmune diabetes mellitus in adults (LADA): the role of antibodies to glutamic acid decarboxylase in diagnosis and prediction of insulin dependency. Diabet Med 11:299-303, 1994.

19. Bottazzo GF, Florin-Christensen A, Doniach D. Islet-cell antibodies in diabetes mellitus with autoimmune polyendocrine deficiencies. Lancet 2:1279-1283, 1974.

20. Levy-Marchal C, Papoz L, de Beaufort C, Doutreix J, Froment V, Voirin J, Czernichow P. Clinical and laboratory features of type I diabetic children at time of diagnosis. Diabetic Med 9:279-284, 1992.

21. Eberhardt MS, Wagener DK, Orchard TJ, LaPorte RE, Cavender DE, Rabin BS, Atchison RW, Kuller LH, Drash AL, Becker DJ. HLA heterogeneity of insulin-dependent diabetes mellitus at diagnosis. The Pittsburgh IDDM Study. Diabetes 34:1247-1252, 1985.

22. Foulis AK, Liddle CN, Farquharson MA, Richmond JA, Weir RS. The histopathology of the pancreas in type I diabetes (insulin dependent) mellitus: a 25-year review of deaths in patients under 20 years of age in the United Kingdom. Diabetologia 29:267-274, 1986.

23. Childhood Diabetes Research Committee Ministry of Health and Welfare-Japan, Polish Diabetes Research Group - Poznan, The Netherlands Institute for Preventive Health Care – Leiden, Diabetes Research Center of Pittsburgh, Pennsylvania. How frequently do children die at the onset of insulin-dependent diabetes? Analyses of registry data from Japan, Poland, the Netherlands, and Allegheny County, Pennsylvania. Diab Nutr Metab 3:57-62, 1990.

24. Kostraba JN, Gay EC, Rewers M, Chase HP, Klingensmith GJ, Hamman RF. Increasing trend of outpatient management of children with newly diagnosed IDDM. Colorado IDDM registry, 1978-88. Diabetes Care 15:95- 100, 1992.

25. Pinkney JH, Bingley PJ, Sawtell PA, Dunger DB, Gale EAM, The Bart's-Oxford Study Group. Presentation and progress of childhood diabetes mellitus: A prospective population-based study. Diabetologia 37:70-74, 1994.

26. Karvonen M, Viik-Kajander M, Moltchanova E, Libman I, LaPorte R, Tuomilehto J. Incidence of childhood type 1 diabetes worldwide. Diabetes Mondiale (DiaMond) Project Group. Diabetes Care 23:1516-1526, 2000.

27. Rewers M, Kostraba JN. Epidemiology of type I diabetes. In *Type 1 diabetes: molecular, cellular, and clinical immunology.* Eisenbarth GS, Lafferty KJ, eds., Oxford University Press, 9:172-208, 1996.

28. Pilcher CC, Dickens K, Elliott RB. ICA only develop in early childhood. Diabetes Res Clin Pract 14(Suppl. 1):s82-s82, 1991.

29. Rewers M, Stone RA, LaPorte RE, Drash AL, Becker DJ, Walczak M, Kuller LH. Poisson regression modeling of temporal variation in incidence of childhood insulin-dependent diabetes mellitus in Allegheny County, Pennsylvania, and Wielkopolska, Poland, 1970-1985. Am J Epidemiol 129:569-581, 1989.

30. Rosenbloom AL, Joe JR, Young RS, Winter WE. Emerging epidemic of type 2 diabetes in youth. Diabetes Care 22:345-354, 1999.

31. Dabelea D, Hanson RL, Bennett PH, Roumain J , Knowler WC, Pettitt DJ. Increasing prevalence of Type II diabetes in American Indian children. Diabetologia 41:904-910, 1998.

32. Joner GSovik O. The incidence of type 1 (insulin-dependent) diabetes mellitus 15- 29 years in Norway 1978-1982. Diabetologia 34:271-274, 1991.

33. Christau B, Kromann H, Andersen OO, Christy M, Buschard K, Arnung K, Kristensen IH, Peitersen B, Steinrud J, Nerup J. Incidence, seasonal and geographic patterns of juvenile-onset insulin-dependent diabetes mellitus is Denmark. Diabetologia 13(4):281-284, 1977.

34. Turner R, Stratton I, Horton V, Manley S, Zimmet P, Mackay IR, Shattock M, Bottazzo GF, Holman R. UKPDS 25: autoantibodies to islet-cell cytoplasm and glutamic acid decarboxylase for prediction of insulin requirement in type 2 diabetes. UK Prospective Diabetes Study Group [published erratum appears in Lancet 1998 Jan 31;351(9099):376]. Lancet 350:1288-1293, 1997.

35. Horton V, Stratton I, Bottazzo GF, Shattock M, Mackay I, Zimmet P, Manley S, Holman R, Turner R. Genetic heterogeneity of autoimmune diabetes: age of presentation in adults is influenced by HLA DRB1 and DQB1 genotypes (UKPDS 43). UK Prospective Diabetes Study (UKPDS) Group. Diabetologia 42:608-616, 1999.

36. Diabetes Epidemiology Research International Group. Geographic patterns of childhood insulin-dependent diabetes mellitus. Diabetes 37:1113-1119, 1988.

37. Kostraba JN, Gay EC, Cai Y, Cruickshanks KJ, Rewers MJ, Klingensmith GJ, Chase HP, Hamman RF. Incidence of insulin-dependent diabetes mellitus in Colorado. Epidemiology 3:232-238, 1992.

38. Siemiatycki J, Colle E, Campbell S, Dewar RA , Belmonte MM. Case-control study of IDDM. Diabetes Care 12:209-216, 1989.

39. Zimmet PZ, Rowley MJ, Mackay IR, Knowles WJ , Chen QY, Chapman LH, Serjeantson SW. The ethnic distribution of antibodies to glutamic acid decarboxylase: presence and levels of insulin-dependent diabetes mellitus in Europid and Asian subjects. J Diabetes Complications 7:1-7, 1993.

40. Gale EAGillespie KM. Diabetes and gender. Diabetologia 44:3-15, 2001.

41. Diabetes Epidemiology Research International Group. Geographic patterns of childhood insulin-dependent diabetes mellitus. Diabetes 37:1113-1119, 1988.

42. Bruno G, Merletti F, Vuolo A, Pisu E, Giorio M, Pagano G. Sex differences in incidence of IDDM in age group 15-29 yr. Higher risk in males in Province of Turin, Italy. Diabetes Care 16(1):133-136, 1993.

43. Gamble DR. The epidemiology of insulin-dependent diabetes, with particular reference to the relationship of virus infection to its etiology. Epidemiol Rev 2:49-70, 1980.

44. Kostraba JN, Gay EC, Cai Y, Cruickshanks KJ, Rewers MJ, Klingensmith GJ, Chase HP, Hamman RF. Incidence of insulin-dependent diabetes mellitus in Colorado. Epidemiology 3:232-238, 1992.

45. Ludvigsson JAfoke AO. Seasonality of type 1 (insulin-dependent) diabetes mellitus: values of C-peptide, insulin antibodies and haemoglobin A_{1c} show evidence of a more rapid loss of insulin secretion in epidemic patients. Diabetologia 32:84-91, 1989.

46. Diabetes Epidemiology Research International Group. Secular trends in incidence of childhood IDDM in 10 countries. Diabetes 39:858-864, 1990.

47. Nystrom L, Dahlquist G, Rewers M, Wall S. The Swedish childhood diabetes study: an analysis of the temporal variation in diabetes incidence, 1978-1987. Int J Epidemiol 19:141-146, 1990.

48. Karvonen M, Pitkaniemi J, Tuomilehto J. The onset age of type 1 diabetes in Finnish children has become younger. The Finnish Childhood Diabetes Registry Group. Diabetes Care 22:1066-1070, 1999.

49. Cordell HJTodd JA. Multifactorial inheritance in type 1 diabetes. [Review]. Trends Genet 11:499-504, 1995.

50. Allen C, Palta M, D'Alessio DJ. Risk of diabetes in siblings and other relatives of IDDM subjects. Diabetes 40:831-836, 1991.

51. Lorenzen T, Pociot F, Hougaard P, Nerup J. Long-term risk of IDDM in first-degree relatives of patients with IDDM. Diabetologia 37:321-327, 1994.

52. O'Leary LA, Dorman JS, LaPorte RE, Orchard TJ, Becker DJ, Kuller LH, Eberhardt MS, Cavender DE, Rabin BS, Drash AL. Familial and sporadic insulin-dependent diabetes: Evidence for heterogeneous etiologies? Diab Res Clin Pract 14:183-190, 1991.

53. Erlich HA, Griffith RL, Bugawan TL, Ziegler R, Alper C, Eisenbarth G. Implication of specific DQB1 alleles in genetic susceptibility and resistance by identification of IDDM siblings with novel HLA-DQB1 allele and unusual DR2 and DR1 haplotypes. Diabetes 40:478-481, 1991.

54. Rewers M, Bugawan TL, Norris JM, Blair A, Beaty B, Hoffman M, McDuffie RS, Hamman RF, Klingensmith G, Eisenbarth GS, Erlich HA. Newborn screening for HLA markers associated with IDDM: Diabetes Autoimmunity Study in the Young (DAISY). Diabetologia 39:807-812, 1996.

55. Greenbaum CJ, Cuthbertson D, Eisenbarth GS, Schatz DA, Zeidler A, Krischer JP. Islet cell antibody positive relatives with HLA-DQA1*0102, DQB1*0602: Identification by the Diabetes Prevention Trial-1. J Clin Endocrinol Metab 85:1255-1260, 2000.

56. Chase HP, Voss MA, Butler-Simon N, Hoops S, O'Brien D, Dobersen MJ. Diagnosis of pre-type I diabetes. J Pediatr 111:807-812, 1987.

57. Levy-Marchal C, Tichet J, Fajardy I, Dubois F, Czernichow P. Follow-up of children from a background population with high ICA titres. Diabetologia 35 Suppl 1:A32-A32, 1992.

58. Cox NJ, Wapelhorst B, Morrison VA, Johnson L, Pinchuk L, Spielman RS, Todd JA, Concannon P. Seven regions of the genome show evidence of linkage to type 1 diabetes in a consensus analysis of 767 multiplex families. Am J Hum Genet 69:820-830, 2001.

59. Kaprio J, Tuomilehto J, Koskenvuo M, Romanov K, Reunanen A, Eriksson J, Stengard J, Kesaniemi YA. Concordance for type 1 (insulin-dependent) and type 2 (non-insulin-dependent) diabetes mellitus in a population-based cohort of twins in Finland. Diabetologia 35:1060-1067, 1992.

60. Pak CY, Hyone-Myong E, McArthur RG, Yoon JW. Association of cytomegalovirus infection with autoimmune type 1 diabetes. Lancet 2:1-3, 1988.

61. Hyoty H, Hiltunen M, Reunanen A, Leinikki P, Vesikari T, Lounamaa R, Tuomilehto J, Akerblom HK. Decline of mumps antibodies in type 1 (insulin-dependent) diabetic children and a plateau in the rising incidence of type 1 diabetes after introduction of the mumps-measles-rubella vaccine in Finland. Childhood Diabetes in Finland Study Group. Diabetologia 36:1303-1308, 1993.

62. Ginsberg-Fellner F, Witt ME, Yagihashi S, Dobersen MJ, Taub F, Fedun B, Mcevoy RC, Roman SH, Davies RG, Cooper LZ, et al. Congenital rubella syndrome as a model for type 1 (insulin-dependent) diabetes mellitus: increased prevalence of islet cell surface antibodies. Diabetologia 27 Suppl:87-89, 1984.

63. Conrad B, Weidmann E, Trucco G, Rudert WA, Behboo R, Ricordi C, Rodriquez-Rilo H, Finegold D, Trucco M. Evidence for superantigen involvement in insulin-dependent diabetes mellitus aetiology. Nature 371:351- 355, 1994.

64. Honeyman MC, Coulson BS, Stone NL, Gellert SA, Goldwater PN, Steele CE, Couper JJ, Tait BD, Colman PG, Harrison LC. Association between rotavirus infection and pancreatic islet autoimmunity in children at risk of developing type 1 diabetes. Diabetes 49:1319-1324, 2000.

65. Oldstone MB, Nerenberg M, Southern P, Price J, Lewicki H. Virus infection triggers insulin-dependent diabetes mellitus in a transgenic model: role of anti-self (virus) immune response. Cell 65:319-331, 1991.

66. Helmke K, Otten A, Willems WR, Brockhaus R, Mueller-Eckhardt G, Stief T, Bertrams J, Wolf H, Federlin K. Islet cell antibodies and the development of diabetes mellitus in relation to mumps infection and mumps vaccination. Diabetologia 29:30-33, 1986.

67. Bodansky HJ, Dean BM, Bottazzo GF, Grant PJ , McNally J, Hambling MH. Islet-cell antibodies and insulin autoantibodies in association with common viral infections. Lancet Dec 13:1351-1353, 1986.

68. Champsaur HF, Bottazzo GF, Bertrams J, Assan R, Bach C. Virologic, immunologic, and genetic factors in insulin-dependent diabetes mellitus. J Pediatr 100:15-20, 1982.

69. Blom L, Nystrom L, Dahlquist G. The Swedish childhood diabetes study. Vaccinations and infections as risk determinants for diabetes in childhood. Diabetologia 34:176-181, 1991.

70. Menser MA, Forrest JM, Bransby RD. Rubella infection and diabetes mellitus. Lancet 1:57-60, 1978.

71. Karounos DG, Wolinsky JS, Thomas JW. Monoclonal antibody to rubella virus capsid protein recognizes a β-cell antigen. J Immunol 150 :3080-3085, 1993.

72. Rewers M, Atkinson M. The possible role of enteroviruses in diabetes mellitus. 353-385, 1996.

73. Graves PM, Norris JM, Pallansch MA, Gerling IC, Rewers M. The role of enteroviral infections in the development of IDDM: limitations of current approaches. Diabetes 46: 161-168, 1997.

74. Jenson AB, Rosenberg HS, Notkins AL. Pancreatic islet-cell damage in children with fatal viral infections. Lancet Aug 16:354-358, 1980.

75. Wagenknecht LE, Roseman JM, Herman WH. Increased incidence of insulin-dependent diabetes mellitus following an epidemic of coxsackievirus B5. Am J Epidemiol 133:1024-1031, 1991.

76. Kaufman DL, Clare-Salzler M, Tian J, Forsthuber T, Ting GS, Robinson P, Atkinson MA, Sercarz EE, Tobin AJ, Lehmann PV. Spontaneous loss of T-cell tolerance to glutamic acid decarboxylase in murine insulin-dependent diabetes [see comments]. Nature 366:69-72, 1993.

77. Scherbaum WA, Hampl W, Muir P, Gluck M, Seibler J, Egle H, Hauner H, Boehm BO, Heinze E, Banatvala JE, Pfeiffer EF . No association between islet cell antibodies and coxsackie B, mumps, rubella and cytomegalovirus antibodies in non-diabetic individuals aged 7-19 years. Diabetologia 34:835-838, 1991.

78. Lonnrot M, Korpela K, Knip M, Ilonen J, Simell O, Korhonen S, Savola K, Muona P, Simell T, Koskela P, Hyoty H. Enterovirus infection as a risk factor for beta-cell autoimmunity in a prospectively observed birth cohort: the Finnish Diabetes Prediction and Prevention Study. Diabetes 49:1314-1318, 2000.

79. Hyoty H, Hiltunen M, Knip M, Laakkonen M, Vahasalo P, Karjalainen J, Koskela P, Roivainen M, Leinikki P, Hovi T, . A prospective study of the role of coxsackie B and other enterovirus infections in the pathogenesis of IDDM. Childhood Diabetes in Finland (DiMe) Study Group. Diabetes 44:652-657, 1995.

80. Dahlquist G, Frisk G, Ivarsson SA, Svanberg L, Forsgren M, Diderholm H. Indications that maternal coxsackie B virus infection during pregnancy is a risk factor for childhood-onset IDDM. Diabetologia 38:1371-1373, 1995.

81. McKinney PA, Parslow R, Gurney KA, Law GR, Bodansky HJ, Williams R. Perinatal and neonatal determinants of childhood type 1 diabetes. A case-control study in Yorkshire, U.K. Diabetes Care 22:928-932, 1999.

82. Rothwell PM, Staines A, Smail P, Wadsworth E , McKinney P. Seasonality of birth of patients with childhood diabetes in Britain. BMJ 312:1456-1457, 1996.

83. Wilberz S, Partke HJ, Dagnaes-Hansen F, Herberg L. Persistent MHV (mouse hepatitis virus) infection reduces the incidence of diabetes mellitus in non-obese diabetic mice. Diabetologia 34:2-5, 1991.

84. McKinney PA, Okasha M, Parslow RC, Law GR, Gurney KA, Williams R, Bodansky HJ. Early social mixing and childhood Type 1 diabetes mellitus: a case- control study in Yorkshire, UK. Diabet Med 17:236-242, 2000.

85. Infections and vaccinations as risk factors for childhood type I (insulin-dependent) diabetes mellitus: a multicentre case-control investigation. EURODIAB Substudy 2 Study Group. Diabetologia 43:47-53, 2000.

86. Graves PM, Barriga KJ, Norris JM, Hoffman MR , Yu L, Eisenbarth GS, Rewers M. Lack of association between early childhood immunizations and beta-cell autoimmunity. Diabetes Care 22:1694-1697, 1999.

87. Atkinson MA, Winter WE, Skordis N, Beppu H, Riley WM, Maclaren NK. Dietary protein restriction reduces the frequency and delays the onset of insulin dependent diabetes in BB rats. Autoimmunity 2:11-20, 1988.

88. Martin JM, Trink B, Daneman D, Dosch H-M, Robinson B. Milk proteins in the etiology of insulin-dependent diabetes mellitus (IDDM). Ann Med 23:447-452, 1991.

89. Couper JJ, Steele C, Beresford S, Powell T , McCaul K, Pollard A, Gellert S, Tait B, Harrison LC, Colman PG. Lack of association between duration of breast-feeding or introduction of cow's milk and development of islet autoimmunity. Diabetes 48:2145-2149, 1999.

90. Borch-Johnsen K, Joner G, Mandrup-Poulsen T, Christy M, Zachau-Christiansen B, Kastrup K, Nerup J. Relation between breast-feeding and incidence rates of insulin-dependent diabetes mellitus. Lancet 2:1083-1086, 1984.

91. Mayer EJ, Hamman RF, Gay EC, Lezotle DC, Savitz DA, Klingensmith GJ. Reduced risk of IDDM among breast-fed children. The Colorado IDDM Registry. Diabetes 37:1625-1632, 1988.

92. Nigro G, Campea L, De Novellis A, Orsini M. Breast-feeding and insulin-dependent diabetes mellitus. Lancet 1:467 (Letter)-1985.

93. Kyvik KO, Green A, Svendsen A, Mortensen K. Breast feeding and the development of type I diabetes mellitus. Diabetic Med 9:233-235, 1992.

94. Virtanen SM, Rasanen L, Aro A, Ylonen K, Lounamaa R, Tuomilehto J, Akerblom HK, the 'Childhood Diabetes in Finland' Study Group. Feeding in infancy and the risk of type 1 diabetes mellitus in Finnish children. Diabetic Med 9:815-819, 1992.

95. Gerstein HC. Cow's milk exposure and type I diabetes mellitus - a critical overview of the clinical literature. Diabetes Care 17:13-19, 1994.

96. Norris JMScott FW. A meta-analysis of infant diet and insulin-dependent diabetes mellitus: do biases play a role? Epidemiology 7:87-92, 1996.

97. Savilahti E, Akerblom HK, Tainio VM, Koskimies S. Children with newly diagnosed insulin dependent diabetes mellitus have incresed levels of cow's milk antibodies. Diabetes Res 7:137-140, 1988.

98. Karjalainen J, Martin JM, Knip M, Ilonen J, Robinson BH, Savilahti E, Akerblom HK, Dosch HM. A bovine albumin peptide as a possible trigger of insulin- dependent diabetes mellitus [see comments]. N Engl J Med 327:302-307, 1992.

99. Hummel M, Fuchtenbusch M, Schenker M, Ziegler AG. No major association of breast-feeding, vaccinations, and childhood viral diseases with early islet autoimmunity in the German BABYDIAB Study. Diabetes Care 23 :969-974, 2000.

100. Virtanen SM, Laara E, Hypponen E, Reijonen H, Rasanen L, Aro A, Knip M, Ilonen J, Akerblom HK. Cow's milk consumption, HLA-DQB1 genotype, and type 1 diabetes: a nested case-control study of siblings of children with diabetes. Childhood diabetes in Finland study group [In Process Citation]. Diabetes 49:912-917, 2000.

101. Paronen J, Knip M, Savilahti E, Virtanen SM, Ilonen J, Akerblom HK, Vaarala O. Effect of cow's milk exposure and maternal type 1 diabetes on cellular and humoral immunization to dietary insulin in infants at genetic risk for type 1 diabetes. Finnish Trial to Reduce IDDM in the Genetically at Risk Study Group. Diabetes 49:1657-1665, 2000.

102. Elias D, Prigozin H, Polak N, Rapoport M, Lohse AW, Cohen IR. Autoimmune diabetes induced by the beta-cell toxin STZ. Immunity to the 60-kDa heat shock protein and to insulin. Diabetes 43:992-998, 1994.

103. Rayfield EJIshimura K. Environmetal factors and insulin dependent diabetes mellitus. Diabetes Metab Rev 3:925-957, 1987.

104. Dahlquist GG, Blom LG, Persson L-Å, Sandström AIM, Wall SGI. Dietary factors and the risk of developing insulin dependent diabetes in childhood. Br Med J 300:1302-1306, 1990.

105. Toniolo A, Onodera T, Yoon JW, Notkins AL. Induction of diabetes by cumulative environmental insults from viruses and chemicals. Nature 288:383-385, 1980.

106. Khoury MJ, Flanders WD, Greenland S, Adams MJ. On the measurement of susceptibility in epidemiologic studies. Am J Epidemiol 129:183-190, 1989.

107. Fohlman J, Bohme J, Rask L, Frisk G, Diderholm H, Friman G, Tuvemo T. Matching of host genotype and serotypes of Coxsackie B virus in the development of juvenile diabetes. Scand J Immunol 26:105-110, 1987.

108. Kostraba JN, Cruickshanks KJ, Lawler-Heavner J, Jobim LF, Rewers MJ, Gay EC , Chase HP, Klingensmith G, Hamman RF. Early exposure to cow's milk and solid foods in infancy, genetic predisposition and risk of IDDM. Diabetes 42:288-295, 1993.

109. Norris JM, Beaty B, Klingensmith G, Yu L, Hoffman M, Chase HP, Erlich HA, Hamman RF, Eisenbarth GS, Rewers M. Lack of association between early exposure to cow's milk protein and β-cell autoimmunity: Diabetes Autoimmunity Study in the Young (DAISY). JAMA 276:609-614, 1996.

110. Ortqvist E, Falorni A, Scheynius A, Persson B, Lernmark A. Age governs gender-dependent islet cell autoreactivity and predicts the clinical course in childhood IDDM. Acta Paediatr 86 :1166-1171, 1997.

111. Wallensteen M, Dahlquist G, Persson B, Landin-Olsson M, Lernmark A, Sundkvist G, Thalme B. Factors influencing the magnitude, duration, and rate of fall of B-cell function in Type I (insulin-dependent) diabetic children followed for two years from their clinical diagnosis. Diabetologia 31:664-669, 1988.

112. Agner T, Damm P, Binder C. Remission in IDDM: prospective study of basal C-peptide and insulin dose in 268 consecutive patients. Diabetes Care 10:164-169, 1987.

113. Fukuda M, Tanaka A, Tahara Y, Ikegami H, Yamamoto Y, Kumahara Y, Shima K. Correlation between minimal secretory capacity of pancreatic beta-cells and stability of diabetic control. Diabetes 37:81-88, 1988.

114. Schiffrin A, Suissa S, Poussier P, Guttmann R, Weitzner G. Prospective study of predictors of beta-cell survival in type I diabetes. Diabetes 37:920-925, 1988.

115. Kolb H, Dannehl K, Gruenklee D, Zielasek J, Bertrams J, Hubinger A, Gries FA. Prospective analysis of islet cell antibodies in children with type I (insulin-dependent) diabetes. Diabetologia 31:189-194, 1988.

116. Knip M, Llonen J, Mustonen A, Akerblom HK. Evidence of an accelerated B-cell destruction in HLA-Dw3/Dw4 heterozygous children with type I (insulin-dependent) diabetes. Diabetologia 29:347-351, 1986.

117. Pipeleers DLing Z. Pancreatic beta cells in insulin-dependent diabetes. Diabetes Metab Rev 8:209-227, 1992.

118. Madsbad S, Faber OK, Binder C, McNair P, Christiansen C, Transbol I. Prevalence of residual beta-cell function in insulin-dependent diabetics in relation to age at onset and duration of diabetes. Diabetes 27(Suppl. 1):262-264, 1978.

119. WHO Study Group. Diabetes Mellitus - Technical Report Series 727. 1985.

120. Songer TJ. Health services and costing in diabetes. Med J Aust 152:115-117, 1990.

121. Dorman JS, LaPorte RE, Kuller LH, Cruickshanks KJ, Orchard TJ, Wagener DK, Becker DJ, Cavender DE, Drash AL. The Pittsburgh insulin-dependent diabetes mellitus (IDDM) morbidity and mortality study. Mortality results. Diabetes 33: 271-276, 1984.

122. Major cross-country differences in risk of dying for people with IDDM. Diabetes Epidemiology Research International Mortality Study Group. Diabetes Care 14:49-54, 1991.

123. Matsushima M, LaPorte RE, Maruyama M, Shimizu K, Nishimura R, Tajima N, for the DERI Mortality Study Group. Geographic variation in mortality among individuals with youth-onset diabetes mellitus across the world. Diabetologia 40:212-216, 1997.

124. International evaluation of cause-specific mortality and IDDM. Diabetes Epidemiology Research International Mortality Study Group. Diabetes Care 14:55-60, 1991.

125. Borch-Johnsen K, Nissen H, Henriksen E, Kreiner S, Salling N, Deckert T, Nerup J. The natural history of insulin-dependent diabetes mellitus in Denmark: 1. Long-term survival with and without late diabetic complications. Diabetic Med 4:201-210, 1987.

126. Chowdhury TA, Dyer PH, Mijovic CH, Dunger DB, Barnett AH, Bain SC. Human leucocyte antigen and insulin gene regions and nephropathy in Type I diabetes. Diabetologia 42:1017-1020, 1999.

127. Doria A, Onuma T, Gearin G, Freire MB, Warram JH, Krolewski AS. Angiotensinogen polymorphism M235T, hypertension, and nephropathy in insulin-dependent diabetes. Hypertension 27:1134-1139, 1996.

128. Garin MC, James RW, Dussoix P, Blanche H, Passa P, Froguel P, Ruiz, J. Paraoxonase polymorphism Met-Leu54 is associated with modified serum concentrations of the enzyme. A possible link between the paraoxonase gene and increased risk of cardiovascular disease in diabetes. J Clin Invest 99:62-66, 1997.

129. Rewers M, Kamboh MI, Hoag S, Shetterly SM, Ferrell RE, Hamman RF. Apolipoprotein A-IV polymorphism associated with myocardial infarction in obese NIDDM patients. The San Luis Valley Diabetes Study. Diabetes 43:1485-1489, 1994.

130. Notkins ALYoon JW. Virus-induced diabetes in mice prevented by a live attenuated vaccine. N Engl J Med 306:486-1982.

131. See DMTilles JG. WIN 54954 treatment of mice infected with a diabetogenic strain of group B coxsackievirus. Antimicrob Agents Chemother 37:1593-1598, 1993.

132. Eisenbarth GS, Verge CF, Allen H, Rewers MJ. The design of trials for prevention of IDDM. Diabetes 42:941 -947, 1993.

133. Gale EA. Theory and practice of nicotinamide trials in pre-type 1 diabetes. J Pediatr Endocrinol Metab 9:375-379, 1996.

134. Knip M, Douek IF, Moore WP, Gillmor HA, McLean AE, Bingley PJ, Gale EA. Safety of high-dose nicotinamide: a review. Diabetologia 43:1337-1345, 2000.

135. Lampeter EF, Klinghammer A, Scherbaum WA, Heinze E, Haastert B, Giani G, Kolb H. The Deutsche Nicotinamide Intervention Study: an attempt to prevent type 1 diabetes. DENIS Group. Diabetes 47:980-984, 1998.

136. Keller RJ, Eisenbarth GS, Jackson RA. Insulin prophylaxis in individuals at high risk of type I diabetes. Lancet 341:927-928, 1993.

137. Pozzilli P, Pitocco D, Visalli N, Cavallo MG, Buzzetti R, Crino A, Spera S, Suraci C, Multari G, Cervoni M, Manca BM, Matteoli MC, Marietti G, Ferrazzoli F, Cassone FM, Giordano C, Sbriglia M, Sarugeri E, Ghirlanda G. No effect of oral insulin on residual beta-cell function in recent-onset type I diabetes (the IMDIAB VII). IMDIAB Group [In Process Citation]. Diabetologia 43:1000-1004, 2000.

138. Lipton R, LaPorte RE, Becker DJ, Dorman JS, Orchard TJ, Atchison J, Drash AL. Cyclosporin therapy for prevention and cure of IDDM. Epidemiological perspective of benefits and risks. Diabetes Care 13:776-784, 1990.

139. Feutren G, Assan G, Karsenty G, DuRostu H , Sirmai J, Papoz L, Vialettes B, Vexiau P, Rodier M, Lallemand A, Bach JF. Cyclosporin increases the rate and length of remissions in insulin dependent diabetes of recent onset. Results of a multicentre double-blind trial. Lancet 2:119-124, 1986.

140. Martin S, Schernthaner G, Nerup J, Gries FA , Koivisto VA, Dupre J, Standl E, Hamet P, McArthur R, Tan MH, et al. Follow-up of cyclosporin A treatment in type 1 (insulin- dependent) diabetes mellitus: lack of long-term effects. Diabetologia 34:429-434, 1991.

141. Shah SC, Malone JI, Simpson NE. A randomized trial of intensive insulin therapy in newly diagnosed insulin-dependent diabetes mellitus. N Engl J Med 320:550-554, 1989.

142. Allen HF, Klingensmith GJ, Jensen P, Simoes E, Hayward A, Chase HP. Effect of BCG vaccination on new-onset insulin-dependent diabetes mellitus: A randomized clinical study. Diabetes Care 22:1703-1707, 1998.

143. Herold KC, Bluestone JA, Montag AG, Parihar A, Wiegner A, Gress RE, Hirsch R. Prevention of autoimmune diabetes with nonactivating anti-CD3 monoclonal antibody. Diabetes 41:385- 391, 1992.

144. Hao L, Chan S-M, Lafferty KJ. Mycophenolate mofetil can prevent the development of diabetes in BB rats. Ann NY Acad Sci 328-332 , 1993.

145. Vincenti F, Kirkman R, Light S, Blumgardner G, Pescovitz M, Halloran P, Neylan J, Wilkinson A, Ekberg H, Gaston R, Backman L, Burdick J, Daclizumab Triple Therapy Study Group. Interleukin-2-receptor blockade with daclizumab to prevent acute rejection in renal transplantation. N Engl J Med 338:161-165, 1998.

Chapter 2. Type 2 Diabetes Mellitus: Etiology, Pathogenesis and Clinical Manifestations

Yolanta T. Kruszynska

INTRODUCTION

Type 2 diabetes mellitus affects about 3% of the population or 100 million people worldwide. The prevalence is higher in Europe and the USA, affecting 5-7% of the population and is increasing. Many cases (30% or more) are undiagnosed. Although common, its pathogenesis remains unclear. There are many reasons for this. Perhaps the most important is the heterogeneity of type 2 diabetes due in part to a variable interplay between genetic and environmental factors. Although the diagnosis rests on documentation of hyperglycemia it is important to appreciate that other metabolic abnormalities, for example disturbances of lipid metabolism, are also present and may precede the emergence of hyperglycemia (see Chapter VI.11). As depicted in Figure 1, overt hyperglycemia and the syndrome of type 2 diabetes is due to a variable combination of insulin resistance affecting the liver and peripheral insulin target tissues and of impaired insulin secretion. Since insulin resistance and abnormalities of insulin secretion may be associated with other pathologies, for example liver disease, renal disease, glucocorticoid, growth hormone or thyroid hormone excess, diabetes may be secondary to these conditions (see Chapter V.5).

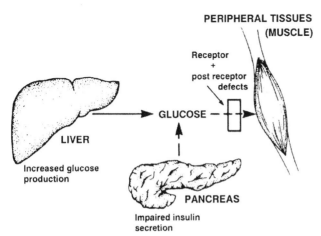

Figure 1. Metabolic abnormalities in type 2 diabetes that contribute to hyperglycemia.

ETIOLOGY OF TYPE 2 DIABETES MELLITUS

Genetic and environmental predictors of type 2 diabetes

Twin studies suggest that genetic makeup explains 60-90% of the susceptibility to type 2 diabetes. The concordance rate in monozygotic twins is 70-90% compared to only 15-25% in dizygotic twins. Because of the age-dependent penetrance of type 2 diabetes, the concordance rate in the monozygotic twin studies increases with age, approaching 100% with life-long follow-up. Type 2 diabetes and impaired glucose tolerance (IGT) cluster in families. Thus, most patients have a positive family history, and the lifetime risk for developing type 2 diabetes is increased up to 40% (more than five times the background rate) by having a first degree relative with the disease. If both parents have type 2 diabetes the risk to the offspring may be as high as 70%. Available evidence supports a polygenic mode of inheritance with a considerable environmental input.[1]

The striking ethnic variation in type 2 diabetes prevalence (see Chapter III.2) supports the importance of genetic factors: in the US the prevalence is 2 to 4 % in Caucasians, 4 to 6 % in American blacks, 10 to 15 % in Mexican-Americans, and 35 % in the Pima Indians in Arizona. In adult Pimas, over 75% of whom are obese, a positive family history of type 2 diabetes is a better predictor of the incidence of type 2 diabetes than the combined effects of obesity, gender and physical fitness.

Environmental influences interact with genetic factors to determine susceptibility to type 2 diabetes by affecting either insulin action, insulin secretion or both. The prevalence of type 2 diabetes has increased markedly in populations that have rapidly adopted a Western lifestyle (for example the Pima Indians) and in many populations that have migrated to regions with a more affluent lifestyle compared to their native country (see Chapter IV.2). Physical inactivity, obesity and dietary influences are all likely factors that may increase the risk of diabetes in a genetically predisposed individual.

Obesity is a strong independent risk factor, and the duration of obesity, is also highly predictive of type 2 diabetes. The distribution of the excess fat within the body is important. Thus, truncal obesity is more strongly associated with insulin resistance, and in several prospective studies measures of abdominal obesity such as the waist-hip ratio or the extent of intraabdominal fat accumulation as measured by computerized tomography have been found to be strong predictors of type 2 diabetes.[2,3] Sedentary persons are more likely to develop type 2 diabetes.[4] The antidiabetogenic effect of moderate regular physical activity is likely related to the beneficial effects on insulin action and prevention of obesity: the protective effect appears to be greatest in those at highest risk for type 2 diabetes such as obese subjects and those with a positive family history.

It is generally assumed, based largely on data from animal studies, that diets high in saturated fat and low in complex carbohydrates and soluble-fibre predispose not only to obesity but also to type 2 diabetes. The prevalence of obesity and diabetes in different populations is positively correlated with the dietary fat content.[5] However, this relationship is complicated because a high fat intake generally implies a high energy intake.[4] In most interventional studies, no change in insulin sensitivity is found when normal subjects are fed an isocaloric diet high in saturated fat compared to a low fat diet high in complex carbohydrates.[6,7] Some have, however, shown effects on insulin secretion and glucose tolerance.[7]

Natural history of type 2 diabetes

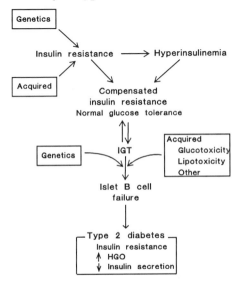

Figure. 2. Proposed etiology for the development of type 2 diabetes mellitus.

Type 2 diabetes evolves in stages (Figure 2). Whether insulin resistance or impaired insulin secretion is the primary abnormality or indeed whether both are independent primary defects has been hotly debated. A major difficulty in resolving the issue has been that insulin resistance can lead to abnormalities of insulin secretion and vice versa. The weight of evidence from prospective studies of high risk populations such as the Pima Indians, before they become hyperglycemic and develop secondary defects, and studies of non-diabetic first degree relatives of type 2 diabetic patients, suggests that in most populations those who develop type 2 diabetes begin with insulin resistance which is present when fasting plasma glucose and glucose tolerance are normal.[3,8,9] Thus, insulin resistance is thought to be an inherited initial defect in most patients (Figure 2). Factors such as obesity,

181

sedentary lifestyle, and aging may be additive. At this early stage fasting insulin levels and glucose-stimulated insulin responses are increased and sufficient to maintain normal glucose tolerance. Some subjects develop IGT. They too typically have increased fasting and postprandial insulin levels, but these do not fully compensate for insulin resistance. In some this is due to more marked insulin resistance, but in many it appears to be due to a poorer insulin response.[10] Eventually, compensation fails in some subjects, because islet β-cell function declines. Why this decline occurs is unclear; it may be due to genetic abnormalities affecting β-cell function, to acquired defects (such as glucotoxicity and lipotoxicity), or a combination of factors.

Abnormalities of hepatic glucose metabolism also become apparent during the transition from IGT to overt type 2 diabetes. Subjects with IGT may display hepatic insulin insensitivity but have normal basal rates of hepatic glucose output (HGO): HGO tends to increase at fasting glucose levels above 140 mg/dl.[11] Thus, excess glucose output by the liver is a contributory factor to the pathogenesis of hyperglycemia in type 2 diabetes.

The proportion of insulin resistant subjects who progress to type 2 diabetes varies between ethnic groups. In most populations the conversion rate from IGT to type 2 diabetes is 2-6 % per year over 10 years.[12] A small percentage of subjects with IGT may revert to normal glucose tolerance while others remain with IGT for many years.

METABOLIC DISTURBANCES IN TYPE 2 DIABETES

Hyperglycemia is often accompanied by increased levels of the gluconeogenic precursors, lactate, alanine, pyruvate and glycerol. Lipolysis is often increased, particularly in obese patients and those with poor insulin secretion resulting in elevated fasting and postprandial plasma free fatty acid (FFA) levels and increased hepatic VLDL production. Under normal circumstances enough insulin is present to prevent unrestrained lipolysis and the development of ketoacidosis, but ketoacidosis may develop during intercurrent illness (trauma, severe infection, myocardial infarction) because of increased counter regulatory hormone levels. Dyslipidemia in type 2 diabetes, like the abnormalities of glucose metabolism, is due to a combination of insulin resistance and inadequate insulin secretion and is discussed in Chapter VI.11.

Tissue protein metabolism is more sensitive to insulin compared with that of glucose so tissue wasting is not typical. Plasma amino acid levels and their suppression by insulin are usually normal. The plasma amino acid response to protein ingestion is also normal without an accompanying increase in glucose levels.[13] The remainder of this chapter will focus on the disturbances of glucose metabolism.

CLINICAL FEATURES OF TYPE 2 DIABETES

The typical patient is overweight and presents with hyperglycemia after age 40. However, in recent years type 2 diabetes has started to appear in children in association with increasing rates of obesity and in some regions the prevalence of type 2 diabetes in children now exceeds that of type 1 diabetes. This trend is particularly evident in certain minority groups in the US such as Hispanic and African-American children.[14] Figure 3 presents the typical mode of presentation of type 2 diabetes. Although most present with hyperglycemic symptoms (thirst, polyuria, tiredness) many are diagnosed incidentally by screening or during medical examinations conducted for unrelated reasons. In some diabetes is diagnosed when they present with infections, especially urinary tract and skin infections and genital candidiasis (especially in women). Some present with complications of the diabetic condition itself, most commonly, macrovascular disease presenting as angina, myocardial infarction, stroke or peripheral vascular disease. A small proportion present with microvascular complications (retinopathy, maculopathy, neuropathy, renal damage). Because diabetic tissue damage can be detected clinically at the time of diagnosis in about 50% of patients,[15] it is clear that many patients may have had significant hyperglycemia for 5-10 years before the diagnosis is made.

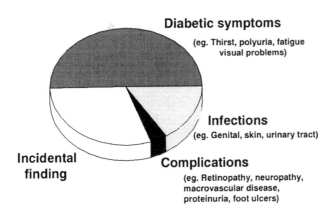

Figure 3. Presentation of patients with type 2 diabetes.

The age adjusted life expectancy of a patient with type 2 diabetes is reduced by 5-10 years compared with the general population. Overall mortality is increased 2-4 fold; over 50% die from ischemic heart disease. Myocardial infarction is both more common and carries a worse prognosis. Stroke and peripheral vascular disease are more common. Retinopathy (especially maculopathy), cataracts and neuropathy are common contributing substantially to morbidity. At least one-third of male patients have some degree of impotence. Diabetic nephropathy is increasing in prevalence and type 2 diabetes is now the leading cause of end stage renal disease in many countries. In several studies over 10% of patients within 1 year of diagnosis already had gross proteinuria. These patients were probably hyperglycemic for several years prior to diagnosis of their diabetes. Microvascular complications and the importance of blood glucose and blood pressure control in their prevention are discussed fully in section VII.

The relationship between macrovascular disease and glycemia has been more difficult to establish than is the case for microvascular complications (see chapters VIII.3 and VIII.5). One reason is the association of type 2 diabetes with a set of cardiovascular risk factors that precede the development of hyperglycemia, being found in subjects with IGT and in the normoglycemic 1st degree relatives of type 2 diabetic patients. They include hypertension (>50% of patients), hypertriglyceridemia, smaller and denser LDL particles, low HDL cholesterol and abnormalities of blood coagulation and fibrinolysis. The association of this cluster of abnormalities with insulin resistance, hyperinsulinemia and often central obesity has been designated syndrome X and is discussed in Chapter VIII.5. Because these risk factors operate in the pre-hyperglycemic phase it is not surprising that about 10% of patients already have macroangiopathy at diagnosis of their diabetes. Because excess mortality in type 2 diabetes is largely due to ischemic heart disease, effective management requires not only near normalization of blood glucose levels but also modification of these risk factors through good blood pressure control, treatment of dyslipidemia, use of antiplatelet agents and lifestyle changes.

INSULIN SECRETION

In IGT insulin secretion may be normal, increased or decreased. This variability is partly due to the heterogeneity of this category, and partly to confounding effects of obesity and insulin resistance, which are associated with enhanced insulin secretion in normoglycemic subjects.[8] However, compared to normoglycemic subjects matched for degree of insulin resistance and obesity, IGT subjects secrete less insulin at any given glucose level.[10] Islet β-cell function declines on going from IGT to diabetes and during established type 2 diabetes.[16,17] This progressive deterioration in β-cell function appears to be the main reason why patients, initially well controlled on a single oral hypoglycemic agent, over the years require escalation of their therapy (e.g. combined oral agents or insulin) to achieve glycemic control (see Chapter VII-6). Qualitative secretory abnormalities may also contribute to impaired glucose homeostasis (Table 1).

Table 1. Islet β-cell and insulin secretory defects in type 2 diabetes

Decreased insulin secretory capacity
Decreased β-cell sensitivity to glucose
Loss of first phase insulin secretion to glucose
Increased release of proinsulin and its split products
Disruption of normal pattern of pulsatile secretion
Morphological changes (decreased β-cell mass; amyloid deposits)

Basal and glucose stimulated insulin secretion

Basal insulin levels are often increased in type 2 diabetes, especially in obese hyperglycemic patients. However, these elevated insulin levels are maintained only in the presence of fasting hyperglycemia; normal subjects, matched for BMI and rendered similarly hyperglycemic by infusion of glucose, have higher circulating insulin levels. In fact the secretory defect may be more marked than suggested by peripheral insulin levels. This is because in many patients, an increased proportion of proinsulin and its major intermediate conversion product, des 31-32 proinsulin are released along with insulin. Proinsulin and its intermediates cross-react with insulin in most immunoassays so that the plasma concentration of 'true insulin' is often overestimated in type 2 diabetic patients.[18] Proinsulin and its derivatives may account for as much as 30-50% of total immunoreactive plasma insulin because in addition to increased release from the β-cell their circulating half-life is longer than that of insulin. Basal levels of 'true insulin' are either normal or moderately elevated in type 2 diabetes.

Insulin secretion in response to a sustained intravenous glucose stimulus is normally biphasic (Chapter II.2). A short lived surge (1st phase) that peaks 1 to 3 minutes after a rise in glucose levels and returns to baseline by 6 to 10 minutes, is followed by a gradual increase (2nd phase). The 1st phase is typically lost once fasting plasma glucose exceeds 126 mg/dl and 2nd phase insulin secretion is markedly reduced at any given glucose level by comparison with age and BMI matched normal subjects (Figure 4). In general, the more severe the diabetes, the lower the 2nd phase response. Insulin secretion to a maximal stimulus is also decreased.

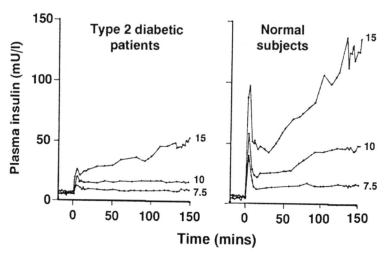

Figure 4. Plasma insulin responses to intravenous glucose in controls and type 2 diabetic patients treated with diet alone. Blood glucose was kept at 7.5 mmol/l (135 mg/dl), 10 mmol/l (180 mg/dl) and 15 mmol/l (270 mg/dl) from 0 until 150 min on 3 separate days in the 2 groups of subjects. First phase insulin secretion is virtually absent and second phase insulin responses are markedly reduced in the diabetic patients. (From Hosker JP, Rudenski AS, Burnett MA, Matthews DR, Turner RC. Similar reduction of first-and-second-phase B-cell responses at three different glucose levels in type II diabetes and the effect of gliclazide therapy. Metabolism 38:767-772, 1989, with permission).

Insulin levels are more variable after oral glucose. The insulin response is usually reduced in patients with obvious fasting hyperglycemia, but may be greater than normal when fasting glucose levels are below 150 mg/dl (Figure 5).

Insulin secretion in response to non-glucose stimuli and mixed meals

The β-cell defects in type 2 diabetes, are relatively (but not completely) specific for glucose. The insulin response to other stimuli, such as arginine, may be near normal if measured in patients when their fasting glucose level is high. However, because the ability of hyperglycemia to enhance the response to various non-glucose stimuli is impaired in parallel with the decline in insulin secretion to glucose per se,[19] the insulin response to non-glucose stimuli is usually subnormal when patients and controls are studied at the same glucose level. The relative preservation of insulin responses to certain amino acids and insulinogenic gut peptides (incretins) released during meal absorption may explain why the insulin response to mixed meals is better than to oral glucose. The patient with mild to moderate hyperglycemia often has an exaggerated insulin response 2 to 4 hours after a

meal (even allowing for increased circulating proinsulin).[20]   Once fasting
plasma glucose exceeds 200-220 mg/dl, decreased insulin levels are more

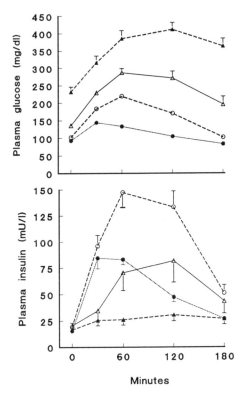

Figure 5. Plasma glucose and insulin responses to oral glucose in 4 subject
groups: (•), normal; (o), impaired glucose tolerance; (Δ), type 2 diabetic with
fasting plasma glucose below 150 mg/dl; (▲) type 2 diabetic with fasting plasma
glucose above 150 mg/dl (From Reaven et al. Am J Med 60:80-88, 1976, with
permission).

common. The insulin response to meals is often delayed and this may
contribute to postprandial hyperglycemia: when insulin is given
intravenously to supplement the early response, both postprandial
hyperglycemia and the delayed hyperinsulinemia are reduced.[21]

Possible causes of β-cell dysfunction
        These include a defect in β-cell glucose metabolism and
glucose-sensing, deficiency of some key stimulatory molecule, reduction in
β-cell mass and deposition of amyloid. The role played by these requires
further studies. Some defects may be hereditary while others are acquired.

The identification of possible "diabetes genes" encoding proteins essential for normal β-cell development and function is an area of intensive study.

The number of β cells may be reduced by 20 to 50% in patients with longstanding type 2 diabetes.[19] However, since in the absence of insulin resistance, more than 80 % of β cells must be lost before insulinopenic diabetes develops, the function of the remaining β cells must be impaired. No data are available on β-cell content early in the course of type 2 diabetes. Fewer β-cells could be a consequence of longstanding diabetes. Conversely, a decrease in β-cell numbers could lead to decreased function of the remaining β cells.

Glucotoxicity and lipotoxicity

The 'glucotoxicity' theory holds that some of the β-cell defects are secondary to chronic hyperglycemia. Support for the theory comes 1) from studies showing that prolonged exposure of rat or human islets to high glucose levels can induce a number of defects, and 2) from the observation that the absent 1st phase insulin response and defective glucose recognition by β-cells in type 2 diabetes may be ameliorated after a period of good glycemic control irrespective of the treatment used (diet, insulin or oral agents).[22,23] This reversibility suggests that the abnormalities may, at least in part, be secondary to hyperglycemia or some other factor associated with uncontrolled diabetes (eg elevated plasma FFA). According to the 'lipotoxicity' theory, chronically increased uptake of FFA by islet β-cells and / or a defect of β-cell FFA metabolism, leads to islet lipid deposition which contributes to the decline in insulin secretion in type 2 diabetes.[24] Genetic factors may influence islet FFA handling and hence susceptibility to β-cell lipotoxicity.[24] It seems likely that glucotoxicity and lipotoxicity play some role in the impaired β-cell function.

Islet amyloid and IAPP

Islet amyloid deposits are found at postmortem in up to 90% of type 2 diabetic patients. They are composed of insoluble fibrils formed from islet amyloid polypeptide (IAPP), also known as amylin. IAPP is a 37 amino acid peptide synthesised by the β-cell, stored in the insulin secretory granules, and co-released with insulin. Although produced at much lower rates than insulin, its production parallels that of insulin being enhanced by hyperglycemia. Amyloid formation could be due to increased IAPP production, decreased IAPP clearance or both. The fibrils are deposited between the capillaries and the endocrine cells and within invaginations of the β-cell membrane. Even small deposits could pose a physical barrier to the diffusion of nutrients from the circulation and of hormones from the islet cells. They might also interfere with membrane function and hence glucose signaling and secretory granule release. Amyloid deposition may play a role in the reduction of β-cell mass.[19]

INSULIN RESISTANCE

Insulin resistance may be defined as a subnormal biologic response to a given concentration of insulin. The most widely used methods of estimating insulin sensitivity with respect to glucose metabolism are the glucose clamp and the minimal model.[25] With both methods type 2 diabetic patients and obese non-diabetic subjects are characteristically less insulin sensitive than normal controls.

The glucose clamp technique entails a constant intravenous infusion of insulin for several hours, while blood glucose is kept at a predetermined level by a feedback - controlled infusion of glucose. As the insulin acts to stimulate tissue glucose uptake and suppress HGO, the amount of glucose needed to maintain the target glucose level increases progressively until a steady state is reached at which time the rate of whole body glucose disposal is the sum of the glucose infusion rate and the rate of any residual output of glucose from the liver. The latter can be quantified if a radioactive or stable isotope of glucose is infused during the study. The more sensitive the subject the higher the glucose disposal rate at any given glucose and insulin level. Bergman's minimal model is easier to perform but the analysis is somewhat more complicated: timed blood samples are collected for measurement of plasma glucose and insulin for about 3 hours following an intravenous glucose bolus. The glucose and insulin values are entered into a computer model to generate an index of insulin sensitivity.[25]

Figure 6 depicts dose response curves for insulin stimulated whole body glucose uptake during glucose clamp studies. Type 2 diabetic patients exhibit both a rightward shift (diminished sensitivity) and a marked decrease in the maximal rate (decreased responsiveness). The changes tend to be more pronounced in obese diabetic patients (Figure 6). Obesity per se is associated with a variable degree of insulin resistance: some subjects are mildly resistant and display only a rightward shift in their dose response curve while others are more resistant and exhibit both a rightward shift and a decreased maximal response. However, even the latter group tend to be less resistant than equally obese type 2 diabetic patients.

When glucose is infused intravenously (e.g. during a glucose clamp) 80 to 85 % of overall insulin-stimulated glucose uptake is accounted for by skeletal muscle. It follows therefore that muscle is resistant to insulin in type 2 diabetes and obesity. Some glucose is oxidised but most (especially at higher insulin doses) is stored as muscle glycogen. In type 2 diabetes defects in both oxidative and non-oxidative glucose Rd (predominantly glycogen

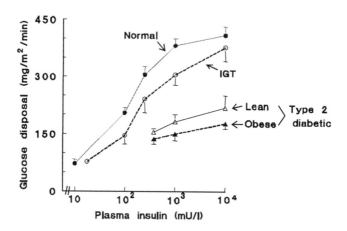

Figure 6. Mean insulin dose response curves for whole body glucose disposal during glucose clamps at the indicated steady state plasma insulin levels. The IGT subjects have a rightward shift in the curve but no change in the maximal response. The lean and obese type 2 diabetic patients have both a rightward shift and a reduced maximal response. (From Kolterman OG, Gray RS, Griffin J, Burstein P, Insel J. Scarlett JA, Olefsky JM. Receptor and postreceptor defects contribute to the insulin resistance in noninsulin-dependent diabetes mellitus. J Clin Invest 68:957-969, 1981, with permission).

storage) are found, although the defect in the latter is greater.[26] A decreased rate of muscle glycogen synthesis in type 2 diabetes has been directly shown[26] and the magnitude of this defect correlates well with the impairment of whole body glucose uptake.

Studies using nuclear magnetic resonance spectroscopy to examine muscle metabolism strongly suggest that the lower rates of muscle glucose uptake and glycogen synthesis in type 2 diabetic patients are due primarily to a defect of glucose transport.[26] This does not preclude additional defects that may affect glucose metabolism. Indeed, a number of abnormalities are demonstrable in muscle of type 2 diabetic patients. These include impaired synthesis of hexokinase II probably due to decreased hexokinase II gene transcription in response to insulin.[27] Since hexokinase phosphorylates glucose to glucose-6-phosphate it augments glucose uptake by maintaining a glucose gradient across the membrane (lower inside). Thus, an impairment of glucose phosphorylation could contribute to decreased glucose uptake. Activation of glycogen synthase (rate limiting enzyme for glycogen synthesis from glucose-6-phosphate) and of pyruvate dehydrogenase (rate limiting for oxidation of pyruvate produced by glycolysis) are also impaired in diabetes.[28,29]

Insulin stimulated glucose transport is decreased in adipocytes and skeletal muscle strips from type 2 diabetic patients and obese subjects.[30] Glucose transport activity in these tissues correlates well with whole body insulin sensitivity in both obese and type 2 diabetic subjects.

Mechanisms of insulin resistance

Decreased numbers of insulin receptors can lead to insulin resistance. However, in adipocytes and skeletal muscle only a fraction (10-20%) of surface receptors need be occupied for maximal stimulation of glucose transport by insulin. The upshot is that with fewer cell surface receptors there is a rightward shift in the insulin dose response curve, but a normal maximal response. A reduced maximal response in diabetes implies a postbinding defect because the number of receptors is unlikely to be reduced below 10-20% of normal. In obesity and subjects with IGT there are fewer insulin receptors on insulin target tissues, probably because of downregulation by hyperinsulinemia. This decrease could contribute to their insulin insensitivity (Figure 6). Insulin receptors are also moderately reduced in most obese and non-obese type 2 diabetic patients, but in these patients insulin resistance is primarily due to post-binding defects.

Much work has been conducted to identify possible post-binding defects of insulin action in obesity and type 2 diabetes. Because resistance is evident in different actions of insulin (e.g. glucose transport, regulation of gene expression) which may involve different signaling elements it is thought that the primary defect(s) responsible for insulin resistance must involve some early common step in the insulin signaling pathway (see Chapter II.3. for a description of normal insulin signaling). The focus of attention has been on three early targets: the insulin receptor itself, the family of insulin receptor substrates (especially IRS-1 and IRS-2) and phosphatidylinositol-3-kinase (PI-3-kinase), a lipid kinase critical for insulin's effects on glucose transport and some other actions of insulin.

The insulin receptor gene sequence is normal in >99% of subjects with typical type 2 diabetes indicating that the receptor is not a diabetes susceptibility gene, except in a tiny fraction of patients. Decreased tyrosine kinase activity of liver, muscle and adipocyte insulin receptors has been found in type 2 diabetes, but this is probably an acquired defect as it is reversible with weight loss and improved glycemic control in obese type 2 diabetic patients.[31]

The insulin receptor substrates, IRS-1 and IRS-2 (see Chapter II.3) play a key role in transmission of the signal from the insulin receptor to downstream proteins. Their function is influenced by their phosphorylation state. In type 2 diabetes the ability of insulin to stimulate IRS-1 phosphorylation on tyrosines is impaired in both adipocytes and skeletal muscle.[31,32] Decreased muscle IRS-2 phosphorylation in response to insulin has also been reported. PI-3-kinase, which is essential for insulin's effects on Glut 4 translocation and glycogen synthase activation, is activated by binding to tyrosine phosphorylated IRS-1 and IRS-2. The insulin induced association of PI-3-kinase with IRS-1 and IRS-2, and hence activation of PI-3-kinase are impaired in muscle of type 2 diabetic patients.[32]

The glucose transport system is a possible site for a postreceptor defect. Skeletal muscle, adipocytes and cardiac muscle express a glucose transporter isoform (Glut 4) that in the basal state is primarily in an intracellular vesicular location. Insulin stimulates glucose transport in these tissues by causing the recruitment of Glut 4 proteins from the intracellular pool to the plasma membrane. In the vast majority of type 2 diabetic patients the Glut 4 gene coding sequence and muscle Glut 4 protein levels are normal but insulin stimulated translocation of Glut 4 to the plasma membrane is impaired.[30,33] The trafficking of Glut 4 to and from the plasma membrane is a complex process: a large number of proteins are involved in the movement of vesicles, membrane fusion, and endocytotic events. Impaired Glut 4 translocation could be due to an abnormality in any of these proteins or it could be due to an impairment of insulin signaling.

Insulin resistance: acquired and genetic components

A combination of inherited and acquired factors contribute to the insulin resistance in type 2 diabetes. Apart from obesity, dietary influences and physical inactivity, the development of type 2 diabetes per se leads to a worsening of insulin resistance.[34,35] Two factors that may contribute to insulin resistance once diabetes has developed are elevated plasma FFA levels and hyperglycemia. Animal and clinical studies suggest that both hyperglycemia and increased FFA availability may play an important role in the acquired component of insulin resistance in type 2 diabetes.[36,37] The component of insulin resistance that appears to be due to the diabetes may be reversible by tight blood glucose control (which also lowers plasma FFA levels). Thus insulin sensitivity is improved (but not normalized) by tight glycemic control: the degree of improvement varies from as little as 10% to as much as 75% in various studies.[2,23,38,39]

Heredity is thought to be a major determinant of the irreversible component of insulin resistance and there has been much work to try and identify the genetic causes of insulin resistance. Several genes, including the insulin receptor, Glut-4, glycogen synthase, and PI-3-kinase have been examined as potential candidate genes in insulin resistance and type 2 diabetes. However, the primary sequences of these proteins have generally been found to be normal, except in patients with rare forms of diabetes. In some populations, polymorphisms of IRS-1 have been found to be two to three times more common in type 2 diabetic than in non-diabetic subjects, and some of these IRS-1 variants were associated with impaired IRS-1 function[40]. Clearly, these findings merit further study as they could contribute to the genetic basis of type 2 diabetes. Gene mapping studies which make use of polymorphic genetic markers or single nucleotide polymorphisms (SNP's) that are distributed throughout the genome have also been employed in the search for genes associated with insulin resistance that may predispose to type 2 diabetes. So far these studies are in their early stages but linkage has been found between a diverse group of genes and either in vivo insulin resistance or the diabetes phenotype in different populations (see Chapter IV.1).

An important conceptual advance in our understanding of potential mechanisms of insulin resistance leading to the development of type 2 diabetes has come from transgenic mouse models in which specific genes thought to play a key role in insulin action have been disrupted either in a specific tissue or at the whole body level. Such studies have shown that whereas even a major disruption of a single gene (for example the insulin receptor or IRS-1) may have little phenotypic effect, combinations of relatively minor defects for example of the insulin receptor and downstream signaling molecules such as IRS-1 and IRS-2 can act synergistically to cause insulin resistance and glucose intolerance.[41] This fits nicely with the polygenic model of type 2 diabetes inheritance and also allows for the synergistic interaction of genetic and acquired defects such as the downregulation of insulin receptors by high circulating insulin levels or defects induced by hyperglycemia and/or elevated fatty acid levels.

GLUCOSE METABOLISM IN TYPE 2 DIABETES

Hyperglycemia is due to a variable combination of overproduction of glucose by the liver and impaired insulin stimulated tissue glucose uptake. Hyperglycemia, through a mass action effect, results in enhanced non-insulin mediated glucose uptake by tissues other than brain (including insulin target tissues), thereby compensating to a variable extent for impaired insulin mediated glucose uptake. The contributions of hepatic glucose overproduction and peripheral tissue insulin resistance to hyperglycemia in type 2 diabetes vary between fasting and postprandial states and are discussed below.

Hepatic glucose output (HGO)

After an overnight fast glucose is produced at about 1.8-2.2 mg/kg/min with about 90% coming from the liver. In type 2 diabetic patients with fasting plasma glucose levels above 140 mg/dl, basal HGO tends to be modestly increased, and fasting glucose levels correlate with HGO.[9] This suggests that in the more severely hyperglycemic patient increased HGO contributes to fasting hyperglycemia. In patients with mildly raised fasting plasma glucose (<140 mg/dl) who have better insulin secretion, HGO may be normal. One could speculate that in these patients an increase in HGO contributes to the initial rise in plasma glucose but as their fasting glucose level rises they secrete more insulin which restores HGO towards normal with establishment of a new steady state in which fasting glucose and insulin levels are elevated but HGO is within the normal range, albeit not normal for the prevailing insulin and glucose levels.

Most studies suggest that gluconeogenesis is increased in diabetic patients with fasting hyperglycemia, and that this explains their increased HGO.[42,43] Factors that may augment gluconeogenesis in diabetes include hepatic insulin resistance, relative insulin deficiency, and increased plasma levels of glucagon, gluconeogenic precursors and FFA. There has been particular interest in the role of FFA. Not only do they supply energy for gluconeogenesis but they also stimulate several gluconeogenic enzymes, and insulin's ability to suppress HGO may be partly indirect and mediated by suppression of fat cell lipolysis and plasma FFA levels.[44]

Suppression of HGO after meals is also impaired. The effect is to deliver more glucose into the systemic circulation (together with that absorbed from the gut) so that hepatic overproduction of glucose also contributes to postprandial hyperglycemia.

Pathogenesis of fasting hyperglycemia

In the fasted state insulin levels are low and 75-85% of glucose uptake is non-insulin mediated. Insulin-independent glucose uptake by the brain accounts for a large part of this basal uptake (50-60%), and is normal in diabetes. Because skeletal muscle accounts for only 15-20% of basal glucose uptake, it follows that insulin resistance causing an impairment of insulin-mediated muscle glucose uptake will have relatively little effect on basal glucose utilization rates or fasting glucose levels; more glucose has to enter the circulation (primarily from the liver) for fasting glucose levels to increase substantially. In the setting of insulin resistance and impaired insulin secretion, insulin mediated glucose uptake cannot increase appropriately in response to an increase in HGO, and small increases in glucose production cause a proportional increase in glucose levels. As the glucose level rises the mass action effect of hyperglycemia promotes glucose disposal and the system re-equilibrates at which point increased glucose entry into the circulation is matched by increased glucose disposal (including urinary glucose loss) in the presence of fasting hyperglycemia.

Pathogenesis of postprandial hyperglycemia

Most ingested glucose enters the systemic circulation (<10% is taken up by the liver on first pass) and is then taken up by peripheral tissues (50-60% is taken up by skeletal muscle) and to a lesser extent the liver. Several factors contribute to postprandial hyperglycemia in type 2 diabetes. Firstly, the total amount of glucose entering the systemic circulation is increased because suppression of HGO is impaired (see above). Secondly, the efficiency of glucose removal is reduced because of muscle insulin resistance and relative or absolute insulin deficiency. Thirdly, hepatic uptake of glucose (newly absorbed and recirculating) is impaired, although this defect makes a relatively small contribution, because the liver normally takes up only 20-35% of a glucose load. The marked increase in plasma glucose levels seen in type 2 diabetes after carbohydrate ingestion promotes glucose uptake by muscle and other tissues by mass action, and this compensates for diminished insulin-mediated glucose uptake. However, the intracellular disposition of the glucose is abnormal. For example, hyperglycemia does not fully compensate for impaired muscle glycogen synthase activation by insulin[28] so less of the glucose taken up by muscle is stored as glycogen and more is metabolised through glycolysis. This in turn leads to increased release of the gluconeogenic precursors, lactate, alanine and pyruvate which are taken up by the liver and help to sustain the increased rates of gluconeogenesis and HGO.

SUMMARY

The development of type 2 diabetes requires the presence of defects of both insulin action and insulin secretion. Epidemiological and clinical evidence suggests that in most (but not all) populations insulin resistance most commonly initiates the sequence of events leading to type 2 diabetes. As long as the islet β-cells can compensate with a high enough insulin output to overcome the insulin resistance, glucose tolerance remains normal or only mildly impaired. However, a progressive decline in β-cell function in a subset of insulin resistant subjects eventually leads to overt hyperglycemia.

Insulin resistance affects the main insulin target tissues, namely, skeletal muscle, the liver and adipose tissue. Metabolic abnormalities in type 2 diabetes resulting from the effects of insulin resistance and impaired insulin secretion on these target tissues include decreased insulin stimulated skeletal muscle glucose uptake, overproduction of glucose by the liver and impaired suppression of adipocyte lipolysis. Impaired insulin stimulated muscle glucose uptake is the main cause of postprandial hyperglycemia. Overproduction of glucose by the liver is the main cause of fasting hyperglycemia and also contributes to postprandial hyperglycemia. Impaired suppression of lipolysis results in higher fasting and 24h circulating plasma

FFA levels which in turn may contribute to both muscle insulin resistance and overproduction of glucose by the liver. Chronically elevated FFA levels may also have adverse effects on islet β cell function. Hyperglycemia as well as being the key determinant for the development of microvascular diabetic complications also has adverse effects on both islet β cell function and may exacerabate the insulin resistant state (glucotoxicity).

Ischemic heart disease is the main cause of the excess mortality in type 2 diabetes. Effective management to ensure immediate well-being and for prevention of both microvascular and macrovascular complications requires near normalization of blood glucose levels by diet, lifestyle changes and glucose lowering therapeutic agents and attention to other risk factors including good blood pressure control, use of antiplatelet agents and treatment of dyslipidemia.

Acknowledgement: Dr Kruszynska is supported by the Whittier Institute for Diabetes.

REFERENCES

1. Froguel P, Velho G. Genetic determinants of type 2 diabetes. Recent Prog Horm Res 56:91-105, 2001.
2. Grundy SM. Metabolic complications of obesity. Endocrine 13:155-165, 2000.
3. Groop LC. Insulin resistance: the fundamental trigger of type 2 diabetes. Diabetes Obes Metab 1(Suppl 1):S1-S7, 1999.
4. Clark DO. Physical activity efficacy and effectiveness among older adults and minorities. Diabetes Care 20:1176-1182, 1997.
5. Jung RT. Obesity and nutritional factors in the pathogenesis of non-insulin-dependent diabetes mellitus. In Pickup J, Williams G, Eds. Textbook of Diabetes, 2nd ed. Blackwell Science, Oxford, UK, pp 19.1-19.23, 1997.
6. Yost TJ, Jensen DR, Haugen BR, Eckel RH. Effect of dietary macronutrient composition on tissue-specific lipoprotein lipase activity and insulin action in normal-weight subjects. Am J Clin Nutr 68:296-302, 1998.
7. Swinburn BA, Boyce VL, Bergman RN, Howard BV, Bogardus C. Deterioration in carbohydrate metabolism and lipoprotein changes induced by modern, high fat diet in Pima Indians and Caucasians. J Clin Endocrinol Metab 73:156-165, 1991.
8. Cavaghan MK, Ehrmann DA, Polonsky KS. Interactions between insulin resistance and insulin secretion in the development of glucose intolerance. J Clin Invest 106:329-333, 2000.

9. Stern MP. Strategies and prospects for finding insulin resistance genes. J Clin Invest 106:323-327, 2000.
10. Polonsky KS, Sturis J, Bell GI. Non-insulin-dependent diabetes mellitus-a genetically programmed failure of the beta cell to compensate for insulin resistance. N Engl J Med 334:777-783, 1996.
11. Ferrannini E, Groop LC. Hepatic glucose production in insulin-resistant states. Diab Metab Rev 5:711-725, 1989.
12. Alberti KGMM. The clinical significance of impaired glucose tolerance. Diabet Med 13:927-937, 1996.
13. Gannon MC, Nuttall JA, Damberg G, Gupta V, Nuttall FQ. Effect of protein ingestion on the glucose appearance rate in people with type 2 diabetes. J Clin Endocrinol Metab 86:1040-1047, 2001.
14. Fagot-Campagna A. Emergence of type 2 diabetes mellitus in children: epidemiological evidence. J Pediatr Endocrinol Metab 13 (Suppl 6):1395-402, 2000.
15. UK Prospective Diabetes Study Group. Intensive blood-glucose control with sulphonylureas or insulin compared with conventional treatment and risk of complications in patients with type 2 diabetes (UKPDS 33). Lancet 352:837-853, 1998.
16. UK Prospective Diabetes Study Group. UK prospective diabetes study 16: Overview of 6 years ' therapy of type II diabetes: A progressive disease. Diabetes 44:1249-1258, 1995.
17. Kahn SE. The importance of the beta-cell in the pathogenesis of type 2 diabetes mellitus. Am J Med 108 (Suppl 6a):2S-8S, 2000.
18. Temple RC, Clark PM, Nagi DK, et al. Radioimmunoassay may overestimate insulin in non-insulin-dependent diabetics. Clin Endocrinol (Oxf)32:689-693,1990.
19. Porte D Jr, Kahn SE. Beta-cell dysfunction and failure in type 2 diabetes: potential mechanisms. Diabetes 50 (Suppl 1):S160-163, 2001.
20. Reaven GM, Chen YDI, Hollenbeck CB, et al. Plasma insulin, C-peptide, and proinsulin concentrations in obese and nonobese individuals with varying degrees of glucose tolerance. J Clin Endocrinol Metab 76:44-48, 1993.
21. Bruce DG, Chisholm DJ, Storlien LH, Kraegen EW. Physiological importance of deficiency in early prandial insulin secretion in non-insulin-dependent diabetes. Diabetes 37:736-744, 1998.
22. Garvey WT, Olefsky JM, Griffin J, et al. The effects of insulin treatment on insulin secretion and action in type II diabetes mellitus. Diabetes 34:222-234, 1985.
23. Henry RR, Wallace P, Olefsky JM. The effects of weight loss on the mechanims of hyperglycemia in obese noninsulin-dependent diabetes mellitus. Diabetes 35:990-998, 1986.

24. McGarry JD, Dobbins RL. Fatty acids, lipotoxicity and insulin secretion. Diabetologia 42:128-138, 1999.
25. Ferrannini E, Mari A. How to measure insulin sensitivity. J Hypertens 16:895-906, 1998.
26. Cline GW, Petersen KF, Krssak M, et al. Impaired glucose transport as a cause of decreased insulin-stimulated muscle glycogen synthesis in type 2 diabetes. N Engl J Med 341:240-246, 1999.
27. Kruszynska YT, Mulford MI, Baloga J, Yu JG, Olefsky JM. Regulation of skeletal muscle hexokinase II by insulin in nondiabetic and NIDDM subjects. Diabetes 47:1107-1113, 1998.
28. Thorburn AW, Gumbiner B, Bulacan F, et al. Multiple defects in muscle glycogen synthase activity contribute to reduced glycogen synthesis in non-insulin dependent diabetes mellitus. J Clin Invest 87:489-495, 1991.
29. DeFronzo RA, Bonadonna RC, Ferrannini E. Pathogenesis of NIDDM. A balanced overview. Diabetes Care 15:318-368, 1992.
30. Kruszynska YT, Olefsky JM. Cellular and molecular mechanisms of non-insulin dependent diabetes mellitus. J Invest Med 44:413-428, 1996.
31. Thies RS, Molina JM, Ciaraldi TP et al. Insulin receptor autophosphorylation and endogenous substrate phosphorylation in human adipocytes from control, obese and non-insulin dependent diabetic subjects. Diabetes 39:250-259, 1990.
32. Cusi K, Katsumi M, Osman A, et al. Insulin resistance differentially affects the PI-3-kinase- and MAP kinase-mediated signaling in human muscle. J Clin Invest 105:311-320, 2000.
33. Kelley DE, Mintun MA, Watkins SC, et al. The effect of non-insulin dependent diabetes mellitus and obesity on glucose transport and phosphorylation in skeletal muscle. J Clin Invest 97:2705-2713, 1996.
34. Vaag A, Henriksen JE, Madsbad S, Holm N, Beck-Nielsen H. Insulin secretion, insulin action, and hepatic glucose production in identical twins discordant for non-insulin-dependent diabetes mellitus. J Clin Invest 95:690-698, 1995.
35. Eriksson J, Franssila-Kallunki A, Ekstrand A, et al. Early metabolic defects in persons at increased risk for non-insulin dependent diabetes mellitus. N Engl J Med 321:337-343, 1989.
36. Yki-Jarvinen H. Glucose toxicity. Endocr Rev 13:415-431, 1992.
37. Shulman GI. Cellular mechanisms of insulin resistance in humans. Am J Cardiol 84:3J-10J, 1999.
38. Henry RR, Gumbiner B, Ditzler T, Wallace P, Lyon R, Glauber HS. Intensive conventional insulin therapy for type II diabetes. Metabolic effects during a 6-mo outpatient trial. Diabetes Care 16:21-31, 1993.

39. Hollenbeck CB, Reaven GM. Treatment of patients with non-insulin-dependent diabetes mellitus: Diabetic control and insulin secretion and action after different treatment modalities. Diabetic Med 4:311-316, 1987.

40. Virkamaki A, Ueki K, Kahn RC. Protein-protein interaction in insulin signaling and the molecular mechanisms of insulin resistance. J Clin Invest 103:931-943, 1999.

41. Kadowaki T. Insights into insulin resistance and type 2 diabetes from knockout mouse models. J Clin Invest 106:459-465, 2000.

42. Gastaldelli A, Baldi S, Pettiti M, et al. Influence of obesity and type 2 diabetes on gluconeogenesis and glucose output in humans: a quantitative study. Diabetes 49:1367-1373, 2000.

43. Wajngot A, Chandramouli V, Schumann WC, et al. Quantitative contributions of gluconeogenesis to glucose production during fasting in type 2 diabetes mellitus. Metabolism 50:47-52, 2001.

44. Bergman RN. Non-esterified fatty acids and the liver: why is insulin secreted into the portal vein? Diabetologia 43:946-952, 2000.

Chapter 3. Maturity-Onset Diabetes of the Young: Molecular Genetics, Clinical Manifestations and Therapy

Markus Stoffel

DEFINITION AND GENETIC CLASSIFICATION OF MODY

Type 2 diabetes accounts for ≥90% of all diabetes. It ranks among the top ten causes of death in western nations and afflicts about 5% of populations in industrialized countries. Type 2 diabetes is a heterogeneous, complex metabolic syndrome in which hyperglycemia results from decreased insulin effectiveness (insulin resistance) and an impaired insulin secretory response to glucose. Genetic and lifestyle factors (e.g. weight, physical activity) predispose to the development of these defects, however, the genetic mechanisms that underlie the pathophysiology of most forms of type 2 diabetes are not completely understood.

Although most forms of type 2 diabetes appear to be polygenic, monogenic forms have also been identified. The diseases collectively termed "maturity-onset diabetes of the young" (MODY) (Table 1), constitute the most common monogenic forms of diabetes, and are characterized by an early age of onset (<25 years of age), autosomal dominant inheritance, and defects in pancreatic β-cell function. Patients with MODY can be distinguished from patients with type 1 diabetes by a lack of glutamic acid decarboxylase antibodies (GAD-Ab). The phenotype of patients with MODY is variable, underlining that this disorder is genetically heterogeneous.

Table 1. Definition of MODY

- Impaired glucose tolerance
- Age of onset <25 years
- Autosomal-dominant inheritance

Using genetic linkage and candidate gene approaches, mutations in genes on chromosomes 2, 7, 12, 13, 19, and 20 have been linked to MODY and collectively may represent up to 3% of all patients with type 2 diabetes (Table 2). The gene on chromosome 7 (MODY2) encodes the glycolytic enzyme glucokinase which plays a key role in generating the metabolic signal for insulin secretion and integrating hepatic glucose uptake.[1] The genes on chromosomes 20 (*MODY1*), 12 (*MODY3*), 19 (*MODY5*), and 13

(*MODY4*) contain mutations in transcription factors hepatocyte nuclear factor (HNF)–4α, HNF-1α, HNF-1β, and PDX-1, respectively.[2-6] Mutations in NEURO-D1/BETA-2 (MODY6) are responsible for an autosomal dominant form of diabetes that may have a more variable age of onset.[7,8] Rare mutations in the insulin gene have also been shown to give rise to a MODY-like phenotype in humans.

Table 2. Genetic classification of MODY:

MODY1: Hepatocyte Nuclear Factor 4α	(HNF-4α)
MODY2: Glucokinase	(GCK)
MODY3: Hepatocyte Nuclear Factor 1α	(HNF-1α)
MODY4: Insulin Promoter Factor	(IPF-1/PDX-1)
MODY5: Hepatocyte Nuclear Factor 1β	(HNF-1β)
MODY6: Neurogenic Differentiation-1	(NEURO-D1/BETA2)
INSULIN Gene Mutations	(INS)

Biochemical and genetic studies have shown that MODY genes are functionally related and form a transcriptional network that is critical for formal pancreatic islet development, differentiation, and metabolism. This chapter will discuss the function and molecular defects of different MODY genes and the clinical manifestations of the various subtypes.

MODY GENES AND PHENOTYPES

Hepatocyte Nuclear Factor-4α (MODY1)

HNF-4α is an orphan member of the superfamily of ligand-dependent transcription factors. It contains a zinc finger region (amino acids 48 to 128) and binds DNA as a homodimer. Two transcriptional activation domains, designated AF-1 and AF-2, flank the DNA binding domain. AF-1 consists of the first 24 amino acids and functions as a constitutive autonomous activator of transcription. The AF2 transactivation domain of HNF-4α, spanning amino acid residues 128-366, includes the dimerization interface and ligand binding domain.

The HNF-4α gene is located on chromosome 20q (20q12-q13.1) and plays a critical role in the normal function of liver, intestine, kidney, and pancreatic islets.[10,11] Clinical studies demonstrated that loss-of-function mutations in HNF-4α (Figure 1) cause diabetes by compromising β-cell function. Prediabetic subjects with HNF-4α mutations have normal sensitivity to insulin and first-phase insulin responses to intravenous glucose.[12] However, compared with normal subjects, MODY1 patients exhibit a decrease in plasma C-peptide concentration, decrease in absolute

Table 3. Clinical Features of MODY 1:

- Decreased insulin secretion
- Decreased glucagon response to arginine
- Variable phenotype:low/normal plasma C-peptide, insulin levels
- Low/normal serum APOAII, CIII, triglyceride levels
- Tendency to develop diabetic complications

---

amplitude of insulin secretory oscillations, and reduced insulin secretion rates in response to intravenous glucose infusions as blood glucose levels increase above 7mmol/l.[12] Furthermore, HNF-4α haploinsufficiency leads to diminished glucagon secretory responses to arginine, suggesting a role of the MODY1 gene in α-cell function.[13]

Clinically, MODY1 patients frequently develop severe diabetes and complications, including micro- and macro-vascular angiopathy and peripheral neuropathy (Table 3). About 30% of cases with MODY1 require insulin therapy and the majority of the remainder are treated with oral anti-diabetic drugs. Molecular studies indicate that the mechanism by which HNF-4α deficiency results in an impairment of insulin secretion involves abnormal pancreatic islet gene expression. Several genes of the glucose-stimulated insulin secretion pathway in pancreatic β-cells are regulated by HNF-4α. They include the glucose transporter-2 (GLUT-2) and enzymes of glycolysis, including aldolase B, glyceraldehyde-3-phosphate dehydrogenase, and L-pyruvate kinase.[11] HNF-4α also regulates the expression of other transcription factors, such as HNF-1α (the MODY3 gene), which itself is a transcriptional activator of the insulin gene.[11] Together, these observations suggest that diminished HNF-4α activity can impair glucose-stimulated insulin secretion by decreasing the expression of genes involved in glucose entry and metabolism in pancreatic β-cells as well as insulin gene transcription.[11] Since HNF-4α proteins are not only expressed in pancreatic β-cells but also play a key role in hepatocyte differentiation, mutations in this gene could be expected to result in pleiotropic phenotypes. Indeed, subjects with HNF-4α haploinsufficiency have diminished serum apolipoprotein (Apo)A2, apoC3, Lp(a) and triglyceride levels compared to normal controls or patients with other forms of early-onset diabetes.[14]

The first HNF-4α/MODY1 mutation was found in R-W pedigree, a family of German ancestry. The affected members of the R-W family have a nonsense mutation, Q268X, in the HNF4α gene.[2] This mutation generates a truncated protein that contains an intact DNA binding domain but lacks part of the AF2 region. Functional studies of this mutation revealed that the mutant protein lacks transcriptional activity and does not interact with the wild-type HNF-4α in a dominant-negative fashion.[11]

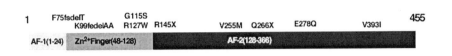

Figure 1. Functional domains and muttions in HNF-4α.

Additional HNF-4α variants associated with MODY1 have since then been identified and include F75fsdelT, K99fsdelAA, R154X, R127W, V255M, E276Q, V393I, and G115S.[15,16] F75fsdelT and K99fsdelAA are frameshift mutations that lead to truncated HNF-4α proteins. HNF-4α(R154X) produces a truncated protein containing only the DNA binding domain and the AF1 transactivation domain. This mutant protein lacks transactivation potential and may exert a mild dominant-negative effect on the activity of wild-type HNF-4α in β-cells. In contrast to the frameshift or nonsense mutants, the functional properties of HNF-4α missense mutants are more varied. HNF-4α(V393I), located in the AF2 domain, leads to a two-fold decrease in transactivation potential.[17] Other sequence variants, such as HNF-4α(R127W) and HNF-4α (V255M), have a modest reduction in transcriptional activation.[18] Only one missense mutation that is located in the DNA binding domain of HNF-4α has been reported. This mutation, HNF-4α(G115S), leads to an impairment in the ability of the mutant protein to bind to HNF4 consensus binding sites, thereby reducing its transactivation activity.

Glucokinase (MODY2)

The phosphorylation of glucose at the sixth carbon position is the first step in glycolysis and is catalyzed by a family of enzymes called hexokinases. Glucokinase (GCK) is expressed mainly in the liver and endocrine pancreas and is a unique member of this family. In contrast to hexokinases 1, 2, and 3, glucokinase (hexokinase 4) is characterized by a high substrate specificity for glucose, a high Km of about 10mM (versus 0.1-0.001mM for the other hexokinases), and a lack of inhibition by metabolites,

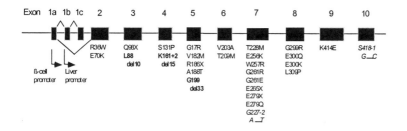

Figure 2. Mutations in the glucokinase gene.

such as glucose 6-phospahate or glucose 1,6 bisphosphate. These unique biochemical properties allow glucokinase to serve as the glucose sensor of the pancreatic β-cell by integrating glucose metabolism and insulin secretion.[1]

Genetic linkage between DNA polymorphisms in the glucokinase gene (Figure 2) on the short arm of chromosome 7 (7p15-p14) and MODY was initially reported in families of French origin. More than 80 different GCK mutations have been identified since then, and, depending on the population, may represent from 11% to 63% of all MODY. Impairment in the enzymatic activity of mutant GCK leads to decreased glycolytic flux in pancreatic β-cells.[19] This translates *in vivo* into a rightward shift in the dose response curve relating blood glucose and insulin secretion rates (ISR) obtained during a graded intravenous glucose infusion. Average ISRs over a glucose range between 5 and 9 mM are 61% lower in MODY2 subjects than in control subjects.[19] The release of insulin in response to arginine in MODY2 is preserved, indicating that the insulin secretion defect in MODY2 patients is due to abnormal glucose sensing. Complete loss of glucokinase activity in subjects with homozygous mutations in the GCK gene (T228M and M210K) causes neonatal diabetes, a rare form of diabetes that requires insulin therapy within the first weeks of life.[20] In contrast, individuals with activating glucokinase mutations (e.g. HNF-4αV455M) develop an autosomal dominant form of familial hyperinsulinism due to a leftward shift of the dose-response curve relating blood glucose and insulin secretion rates.[21] These genetic findings highlight the importance of glucokinase as a glucose sensor and critical regulator for insulin secretion in pancreatic β-cells.

Glucokinase-deficient mice have been shown to be an excellent animal model for the genetic defect in humans. Mice that lack glucokinase activity die perinatally with severe hyperglycemia and phenotypically resemble rare forms of neonatal diabetes. Heterozygous mice have elevated blood glucose levels and reduced insulin secretion. Expression of GCK in β-cells in the absence of expression in the liver can prevent perinatal death of GCK null mice, providing strong evidence for the need of β-cells GCK in glucose sensing and for maintaining normal glucose levels.[22]

13C nuclear magnetic spectroscopy studies have revealed that a hepatic glucose cycling defect also contributes to the molecular etiologies of MODY2 phenotype. MODY 2 patients have decreased net accumulation of hepatic glycogen and augmented hepatic gluconeogenesis after a meal.[23] These results suggest that, in addition to β-cell dysfunction, abnormalities in liver glycogen metabolism contribute to the hyperglycemia in patients with glucokinase-deficient diabetes.[23]

Fetal insulin secretion in response to maternal glycemia is an important determinant for intrauterine growth. Glucose sensing defects in pancreatic β-cells, caused by a heterozygous mutation in the glucokinase gene, can reduce fetal growth and birth weight in addition to causing hyperglycemia after birth.[24] Fetuses that have inherited a glucokinase mutation from the mother or father have a reduced birth weight of 521 g ($p = 0.0002$) compared to unaffected siblings.[24] Maternal hyperglycemia due to glucokinase mutations results in a mean increase in birth weight of 601 g ($P = 0.001$).[24] Since glucose, but not insulin, crosses the placenta, it is likely that these changes in birth weight reflect changes in fetal insulin secretion that are influenced directly by the fetal genotype and indirectly, through maternal hyperglycemia, by the maternal GCK-genotype.[24]

In contrast to MODY1 and MODY3 patients, who frequently develop diabetes at the time of puberty, hyperglycemia in subjects with GCK mutations frequently manifests in the neonatal period and invariably develops before adolescence.[24,25] Glucokinase deficiency is not associated with an increased incidence of diabetic complications, including proliferative retinopathy, neuropathy, or proteinuria, and other manifestations of the metabolic syndrome such as hypertension, obesity, or dyslipidemia.[25, 26] This finding is also consistent with the low frequency of coronary heart disease in MODY2 patients.

Clinical features of MODY 2 are summarized in Table 4.

Table 4. Clinical Features of MODY2:

- Mild defect in insulin secretion
- Mild fasting and postprandial hyperglycemia
- Low/normal plasma C-peptide, insulin levels
- Little tendency for disease progression
- Age of onset: perinatal
- Low birth weight of affected newborns
- Homozygous GCK-mutation: Neonatal (insulin-dependent) diabetes
- Activating GCK mutations: Autosomal dominant familial hyperinsulinism

Hepatocyte Nuclear Factor-1α (MODY3)

HNF-1α is a homeodomain transcription factor composed of an N-terminal dimerization domain, a POU-homeobox DNA binding domain, and a C-terminal transactivation domain. HNF-1α is expressed in liver, kidney, intestine, and pancreatic islets where it directs tissue-specific gene expression. The gene encoding HNF-1α is located on the long arm of chromosome 12 (12q24.2) and was identified as the MODY3 gene through a combination of genetic linkage analysis and positional cloning.[5] Depending on the population, MODY3 accounts for 21%-73% of all MODYs. More than 60 different HNF-1α mutations have been found to co-segregate with diabetes in U.K., German, French, Danish, Italian, Finnish, North American, and Japanese families (Figure 3). They include missense, nonsense, deletion, insertion, and frame shift mutations. Most HNF-1α mutations can be predicted to result in loss-of-function. However, mutant HNF-1α proteins with an intact dimerization domain may impair pancreatic β-cell function by forming nonproductive dimers with wild-type protein, thereby exhibiting dominant negative activity. This mechanism has been shown for frameshift mutation HNF1α-P291fsinsC. Overexpression of HNF1α-P291fsinsC in MIN6 cells, a murine β-cell line, resulted in 40% inhibition of the endogenous HNF-1α activity in a dose-dependent manner.[33] Furthermore, the formation of heterodimers between wild type and HNF1α-P291fsinsC mutant proteins has been observed, indicating that this mutant protein has dominant-negative activity.[33] Codon 291, in the poly-C tract of exon 4, is a frequent site for mutations in the HNF-1α gene. This is likely due to slipped mispairing during DNA replication, thereby causing this region to be a mutation hotspot.[34]

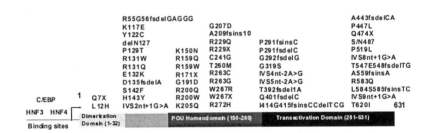

					A443fsdelCA
					P447L
R55G56fsdelGAGGG					Q474X
K117E			G207D		S/N487
Y122C			A209fsins10		P519L
delN127			R229Q		IVS8nt+1G>A
P129T	K150N		R229X	P291fsinsC	T547E548fsdelTG
R131W	R159Q		C241G	P291fsdelC	A559fsinsA
R131Q	R159W		T260M	G292fsdelG	R583Q
E132K	R171X		R263C	G319S	L584S585fsinsTC
D135fsdelA	G191D		R263G	IVS4nt-2A>G	IVS9nt+1G>A
S142F	R200Q		W267R	IVS5nt-2A>G	T620I
H143Y	R200W		W267X	T392fsdel1A	631
IVS2nt+1G>A	K205Q		R272H	Q401fsdelC	
				I414G415fsinsCCdelTCG	

C/EBP — 1 — Q7X
HNF3 HNF4 — L12H

| Binding sites | Dimerization Domain (1-32) | POU Homeodomain (150-280) | Transactivation Domain (281-631) |

Figure 3. Functional domains and mutations in HNF-1α.

Hypomorphic HNF-1α mutations may also contribute to the development of type 2 diabetes in some populations. The HNF-1α(G319S) variant is associated with type 2 diabetes in the Canadian Oji-Cree population with odd ratios of 4.0 and 1.97 in individuals with homozygous and heterozygous G319S mutation, respectively.[35] This mutation is located in the proline-rich transactivation domain and substitutes a conserved glycine residue. Clinical studies indicate that the G319S variant in the Canadian Oji-Cree population is associated with earlier onset of diabetes in women, lower body mass index and higher plasma glucose after oral glucose challenge.[35]

Table 5. Clinical Features of MODY 3:

- Defect in insulin secretion
- Fasting and postprandial hyperglycemia
- Low plasma C-peptide, insulin levels
- Tendency for disease progression
- Increased sensitivity to sulphonylurea therapy

HNF-1α mutations lead to β-cell dysfunction and result in elevated fasting glycemia and impaired glucose stimulated insulin secretion.[36] Other clinical features of MODY3 (Table 5) include increased proinsulin-to-insulin ratios, increased responsiveness to sulfonylureas, and lower body mass index (BMI).[25, 36, 37] HNF-1α mutations are highly penetrant, with 63% of MODY3 diagnosed by the age of 25 years, 78.6% by 35 years, and 95.5% by 55 years.[38] Subjects with HNF-1α mutations have a more rapid deterioration in β-cell function than MODY2 subjects.[25] Heterozygous HNF-1α patients frequently require treatment with oral hypoglycemic agents or insulin.[25]

Mice lacking Hnf-1α develop diabetes within the first month of life due to defects in insulin secretion. Pancreatic islets from Hnf-1α null mice have impaired β-cell glycolytic signaling due to decreased expression of glucose transporter-2 and glycolytic enzymes, such as L-pyruvate kinase and glycokinase.[31,32] Mutant Hnf-1α mice also exhibit dwarfism, renal Fanconi-like syndrome, glycogen storage disease 1b, and defects in bile acid and plasma HDL-cholesterol metabolism.[27-30] However, the hepatic and renal manifestations only develop in the absence of HNF-1α but are not a feature of heterozygous mice.

Insulin Promoter Factor-1 (MODY4)

Insulin promoter factor-1 or pancreatic and duodenal homeobox gene-1 (IPF-1, PDX-1) (Figure 4) is a homeodomain transcription factor that is required for endocrine and exocrine pancreas development as well as insulin gene expression in the adult islet. PDX-1 binds to promoters of target genes as a heterodimer with the ubiquitously expressed homeodomain protein PBX.[39] PDX-1 is an essential gene for early pancreas development. During development in mice, Pdx-1 is initially expressed at 8.5 days post coitum (dpc) in the dorsal and ventral gut epithelium that will later develop into a pancreas. At 9.5 dpc, Pdx-1 expression marks the dorsal and ventral pancreatic buds of the gut and later is restricted to differentiating insulin producing β-cells and somatostatin producing δ-cell.[40] Targeted disruption of the Pdx-1 gene results in a failure of the pancreas to develop.[41] Furthermore, β-cell-specific inactivation of the mouse Pdx-1 gene leads to β-cell dedifferentiation, loss of proper glucose sensing, insulin processing,

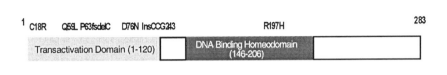

Figure 4. Functional domains and mutations in PDX-1.

and the development of diabetes.[42] Thus, Pdx-1 appears to be a key regulator in early pancreas formation and later in maintaining islet pattern of hormone expression and normoglycemia.

The PDX-1 gene maps to human chromosome 13 (13q12.1) and is involved in several human disorders including pancreatic agenesis and diabetes.[3,4] A single nucleotide deletion within codon 63 (Pro63fsdelC) of the human PDX-1 gene has been reported to cause pancreatic agenesis. This patient inherited the mutant allele from his parents who were heterozygous for the same mutation.[3] Heterozygous family members have early-onset diabetes (range, 17 to 67 years) (Table 6).[4] The point deletion leads to an out-of-frame protein downstream of the PDX-1 transactivation domain, resulting in a non-functional protein lacking the homeodomain that is essential for DNA binding.[3] Expression studies of the mutant PDX1(Pro63fsdelC) protein in eukaryotic cells revealed a second PDX-1 isoform that resulted from an internal translation initiating at an out-of-frame AUG.[44] The reading frame crosses over to the wild type IPF1 reading frame at the site of the point deletion just carboxy-proximal to the transactivation domain, resulting in a second PDX1 isoform that contains the COOH-terminal DNA-binding domain but lacks the amino-terminal transactivation domain.[44] This terminal domain PDX-1 isoform may inhibit the transactivation functions of wild type PDX-1, suggesting that a dominant negative mechanism may contribute to the development of diabetes in individuals with this mutation. Six of eight affected heterozygotes in this pedigree were treated with diet or oral hypoglycemic agents. None of the family members carrying the PDX-1(Pro63fsdelC) mutation showed ketosis or other indications of severe insulin deficiency.[4]

Table 6. Clinical Features of MODY4:

- Defect insulin secretion
- Fasting and posprandial hyperglycemia
- Low plasma C-peptide, insulin levels
- Tendency for disease progression
- Homozygous PDX-1 mutation: Pancreatic agenesis

Other PDX-1 mutations that predispose carriers to diabetes include D76N, C18R, R197H, Q59L, and InsCCG243.[45,46] The PDX-1(InsCCG243) mutation is linked in two French families with a late-onset form of type 2 diabetes and autosomal inheritance, in which insulin secretion becomes progressively impaired over time. The non-diabetic carriers have lower than normal insulin levels at high glucose levels.[45] The InsCCG243 mutation occurs at the COOH-terminal border of PDX-1 homeodomain required for transactivation. Three PDX-1 missense mutations (C18R, D76N, and R197H) were found in diabetic subjects from Great Britain. Functional analysis of these mutations suggest that they exhibit decreased binding activity to the human insulin gene promoter and reduced activation of the insulin gene in response to hyperglycemia.[46] These mutations are estimated to have a frequency of 1% in the English population and may predispose to type 2 diabetes (relative risk of 3.0).[45] The PDX-1 mutations (D76N) and (Q59L) were also found in French, late-onset type 2 diabetic families with a relative risk of 12.6 for diabetes and with decreased glucose-stimulated insulin-secretion in non-diabetic individuals.[45] These mutations are located in the amino-terminal transactivation region that mediates insulin transcription. In summary, hypomorphic PDX-1 variants may lead to a progressive impairment of β-cell function and glucose homeostasis in concert with other inherited metabolic abnormalities and risk factors such as age, obesity-related insulin resistance and physical inactivity. Therefore, PDX-1 mutations may also be involved in the polygenic basis of late-onset type 2 diabetes.[45, 46]

Hepatocyte Nuclear Factor-1β (MODY5)

HNF-1α and -1β are homologous proteins belonging to a large superfamily of homeodomain-containing transcription factors. As such, HNF-1β is structurally similar to HNF-1α with an N-terminal dimerization domain, a POU-homeobox DNA binding domain, and a C-terminal transactivation domain. HNF-1α and -1β bind to DNA as homo- and/or heterodimers. The HNF-1 genes have an overlapping tissue distribution but HNF-1α/HNF1β ratios differ from one organ to another with HNF-1α being the predominant form in the liver and HNF-1β the major form in the kidney. Inactivation of the HNF-1β gene in mice results in early embryonic lethality by day 7.5 of development. HNF-1β-deficient embryos exhibit an abnormal extraembryonic region, poorly organized ectoderm, and no discernible visceral endoderm.[47, 48]

Table 7. Functional domains and mutations in HNF-1β

- Renal dysfunction and early-onset diabetes
- Variable renal phenotype: nephron agenesis,cysts, familial hypoplastic Glomerulocystic kidney disease, Müellerian aplasia
- Low plasma C-peptide, insulin levels
- Tendency for disease progression, progressive hypoplastic glomerulocystic nephropathy

The gene encoding HNF-1β (Figure 5) maps to chromosome 17q (17cen-q21.3) and genetic variation in this gene is responsible for several human disorders including MODY5 (Table 7), familial hypoplastic glomerulocystic kidney disease, and Müllerian aplasia.[6, 49-51] HNF-1β mutations are rare causes of MODY and only a few MODY5 families have been identified and studied. MODY5 develops early in life (10-25 years) and ultimately requires insulin replacement therapy to control hyperglycemia. The first HNF-1β mutation found to be associated with MODY was HNF-1β(R177X).[6] Nephropathy, in addition to diabetes, was found in this pedigree suggesting that decreased expression levels of HNF-1β in the kidney contribute to renal dysfunction.[6] This loss-of-function mutation generated a truncated protein lacking the C-terminal transactivation domain.[6]

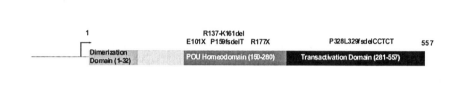

Figure 5. Functional domains and mutations in HNF-1β.

Diabetes, renal dysfunction progressing to end-stage renal disease, and Müllerian aplasia were found in a Norwegian family.[49] This syndrome was caused by a 75-bp deletion in exon 2 of the HNF-1β gene. The deletion is located in the POU DNA binding homeodomain and functional studies revealed that the HNF1β(R137-K161del) mutant lost its DNA binding property and could not activate a reporter gene, indicating that this mutant is functionally inactive.[49]

In contrast to other MODY types, patients with mutations in the HNF-1β gene have early and rapidly progressing familial hypoplastic glomerulocystic kidney disease that is distinct from the diabetic nephropathy in type 1 or type 2 diabetes. Three other HNF-1β mutations, P328L329fsdelCCTCT, P159fsdelT, and E101X, were found in families with a history of renal dysfunction and early-onset diabetes.[50, 51] Both frameshift P159fsdelT and nonsense E101X mutations lack the POU DNA binding domain and result in inactive protein.[50] HNF-1β(P328L329fsdelCCTCT) is a 5-bp deletion resulting in a truncated protein that retains the DNA-binding domain. This mutation is associated with

212

nephron agenesis and exhibits gain-of-function activity with increased transcriptional activation potential *in vitro*.[51] In summary, there is increasing evidence that normal expression levels and activity of HNF-1β are critical for β-cell function and kidney development and that both loss-of-function and gain-of-function mutations can lead to disease in these organs.

Neurogenic Differentiation Factor 1 (MODY6)

NEURO-D1/Beta2 (Figure 6) belongs to the basic helix-loop-helix (bHLH) family of transcription factors that is involved in determining cell type during development. Neuro-D1 is composed of a bHLH DNA binding domain and a C-terminal transactivation domain that interacts with the cellular co-activator p300 and CBP. NEURO-D1 is expressed in pancreatic islets, intestine, and the brain.[52] Mice deficient for Neuro-D1 function have abnormal islet morphology, overt diabetes, and die after birth.[52]

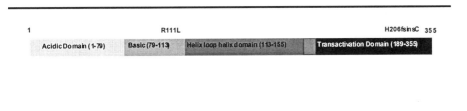

Figure 6. Functional domains and mutations in NEURO-D1/BETA2.

Mutations in the NEURO-D1 gene have recently been reported as being associated with diabetes in two families with autosomal dominant inheritance.[7] One of the families had a G to T substitution in codon 111, causing a substitution of Arg to Leu (R111L) in the proximal bHLH domain. *In vitro* studies suggest that Neuro-D1(R111L) has lost its DNA binding activity and is less effective in transactivating the insulin promoter. Clinical features of subjects with this mutation are similar to type 2 diabetes with high fasting serum insulin levels, elevated levels of insulin two hours after oral glucose, and an average age of diagnosis of 40 (range 30-59 years).[7]

The second mutation in the NEURO-D1 gene consists of an insertion of a cytosine residue in a polyC tract in codon 206 (206+C).[7] NeuroD (H206fsinsC) gives rise to a truncated polypeptide lacking the C-terminal transactivation domain, a region that associates with the co-activators CBP and p300. This mutant retains its ability to bind to DNA, however, it has lost its ability to activate transcription through the deletion of the protein domain that interacts with co-activator p300.[7] The clinical profile of patients with this truncated protein is more severe and shares clinical features of MODY such as low endogenous insulin secretion and early age of onset (range 17-56 years).[7]

Insulin gene mutations

Insulin is synthesized in β-cells of the islets of Langerhans and is a central hormone that maintains glucose homeostasis. Insulin-deficient mice die shortly after birth due to severe hyperglycemia.[53] All cell types of the endocrine pancreas are present in insulin deficient mice suggesting that insulin is not required for development and differentiation of the endocrine pancreas.[53]

Naturally occurring mutations in the insulin gene that result in the synthesis of abnormal insulin proteins have been found in humans to result in a MODY-like phenotype.[9] These abnormal insulin proteins have altered metabolic properties and usually present with inappropriate high serum insulin levels and high insulin/C-peptide ratios due to abnormal post-translational processing and an increased half-life. In many cases, diabetes develops only in individuals with underlying insulin resistance or other risk factors for diabetes. Some mutations in the insulin gene have been reported to segregate with early-onset diabetes with incomplete penetrance and are inherited in an autosomal dominant manner.[9]

SUMMARY

Maturity-onset diabetes of the young (MODY) is a group of monogenic forms of type 2 diabetes that are characterized by an early disease-onset, autosomal dominant inheritance, and defects in insulin secretion. Genetic studies have identified mutations in at least six genes associated with different forms of MODY. The majority of the MODY subtypes are caused by mutations in transcription factors that include hepatocyte nuclear factor (HNF)–4α, HNF-1α, PDX-1, HNF-1β, and NEURO-D1/BETA-2. In addition, genetic defects in the glucokinase gene, the glucose sensor of the pancreatic β-cells, and the insulin gene, also lead to impaired glucose tolerance. The genetic heterogeneity of MODY is reflected in the phenotypic spectrum of the disease. MODY is caused by impaired glucose-stimulated insulin secretion due to defects in pancreatic β-cells and can be discriminated from type 1 diabetes by lack of glutamic acid decarboxylase antibodies. Insulin sensitivity in MODY is normal or increased and insulin resistance is generally not associated with MODY. Glucokinase-deficient diabetes (MODY2) has little tendency to progress, whereas all other forms can develop severe diabetic complications. Restoration of normoglycemia should be attempted with diet and exercise (to maximize insulin sensitivity), oral antidiabetic therapy (insulin secretagogues such as sulphonylureas) and/or insulin.

REFERENCES

1.	Matschinsky FM: Glucokinase as glucose sensor and metabolic signal generator in pancreatic beta-cells and hepatocytes. Diabetes 39:647-652, 1990.
2.	Yamagata K, Furuta H, Oda N, Kaisaki PJ, Menzel S, Cox NJ, Fajans SS, Signorini S, Stoffel M, Bell GI: Mutations in the hepatocyte nuclear factor-4alpha gene in maturity-onset diabetes of the young (MODY1). [see comments]. Nature 384:458-460, 1996.
3.	Stoffers DA, Zinkin NT, Stanojevic V, Clarke WL, Habener JF: Pancreatic agenesis attributable to a single nucleotide deletion in the human IPF1 gene coding sequence. Nature Genetics 15:106-110, 1997.
4.	Stoffers DA, Ferrer J, Clarke WL, Habener JF: Early-onset type-II diabetes mellitus (MODY4) linked to IPF1. Nature Genetics 17:138-139, 1997.
5.	Yamagata K, Oda N, Kaisaki PJ, Menzel S, Furuta H, Vaxillaire M, Southam L, Cox RD, Lathrop GM, Boriraj VV, Chen X, Cox NJ, Oda Y, Yano H, Le Beau MM, Yamada S, Nishigori H, Takeda J, Fajans SS, Hattersley AT, Iwasaki N, Hansen T, Pedersen O, Polonsky KS, Bell GI: Mutations in the hepatocyte nuclear factor-1alpha gene in maturity-onset diabetes of the young (MODY3). [see comments]. Nature 384:455-458, 1996.
6.	Horikawa Y, Iwasaki N, Hara M, Furuta H, Hinokio Y, Cockburn BN, Lindner T, Yamagata K, Ogata M, Tomonaga O, Kuroki H, Kasahara T, Iwamoto Y, Bell GI: Mutation in hepatocyte nuclear factor-1 beta gene (TCF2) associated with MODY. Nature Genetics 17:384-385, 1997.
7.	Malecki MT, Jhala US, Antonellis A, Fields L, Doria A, Orban T, Saad M, Warram JH, Montminy M, Krolewski AS: Mutations in NEUROD1 are associated with the development of type 2 diabetes mellitus. Nature Genetics 23:323-328, 1999.
8.	Waeber G, Delplanque J, Bonny C, Mooser V, Steinmann M, Widmann C, Maillard A, Miklossy J, Dina C, Hani EH, Vionnet N, Nicod P, Boutin P, Froguel P: The gene MAPK8IP1, encoding islet-brain-1, is a candidate for type 2 diabetes. Nature Genetics 24:291-295, 2000.
9.	Vinik A, Bell G: Mutant insulin syndromes. [erratum appears in Horm Metab Res 1988 Mar;20(3):191]. Hormone Metab Res 20:1-10, 1988.

10. Chen WS, Manova K, Weinstein DC, Duncan SA, Plump AS, Prezioso VR, Bachvarova RF, Darnell JE: Disruption of the HNF-4 gene, expressed in visceral endoderm, leads to cell death in embryonic ectoderm and impaired gastrulation of mouse embryos. Genes & Development 8:2466-2477, 1994.

11. Stoffel M, Duncan SA: The maturity-onset diabetes of the young (MODY1) transcription factor HNF4alpha regulates expression of genes required for glucose transport and metabolism. Proc Natl Acad Sci USA 94:13209-13214, 1997.

12. Byrne MM, Sturis J, Fajans SS, Ortiz FJ, Stoltz A, Stoffel M, Smith MJ, Bell GI, Halter JB, Polonsky KS: Altered insulin secretory responses to glucose in subjects with a mutation in the MODY1 gene on chromosome 20. Diabetes 44:699-704, 1995.

13. Herman WH, Fajans SS, Smith MJ, Polonsky KS, Bell GI, Halter JB: Diminished insulin and glucagon secretory responses to arginine in nondiabetic subjects with a mutation in the hepatocyte nuclear factor-4alpha/MODY1 gene. Diabetes 46:1749-1754, 1997.

14. Shih DQ, Dansky HM, Fleisher M, Assmann G, Fajans SS, Stoffel M: Genotype/phenotype relationships in HNF-4alpha/MODY1: haploinsufficiency is associated with reduced apolipoprotein (AII), apolipoprotein (CIII), lipoprotein(a), and triglyceride levels. Diabetes 49:832-837, 2000.

15. Moller AM, Urhammer SA, Dalgaard LT, Reneland R, Berglund L, Hansen T, Clausen JO, Lithell H, Pedersen O: Studies of the genetic variability of the coding region of the hepatocyte nuclear factor-4alpha in Caucasians with maturity onset NIDDM. Diabetologia 40:980-983, 1997.

16. Malecki MT, Yang Y, Antonellis A, Curtis S, Warram JH, Krolewski AS: Identification of new mutations in the hepatocyte nuclear factor 4alpha gene among families with early onset Type 2 diabetes mellitus. Diabetic Medicine 16:193-200, 1999.

17. Hani EH, Suaud L, Boutin P, Chevre JC, Durand E, Philippi A, Demenais F, Vionnet N, Furuta H, Velho G, Bell GI, Laine B, Froguel P: A missense mutation in hepatocyte nuclear factor-4 alpha, resulting in a reduced transactivation activity, in human late-onset non-insulin-dependent diabetes mellitus. J Clin Invest 101:521-526, 1998.

18. Navas MA, Munoz-Elias EJ, Kim J, Shih D, Stoffel M: Functional characterization of the MODY1 gene mutations HNF4(R127W), HNF4(V255M), and HNF4(E276Q). Diabetes 48:1459-1465, 1999.

19. Byrne MM, Sturis J, Clement K, Vionnet N, Pueyo ME, Stoffel M, Takeda J, Passa P, Cohen D, Bell GI: Insulin secretory abnormalities in subjects with hyperglycemia due to glucokinase mutations. J Clin Invest 93:1120-1130, 1994.

20. Njolstad PR, Sovik O, Cuesta-Munoz A, Bjorkhaug L, Massa O, Barbetti F, Undlien DE, Shiota C, Magnuson MA, Molven A, Matschinsky FM, Bell GI: Neonatal Diabetes Mellitus Due to Complete Glucokinase Deficiency. N Engl J Med 344:1588-1592, 2001.

21. Glaser B, Kesavan P, Heyman M, Davis E, Cuesta A, Buchs A, Stanley CA, Thornton PS, Permutt MA, Matschinsky FM, Herold KC: Familial hyperinsulinism caused by an activating glucokinase mutation. N Engl J Med 338:226-230, 1998.

22. Grupe A, Hultgren B, Ryan A, Ma YH, Bauer M, Stewart TA: Transgenic knockouts reveal a critical requirement for pancreatic beta cell glucokinase in maintaining glucose homeostasis. Cell 83:69-78, 1995.

23. Velho G, Petersen KF, Perseghin G, Hwang JH, Rothman DL, Pueyo ME, Cline GW, Froguel P, Shulman GI: Impaired hepatic glycogen synthesis in glucokinase-deficient (MODY-2) subjects. J Clin Invest 98:1755-1761, 1996.

24. Hattersley AT, Beards F, Ballantyne E, Appleton M, Harvey R, Ellard S: Mutations in the glucokinase gene of the fetus result in reduced birth weight. [see comments]. Nature Genetics 19:268-270, 1998.

25. Pearson ER, Velho G, Clark P, Stride A, Shepherd M, Frayling TM, Bulman MP, Ellard S, Froguel P, Hattersley AT: beta-cell genes and diabetes: quantitative and qualitative differences in the pathophysiology of hepatic nuclear factor-1alpha and glucokinase mutations. Diabetes 50 (Suppl 1):S101-107, 2001.

26. Froguel P, Zouali H, Vionnet N, Velho G, Vaxillaire M, Sun F, Lesage S, Stoffel M, Takeda J, Passa P: Familial hyperglycemia due to mutations in glucokinase. Definition of a subtype of diabetes mellitus. [see comments]. N Engl J Med 328:697-702, 1993.

27. Pontoglio M, Barra J, Hadchouel M, Doyen A, Kress C, Bach JP, Babinet C, Yaniv M: Hepatocyte nuclear factor 1 inactivation results in hepatic dysfunction, phenylketonuria, and renal Fanconi syndrome. Cell 84:575-585, 1996.

28. Lee YH, Sauer B, Gonzalez FJ: Laron dwarfism and non-insulin-dependent diabetes mellitus in the Hnf-1alpha knockout mouse. Mol Cell Biol 18:3059-3068, 1998.

29. Hiraiwa H, Pan C-J, Lin B, Akiyama TE, Gonzalez FJ, Chou JY: A molecular link between the common phenotypes of type 1 glycogen storage disease and HNF1-alpha-null mice. J Biol Chem 276:7963-7967, 2001.

30. Shih DQ, Bussen M, Sehayek E, Ananthanarayanan M, Shneider BL, Suchy FJ, Shefer S, Bollileni JS, Gonzalez FJ, Breslow JL, Stoffel M: Hepatocyte nuclear factor-1alpha is an essential regulator of bile acid and plasma cholesterol metabolism. Nature Genetics 27:375-382, 2001.

31. Dukes ID, Sreenan S, Roe MW, Levisetti M, Zhou YP, Ostrega D, Bell GI, Pontoglio M, Yaniv M, Philipson L, Polonsky KS: Defective pancreatic beta-cell glycolytic signaling in hepatocyte nuclear factor-1alpha-deficient mice. J Biol Chem 273:24457-24464, 1998.

32. Shih DQ, Screenan S, Munoz KN, Phillipson L, Pontoglio M, Yaniv M, Polonsky KS, Stoffel M: Loss of HNF-1a function in mice leads to abnormal expression of genes involved in pancreatic islet development and metabolism. Diabetes 50:2472-2480, 2001.

33. Yamagata K, Yang Q, Yamamoto K, Iwahashi H, Miyagawa J, Okita K, Yoshiuchi I, Miyazaki J, Noguchi T, Nakajima H, Namba M, Hanafusa T, Matsuzawa Y: Mutation P291fsinsC in the transcription factor hepatocyte nuclear factor-1alpha is dominant negative. Diabetes 47:1231-1235, 1998.

34. Kaisaki PJ, Menzel S, Lindner T, Oda N, Rjasanowski I, Sahm J, Meincke G, Schulze J, Schmechel H, Petzold C, Ledermann HM, Sachse G, Boriraj VV, Menzel R, Kerner W, Turner RC, Yamagata K, Bell GI: Mutations in the hepatocyte nuclear factor-1alpha gene in MODY and early-onset NIDDM: evidence for a mutational hotspot in exon 4. [erratum appears in Diabetes 1997 Jul;46(7):1239]. Diabetes 46:528-535, 1997.

35. Hegele RA, Cao H, Harris SB, Hanley AJ, Zinman B: The hepatic nuclear factor-1alpha G319S variant is associated with early-onset type 2 diabetes in Canadian Oji-Cree. J Clin Endocrinol Metab 84:1077-1082, 1999.

36. Lehto M, Tuomi T, Mahtani MM, Widen E, Forsblom C, Sarelin L, Gullstrom M, Isomaa B, Lehtovirta M, Hyrkko A, Kanninen T, Orho M, Manley S, Turner RC, Brettin T, Kirby A, Thomas J, Duyk G, Lander E, Taskinen MR, Groop L: Characterization of the MODY3 phenotype. Early-onset diabetes caused by an insulin secretion defect. J Clin Invest 99:582-591, 1997.

37. Hansen T, Eiberg H, Rouard M, Vaxillaire M, Moller AM, Rasmussen SK, Fridberg M, Urhammer SA, Holst JJ, Almind K, Echwald SM, Hansen L, Bell GI, Pedersen O: Novel MODY3 mutations in the hepatocyte nuclear factor-1alpha gene: evidence for a hyperexcitability of pancreatic beta-cells to intravenous secretagogues in a glucose-tolerant carrier of a P447L mutation. Diabetes 46:726-730, 1997.

38. Frayling TM, Evans JC, Bulman MP, Pearson E, Allen L, Owen K, Bingham C, Hannemann M, Shepherd M, Ellard S, Hattersley AT: beta-cell genes and diabetes: molecular and clinical characterization of mutations in transcription factors. Diabetes 50 (Suppl 1):S94-100, 2001.

39. Dutta S, Gannon M, Peers B, Wright C, Bonner-Weir S, Montminy M: PDX:PBX complexes are required for normal proliferation of pancreatic cells during development. Proc Natl Acad Sci USA 98:1065-1070, 2001.

40. Ohlsson H, Karlsson K, Edlund T: IPF1, a homeodomain-containing transactivator of the insulin gene. EMBO Journal 12:4251-4259, 1993.

41. Jonsson J, Carlsson L, Edlund T, Edlund H: Insulin-promoter-factor 1 is required for pancreas development in mice. Nature 371:606-609, 1994.

42. Ahlgren U, Jonsson J, Jonsson L, Simu K, Edlund H: beta-cell-specific inactivation of the mouse Ipf1/Pdx1 gene results in loss of the beta-cell phenotype and maturity onset diabetes. Genes & Development 12:1763-1768, 1998.

43. Hart AW, Baeza N, Apelqvist A, Edlund H: Attenuation of FGF signalling in mouse beta-cells leads to diabetes. Nature 408:864-868, 2000.

44. Stoffers DA, Stanojevic V, Habener JF: Insulin promoter factor-1 gene mutation linked to early-onset type 2 diabetes mellitus directs expression of a dominant negative isoprotein. J Clin Invest 102:232-241, 1998.

45. Hani EH, Stoffers DA, Chevre JC, Durand E, Stanojevic V, Dina C, Habener JF, Froguel P: Defective mutations in the insulin promoter factor-1 (IPF-1) gene in late-onset type 2 diabetes mellitus. J Clin Invest 104:R41-48, 1999.

46. Macfarlane WM, Frayling TM, Ellard S, Evans JC, Allen LI, Bulman MP, Ayres S, Shepherd M, Clark P, Millward A, Demaine A, Wilkin T, Docherty K, Hattersley AT: Missense mutations in the insulin promoter factor-1 gene predispose to type 2 diabetes. J Clin Invest 104:R33-39, 1999.

47.   Coffinier C, Thepot D, Babinet C, Yaniv M, Barra J: Essential role for the homeoprotein vHNF1/HNF1beta in visceral endoderm differentiation. Development 126:4785-4794, 1999.

48.   Barbacci E, Reber M, Ott MO, Breillat C, Huetz F, Cereghini S: Variant hepatocyte nuclear factor 1 is required for visceral endoderm specification. Development 126:4795-4805, 1999.

49.   Lindner TH, Njolstad PR, Horikawa Y, Bostad L, Bell GI, Sovik O: A novel syndrome of diabetes mellitus, renal dysfunction and genital malformation associated with a partial deletion of the pseudo-POU domain of hepatocyte nuclear factor-1beta. Hum Mol Genetics 8:2001-2008, 1999.

50.   Bingham C, Bulman MP, Ellard S, Allen LI, Lipkin GW, Hoff WG, Woolf AS, Rizzoni G, Novelli G, Nicholls AJ, Hattersley AT: Mutations in the hepatocyte nuclear factor-1beta gene are associated with familial hypoplastic glomerulocystic kidney disease. Am J Hum Gen 68:219-224, 2001.

51.   Bingham C, Ellard S, Allen L, Bulman M, Shepherd M, Frayling T, Berry PJ, Clark PM, Lindner T, Bell GI, Ryffel GU, Nicholls AJ, Hattersley AT: Abnormal nephron development associated with a frameshift mutation in the transcription factor hepatocyte nuclear factor-1 beta. [see comments]. Kid Intl 57:898-907, 2000.

52.   Naya FJ, Huang HP, Qiu Y, Mutoh H, DeMayo FJ, Leiter AB, Tsai MJ: Diabetes, defective pancreatic morphogenesis, and abnormal enteroendocrine differentiation in BETA2/neuroD-deficient mice. Genes & Development 11:2323-2334, 1997.

53.   Duvillie B, Cordonnier N, Deltour L, Dandoy-Dron F, Itier JM, Monthioux E, Jami J, Joshi RL, Bucchini D: Phenotypic alterations in insulin-deficient mutant mice. Proc Natl Acad Sci USA 94:5137-5140, 1997.

Chapter 4. Diabetes in Pregnancy

Adina E. Schneider and Elliot J.Rayfield

INTRODUCTION

Diabetes complicates 4% of all pregnancies is the United States and is a significant cause of maternal and fetal morbidity.[1] The majority (88%) of diabetes cases in pregnancy are due to gestational diabetes which is associated with increased BMI and increased age. The remaining 12% are due to type 1 and type 2 diabetes, often referred to as pregestational diabetes. Patients with gestational diabetes usually develop hyperglycemia during the second half of pregnancy. Hyperglycemia at this stage of gestation clearly causes   fetal macrosomia and neonatal hypoglycemia.   Patients with pregestational diabetes are at risk for hyperglycemia early in pregnancy; this hyperglycemia is associated with significantly increased rates of fetal loss and fetal malformation. The evidence that has accrued over the past twenty years reveals that tight glycemic control can prevent most of the maternal and fetal complications of diabetes. The neonatal death rate in pregnancies complicated by diabetes was 50% prior to the introduction of insulin, 10% in 1939 after the introduction of insulin, and approached that in non-diabetic pregnancies by the 1980s.[2]

PATHOPHYSIOLOGY OF PREGNANCY

The first trimester of pregnancy is associated with increased insulin sensitivity which may be due to increased adipocyte binding of insulin in the presence of increased estradiol levels.[3] In addition, insulin secretion in response to glucose appears to be enhanced during the first twenty weeks of pregnancy.[4] During normal pregnancy fasting and postprandial glucose levels are lower than in the nonpregnant state and HBA1C falls approximately 20%. This is also explained by fetal utilization of glucose. However, as the levels of cortisol, progesterone, estrogen, prolactin, and human placental lactogen rise later in pregnancy, a state of insulin resistance ensues (Figure 1). Fasting insulin levels rise and C-peptide peaks at about 28-32 weeks gestation. Human placental lactogen, which is homologous to growth hormone, is an insulin antagonist and is likely responsible for most of the observed insulin resistance.[3]

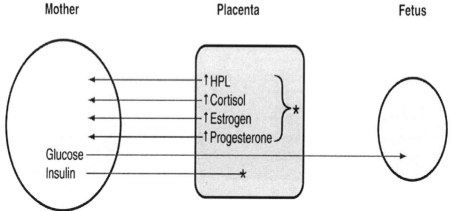

Figure 1. Movement of hormones and glucose across the placental barrier.

GESTATIONAL DIABETES

Gestational diabetes (GDM) is defined as glucose intolerance of varying severity with onset or first recognition during pregnancy. As discussed above, insulin resistance is a normal consequence of pregnancy. Women with GDM, in contrast to normal pregnant women, have an impaired ability to secrete insulin.[5] Beta cells of women with GDM appear to compensate poorly for insulin resistance.[6] Mention is made of GDM as early as 1946, when Miller observed an 8% neonatal mortality among infants born to mothers who subsequently developed diabetes.[7]

Diagnosis

The diagnosis of GDM is determined by the results of an oral glucose tolerance test (OGTT). The currently used values for the 100g test are based on the calculations of O'Sullivan and Mahan who performed the 100g OGTT on 752 pregnant women and set the diagnostic threshold at greater than 2 standard deviations above the mean.[8] This cutoff was based on a retrospective evaluation of 1,013 subjects; 22% of the women who had a glucose tolerance test of greater than 2 SD above the mean developed diabetes in the next 7-8 years. In 1978 ACOG (American Congress of Obstetricians and Gynecologists) recommended the use of the O'Sullivan-Mahan criteria for the diagnosis of gestational diabetes. Coustan and Carpenter revised these criteria in 1982 to account for the shift from venous to plasma blood glucose levels and for changes in technology.[9] Table 1 shows the criteria for diagnosis of GDM after a 100 gram or 75 gram oral glucose load. The 75 g load is advocated by the World Health Organization (WHO) and is more sensitive and less specific than the 100g load which is advocated by the American Diabetes Association (ADA). Either test should be performed in the morning with the patient seated after an overnight fast of 8-14 hours. Over the preceding 3 days the patient should have unrestricted carbohydrate intake and unrestricted physical activity. Two or more positive values are necessary for the diagnosis of GDM.

Table 1. Diagnostic Criteria for GDM

	ADA	WHO
Glucose load	100g	75g
Fasting	95	95
1 hr	180	180
2 hr	155	155
3 hr	140	

Screening

It is essential that all women presenting for the first prenatal visit be assessed for their risk of developing gestational diabetes. The ADA and ACOG advocate a 2 step approach to screening. A 50 gm glucose test is performed on all average risk patients at 24-28 weeks. If the threshold level (>140mg/dl at 1 hr) is met, the above 100gm oral glucose tolerance test is performed.[10]

Women who are deemed to be at high risk should undergo blood glucose testing as early as possible in the pregnancy using the 1 or 2 step procedure. If they do not meet the diagnostic threshold the testing should be repeated at 24- 28 weeks. High risk characteristics include: obesity, family history of type 2 DM, personal history of prior GDM, glucose intolerance, or glucosuria.[10]

An area of continued controversy is whether low risk women should undergo screening. Low risk characteristics include: age <25, normal weight before pregnancy, no known diabetes in first degree relatives, no history of poor obstetric outcome, no history of abnormal glucose metabolism, and member of an ethnic group with a low prevalence of GDM. The ADA does not recommend screening women who meet all of the aforementioned criteria. In a study of 573 low risk pregnant women, a 2.8% prevalence of GDM was found using the 75g glucose tolerance test. There was no difference in pregnancy outcomes in this group when compared to other patients with GDM. 10% of all cases of GDM would have been missed if low risk patients had not been screened.[11] Thus, many experts advocate continued screening of all pregnant women.[12]

Morbidity

The consequences of untreated gestational diabetes have been well described. Maternal glucose crosses the placenta, while insulin does not. Thus, maternal hyperglycemia leads to fetal hyperinsulinemia which results in macrosomia and neonatal hypoglycemia. Maternal consequences of gestational diabetes include: preeclampsia, polyhydramnios, operative delivery, and future development of overt diabetes. Fetal and infant consequences include: macrosomia, shoulder dystocia, polycythemia, hyperbilirubinemia, and increased risk of developing obesity and diabetes in later life.[13]

Table 2. Morbidity of Gestational Diabetes

Maternal	Fetal and Newborn
Preeclampsia Macrosomia	Neonatal hypoglycemia
C section	Shoulder dystocia
Polyhydramnios	Polycythemia
	Hypocalcemia
	Hyperbiliribinemia
	Future DM, obesity

There is now ample evidence that identification and treatment of women who meet the above diagnostic criteria is associated with decreased perinatal morbidity. It appears that strict metabolic control is necessary to reduce macrosomia and mortality. A reduction in macrosomia has been shown to occur only in patients who achieve a FBG of <95 mg/dl.[14] A prospective controlled trial compared the pregnancy outcomes of 102 women with gestational diabetes who were under strict control with 102 nondiabetic controls. The women with gestational diabetes were treated with diet or diet and insulin to achieve a BG < 130mg/dl one hour after breakfast. The perinatal outcomes in the pregnancies complicated by gesational diabetes were equal to the control pregnancies.[15] In an important study, De Veciana showed that postprandial, rather than preprandial, blood glucose monitoring resulted in improved glycemic control and decreased the risk of macrosomia, cesarean delivery (12% vs 36%, p=0.04) and neonatal hypoglycemia (3% vs 25%, p=0.05).[16]

Target glucose levels

Blood glucose goals for diabetic pregnancy have been determined with previously mentioned studies in mind.[17]

Fasting	60-90 mg/dl
Premeal	60-105 mg/dl
1 hour postprandial	100-140 mg/dl
2 hours postprandial	60-120 mg/dl
HBA1C	<6 %

In order to meet the above goals for normoglycemia in pregnancy, self monitoring of blood glucose is essential. Weekly monitoring of blood glucose levels is unlikely to identify women at risk for perinatal complications. Self monitoring of blood glucose levels is necessary in patients treated with diet therapy alone so that those failing to meet euglycemic goals can be identified as early as possible. We advocate blood glucose testing before meals, after meals and at bedtime to ensure attainment of ideal glycemic control.

Diet therapy and exercise

Diet therapy for gestational diabetes should be provided by a nutritionist or other professional with experience in treating pregnant women with diabetes. Limiting carbohydrate intake to 35-45% of total calories is the cornerstone of this therapy.[18] The avoidance of simple carbohydrates is advocated as they lead to high postprandial glucose values. In addition caloric restriction should be imposed on obese patients. A wait gain of only 7 kg is permitted for patients with a BMI of >29 kg/m2, while patients with a BMI of <19 kg/m2 should gain up to 18 kg.[19] Physical exercise has been shown to improve maternal glucose control and is advocated by the ADA for patients with gestational diabetes.[17]

Insulin

Patients who fail to meet the above stated glycemic goals or who show signs of excess fetal growth should be started on insulin. Since pregnancy is an insulin resistant state, high doses of insulin are often required to maintain euglycemia. An initial starting dose of insulin can be estimated as 0.7 Units/kg/day. Most patients will require at least three injections (prebreakfast, predinner, bedtime) to achieve the previously described goals. The new synthetic human insulin analog, Humalog, is now in common use during pregnancy. Its rapid onset of action has been shown to improve postprandial blood glucose levels, which is particularly important in pregnant diabetics. Oral agents are not approved for use in pregnancy. A recent study showed similar outcomes in a group of 201 patients with gestational diabetes treated with glyburide compared with a group of 203 insulin treated patients.[20] Larger studies are needed before the use of sulfonylureas can be recommended during pregnancy.

Labor and delivery

It is very important to prevent maternal hyperglycemia late in gestation as this results in fetal hyperinsulinemia and neonatal hypoglycemia. Blood glucose should be maintained in the range of 70-110. Most women with GDM will not require insulin once active labor begins and rarely require insulin after delivery.

Fetal Surveillance

The intensity of fetal monitoring is determined by the severity of GDM. At a minimum, patients treated with diet alone should be taught to measure fetal movements during the last 8-10 weeks of pregnancy. Patients who are being treated with insulin should undergo non-stress testing beginning at 32 weeks gestation. Fetal ultrasound may be used to assess fetal size at 29-33 weeks and should be used for detection of fetal anomalies in patients who had GDM diagnosed during the first trimester or who have fasting glucose of >120 mg/dl.[19]

Long term consequences to mother and offspring

Women who have had GDM at are at high risk for developing type 2 diabetes. Risk factors for development of diabetes in these women are: gestational age at diagnosis, severity of GDM, level of glycemia at the first post partum visit, obesity and further pregnancy.[17] A cohort of 666 Latino women with GDM was followed for up to 7.5 years; women with an additional pregnancy had an increased risk (rate ratio 3.34) of developing type 2 DM compared to women without an additional pregnancy.[21] Women with GDM should be evaluated for glucose intolerance 6-12 weeks post partum and annually thereafter. Counseling women on the risks of glucose intolerance and future diabetes is essential.

The children of women who have had GDM have increased risk of developing obesity and abnormal glucose tolerance by the time of puberty. The healthcare providers of these children should be aware of this risk so that they can encourage their patients to make appropriate lifestyle changes. [19]

PREGESTATIONAL DIABETES

Type 1 and type 2 diabetes complicate 0.15 % and 0.33 % of pregnancies in the United States, respectively.[1] When treating these patients, it is not only essential to assess the effect the diabetes has on the pregnancy, but also the impact the pregnancy has on diabetic complications, such as retinopathy and nephropathy.[3]

Unlike most patients with gestational diabetes who develop hyperglycemia during the second half of pregnancy, patients with pregestational diabetes may be hyperglycemic from conception. The presence of poor glycemic control during the first 7 weeks of fetal development results in significant rates of congenital malformations and fetal mortality.[22] It cannot be overemphasized that women with pregestational diabetes receive intensive preconception counseling and achieve tight glycemic control before becoming pregnant.

Congenital malformations

Before the introduction of insulin diabetic women were rarely able to produce viable offspring. The introduction of insulin and improvement in glycemic control has led to decreased rates of fetal death and congenital malformations. Malformations appear to be a result of metabolic derangements, predominantly hyperglycemia, early in organogenesis The exact mechanism by which hyperglycemia causes anomalies remains undetermined, but likely involves generation of oxygen free radicals and the disruption of the embryonic yolk sac.[37] Alterations in other metabolites such as myo-inositol[38], arachidonic acid[39], prostaglandins[37], have also been postulated to play a role in the dysmorphogenesis. These data are largely derived from animal studies and further work will need to be done to more fully understand the pathogenesis of the malformations

The level of glycemic control early in organogenesis has been shown to impact rates of malformations. Miller et al showed that a HBA1C in the first trimester of >8.5% was associated with a malformation rate of 22.4%, a HBA1C 7- 8.4% was associated with a rate of 5%, while a HBA1C <6.9% was associated with no malformations.[23] The duration of diabetes and presence of vasculopathy have also been shown to be associated with an increased risk of anomalies.[24]

Clinical trials have clearly shown that attainment of euglycemia before conception almost eliminates the excessive risk of congenital malformations. The incidence of major malformations in women with careful preconception care has been reported to be 0.8-1.6 %, compared with 6.5-8.2 % in women who did not receive preconception care.[25, 26, 27]

Preconception care

Pregnancy must be a planned event for women with type 1 and 2 diabetes. Jovanovic points out that women with type 2 diabetes are less likely to receive preconception care because the disease has often gone undiagnosed.[22] In addition, type 2 diabetes is also more prevalent in minority groups who may have less access to care.

The goals of preconception care are to achieve a HBA1C as low as possible without the development of hypoglycemia:[28] Patients with type 2 diabetes who are being treated with oral agents must be switched to insulin, as there are currently no oral agents approved for use in pregnancy. Patients should become facile with frequent blood glucose monitoring and self adjustment of insulin. Conception should be deferred until the patient is normoglycemic:

Fasting BG <95 mg/d
1 hr post prandial BG <140 mg/dl
2 hr post prandial BG <120 mg/dl

Another important aspect of preconception care is the identification of diabetic complications that might be aggravated by pregnancy. A dilated retinal exam, blood pressure measurement, cardiovascular exam and lower extremity exam are imperative. Evaluation of renal function, via a 24 urine collection for microablumin/creatinine, and thyroid function, via TSH, are essential components of the initial visit. Hypertensive women should be treated with agents such as aldomet, which have been shown to be safe in pregnancy; ACE inhibitors, diuretics and beta blockers should be avoided.[28]

Table 3. Preconception Care – Initial Visit

HbA1c
BG record
24 hour Urine microalbumin/creat
TSH
Blood pressure
Retinal Exam
Cardiovascular evaluation
Neurologic exam
Nutritional Evaluation
Counseling on risks of pregnancy

Diabetic retinopathy

Progression of diabetic retinopathy is a risk of tightened metabolic control in early pregnancy. A prospective study of 140 diabetic women without proliferative retinopathy revealed progression of retinopathy in 10.3% of patients with no retinopathy, 21.1% of patients with microaneurysms, 54.8% of patients with moderate to severe nonproliferative retinopathy. Proliferative retinopathy developed in 6.3% of patients with mild and 29% of patients with moderate to severe retinopathy. The odds ratio of developing proliferative disease in patients with HBA1C >6 SD above the mean versus 2 SD above the mean was 2.7.[29] Risk factors for progression to proliferative retinopathy are: baseline retinopathy, elevated HBA1C at conception, rapid normalization of blood glucose, duration of diabetes greater than 6 years and proteinuria.[22]

Diabetic nephropathy

Careful assessment of renal function is mandatory in all diabetic women planning a pregnancy. The increased glomerular filtration rate seen in pregnancy often results in increased proteinuria; thus, a 24 hour urine for microalbumin and creatinine should be collected prior to conception. Although pregnancy is associated with a transient decline in renal function, it does not appear to hasten the onset of end stage renal disease in women with nephropathy.[30] The ideal medical therapy for diabetic nephropathy, ACE inhibitors, are contraindicated during pregnancy. Alpha methyl-dopa is considered safe during early pregnancy. Diltiazem, which is a more effective agent in preventing progression of nephropathy, can be used at the end of the first trimester.[31] Pre-eclampsia is the most common complication in patients with overt nephropathy; other maternal complications include anemia and nephrotic syndrome. Fetal complications include: fetal distress, intrauterine growth retardation, preterm delivery, and stillbirth. Diabetic nephropathy, in the absence of HTN, impacts fetal outcome when renal function is impaired by at least 50%.[22] With improved preconception and perinatal glycemic and blood pressure control, perinatal mortality has decreased to 5%.[22]

Treatment

Close follow up by a diabetic team is required throughout gestation to assure maintenance of strict glycemic control. Office visits every 2-3 weeks are usually necessary with more frequent telephone contact as needed.

Table 4. Neonatal care

5-9 blood glucose measurements/d
HBA1C every 4-6 weeks
Office Visits every 2-3 weeks
Telephone Contact (as needed)
Fetal Surveillance

Multiple blood glucose measurements and insulin injections are required to achieve tight glycemic control. As noted previously, postprandial monitoring seems to result in improved fetal outcome. Postprandial blood glucose levels are the most important predictor of fetal macrosomia.[32] HBA1C should be monitored to confirm the level of control. The usual insulin requirement in type 1 patients early in pregnancy is 0.7U/kg/dy divided into 3-4 injections. As human placental lactogen rises, the requirements increase to 0.8U/kg/dy (week 18-26), 0.9U/kg/dy (week 26-36), and 1.0U/kg/dy (week 36 - term). Insulin pump therapy can achieve glucose control and perinatal outcomes equal to multiple injection regimens.[33]

As discussed for women with gestational diabetetes, women with type 2 diabetes must be treated with insulin during pregnancy. Again, insulin requirements in these patients are often high due to obesity and insulin resistance.

Diet and exercise

As discussed for gestational diabetics, patients with type 1 or type 2 diabetes should be followed closely by a nutritionist or other professional with experience in treating pregnant diabetics. Recommended caloric intake should be determined by pregestational weight. 24kcal/kg/d is recommended for women at ideal body weight. 40-50% of calories should be from carbohydrate, 20 % from protein and 30-40 % from fat. Calories are distributed over the course of the day as follows: 10% for breakfast, 30 % for lunch, 30% for dinner, and 30% for snacks.[22] Similar to gestational diabetics, exercise may be beneficial for pregnant patients with type 2 diabetes. Exercise in pregnant women with type 1 diabetes may lead to increased hypoglycemic episodes and is only permitted in women who participated in an exercise program prior to becoming pregnant.[22]

Hypoglycemia

Hypoglycemia is an important complication of tight glucose control during pregnancy. Early pregnancy is associated with decreased fasting glucose levels due to increased glucose uptake by the placental fetal unit and decreased hepatic glucose production. 33% of all pregnant women treated with insulin have at least one episode of hypoglycemia.[34] The majority of these episodes occur during the first trimester. Recurrent episodes of hypoglycemia may be associated with small for gestational age infants[19] and severe prolonged episodes of hypoglycemia can result in intrauterine fetal demise.[35]

Diabetic ketoacidosis (DKA)

Although its frequency has decreased markedly, diabetic ketoacidosis remains a serious emergency in the pregnant woman with type 1 diabetes and is associated with increased fetal morbidity and mortality. Ketogenesis appears to be accelerated during the third trimester. The mechanism by which DKA results in poor fetal outcome is not clear but is hypothesized to be due to fetal hypoxia. Another possibility is that the fetus becomes acidotic and develops hypokalemia with subsequent cardiac arrest.[36] The fetal heart rate should be continuously monitored while the mother is undergoing intensive treatment of DKA. It is also prudent to alert a neonatalogist.

Labor and delivery

The maintenance of maternal euglycemia at delivery is necessary in order to prevent neonatal hypoglycemia. The goal of insulin therapy is to keep the blood glucose between 70- 90mg/dl.[22] This can best be accomplished via an insulin drip. When active labor begins the insulin requirement of the mother usually declines and drops even further as the placenta is expelled. Thus, intravenous glucose should be started once active labor begins. After the delivery the mother may not require any insulin therapy for 24 –72 hours. The cause of this clinical observation remains speculative but may be attributed to a state of functional hypopituitarism after delivery of the placenta.[40]

Fetal surveillance

Fetal surveillance may be deferred until the 35th week in patients with pregestational diabetes who have been under strict metabolic control. Those patients with poor control, nephropathy, hypertension, or vascular disease should begin surveillance at week 26.   The best method of surveillance is via fetal ultrasound which can estimate gestational age, screen for anomalies, determine amniotic fluid volume and asses fetus status through doppler and biophysical profiles.[22]

SUMMARY

The presence of diabetes in a pregnant woman can result in serious maternal and neonatal morbidity and mortality if not treated appropriately. Screening pregnant women for gestational diabetes and attainment of euglycemia, either by diet or insulin therapy, clearly prevents potentially catastrophic maternal and fetal events. Pregnancies that suffer from hyperglycemia early in gestation are at high risk for fetal loss and malformations. Thus, preconception care is essential for all type 1 and type 2 diabetic women. Diabetic women of reproductive age must be continually reminded of the need to plan their pregnancies. Maintenance of strict glycemic control requires tremendous effort on the part of the patient and the health care team. This should be considered an achievable goal in all pregnant diabetics.

REFERENCES

1. Engelgau M. Herman W, Smith P, German R, Aubert R. The epidemiology of diabetes and pregnancy in the US, 1988. Diabetes Care 18:1029-1033, 1995.
2. Tyrala E. The infant of the diabetic mother. Obstetrics and Gynecology Clinics 23:221-241, 1996.
3. Ryan EA. Prevention and treatment of diabetes and its complications: Pregnancy and Diabetes. Medical Clinics of North America 82:823-845, 1998.
4. Boden G. Fuel Metabolism in pregnancy and gestational diabetes mellitus. Obstetr and Gynecol Clinics 23:1-10, 1996.
5. Kuhl C. Etiology and pathogenesis of gestational diabetes. Diabetes Care 21(S2):B19, 1998.
6. Buchanan TA. Pancreatic B cell defects in gestational diabetes: implications for pathogenesis and prevention of type 2 diabetes. J Clin Endocrinol Metab 86:989-993, 2001.
7. Miller HC. The effect of diabetic and prediabetic pregnancies on the fetus and newborn infant. J Pediatr 26: 455-461, 1946.
8. O'Sullivan JB, Mahan CM. Criteria for the oral glucose tolerance test in pregnancy. Diabetes 13:285, 1964.
9. Coustan DR, Carpenter MW. The diagnosis of gestational diabetes. Diabetes Care 21:B5-B8, 1998.
10. ADA position statement. Diabetes Care 24(S1):S77-S79, 2001.
11. Moses R, Moses J, Davis W. Gestational diabetes: Do lean young caucasian women need to be tested? Diabetes Care 21:1803-1807, 1998.
12. Pettitt D. GDM: Who to test, how to test. Diabetes Care 21: 1789-1790, 1998.

13. Jovanovic L. American Diabetes Association's Fourth International Workshop—Conference on Gestational Diabetes Mellitus: summary and discussion. Therapeutic interventions. Diabetes Care 21(S2):B131-137, 1998.

14. Opperman W et al. Gestation diabetes and macrosomia. In Early Control in Early Life, NY Academic; New York, 455-468, 1975.

15. Drexel H, Alefred B, Sigurd S, et al. Prevention of perinatal morbidity by tight metabolic control in gestational diabetes. Diabetes Care 11:761-776, 1988.

16. De Veciana M, Major C, Morgan M, Asrat T, et al. Postprandial versus preprandial blood glucose monitoring in women with gestational diabetes mellitus requiring insulin therapy. N Engl J Med 333:1237-1241, 1995.

17. Jovanovic-Peterson L, Medical management of pregnancy complicated by diabetes. American Diabetes Association, Alexandria, VA, 1995.

18. Major CA, Henry MH, De Veciana M, Morgan MA. The effects of carbohydrate restriction in patients with diet controlled gestational diabetes. Obstet Gynecol 91:600-604, 1998.

19. Metzger B, Coustan D. Summary and recommendations of the fourth International workshop--conference on gestational diabetes mellitus. Diabetes Care 21 (S2):B161, 1998.

20. Langer et al. A comparison of glyburide and insulin in women with gestational diabetes mellitus. N Engl J Med 343:1134-1138, 2000.

21. Peters RK. long term effect of single pregnancy in women with previous gestional diabetes mellitus. Lancet 347:227-230, 1996.

22. Jovanovic L. Medical emergencies in the patient with diabetes during pregnancy. Endocrinol Metabol Clin 29, 2000.

23. Miller E, Hare JW, Cloherty JP, et al. Elevated maternal HBA1c and major congenital anomalies in infants of diabetic mothers. N Engl J Med 304: 1331-1334, 1998.

24. Karlsson K, Kjeller I. The outcome of diabetic pregnancies in relation to the mother's blood glucose level. Am J Obstet Gynecol 112:213-220, 1972.

25. Fuhrmann K, Reiker H, Semmler K, et al. The effect of intensified conventional insulin therapy before and during pregnancy on the malformation rate in offspring of diabetic mothers. Exp Clin Endocrinol 83:173-177, 1984.

26. Damm P, Molsted-Pederson L. Significant decrease in congenital malformations in newborn infants of an unselected population of diabetic women. Am J Obstet Gynecol 161: 1163-1167, 1989.

27. Willhoite MB, Benvert HW, Palomaki GE, et al. The impact of preconception counseling on pregnancy outcomes: the experience of the Maine Diabetes in Pregnancy Program. Diabetes Care 16:450-455, 1993.

28. ADA position statement: preconception care of women with diabetes. Diabetes Care 24 (S1, 2001.
29. Chew E et al. Metabolic control and progression of retinopathy, the diabetes in early pregnancy study. Diabetes Care 18:631-637, 1995.
30. Leguizamon G, Reece EA. Effect of medical therapy on progressive nephropathy: influence of pregnancy, diabetes, and hypertension. J Maternal Fetal Med 9:70-78, 2000.
31. Kitzmiller JL, Combs CA. Diabetic nephropathy and pregnancy. Obstetrics and Gynecology Clinics 23:173, 1996.
32. Jovanovic-Peterson L, Peterson CM, Reed GF, et al. Maternal postprandial glucose levels predict birth weight: the diabetes in early pregnancy study. Am J Obstet Gynecol 164:103-111, 1991.
33. Gabbe S. New concepts and applications in the use of the insulin pump during pregnancy. J Maternal Fetal Medicine 9:42-45, 2000.
34. Coustan DR, Reece RA, Sherwin RS, et al. A randomized trial of the insulin pump vs intensive conventional therapy in diabetic pregnancies. JAMA 255:631-636, 1986.
35. Whiteman VE, Homko CJ, Reece EA. Management of hypoglycemia and diabetic ketoacidosis in pregnancy. Obstet Gynecol Clin 23:87-107, 1996
36. Kitzmiller JL. Diabetic ketoacidosis and pregnancy. Contemp Obster Gynecol 20:141-148, 1982.
37. Reece EA, Eriksson UJ. The pathogenesis of diabetes associated congenital malformations. Obstetr and Gynecol Clinics 23:29-45, 1996.
38. Hod M, Star S, Passoneau J, et al. Effect of hyperglycemia on sorbitol and myo-inositol content of cultured rat conceptus: Failure of aldose reductase inhibitors to modify myo-inositol and dysmorphogeneis. Biochem Biophys Res Commun 140: 974-980, 1986.
39. Pinter E, Reece EA, Ogbum P, et al. Relative essential fatty acid deficiency in hyperglycemia – induced embryopathy. Am J Obstet Gynecol 159:1484-1490, 1988.
40. Personal communication. Lois Jovanovic , September 2001.

Chapter 5. Secondary Causes of Diabetes Mellitus

Tamer N. Sargios and Adrienne M. Fleckman

INTRODUCTION

The diabetic syndromes include type 1 diabetes with immune destruction of the pancreatic islets, type 2 diabetes with a complex pathophysiology of insulin resistance combined with insulin secretory failure, distinct monogenetic abnormalities (maturity onset diabetes of the young – MODY), and extreme insulin resistance of several different etiologies. In addition, secondary causes of diabetes mellitus refer to a category in which diabetes is associated with other diseases or conditions. Presumably, the diabetes is caused by those conditions, and could be reversed if those conditions were cured.

Secondary causes constitute less than 2% of total cases of diabetes mellitus. Mechanistically they can be considered in the broad categories of decreased insulin secretion, insulin resistance, and increased counter-regulation, although classification schemes are typically anatomical and pathophysiologic (Table 1). Decreased insulin secretion is generally seen in pancreatic diabetes following destruction of the endocrine pancreas with loss or impairment of insulin secretion, and in somatostatinoma. Liver disease causes insulin resistance via unknown mechanisms. Counter-regulatory hormones balance the glucose-lowering action of insulin. Excess levels of the counter-regulatory hormones glucagon, catecholamines, cortisol, and growth hormone seen with exogenous administration or excess secretion by their respective tumors, can elevate the blood glucose level. The pathogenesis of secondary diabetes is sometimes defined to include autoimmune mechanisms and antagonism of insulin action (discussed in other chapters). There are also a variety of infections (congenital rubella, cytomegalovirus) and rare genetic syndromes that are associated with insulin resistance or diabetes mellitus through unknown mechanisms.[1]

Table 1. Classification of secondary causes of diabetes mellitus

Diseases of the Exocrine Pancreas	Endocrinopathies
Pancreatectomy	Acromegaly
Acute pancreatitis	Cushing's syndrome
Chronic pancreatitis	Pheochromocytoma
Hemochromatosis	Hyperthyroidism
Carcinoma	Hyperparathyroidism
Cystic fibrosis	Hyperaldosteronism

Abnormalities of the Endocrine Pancreas And Endocrine Gut	Genetic Syndromes
Glucagonoma	Klinefelter's syndrome
Somatostatinoma	Turner's syndrome
Gastrinoma	Wolfram's syndrome
VIPoma (Vasoactive intestinal peptide tumor)	Friedreich's syndrome
Carcinoid Syndrome	Huntington's chorea
	Lawrence-Moon-Biedl syndrome
	Myotonic dystrophy
	Porphyria
Liver Disease	Prader-Willi syndrome
Chronic liver disease and cirrhosis	
Hepatitis C	
Acute hepatitis	

DISEASES OF THE EXOCRINE PANCREAS

Acute Pancreatitis

Acute inflammation of the pancreas can cause a transient elevation of the blood and urine glucose levels. The incidence of abnormal carbohydrate metabolism in acute pancreatitis varies from 9% to 70%[2] (Table 2). The wide range is related to the cause of the acute inflammation, with alcohol having a more damaging effect to the pancreatic tissue and higher incidence of glucose intolerance.[3] Hyperglycemia usually subsides within 3-6 weeks after the acute attack. In recent studies, when the National Diabetes Data Group criteria have been applied, 15% and 18% of the patients with a single bout of acute pancreatitis were diagnosed to have overt diabetes mellitus and glucose intolerance respectively.[4] In patients with acute pancreatitis, the plasma insulin concentration is lower than in healthy control subjects and is associated with impaired insulin stimulation in response to glucose or glucagon. Glucagon concentration is usually elevated and tends to remain high for at least one week.[5,6]

Chronic pancreatitis

Chronic pancreatitis is an inflammatory condition that influences both exocrine (digestive) and endocrine function of the pancreas. Although glucose intolerance is frequent in patients with chronic pancreatitis, overt diabetes mellitus usually occurs late in the course of the disease. Patients with chronic calcifying pancreatitis are at higher risk (60-70%) of developing diabetes and glucose intolerance than patients with non-calcifying disease (15-30%).[7] Diabetes caused by chronic pancreatitis requires insulin therapy because of destruction of β-cells. Concomitant damage to alpha cells (secreting glucagon) causes a high incidence of hypoglycemia. Neuropathy and retinopathy occurs in increased frequency in these patients while nephropathy and diabetic ketoacidosis are rare.[8]

Pancreatic cancer

Diabetes mellitus may appear as an early manifestation of pancreatic cancer, even before the tumor becomes apparent. It has been postulated that pancreatic cancer may stimulate the secretion of islet amyloid polypeptide

IAPP) from the β-cells of the pancreas, although the mechanism of IAPP secretion is not yet determined. IAPP causes insulin resistance. It was found that the resection of pancreatic cancer in patients with diabetes mellitus and high level of IAPP is associated with the cure of diabetes and the disappearance of IAPP.[9]

Pancreatectomy

Total pancreatectomy, primarily used for treatment of pancreatic cancer with large lesions in the head of the pancreas, is associated with a high incidence of glucose intolerance. This form of glucose intolerance, which results from pancreatic resection, is termed pancreatogenic diabetes. Pancreatic resections that spare the duodenum, such as distal pancreatectomy, are associated with a lower incidence of new or worsened diabetes than the standard or pylorus-preserving pancreaticoduodenectomy (Whipple procedure) or total pancreatectomy.

In addition to insulin deficiency, the endocrine abnormalities that accompany pancreatic resection can include pancreatic polypeptide (PP) deficiency with preservation of glucagon production if the resection is proximal or glucagon deficiency if the resection is distal. Glucagon deficiency increases susceptibility to hypoglycemia through loss of counterregulation, and PP deficiency is considered to impair hepatic insulin action, thereby contributing to hyperglycemia. The resulting hepatic insulin resistance with persistent endogenous glucose production and enhanced peripheral insulin sensitivity result in a brittle form of diabetes, which can be difficult to manage.[10]

Cystic fibrosis

Cystic fibrosis comprises a clinical triad of abnormalities involving the sweat glands, the exocrine pancreas and the respiratory epithelium. Diabetes mellitus develops in as many as 13% of adults with cystic fibrosis and up to 1% of children with the disease.[11] Early in the course of the disease, the β-cells of the islets of Langerhans appear normal. With disease progression, the exocrine glands are replaced with fibrous tissue, causing the gradual decrease of the number of islet cells.

Pancreatic infiltrative diseases

Primary/ Secondary Hemochromatosis

Hemochromatosis (bronze diabetes) is a state of iron overload due to either a primary (hereditary) or secondary (acquired) causes. The acquired causes include iron loading anemias (thalassemia major, sideroblastic anemia and chronic hemolytic anemia), chronic liver diseases (Hepatitis C, Alcoholic liver disease, nonalcoholic fatty liver)[12], dietary and or parenteral iron overload. Chronic iron deposition in different tissues will eventually cause fibrosis and organ failure. Deposition of iron in the pancreas causes fibrosis and secondary diabetes.

Diabetes mellitus develops in 30% to 60% of patients with advanced disease. Contributing factors include an inherited predisposition for diabetes mellitus, cirrhosis, and direct damage to the pancreas by deposition of iron.[13]

Table 2. **Frequency of diabetes mellitus in pancreatic diseases**

Disease	Frequency	Disease	Frequency
Acute Pancreatitis	9-70 %	Partial Pancreatectomy	20 %
Chronic Pancreatitis	15 %	Total Pancreatectomy	100%
Chronic Calcific Pancreatitis	60-70 %	Cystic Fibrosis	13%
Pancreatic Cancer	40-50 %	Hemachromatosis	30-60%

ABNORMALITIES OF THE ENDOCRINE PANCREAS AND ENDOCRINE GUT

β-cells of the pancreas are responsible for insulin secretion and glucose homeostasis. Abnormalities in the non β-cells of the pancreas can be associated with abnormalities in glucose metabolism and cause glucose intolerance or secondary diabetes. Endocrine tumors of the non-β-cells of the pancreas and or the gut that cause glucose intolerance include:
1- Hypersecretion of glucagon (glucagonoma)
2- Hypersecretion of Somatostatin (somatostatinoma)
3- VIPoma (vasoactive intestinal peptide tumor)
4- Hypersecretion of gastrin (gastrinoma)
5- Carcinoid syndrome

Glucagonoma

The glucagonoma syndrome is a rare disorder with a reported incidence of 0.2 cases per million per year.[14] These tumors secrete glucagon resulting in the "4D syndrome" of diabetes, dermatitis (necrolytic migratory erythema), deep-vein thrombosis, and depression. Glucose intolerance with or without frank diabetes mellitus occurs in 83% to 90% of patients.[15,16] It is due to hypersecretion of glucagon. Glucagon is one of the "counter-regulatory" hormones that counter balance the glucose lowering action of insulin with actions to raise the circulating glucose levels. Glucagon stimulates glycogenolysis, gluconeogenesis, ketogenesis, lipolysis, and insulin secretion; it also inhibits pancreatic and gastric secretion and gut motility.[17] Hyperglycemia results from increased hepatic glycogenolysis and gluconeogenesis. These tumors arise almost exclusively in the pancreas and are malignant in behavior, presenting as metastatic disease at the time of the diagnosis.[18] Postmenopausal women are commonly affected.

Somatostatinoma

Somatostatinomas are neuroendocrine tumors that usually originate in the pancreas or intestine. The release of large amounts of somatostatin causes a distinct clinical syndrome characterized by diabetes mellitus, gallbladder disease, diarrhea, and weight loss. The development of diabetes mellitus is likely secondary to the inhibitory action of somatostatin on insulin release as well as replacement of functional pancreatic tissue.[19, 20]

VIPoma Syndrome

The VIPoma syndrome is due to pancreatic endocrine tumor that secretes excessive amounts of vasoactive intestinal peptide (VIP). This causes a distinct syndrome of fasting large volume diarrhea, hypokalemia and hypochlorhydria. Hyperglycemia is noted in 25 to 50% of patients with VIPomas. It has been attributed to the glycogenolytic effects of VIP on the liver.[21]

Gastrinoma (Zollinger-Ellison) Syndrome

Zollinger-Ellison (ZE) syndrome is characterized by gastrin producing tumors (gastrinoma), hypersecretion of gastric acid, and recurrent peptic ulcers. The tumors usually originate from the pancreas and less frequently from the duodenum. Glucose intolerance and diabetes have been reported in patients with ZE syndrome. It is unclear if gastrin overproduction is the cause of glucose intolerance. Twenty to sixty percent of patients with ZE syndrome have the gastrinoma as part of the genetic multiple endocrine neoplasia (MEN) syndrome.

Carcinoid Syndrome

One report focuses on the link between diabetes mellitus and carcinoid tumors, relating a 50-80% incidence of diabetes or glucose intolerance to active secretion of serotonin.[22] It is more probable that diabetes seen with carcinoid syndrome is related to tumor secretory products such as somatostatin or ACTH causing Cushings' syndrome.

LIVER DISEASE

Chronic liver diseases as a secondary cause of diabetes mellitus

The liver has a major role in glucose homeostasis.[23] It produces glucose by both glycogenolysis (breakdown of glycogen) and gluconeogenesis (newly synthesized glucose). It is a major organ in glucose storage in the form of glycogen.

Insulin increases hepatic glucose uptake and suppresses glucose production by the liver. This results in increase glycogen synthesis and deposition in the liver. Opposing this action, glucagon decreases hepatic glucose uptake from the portal system.

Chronic hepatitis and cirrhosis

Chronic liver disease is associated with an increased incidence of impaired glucose tolerance and diabetes.[24] Multiple studies have demonstrated that insulin resistance is a characteristic feature of patients with liver cirrhosis.[25] Even in the absence of cirrhosis, portal hypertension is associated with increased insulin resistance.[26] This is manifested as glucose intolerance in 60% of cirrhotic patients, while 20% develop overt diabetes mellitus.[27, 28, 29] Both insulin resistance in the muscle and inadequate insulin secretion by the β-cells account for the glucose intolerance in patients with cirrhosis.[30] Insulin resistance is characterized by decreased glucose uptake and decreased non-oxidative glucose metabolism in skeletal muscle, which is accounted for by decreased muscle glycogen synthesis.[31, 32] Hyperglycemia in chronic liver disease may also occur as a result of the therapeutic administration of various medications including interferons and corticosteroids. Cirrhotic patients with overt diabetes have a high mortality rate, which is secondary to an increased risk of liver cell failure and not to diabetes complications per se. This makes the presence of diabetes in cirrhotic patients a risk factor for long-term survival.[33]

Hepatitis C

Overt diabetes mellitus is more prevalent in patients with chronic hepatitis C than in patients with other liver diseases and usually occurs without risk factors.[34,35,36,37] The mechanism by which hepatitis C virus (HCV) infection induces glucose intolerance and diabetes is unknown. Many theories, including cytopathic and immunological mechanisms have been proposed for the effect of HCV on extrahepatic tissues.[38] None of these pathogenic mechanisms has been proven. Virus-induced autoimmunity has been postulated as an explanation of the extrahepatic manifestations of HCV infection including diabetes and glucose intolerance. HCV infection may trigger latent autoimmunity or induce an autoimmune disease *de novo*. The autoimmune possibilities include those of molecular mimicry and immunological dysregulation. Molecular mimicry finds support in that chronic hepatitis C infection shares features with autoimmune hepatitis type 2, which is positive for anti-liver kidney microsomal antibodies.[38,39,40] Proponents of the immune dysregulation theory point to similarities between extrahepatic manifestations of HCV infection and other autoimmune diseases such as thyroiditis, thrombocytopenia.[38,41]

Acute hepatitis

Acute hepatitis is associated with transient glucose intolerance or hypoglycemia,[42] with normalization of glucose homeostasis after recovery.[43]

DRUG-INDUCED OR CHEMICAL-INDUCED DIABETES

Many drugs are known to cause glucose intolerance or diabetes mellitus (Table 3).[44]

Table 3. Drugs causing impaired glucose tolerance and diabetes.

Alcohol	Pentamidine
Nicotinic acid (Niacin)	Steroids, particularly glucocorticoids and OCPS**
Thiazides	Thyroid hormone
B-Blockers	Diazoxide
Calcium Channel Blockers	Cyclosporin
Clonidine	Interferon
Dilantin	Vacor
HIV* protease inhibitors	Others

*Human Immunodeficiency Virus   **Oral Contraceptive Pills

Alcohol, when ingested acutely, has been associated with hypoglycemia due to its inhibitory effect on gluconeogenesis. This effect is mostly seen in fasted individuals with depleted glycogen stores who are dependent on gluconeogenesis to maintain hepatic glucose production. Acute large alcohol intake can cause insulin resistance in peripheral tissues, particularly in the muscles. When ingested on chronic basis, excessive alcohol intake has been associated with moderate to severe insulin resistance and glucose intolerance.

β-adrenergic blockers are widely used in clinical practice. They are considered, along with diuretics, the first line of therapy for hypertension. They are known to promote hypoglycemia both by inhibiting hepatic glucose production directly and by blocking the counter-regulatory hormonal response to hypoglycemia. Studies have shown that nondiabetic patients on β-blockers (particularly the non-selective) may exhibit disturbance in their glucose homeostasis in the form of worsening glucose tolerance. This might be due to worsening insulin secretion or insulin action.

Pentamidine has multiphasic effect on the β-cell of the pancreas. Initially, pentamidine causes β-cells degranulation with release of insulin, which results in hypoglycemia. Later, it causes β-cell destruction and impaired insulin secretion, resulting in hyperglycemia and even diabetic ketoacidosis.[45] Intravenous pentamidine can permanently destroy pancreatic β-cells and has been incriminated in the development of secondary diabetes in multiple cases.[46,47] These reactions, however, are considered rare. Impairment of insulin action can result from the administration of multiple drugs and hormones, such as nicotinic acid and steroids.[48, 49]

Patients on α-interferon treatment for chronic hepatitis C are reported to develop diabetes with islet cell antibodies and, in some cases, insulin deficiency.[41,50] Vacor (Pyriminil) poisoning (synthetic organic rodenticide) can cause hyperglycemia, ketoacidosis and irreversible diabetes, in addition to its toxic effect on the central and peripheral nervous system.[51,52]

Protease Inhibitors, Human Immunodeficiency Virus (HIV) and Glucose Intolerance

Undesirable physical and metabolic changes associated with HIV infection and therapy assume greater importance as life expectancy improves. An acquired lipodystrophy syndrome occurs in a high proportion of chronically HIV infected individuals and variably includes central obesity, dorsal fat pad, facial wasting and wasting of the extremities. Insulin resistance, frank diabetes, and hyperlipidemia are associated with this lipodystrophy.[53] Presumably these metabolic changes carry an increased risk of premature cardiovascular mortality. The metabolic syndrome can occur in HIV-infected individuals in the absence of HIV-specific medications, increases in incidence with the use of some classes of drugs including reverse transcriptase inhibitors, and is greatest in those patients on protease inhibitors.[54] Investigation into mechanisms has included the role of mitochondrial toxicity in producing the syndrome, protection of lipid particles from degradation[55], increased fatty acid and cholesterol biosynthesis[56], inhibition of fat cell differentiation[57], and inhibition of glucose transport into fat and muscle.[58] There is no accepted or proven safe therapy. Reports suggest that other forms of lipodystrophy may be attenuated by treatment with peripheral insulin sensitizers, in particular the thiazolidenedione class of peroxisome-proliferator-γ (PPAR-γ) agonists.[59] A large trial in HIV lipodystrophy has shown modest favorable results with metformin, which decreases hepatic glucose production and may have beneficial effects on the mitochondria.[60]

ENDOCRINOPATHIES

Acromegaly, a state of growth hormone excess, is associated with hyperglycemia and insulin resistance

The major players in the growth hormone (GH) system are GH and IGF-1 (insulin-like growth factor-1). GH and IGF-1 affect glucose and fat metabolism, as well as growth. They have opposing effects on carbohydrate metabolism (Figure 1). A family of IGF binding proteins (IGF-BPs) affects tissue delivery, availability of IGF-1, and gene transcription, thereby altering the balance between growth hormone and IGF-1. In some tissues, the IGF effects cooperate with the GH effects (for example, growth of long bones) and in other tissues, they are antagonistic (the metabolic effects).

Growth, mediated by IGF-1, is an anabolic process that requires cellular uptake of building components, such as amino acids and glucose. Administered separately from growth hormone, IGF-1 lowers elevated blood glucose levels and can cause hypoglycemia. In fact, IGF-1 has been used to treat diabetic ketoacidosis in insulin resistant individuals.[61]

Growth hormone can be regarded as the metabolic partner of IGF-1 because growth hormone provides adequate substrate for the effects of IGF-1 (Figure 1). GH-stimulated fat mobilization and new glucose formation (gluconeogenesis) are required to make building components (substrate) available. Growth hormone acts on the fat cell to stimulate the hormone sensitive lipase, causing lipolysis (breakdown of fat) with the release of glycerol and free fatty acids (FFA). Glycerol is a precursor for hepatic gluconeogenesis. FFA stimulate gluconeogenesis and are the precursors for ketogenesis.[62] FFA elevation also increases output of the lipoprotein VLDL, thereby elevating triglyceride levels.[63] FFA become the preferred substrate for muscle uptake and oxidation. GH also causes inhibition of muscle uptake and oxidation of glucose, even though insulin concentrations are increased because of insulin resistance secondary to GH action.[64] The actions of GH to mobilize FFA, stimulate gluconeogenesis and inhibit insulin action may lead to elevation of blood glucose levels and, sometimes, cause frank diabetes mellitus.

GH excess in children and adolescents prior to closure of the growth plate of the long bones results in continued growth (gigantism). In adults, GH excess causes acromegaly (acral overgrowth). Acromegaly occurs with GH secreting pituitary tumors and rarely with ectopic production of growth hormone releasing hormone, usually by bronchial carcinoids or pancreatic neuroendocrine tumors. Even though GH stimulates IGF-1 secretion and IGF-1 levels are elevated in acromegaly, GH excess is potentially diabetogenic. Twenty-five percent of patients with acromegaly develop diabetes mellitus.[65]

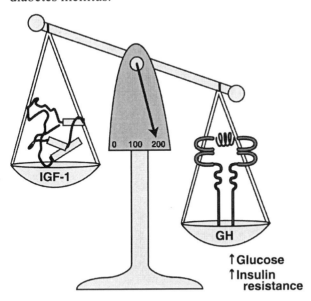

Figure 1. Growth Hormone (GH) and IGF-1 have opposite effects on glucose metabolism. Hepatic IGF-1 appears to be an insulin sensitizer and can lower blood glucose levels, while elevated GH raises blood glucose and is associated with insulin resistance.[66]

Cushing's syndrome, glucocorticoids, and 11-β hydroxysteroid dehydrogenase

Glucocorticoids were named for their ability to raise blood glucose.[67] Excess glucocorticoid secretion or administration can lead to diabetes mellitus. Glucose intolerance and diabetes mellitus are common in Cushing's syndrome (cortisol excess), with frank diabetes or impaired glucose tolerance occurring in 50-90% of affected individuals. Cushings' syndrome results from excess cortisol secretion from adrenal gland tumors; from pituitary or other tumors secreting ACTH, which stimulates adrenal cortisol production; or from exogenously administered glucocorticoids used in the treatment of asthma or auto-immune disorders. Cortisol is one of the counter-regulatory hormones and diabetes mellitus is one of the most common sequelae of Cushings' syndrome. The major actions of cortisol, like those of growth hormone, lead to extra-hepatic mobilization of substrate. Cortisol acts at many steps. One action is to increase the appetite, thereby increasing energy intake with an initial rise in blood glucose level. If stored in visceral fat tissue (lipogenic action of cortisol), this energy contributes to insulin resistance. If mobilized, increased energy intake contributes to increased hepatic glucose production (lipolytic action of cortisol).[68] Cortisol antagonizes the effects of insulin in muscle, preventing protein synthesis and inhibiting glucose utilization; further, its catabolic actions include muscle breakdown[69], with the effect of delivering gluconeogenic precursors to the liver. In the liver, cortisol stimulates both gluconeogenesis and glycogen breakdown.

The pivotal role that cortisol may play in insulin resistance and type 2 diabetes mellitus is highlighted by recent observations that increased cortisol production in visceral fat can be shown in a transgenic mice to recreate the metabolic syndrome of insulin resistance, diabetes and hypertension (Figure 2).[70]

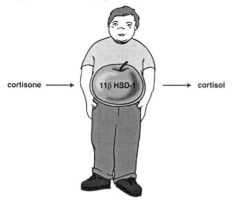

cortisone ⟶ 11β HSD-1 ⟶ cortisol

Figure 2. Increased activity of 11-β hydroxy-steroid dehydrogenase type 1 in transgenic mice increases cortisol production in visceral fat and causes abdominal obesity and the metabolic syndrome resembling that seen in "apple-shaped" people.[71]

Pheochromocytoma

Pheochromocytomas, a general term applied to tumors of the adrenal medulla and extra-adrenal chromaffin tissue, secrete catecholamines, especially nor-epinephrine. Headache (related to extreme elevations of the blood pressure), palpitations and anxiety reflect $alpha_1$-adrenergic stimulation and dominate the clinical presentation. Diabetes occurs in up to 65% of pheochromocytomas, may mirror the paroxysmal rises in blood pressure and has been demonstrated to resolve following tumor resection.[72] Pheochromocytomas whose major secretory product is epinephrine are much more likely than norepinephrine-secreting tumors to present with arrhythmias, non-cardiac pulmonary edema, hypotension and hyperglycemia. This distinct presentation reflects the combined α- and β-adrenergic stimulation of epinephrine (Figure 3). The more common norepinephrine secreting tumors may also cause hyperglycemia since it too is a mixed agonist, although with less β activity than epinephrine.[73]

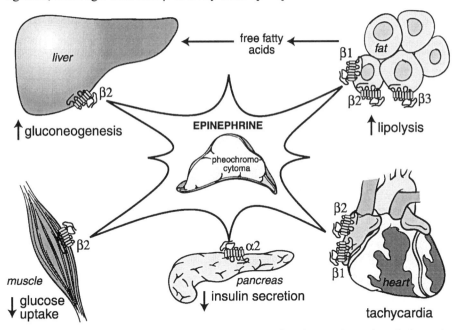

Figure 3. The coordinated actions of elevated epinephrine in pheochromocytoma raise blood glucose.[74]

Hyperthyroidism

Thyroid hormone increases glucose transporters 4 (GLUT 4) in fat tissue and muscle, thereby enhancing the stimulatory effect of insulin.[75] Given the increase in metabolic rate caused by thyroid hormones, it is logical that increased fuel would be made available to tissues. It is paradoxical then that hyperthyroidism is sometimes associated with deterioration of glucose control or with onset of frank diabetes mellitus. Partial explanations implicate increased growth hormone secretion[76], increased hepatic gluconeogenesis and increased hepatic GLUT 2 transporters, through which glucose effluxes out of the liver.[77]

Hyperaldosteronism

Primary hyperaldosteronism, the elevated secretion of the mineralcorticoid aldosterone resulting from adrenal cortical tumors, genetic mutations or idiopathic hyperaldosteronism, is classified with the endocrinopathies that cause secondary diabetes mellitus.[1] Yet, remarkably little literature exists to define the prevalence, mechanism, or resolution of the glucose intolerance seen with hypersecretion of aldosterone. One retrospective study found a prevalence of diabetes of 5-24% in hyperaldosteronism.[78] Physiologic potassium levels play a fundamental role in insulin secretion (Chapter III.2). Potassium stimulates glucose-induced insulin secretion, and insulin lowers serum potassium by driving the cation intracellularly.[79] The hypokalemia that occurs with renal potassium wasting in primary aldosteronism presumably has a restraining or inhibiting effect on insulin secretion and leads to glucose intolerance and diabetes in susceptible individuals. The diabetes that occurs with hyperaldosteronism resolves with cure of the hyperaldosteronism (personal observation).

CONCLUSIONS

Diverse organs and drugs are implicated in secondary diabetes mellitus. Pancreatic destruction is only treatable with insulin replacement. Sometimes medications causing diabetes may be changed, but some are life saving and cannot be discontinued. The lipodystrophy and metabolic consequences of the acquired immunodeficiency syndrome and its therapies are under active investigation. The link between liver disease and diabetes is poorly understood. Cure of the endocrinopathies that cause diabetes ameliorates or cures the associated diabetes. Ultimately, the explanation for the mechanisms that cause secondary diabetes mellitus can be sought in the basic physiology and pathophysiology of the secretion of insulin and its action on target tissues.

REFERENCES

1. Report of the expert committee on the diagnosis and classification of diabetes mellitus. Diabetes Care 24, Suppl 1: 1-32, 2001.
2. Thow J, Semad A, Alberti KGMM. Epidemiology and general aspects of diabetes secondary to pancreatopathy. In: Diabetes secondary to pancreatopathy. Tiengo A, Alberti KGMM, Del Prato S, Vranic M Eds; Excerpta Medica, Amsterdam, 7-20, 1988.

246

3. Del Prato S, Tiengo A. Diabetes secondary to acquired disease of the pancreas. In: International Textbook of Diabetes Mellitus. Alberti KGMM, DeFronzo RA, Keen H, Zimmet P, Eds; John Wiley & Sons, Inc., New York, 199, 1992.

4. Scuro LA, Angelini G, Cavallini G, Vantini I. The late outcome of acute pancreatitis. In: Pancreatitis: concepts and classification.Gyr KL, Singer MV, Sarles H, Eds; Excerpta Medica, Amsterdam, 403-408, 1984.

5. Drew SI, Joffe B, Vinik AI, Seften H, Singer F. The first 24 hours of acute pancreatitis. Changes in biochemical and endocrine homeostasis inpatients with pancreatitis compared to those in control subjects undergoing stress for reasons other than pancreatitis. Amer J Med 64:795-803, 1978.

6. Donowitz M, Hendeler R, Spiro HM, Binder H, Felig P. Glucagon secretion in acute and chronic pancreatitis. J Intern Med 83:778-781, 1975.

7. Mlka D, Hammel P, Sauvanet A, Rufat P, O'toole D, Bardet P, Belghiti J, Pierre Bernades, Ruszniewski P, Lévy P. Risk factors for Diabetes mellitus in chronic pancreatitis. Gastroenterology 119:1324-1322, 2000.

8. Mergener, K, Baillie, J. Chronic pancreatitis. Lancet 350:1379-1385, 1997.

9. Permert J, Larsson J, Fruin AB, Tatemoto K, Herrington MK, von Schenck H, Adrian TE. Islet hormone secretion in pancreatic cancer patients with diabetes. Pancreas 15:60-68, 1997.

10. Slezak LA, Andersen DK. Pancreatic resection: effects on glucose metabolism. World journal of Surgery 25: 452-460, 2001.

11. Shwachman H, Kowalski M, Khaw KT. Cystic fibrosis: a new outlook, 70 patients above 25 years of age. Medicine 56:24-49, 1977.

12. Williams R., Williams HS, Scheuer PJ, Pitcher CS, Loiseau E, Sherlock S. Iron absorption and siderosis in chronic liver disease. Quart J Med 35:151-166, 1967.

13. Powell LW, Yapp TR. Hemochromatosis. Clinics in Liver Disease 4: 211-228, 2000.

14. Norton JA. Neuroendocrine tumors of the pancreas and duodenum. Curr Probl Surg 31:77-156, 1994.

15. Holst JJ. Glucagon-producing tumors. In: Hormone-producing tumors of the gastrointestinal tract. Cohen S, Soloway RD, Ed; Churchill Livingstone, New York, 57, 1985.

16. Guillausseau PJ, Guillausseau-Scholer C. Glucagonomas: Clinical presentation, diagnosis, and advances in management. In: Endocrine Tumors of the Pancreas: Recent Advances in Research and Management. Frontiers of Gastrointestinal Research, Vol. 23. Mignon M, Jensen RT, Eds; S. Karger, Basel, Switzerland, 183, 1995.

17. Holst JJ, Orskov C. Glucagon and other proglucagon-derived peptides. In: Gut Peptides. Walsh JH, Dockray GJ, Eds; Raven Press, New York, 305, 1994.

18. Delcore R, Friesen SR. Gastrointestinal neuroendocrine tumors. J Amer Coll Surg 178:187-211, 1994.

19. Vinik AI, Strodel WE, Eckhauser FE, Moattari AR, Lloyd R. Somatostatinomas, PPomas, neurotensinomas. Semin Oncol 14:263-281, 1987.

20. Sassolas G, Chayvialle JA. GRFomas, somatostatinomas: clinical presentation, diagnosis, and advances in management. In: Endocrine Tumors of the Pancreas: Recent Advances in Research and Management. Frontiers of Gastrointestinal Research, Vol. 23. Mignon M, Jensen RT, Eds; S. Karger, Basel, Switzerland, 194, 1995.

21. Matuchansky C, Rambuaud JC. VIPomas and endocrine cholera: clinical presentation, diagnosis, and advances in management. In: Endocrine Tumors of the Pancreas: Recent Advances in Research and Management. Frontiers of Gastrointestinal Research, Vol. 23. Mignon M, Jensen RT, Eds; S. Karger, Basel, Switzerland, 166, 1995.

22. Feldman JM, Plonk JW, Bivens CH, Levobitz HE. Glucose intolerance in the carcinoid syndrome. Diabetes 24:664-671, 1975.

23. DeFronzo RA, Ferrannini E. Regulation of hepatic glucose metabolism in humans. Diabetes Metab Rev 3:415-459, 1987.

24. Zein NN. Prevalence of diabetes mellitus in patients with end-stage liver cirrhosis due to hepatitis C, alcohol, or cholestatic disease. J Hepatol 32: 209-217, 2000.

25. Petrides AS. Liver disease and diabetes mellitus. Diab Rev 2:2-18, 1994.

26. Cavallo-Perin P, Cassader M, Bozzo C Bruno A, Nuccio P, Dall'Omo AM, Marucci M, Pagano G. Mechanism of insulin resistance in human liver cirrhosis: evidence of combined receptor and postreceptor defect. J Clin Invest 75:1659-1665, 1985.

27. Kingston ME, Ali MA, Atiyeh M, Donnelly RJ. Diabetes mellitus in chronic active hepatitis and cirrhosis. Gastroenterology 87:688-694, 1984.

28. Del Vecchio Blanco C, Gentile S, Marmo R, Carbone L, Coltorti M. Alterations of glucose metabolism in chronic liver disease. DiabetesRes Clin Pract 8:29-36, 1990.

29. Gentile S, Loguerico C, Gentile S, Marmo R, Carbone L, Del Vecchio Blanco C. Incidence of altered glucose tolerance in liver cirrhosis. Diabetes Res Clin Pract 22:37-44, 1993.

30. Marks JB, Skyler JS. The liver and the endocrine system. In: Schiff's Diseases of the Liver. Eighth Edition. Schiff ER, Sorrell MF, Maddrey WC, Eds; Lippincott Williams & Wilkins, Philadelphia, 477-488, 1999.

31. Petrides AS, Groop LC, Riely CA, DeFronzo RA. Effect of physiologic hyperinsulinemia on glucose and lipid metabolism in cirrhosis. J Clin Invest 88:561-570, 1991.
32. Petrides AS, DeFronzo RA. Glucose and insulin metabolism in cirrhosis. J Hepatol 8:107-114, 1989.
33. Fraser GM, Harman I, Meller N, Niv Y, Porath A. Diabetes mellitus is associated with chronic hepatitis C but not chronic hepatitis B infection. Isr J Med Sci 32:526-530, 1996.
34. Marchesini G, Melli A, Checchia GA, Capelli M, Cassarani S, Zoli M, Pisi E. Pancreatic beta-cell function in cirrhotic patients with and without overt diabetes: c-peptide response to glucagons and to meal. Metabolism: Clinical & Experimental 34:695-701, 1985.
35. Allison ME, Wreghitt T, Palmer CR, Lexander GJ. Evidence for a link between hepatitis C virus infection and diabetes mellitus in cirrhotic population. J Hepatol 21:1135-1139, 1994.
36. Grimbert S, Valensi P, Lévy- Marchal C, Perret G, Richardet JP, Raffoux C, Trinchet JC, Beaugrand M. High prevalence of diabetes mellitus in patients with chronic hepatitis C: a case-control study. Gastroenterol Clin Biol 20:544-548, 1996.
37. Knobler H. Schihmanter R. Zifroni A. Fenakel G. Schattner A. Increased risk of type 2 diabetes in noncirrhotic patients with chronic hepatitis C virus infection. Mayo Clinic Proceedings 75:355-359, 2000.
38. Hadziyannis SJ. The spectrum of extrahepatic manifestations in hepatitis C virus infection. J Vir Hepat 4:9-28, 1997.
39. Hadziyannis S, Karamanos B. Diabetes mellitus and chronic hepatitis C virus infection [editorial]. Hepatology 29:604-605, 1999.
40. Strassburg CP, Obermayer-Straub P, Manns MP. Autoimmunity in hepatitis C and D virus infection. J Viral Hepatitis 3:49-59, 1996.
41. Farbis P, Betterle C, Floreani A, Greggio NA, De Lazzari F, Naccarato R, Chiaramonte M. Development of type 1 diabetes mellitus during interferon alfa therapy for chronic HCV hepatitis. Lancet 340:548, 1992.
42. Bianchi G, Marchesini G, Zoli M, Bugianesi E, Fabbri A, Pisi E. Prognostic significance of diabetes in patients with cirrhosis. Hepatology 20:119-125, 1994.
43. Record CO, Alberti KG, Williamson DH, Wright R. Glucose tolerance and metabolic changes in human viral hepatitis. Clin Sci Mol Med 45:677-690, 1973.
44. Bressler P, DeFronzo RA. Drugs and diabetes. Diabetes Reviews 2:53-83, 1994.
45. Lambertus MW, Murthy AR, Nagami P, Bidwell Goetz M. Diabetic ketoacidosis following pentamidine therapy in a patient with the acquired immunodefiency syndrome. West J Med 149:602-604, 1988.

46. Bouchard P, Sai P, Reach G, Caubarrere I, Ganeval D, Assan R. Diabetes mellitus following pentamidine-induced hypoglycemia in humans. Diabetes 31:40-45, 1982.
47. Assan R, Perronne C, Assan D, Chotard L, Mayaud C, Matheron S, Zucman D. Pentamidine-induced derangements of glucose homeostasis. Diabetes Care 18:47-55, 1995.
48. Pandit MK, Burke J, Gustafson AB, Minocha A, Peiris AN. Drug-induced disorders of glucose tolerance. Ann Intern Med 118:529-540, 1993.
49. O'Byrne S, Feely J. Effects of drugs on glucose tolerance in non-insulin-dependent diabetes (parts I and II). Drugs 40:203-219, 1990.
50. Shiba T, Morino Y, Tagawa K, Fujino H, Unuma T. Onset of diabetes with high titer anti-GAD antibody after IFN therapy for chronic hepatitis. Diabetes Res Clin Pract 30:237-241, 1996.
51. Trujillo MH. Pharmacologic antidotes in critical care medicine: a practical guide for drug administration. Crit Care Med 26: 377-391, 1998.
52. Gallanosa AG, Spyker DA, Curnow RT. Diabetes mellitus associated with autonomic and peripheral neuropathy after Vacor poisoning: a review. Clin Toxicol 18:441-449, 1981.
53. Tsiodras S, Mantzoros C, Hammer S, Samore M. Effects of protease inhibitors on hyperglycemia, hyperlipidemia, and lipodystrophy: a 5-year cohort study. Arch Intern Med 160:2050-2056, 2000.
54. Martinez E, Mocroft A, Garcia-Viejo MA, Perez-Cuevas JB, Blanco JL, Mallolas J, Bianchi L, Conget I, Blanch J, Phillips A, Gatell JM. Risk of lipodystrophy in HIV-1-infected patients treated with protease inhibitors: a prospective cohort study. Lancet 357:592-598, 2001.
55. Liang J, Distler O, Cooper DA, Jamil H, Deckelbaum RJ, Ginsberg HN, Sturley SL. HIV protease inhibitors protect apolipoprotein B from degradation by the proteasome: a potential mechanism for protease inhibitor-induced hyperlipidemia. Nature Med 7:1327-1331, 2001.
56. Riddle TM, Kuhel DG, Woollett LA, Fichtenbaum CJ, Hui DY. HIV protease inhibitor induces fatty acid and sterol biosynthesis in liver and adipose tissues due to the accumulation of activated sterol regulatory element-binding proteins in the nucleus. J Biol Chem 276:37514-37519, 2001.
57. Martine C, Auclair M, Vigouroux C, Glorian M, Forest C, Capeau J. The HIV protease inhibitor indinavir impairs sterol regulatory element-binding protein-1 intranuclear localization, inhibits preadipocyte differentiation, and induces insulin resistance. Diabetes 50:1378-1388, 2001.

58. Murata H, Hruz PW, Mueckler M. The mechanism of insulin resistance caused by HIV protease inhibitor therapy. J Biol Chem 275:20251-20254, 2000.

59. Arioglu E, Duncan-Morin J, Segring N, Rother KI, Gottlieb N, Lieberman J, Herion D, Kleiner DE, Reynolds J, Premkumar A, Sumner AE, Hoofnagle J, Reitman ML, Taylor SI. Efficacy and safety of troglitazone in the treatment of lipodystrophy syndromes. [see comments]. Ann Intern Med 133:263-274, 2000.

60. Hadigan C, Corcoran C, Basgoz N, Davis B, Sax P, Grinspoon S. Metformin in the treatment of HIV lipodystrophy syndrome: a randomized controlled trial. JAMA 284:472-477, 2000.

61. Usala AL, Madigan T, Burguera B, Sinha MK, Caro JF, Cunningham P, Powell JG, Butler PC. Treatment of insulin-resistant diabetic ketoacidosis with insulin-like growth factor I in an adolescent with insulin-dependent diabetes [Brief report]. N Engl J Med 327:853-857, 1992.

62. Boden G. Role of fatty acids in the pathogenesis of insulin resistance and NIDDM. Diabetes 46:3-10, 1997.

63. Leung KC, Ho KKY. Stimulation of mitochondrial fatty acid oxidation by growth hormone in human fibroblasts. J Clin Endocrinol Metab 82:4208-4213, 1997.

64. Goodman HN. The metabolic actions of growth hormone. In: Handbook of Physiology, Section, 7; The Endocrine System, Vol. 2. The endocrine pancreas and regulation of metabolism. Jefferson LS, Cherrington AD, Goodman HM, Eds; Oxford University Press, Inc., New York, 849-906, 2001.

65. Kopchick JJ. Growth hormone. In: Endocrinology. Fourth Edition. DeGroot LJ, Jameson LJ, Burger HG, Loriaux DL, Marschall JC, Melmed Shlomo, Odell WD, Potts JT Jr., Rubenstein AH, Eds; W.B. Saunders, New York, 389-404, 2001.

66. Butler AA, LeRoith D. Minireview: tissue-specific versus generalized gene targeting of the igf1 and igf1r genes and their roles in insulin-like growth factor physiology. Endocrinol 142:1685-1688, 2001.

67. Munck A, Naray-Fejes-Toth A. Glucocorticoid action: physiology. In: Endocrinology. Fourth Edition. DeGroot LJ, Jameson LJ, Burger HG, Loriaux DL, Marschall JC, Melmed Shlomo, Odell WD, Potts JT Jr., Rubenstein AH, Eds; W.B. Saunders, New York, 1632-1646, 2001.

68. Salati LM. Regulation of fatty acid biosynsthesis and lipolysis. In: Handbook of Physiology, Section, 7; The Endocrine System, Vol. 2. The endocrine pancreas and regulation of metabolism. Jefferson LS, Cherrington AD, Goodman HM, Eds; Oxford University Press, Inc. New York, , 495-527, 2001.

69. Jefferson LS, Vary TC, Kimball SR. Regulation of protein metabolism in muscle. In: Handbook of Physiology, Section, 7; The Endocrine System, Vol. 2. The endocrine pancreas and regulation of metabolism. Jefferson LS, Cherrington AD, Goodman HM, Eds; Oxford University Press, Inc., New York, 536, 2001.

70. Masuzaki H, Paterson J, Shinyama H, Morton NM, Mullins JJ, Seckl JR, Flier JS. A transgenic model of visceral obesity and the metabolic syndrome. Science 294:2166-2170, 2001.

71. Gura T. Pot-bellied mice point to obesity enzyme [News of the Week]. Science 294:2071-2072, 2001.

72. Manger WM, Gifford RW. Clinical and Experimental Pheochromocytoma. Second Edition. Blackwell Science Inc., Cambridge, 209, 1996.

73. Cryer PE: The prevention and correction of hypoglycemia. In: Handbook of Physiology, Section, 7; The Endocrine System, Vol. 2. The endocrine pancreas and regulation of metabolism. Jefferson LS, Cherrington AD, Goodman HM, Eds; Oxford University Press, Inc., New York, 1057-1092, 2001.

74. Cryer PE. Catecholamines, pheochromocytoma and diabetes. Diabetes Reviews 1:309-317, 1993.

75. Romero R, Casanova B, Pulido N, Suarez AI, Rodriguez E, Rovira A. Stimulation of glucose transport by thyroid hormone in 3T3-L1 adipocytes: increased abundance of GLUT1 and GLUT4 glucose transporter proteins. J Endocrinol 164:187-195, 2000.

76. Tosi F, Moghetti P, Castello R, Negri C, Bonora E, Muggeo M. Early changes in plasma glucagon and growth hormone response to oral glucose in experimental hyperthyroidism. Metabolism: Clinical and Experimental 45:1029-1033, 1996.

77. Mokuno T, Uchimura K, Hayashi R, Hayakawa, Makino M, Nagata M, Kakizawa H, Sawai Y, Kotake M, Oda N, Nakai A, Nagasaka A, Itoh M. Glucose transporter 2 concentrations in hyper- and hypothyroid rat livers. J Endocrinol 160:285-289, 1999.

78. Kreze A Sr., Kreze-Spirova E, Mikulecky M. Diabetes mellitus in primary aldosteronism. Bratislavske Lekarske Listy 101:187-190, 2000.

79. Ferrannini E, Galvan AQ, Santoro D, Natali A. Potassium as a link between insulin and the renin-angiotensin-aldosterone system. J Hypertension, Suppl 10:S5-10, 1992.

Chapter 6. Syndromes of Extreme Insulin Resistance

George Grunberger and Hisham Alrefai

INTRODUCTION

This group of syndromes shares severe insulin resistance and hyperinsulinemia with variable clinical manifestations.[1,2] Attention has been paid to these rare disorders because they provide insight into several aspects of insulin action at the molecular level and advance our understanding of the more common insulin resistant disorders, such as polycystic ovarian syndrome[3] and type 2 diabetes mellitus.[4]

Insulin resistance is defined as a state of suboptimal biological response to a given concentration of insulin.[2] It is possible, therefore, to overcome the resistance by increasing quantity of insulin secreted. Mild to moderate insulin resistance is seen in such clinical conditions as obesity, hypertension, and type 2 diabetes. These are discussed in details in other chapters.

In *extreme* insulin resistance syndromes, hereditary and/or acquired defects in insulin action at different molecular levels result in the diseases described below. In this chapter we review the pathogenesis and classification of syndromes of extreme insulin resistance, and then follow by describing the general and specific features of these conditions.

LABORATORY ASSESSMENT OF INSULIN RESISTANCE

Various tests can be used to assess the presence and/or the level of insulin resistance.

1. *Fasting serum/plasma glucose* may be normal or elevated. This is primarily determined by the magnitude of the basal insulin response.
2. *Glucose tolerance test* may be normal or severely impaired. This is primarily determined by the magnitude of insulin response to carbohydrate or other secretagogue stimulus.
3. *Serum insulin* level, in conjunction with serum glucose, in fasting state or after oral glucose tolerance.
4. The *homeostasis model assessment (HOMA) index,* which is calculated using the formula described by Matthews and associates: fasting serum insulin (μU/ml) multiplied by fasting plasma glucose (mmol/l) and then divided by 22.5. The higher the HOMA index, the lower the insulin sensitivity (i.e. more severe insulin resistance). This method is an inexpensive and validated way for evaluating the insulin resistance.

5. Assessment of sequential plasma glucose levels after intravenous administration of insulin *(insulin tolerance test)* showing decreased response to exogenous insulin.
6. Estimation of the insulin sensitivity index from the *frequently sampled intravenous glucose tolerance test.*
7. Measurement of *in vivo* insulin-mediated glucose disposal by the *euglycemic hyperinsulinemic clamp.*

PATHOGENESIS AND CLASSIFICATION

Significant progress has been made in our understanding of the molecular basis underlying the syndromes of extreme insulin resistance. Some of these diseases are due to genetic defects or mutations in the insulin receptor gene, as seen in the type A syndrome, leprechaunism as well as in the Rabson-Mendenhall syndrome, while circulating antibodies against the insulin receptor are detected in the type B syndrome. The etiology of some of the extreme insulin resistance syndromes is still a mystery, as is the case in many lipodystrophic syndromes.

It is important to mention that some conditions should not be mistakenly categorized under extreme insulin resistance syndromes. These conditions are discussed below.

Conditions that mimic insulin resistance
Although hyperinsulinemia is seen in these genetic diseases, insulin resistance is not present. In fact individuals with these disorders respond appropriately to exogenous insulin.
1) Familial hyperproinsulinemia. This trait is inherited as an autosomal dominant pattern and leads to the inability to convert proinsulin to insulin.[5,6]
2) Mutant insulin molecules. These molecules may act as weak insulin agonists with lower affinity for the insulin receptors.
3) Increased insulin degradation. This phenomenon has been observed in insulin-treated diabetic patients. They respond to exogenous insulin given intravenously but are resistant to subcutaneous insulin.[7] It seems that insulin may be degraded in, or prevented from getting absorbed from, the subcutaneous tissue.

In this chapter we classify the extreme insulin resistance syndromes according to the underlying etiology.
1) Anti-insulin antibodies
Anti-insulin antibodies have been reported in patients with diabetes who were on poorly purified or animal intermittent insulin.[8] This complication was remarkably minimized after the introduction of human or highly purified insulin. In diabetic patients using human insulin only few develop very high capacity immunoglobulins that might lead to extreme insulin resistance.

2) Autoantibodies against insulin receptors

This condition is characterized by spontaneous development of antibodies against insulin receptor. These antibodies can interfere with the ability of insulin to bind to its receptors resulting in insulin resistance. However, hypoglycemia due to direct activation of insulin receptors by these antibodies, has also been described.[9]

3) Mutation in insulin receptor genes

Insulin receptor is composed of two α and two β subunits. Insulin activates, by binding to its α–subunit, the intrinsic tyrosine kinase of the receptor's transmembrane β subunit. Subsequently, activation of several downstream signaling pathways takes place. The end results of this activation and signal transduction are the well-known biological effects of insulin on its target cells, including glucose and aminoacid uptake, glycogenesis, antilipolysis, and others.[10]

The abovementioned cascade of molecular events can be interrupted at various steps, resulting in an impaired insulin action and potential development of extreme insulin resistant clinical conditions. Many mutations have been identified in the insulin receptor gene. These mutations may lead to:

- Decreased insulin receptor biosynthesis
- Premature chain termination in extracellular or intracellular domain
- Accelerated receptor degradation
- Defect in the receptor transport to plasma membranes
- Decreased insulin binding affinity
- Impaired tyrosine kinase activity
- Impaired binding interactions with signaling molecules

4) Defects in target cell

When adequate amounts of insulin are synthesized, secreted into the extracellular space, and gain access to the target tissues, abnormal function is then attributed to the target cell. Since the first step in insulin action is binding to specific cell surface receptors, we must first consider the receptor as a potential site of dysfunction. Studies in the past have revealed a number of general principles regarding the insulin receptor:

a) Using direct binding techniques, estimates can be obtained of both the affinity and concentration of cell surface receptors.

b) Affinity is a complex function and is determined both by multiplicity of binding sites and by negatively cooperative interactions (which are interactions among the receptor sites so that the affinity of the receptors for the hormone progressively decreases as more sites are occupied by insulin).

c) The receptor is highly regulated. Temperature, pH, and ligand concentration are among the various factors that regulate the receptor.

d)   At physiologic temperatures, both the ligand and receptor are internalized by the cell. This receptor-mediated process provides a mechanism to remove the ligand from the cell surface and terminate its signal and a mechanism that may regulate the concentration of receptors on the cell surface.[11]

Interestingly, in target and non-target tissue, insulin is processed in a similar manner.[12] This suggests that biologic activity and receptor regulation are separate functions; however, when target and non-target cells are exposed to a similar environment, their cell surface receptors are regulated in a similar fashion.

5) Decreased insulin clearance

Insulin clearance from the circulation may become impaired in some conditions due to certain insulin receptor defects.[13] So, hyperinsulinemia seen in patients with extreme insulin resistance may result both from increased β– cell secretion as well as from decreased insulin clearance.

6) Other causes of extreme insulin resistance

Some hormonal or metabolic abnormalities may lead, occasionally, to extreme insulin resistance.   These abnormalities include excess of glucocorticoids, growth hormone, catecholamines, glucagon, and free fatty acids.

Specific syndromes of insulin resistance are summarized in table 1 and discussed below.

Table 1. Specific syndromes of extreme insulin resistance

Familial lipodystrophy syndromes
   1. Familial generalized lipodystrophy
   2. Familial partial lipodystrophy
      • Kobberling variety
      • Dunnigan variety
      • Mandibuloacral dysplasia variety
Acquired lipodystrophy syndromes
   1. Acquired generalized lipodystrophy
   2. Acquired partial lipodystrophy
      • Cephalothoracic lipodystrophy
      • Lipodystrophy in HIV patients
Type A insulin resistance syndrome
Leprechaunism
Rabson-Mendenhall syndrome
Type B insulin resistance syndrome

GENERAL CLINICAL FEATURES OF EXTREME INSULIN RESISTANCE

General clinical manifestations of these syndromes can be classified into two main categories: features related to deficiency of insulin action, and those secondary to the effects of high levels of insulin in some relatively insulin sensitive tissues (Table 2).

Table 2. Common features of extreme insulin resistance syndromes

Glucose homeostasis	Impaired glucose tolerance, diabetes, hypoglycemia
Lipid metabolism	Hypertriglyceridemia
Reproductive	Hirsutism, virilization, PCO, amenorrhea
Adipose tissue	Lipoatrophy, lipohypertrophy, obesity
Developmental	Decreased or increased linear growth, mental retardation
Musculoskeletal	Muscle hypertrophy, acromegalic features, muscle cramps
Dermatologic	Acanthosis nigricans, eruptive xanthoma
Abdominal	Fatty liver, cirrhosis, pancreatitis
Cardiac	Cardiomegaly, hypertension

1) Features related to deficiency of insulin action.

In extreme insulin resistant states, the effect of insulin at the target tissue is diminished. Therefore, pancreatic β–cells try to compensate by producing more insulin. If the pancreatic islets are unable to keep up with the increased demand, pathologies will occur including impaired glucose homeostasis and possibly lipodystrophy.

- **Glucose Homeostasis**

Hyperinsulinemia is the hallmark of extreme insulin resistance. The consequences of extreme insulin resistance on glucose homeostasis can range from normal fasting glucose with impaired glucose tolerance to frank type 2-like diabetes mellitus. Diabetes mellitus can sometimes be the presenting complaint in patients with extreme insulin resistance. Tens of thousands of units of insulin administered each day may only have a small or no effect on glucose lowering in some diabetic patients affected by these devastating syndromes. Lastly, hypoglycemia may rarely result from insulin receptor activation by insulin receptor autoantibodies as mentioned above.[9]

- **Lipoatrophy**

Lipoatrophy is manifested by an adipose tissue loss. It is seen in some of extreme insulin resistance syndromes as is detailed below. It is thought that the lack of the lipogenic effect of insulin may be contributing to the loss of adipose tissue.

2) Features directly related to high circulating insulin.

Although many tissues are resistant to insulin action in the extreme insulin resistance syndromes, some tissues that remain relatively sensitive to insulin may show the characteristic features of hyperinsulinemia.

- **Acanthosis nigricans**

Acanthosis nigricans is a hyperpigmented velvety lesion found usually in the neck and the axillary areas (Fig. 1A), and occasionally elsewhere. The palms and soles are typically not involved. Pathologically, it is characterized by an increased number of melanocytes associated with hypekeratotic epidermal papillomatosis. Acanthosis nigricans is strongly associated with insulin resistance. However, the condition is nonspecific, also occurring in obesity, endocrine diseases (such as Cushing's syndrome and acromegaly) as well as in association with malignant tumors.

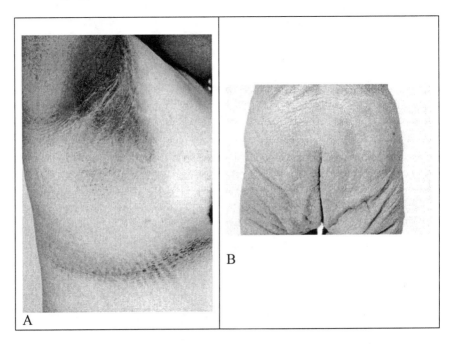

Figure 1. Acanthosis nigricans severity correlates with insulin resistance level.

Acanthosis nigricans is present in all patients with congenital syndromes of extreme insulin resistance syndromes,[14] and in many patients with acquired forms. The severity of acanthosis nigricans correlates with the degree of insulin resistance and the level of serum insulin. Thus, the condition ranges from mild and limited lesions to diffuse skin involvement (Fig. 1B). The exact mechanism leading to acanthosis nigricans in extreme insulin resistance syndromes is still unclear. It is speculated that the related IGF-1 receptors in the skin are activated by the ambient hyperinsulinemia[15] through receptor "specificity spillover".[16] The presence of acanthosis nigricans may warrant an evaluation for an insulin resistant state.

- **Ovarian hyperandrogenism**

    Increased androgen level in females with extreme insulin resistance syndromes is not an uncommon feature. This abnormality may cause amenorrhea, hirsutism, or frank virilization along with polycystic changes in the ovaries. However, these abnormalities are not specific and can be seen in other conditions. The high levels of insulin in extreme insulin resistance syndromes stimulate androgen–producing cells in the ovary[3] where receptors for both insulin and IGF-1 are present. Fasting insulin correlates significantly with mean ovarian volume.[17]

SPECIFIC SYNDROMES OF INSULIN RESISTANCE

Lipodystrophic Syndromes

Lipodystrophic syndromes are a heterogeneous group of disorders characterized by an absence of an adipose tissue as well as an extreme insulin resistance state in most cases. The adipose tissue loss can be familial or acquired, generalized or focal. Several modalities used to evaluate the adipose tissue status include CT scan, MRI, or dual energy x-ray absorptiometry. The etiology of the fat loss is still incompletely understood. The absence of fat and leptin deficiency may contribute to the insulin resistance in these syndromes as will be discussed later.

Familial Generalized Lipodystrophy (Berardinelli-Seip syndrome)

Berardinelli and Seip have separately initially described this autosomal recessive syndrome.

Clinical Manifestations: The loss of adipose tissue is diffuse and affects visceral as well as subcutaneous tissue. The lack of fat is seen at birth or within 2 years of life. Although extreme insulin resistance state is apparent in first decade of life, diabetes is usually manifested in the second decade. The characteristic muscular phenotype observed in many patients with this syndrome is attributed to the adipose tissue loss, high muscular glycogen stores, and possible hyperinsulinemia-mediated changes as described earlier. Various complications have been described, including acute pancreatitis associated with profound hypertriglyceridemia, fatty liver and cirrhosis which may recur after liver transplant,[18] hyperandrogenic state with PCOS, accelerated early growth in children with final short stature, different degrees of mental retardation, cardiac hypertrophy, and arterial hypertension.

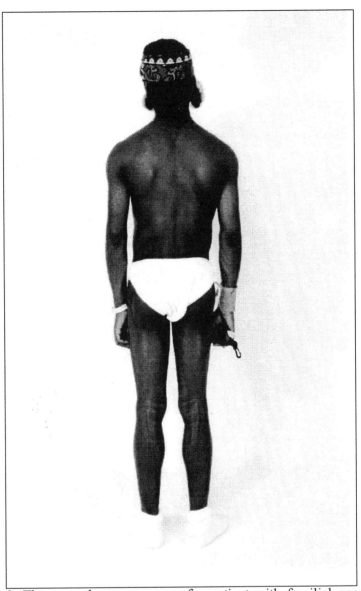

Figure 2. The muscular appearance of a patient with familial generalized lipodystrophy.

Etiology: Recently, a locus for one gene was found to map to human chromosome 9q34.[19] Parental consanguinity is found to be high in this syndrome. The exact mechanism of adipose tissue loss is unclear and different suggestions are available including impaired lipogenesis, increased lipolysis, and underdevelopment of adipocytes. Finally, the pathogenesis of insulin resistance is also unknown and the available data suggest insulin binding defects, insulin receptor defects, and post-receptor defect. Elevated free fatty acids seen in this syndrome may contribute to the severe insulin resistance.

Familial Partial Lipodystrophy Syndromes

- **Kobberling variety**
  The adipose tissue loss is limited to the extremities with normal or even remarkable accumulation of adipose tissue in other subcutaneous as well as visceral areas. The face is spared in this syndrome.
- **Dunnigan variety**
  Patients are born with normal fat distribution but after puberty the fat loss involves the extremities and trunk and spares the face and neck (Fig. 3). An autosomal dominant disease was mapped to chromosome 1q21-22[20,21] which harbors the LMNA gene encoding nuclear lamins A and C. Nuclear lamin A/C R482Q mutation is found in this variety.[22]

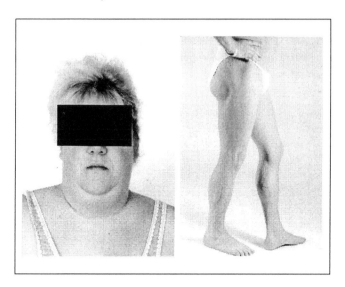

Figure 3. Some phenotypic features of a patient with Dunnigan variety.

- **Mandibuloacral dysplasia variety**
  This is an autosomal recessive condition with stiff joints, mandibuloacral dysplasia, dental and dermal abnormalities.

Acquired Generalized Lipodystrophy (Lawrence syndrome)

The disease is usually manifested in first or second decade of life with insulin resistance syndrome. No similar family history is found and adipose tissue is healthy at birth. The acquired syndrome shares many of the features described in the familial form. Viral infection preceded the relatively rapid appearance of the syndromes in several cases. Inflammatory cells and panniculitis[23] are seen on skin biopsy. Therefore, inflammatory destructive process involving the adipose tissue may play a role in the pathogenesis of this syndrome. In fact, antibodies against adipocyte membranes have been found in one study.[24]

Cephalothoracic lipodystrophy (Barraquer-Simons syndrome)

The characteristic feature of this disorder is fat loss in the trunk and face, with excessive fat accumulation immediately below the waist (Fig. 4).

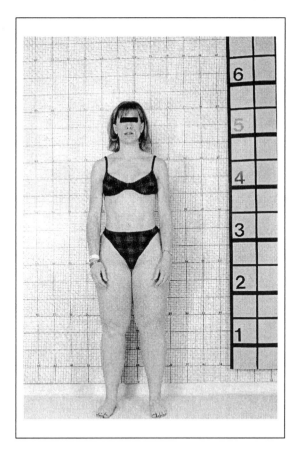

Figure 4. The fat accumulation below the waist is associated with fat loss in other locations in a patient with cephalothoracic lipodystrophy.

It is seen mainly in women and may follow a viral infection. The etiology is still unknown. However, an association between cephalothoracic lipodystrophy and the nephritic factor, low complement in type II mesangioproliferative glomerulonephritis has been documented. Rarely patients develop insulin resistance with its manifestations, or dyslipidemia. Other autoimmune syndromes can be seen. Majority of patients have C3 nephritic factor immunoglobulin, which is suggested to cause lysis of adipose tissue.[25]

Lipodystrophy in HIV patients

This increasingly recognized serious condition is characterized by lipoatrophy in the face and limbs, dorsocervical and visceral adiposity,[26] associated with hypertriglyceridemia, and severe insulin resistance with potentially increased risk of cardiovascular disease. No clear explanation for the syndrome has been confirmed, but emergence of this syndrome has been correlated with the widespread introduction of protease inhibitors to the highly active antiretroviral therapy (HAART) regimens. The risk is also increased if nucleoside analogue reverse transcriptase inhibitors are combined with protease inhibitors.[27] The lipodystrophic changes could be reversed upon stopping protease inhibitors.[28] The precise molecular mechanism of fat redistribution is still unknown. It is suggested that protease inhibitors impair preadipocyte differentiation,[29,30] and promote apoptosis[30] via inhibition of glucose transport,[31] thereby rendering the adipose tissue resistant to insulin. Altered insulin signaling at the level of phosphatidylinositol 3-kinase is suggested to be causing or contributing to insulin resistance state.[32]

Type A Insulin Resistance Syndrome

The transmission of type A syndrome is found to follow autosomal dominant or autosomal recessive pattern with variable penetrance.[1,2]
Clinical manifestations: This syndrome was originally described in young nonobese women with extreme hyperinsulinemia, variable resistance to exogenous insulin, hirsutism, polycystic ovaries, and android habitus.[1] All have had acanthosis nigricans. Only about a third, however, have had fasting hyperglycemia. Most have glucose intolerance, but some patients have normal glucose tolerance, and these patients demonstrate the greatest degree of basal and glucose-stimulated hyperinsulinemia. All of these patients have had elevated plasma testosterone values usually associated with normal concentration of gonadotropins and all have had PCOS. Acromegalic features have been reported in some patients with type A extreme insulin resistance syndrome.[33] Although both GH and IGF-1 levels are normal, IGF-1 receptor activation by the high levels of insulin has been speculated to contribute to "pseudoacromegaly". Weight reduction may help to reduce the insulin levels and some of its manifestations to some extent.

The remarkable muscular pattern seen in these patients may be related to the hyperandrogenic state and/or to insulin-mediated IGF-1 stimulation. In one study, Type A syndrome was associated with increased intraocular pressure and retinal vascular permeability, which improved by IGF-1 administration.[34]

Etiology: Several types of insulin receptor defects have been described. Typically, insulin binding to freshly obtained circulating monocytes and erythrocytes has been decreased. Less commonly, insulin binding has been completely normal. Thus, insulin resistance is a fixed feature of the type A syndrome but insulin binding is either low or normal. Studies of the function of the β-subunit of the monocyte insulin receptors showed concomitant decrease of the receptor autophosphorylation and tyrosine kinase activity with the binding activity in patients with low insulin binding. Interestingly, in one of the patients with normal insulin binding, insulin receptor autophosphorylation and tyrosine kinase activity from circulating monocytes and erythrocytes as well as cultured fibroblasts were greatly decreased.[35] Uncoupling of the receptor binding and phosphorylation thus exists in cells of some patients with type A syndrome. A variant of this syndrome has been seen in a brother and sister who also exhibited muscle cramps, and another family with features of this syndrome has also been described. Another variation of this syndrome seen with precocious puberty, pineal tumors, and developmental defects is referred to as the **Rabson-Mendenhall syndrome (see below)**. It has been reported that PC-1 transmembrane glycoprotein inhibits insulin receptor function by interacting with the α–subunit of the insulin receptor in patients with type A syndrome.[36]

Leprechaunism (Donohue Syndrome)
Leprechaunism is a complex congenital insulin resistance syndrome. Clinical manifestations: These infants are small for gestational age and continue to grow slowly in extrauterine life. They have a characteristically abnormal appearance (Fig. 5) with such features as low-set ears, saddle nose deformity, hypertrichosis, decreased subcutaneous fat, and, occasionally, acanthosis nigricans. Curiously, in these infants a tendency to fasting hypoglycemia coexists with extreme resistance to insulin. Typically, the patients die within the first year of life, although an occasional child may live significantly longer.

Etiology: Insulin binding studies have revealed significant heterogeneity. Leprechaunism appears to be caused by defects in the insulin receptor. Over twenty kinds of mutations in the insulin receptor gene have been reported in patients with leprechaunism thus far. Frequent small feeding may help in reducing the risk of hypoglycemia and the postprandial hyperglycemia.

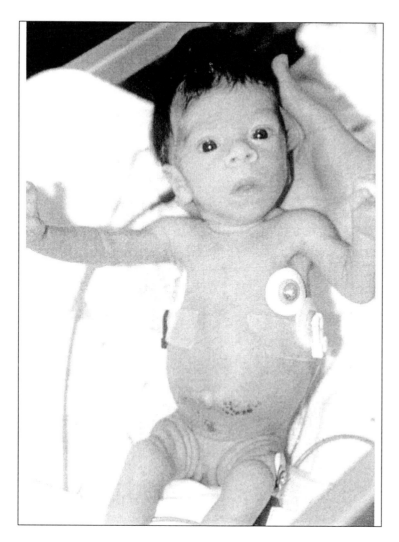

Figure 5. The fat loss is apparent at birth with other features of Leprechaunism.

Rabson-Mendenhall Syndrome

This autosomal recessive syndrome was described in 1956 in a family with hyperplasia of pineal gland and diabetes mellitus. Further characteristic features are low birth weight, thickened nails, hirsutism, acanthosis nigricans, dental precosity and dysplasia, polycystic ovaries, abdominal protuberance, and phallic enlargement. Most affected children die of ketoacidosis and intercurrent infections associated with extreme insulin resistance. Rabson-Mendenhall syndrome appears to lie between the type A syndrome and leprechaunism on the spectrum of severity of insulin receptor dysfunction.

Type B Insulin Resistance Syndrome

This syndrome was initially described in three female patients and shown to be associated with a plasma inhibitor of insulin binding.[37] Subsequently, about twenty patients have been studied. Most have been women of variable age; only two are male patients in the sixth decade of life. *Clinical manifestations:* Patients exhibit acanthosis nigricans, and in one patient this disorder involved the entire body. Almost all patients have fasting hyperglycemia, and in these patients up to 100,000 U insulin/day may be required to normalize the blood glucose. All of these patients have features typical of autoimmune diseases, such as pancytopenia and increased erythrocyte sedimentation rate. In some, a lupus or Sjögren-like syndrome is present with arthralgias, proteinuria, parotid enlargement, and positive antinuclear antibody. About half the patients have anti-DNA antibodies but positive lupus preparations are uncommon. The symptoms may wax and wane reflecting the levels of antibodies, and in some cases spontaneous remission has been described.[38,39]

Etiology: In patients with suggestive clinical features the diagnosis is confirmed by demonstrating an inhibitor of insulin binding. The circulating inhibitor has been shown to be a polyclonal immunoglobulin behaving as an antibody to the insulin receptor.

These antireceptor autoantibodies can mimic insulin action *in vitro*. We have studied one patient who only manifested hypoglycemia.[9] Administration of corticosteroids resulted in a prompt increase in plasma glucose levels in all of similar patients reported to date. Thus, autoantibodies to the insulin receptor must be considered in the differential diagnosis of hypoglycemia. Most patients, however, demonstrate hyperglycemia and insulin resistance. Insulin binding is qualitatively abnormal in circulating cells from these patients. Abnormal insulin binding results from antibody binding on or near the insulin receptor. This yields a competition curve that has decreased specific tracer binding but also a marked increase in the amount of insulin necessary for 50% competition of binding. The net outcome is a major alteration in the affinity of the receptor for insulin. This abnormality can be reversed by removal of the circulating antibody by plasma exchange or by an acid wash procedure, indicating that the underlying receptor is normal. Furthermore, insulin receptors in cultured cells from these patients exhibit normal binding. Analysis of the function of the β–subunit of the receptor from cells of patients with the type B syndrome revealed a generally proportional decrease of the receptor kinase activity and insulin binding. Therefore, the phosphorylating activity expressed per receptor appears to be normal.

A variant of type B syndrome is seen in some ataxia telangectasia patients with the anti-receptor antibodies of IgM subtype.[40]

Although initially the type A and B syndromes were described as distinctly different, we now know that patients with typical clinical and laboratory features of the type B syndrome may manifest the major features

266

of the type A syndrome, including polycystic ovaries, elevated plasma testosterone, and hirsutism. Thus, it is apparent that the type A and B syndromes have overlapping phenotypic features. Furthermore, it is clear that all of the syndromes of severe insulin resistance and acanthosis nigricans have many common clinical features.

THERAPEUTIC MODALITIES

Many patients with extreme insulin resistance are refractory to therapeutic maneuvers and various agents produce variable results. Common modalities include treating the individual manifestations of different diseases such as dyslipidemia (drugs or plasmapheresis), PCOS and hyperandrogenemia, diabetes (including diet, exercise and weight reduction if appropriate), cosmetic surgery (such as liposuction of lipohypertrophic lesions), and so forth.

Thiazolidinediones and metformin

Thiazolidinediones act by activating PPAR-γ and inducing adipocyte differentiation.[41] Thiazolidinediones may improve insulin resistance, diabetes, hyperlipidemia and lipodystrophy.[41,42] Metformin acts in early steps of insulin signal transduction and decreases ovarian and adrenal cytochrome P450c17 activity. Metformin may improve insulin resistance and lipodystrophy[43,44] and decrease hyperandrogenemia.[45]

Insulin

Often, very high doses of insulin may be needed in extreme insulin resistance syndromes. Life style modifications and   insulin sensitizers may help to decrease the insulin requirements.

Growth hormone and IGF-1

IGF-1 shares homology with insulin and has the ability to bind to insulin receptors. IGF-1 has been used in some patients with leprechaunism and found to be effective in preventing the growth retardation as well as in improving hyperglycemia in some cases.[46] IGF-1 has been also used in other types of insulin resistance syndrome.[47,48,49] In HIV lipodystrophy, recombinant human growth hormone has been reported to reverse the buffalo hump and truncal adiposity but not the peripheral lipoatrophy.[50]

Immunomodulation

This modality has been used in antibody-mediated extreme insulin resistance syndromes. Steroids, cyclosporine and cyclophosphamide and plasmapheresis have been used.[38,51,56] A combination of a short-term suppression of autoantibodies with plasmapheresis and cyclophosphamide, followed by a chronic maintenance approach with cyclosporin A and azathioprin offers a promise of prevention of relapses. However, immunosuppressive therapy may not have an impact on the natural history of the disease.[38]

Leptin replacement and adipose tissue implant

In animal studies, it was shown that fat transplantation reversed the hyperglycemia and lowered insulin levels.[52,53] Additionally, leptin replacement improved insulin resistance and hyperlipidemia,[53] which was not seen in another study.[54]

Insulin receptor activators

Insulin mimetics, such as L-783,281 and vanadate, seem to act by stimulating insulin receptor activity. Thus, they may potentially have beneficial effect in some types of extreme insulin resistance syndromes.[55]

SUMMARY

Recent explosion of our knowledge of insulin signal transduction at the molecular level gathered from studies of patients with extreme insulin resistance syndromes has allowed us to rapidly translate the findings to the therapeutic area dealing with the much more common insulin-resistant conditions. Because of the rapid progress in this area, it is expected that students of these conditions get into the habit of frequently updating their knowledge from reviewing general science (such as Nature, Cell, Science) and specific diabetes/metabolism journals (Diabetes, Diabetes Care, Diabetologia, Molecular Endocrinology, Endocrinology, Journal of Clinical Endocrinology and Metabolism, Journal of Clinical Investigation, etc.). Additionally, several professional organizations maintain excellent websites with useful web links on the Internet, allowing a quick search for the updated information.

REFERENCES

1. Kahn CR, Flier JS, Bar RS, et al. The syndrome of insulin resistance and acanthosis nigricans: insulin receptor disorders in man. N Engl J Med; 294:739-745, 1976.
2. Moller DE, Flier JS. Insulin resistance: Mechanisms, syndromes, and implications. N Eng J Med; 325:938-948, 1991.
3. Barbieri RL, Smith S, Ryan KJ, et al. The role of hyperinsulinemia in the pathogenesis of ovarian hyperandrogenism. Fertil Steril 50:197-212, 1988.
4. Barroso I, Curnell M, Crowley VE, et al. Dominant negative mutation in human PPAR gamma associated with severe insulin resistance, diabetes mellitus, and hypertension. Nature 402:880-883, 1999.

5. Collinet M, Berthelon M, Benit P, et al. Familial hyperinsulinemia due to a mutation substituting histidine for arginine at position 65 in proinsulin: identification of the mutation by restriction enzyme mapping. Eur J Pediatr 157:450-460, 1998.

6. Hanede M, Polonsky KS, Bergenstal RM, et al. Familial hyperinsulinemia due to a structurally abnormal insulin. Definition of an emerging new clinical syndrome. N Eng J Med 310:1288-1294, 1984.

7. Duckworth WC, Bennet RG, Hamel FG . Insulin degradation: Progress and potential. Endo Rev 19:608-624, 1998.

8. Francis A, Hanning I, Alberti KG. The influence of insulin antibody levels on the plasma profile and action of subcutaneously injected human and bovine short acting insulins. Diabetologia 28:330-334, 1985.

9. Taylor SI, Grunberger G, Marcus-Samuels B, et al. Hypoglycemia associated with antibodies to the insulin receptor. N Eng J Med 307:1422-1426, 1982.

10. Virkamaki A, Ueki K, Kahn CR. Protein-protein interaction in insulin signaling and the molecular mechanisms of insulin resistance. J Clin Invest 103:931-943, 1999.

11. Gorden P, Carpentier JL, Frechet PO, et al. Internalization of polypeptide hormones: mechanism, intracellular localization and significance. Diabetologia 18:263-274, 1980.

12. Grunberger G, Robert A, Carpentier JL, et al. Human circulating monocytes internalize 125I-insulin in a similar fashion to rat hepatocytes: relevance to receptor regulation in target and non-target tissue. J Lab Clin Med. 106:211-217, 1985.

13. Flier JS, Minaker KL, Landsburg L, et al. Impaired in vivo insulin clearance in patients with target cell resistance to insulin. Diabetes 31:132-135, 1982.

14. Flier JS. Metabolic importance of acanthosis nigricans. Arch Derm 121:193-194, 1985.

15. Cruz PD, Hud JA Jr. Excess insulin binding to insulin-like growth factor receptors: proposed mechanism for acanthosis nigricans. J Invest Dermatol 98 (suppl):82S-85S, 1992.

16. Fradkin JE, Eastman RC, Lesniak MA, et al. Specificity spillover at the hormone receptor: exploring its role in human disease. N Engl J Med; 320:640-645, 1989.

17. Rotman-Pikielny P, Andewelt A, Ozyavuzligil A, et al. Polycystic ovarian syndrome (PCOS): Lessons from patients with severe insulin resistance syndromes. The Endocrine Society's 83rd Annual Meeting p80, 2001.

18. Cauble MS, Gilroy R, Sorrel MF, et al. Lipoatrophic diabetes and end-stage liver disease secondary to nonalcoholic steatohepatitis with recurrence after liver transplantation. Transplantation 71:892-895, 2001.

19. Garg A, Wilson R, Barnes R, et al. A gene for congenital generalized lipodystrophy maps to human chromosome 9q34. J Clin Endocrinol Metab 84:3390-3394, 1999.

20. Peters JM, Barnes R, Bennett L, et al. Localization the gene for familial partial lipodystrophy (Dunnigan Variety) to chromosome 1q21-22. Nat Genet 18:292-295, 1998.

21. Jackson SN, Pinkney J, Bargiotta A, et al. A defect in the regional deposition of adipose tissue (partial lipodystrophy) is encoded by a gene at chromosome 1q. Am J Hum Genet 63:534-540, 1998.

22. Cao H, Hegele RA. Nuclear lamin A/ C R482Q mutations in Canadian kindreds with Dunnigan type familial partial lipodystophy. Hum Molec Genet 9:109-112, 2000.

23. Billings JK, Milgraum SS, Gupta AK, et al. Lipoatrophic panniculitis: a possible autoimmune inflammatory disease of fat report of three cases. Arch Dermatol 123:1662-1666, 1987.

24. Hubler A, Abendroth K, Keiner T, et al. Dysregulation of insulin-like growth factors in a case of generalized acquired lipoatrophic diabetes mellitus (Lawrence syndrome) connected with autoantibodies against adipocytes membranes. Exp Clin Endocrinol Diabetes 106:79-84, 1998.

25. Mathieson PW, Wurzner R, Oliveria DB, et al. Complement mediated adipocytes lysis by nephritic factor sera. J Exp Med 177:1827-1831, 1993.

26. Tsiodras S, Mantzoros C, Hammer S, et al. Effects of protease inhibitors on hyperglycemia, hyperlipidemia and lipodystrophy. A 5-year cohort study. Arch Int Med 160:2050-2056, 2000.

27. Van Der Valk M, Gisolf EH, Reiss P, et al. Increased risk of lipodystrophy when nucleoside analogue reverse trancriptase inhibitors are included with protease inhibitors in the treatment of HIV-1 infection. AIDS 15:847-855, 2001.

28. Panse I, Vasseur E, Raffin-Sanson ML, et al. Lipodystrophy associated with protease inhibitors. Br J Dermatol 142:496-500, 2000.

29. Caron M, Auclair M, Vigouroux C, et al. The HIV protease inhibitor indinavir impairs sterol regulatory element-binding protein −1 intranuclear localization, inhibits preadipocyte differentiation, and induces insulin resistance. Diabetes 50:1378-1388, 2001.

30. Dowell P, Flexner C, Kwiterovich PO, et al. Suppression of preadipocyte differentiation and promotion of adipocytes death by HIV protease inhibitors. J Biol Chem 275:41325-41332, 2000.

31. Murata H, Hruz PW, Mueckler M. The mechanism of insulin resistance caused by HIV protease inhibitor therapy. J Biol Chem 275:20251-20254, 2000.

32. Meyer MM, Schuett M, Jost P, et al. Indinavir decreases insulin-stimulated phosphatidylinositol 3-kinase activity and stimulates leptin secretion in human adipocytes. Diabetes 50 (Suppl 2):A414, 2001.

33. Flier JS, Moller DE, Moses AC, et al. Insulin–mediated pseudoacromegaly: Clinical and biochemical characterization of a syndrome of selective insulin resistance. J Clin Endocrinol Metab 76:1533-1541, 1993.

34. Martin XD, Zenobi PD. Type A syndrome of insulin resistance: anterior chamber anomalies of the eye and effects of insulin – like growth factor-1 on the retina. Ophthalmologica 215:117-123, 2001.

35. Grunberger G, Zick Y, Gorden P. Defect in phosphorylation of insulin receptors in cells from an insulin-resistant patient with normal insulin binding. Science 223:832-934, 1984.

36. Maddux BA, Goldfine ID. Membrane glycoprotein PC-1 inhibition of insulin receptor function occurs via direct interaction with receptor alpha subunit. Diabetes 49:13-19, 2000.

37. Flier JS, Kahn CR, Roth J, et al. Antibodies that impair insulin receptor binding in an unusual diabetic syndrome with severe insulin resistance. Science 190:63-65, 1975.

38. Arioglu E, Andewelt A, Diabo C, et al. Clinical course of autoantibody to the insulin receptor syndrome. The Endocrine Society's 83rd Annual Meeting p113, 2001.

39. Flier JS, Bar RS, Muggeo M, et al. The evolving clinical course of patients with insulin receptor autoantibodies: Spontaneous remission or receptor proliferation with hypoglycemia. J Clin Endocrinol Metab 47:985-995, 1978.

40. Bar RS, Levis WR, Rechler MM, et al. Extreme insulin resistance in ataxia telangectasia: defect in affinity of insulin receptors. N Engl J Med 298:1164-1171, 1978.

41. Burant CF, Sreenan S, Hirano K, et al. Troglitazone action is independent of adipose tissue. J Clin Invest 100:2900-2908, 1997.

42. Arioglu E, Duncan-Morin J, Sebring N, et al. Efficacy and safety of troglitazone in the treatment of lipodystrophy syndrome. Ann Int Med 133:263-274, 2000.

43. Hadigan C, Corcoran C, Basgoz N, et al. Metformin in the treatment of HIV lipodystrophy syndrome. JAMA 284:472-477, 2000.

44. Di Paolo S. Metformin ameliorates extreme insulin resistance in a patient with anti-insulin receptor antibodies: Description of insulin receptor and postreceptor effects in vivo and vitro. Acta Endocrinol 126:117-123, 1992.

45. Rique S, Ibanez L, Marcos MV, et al. Effect of metformin on androgen and insulin concentration in type A insulin resistance syndrome. Diabetologia 43:385-386, 2000.

46. Nakae J, Kato M, Murashita M, et al. Long-term effect of recombinant human insulin – like growth factor1 on metabolic and growth control in a patient with leprechaunism. J Clin Endocrinol Metab 83:542-549, 1998.

47. Morrow LA, O'Brien MB, Moller DE, et al. Recombinant human insulin like growth factor −1 therapy improves glycemic control and insulin action in type A syndrome insulin resistance. J Clin Endocrinol Metabol 79:205-210, 1994.

48. Quin JD, Fisher BM, Paterson KR, et al. Acute response to recombinant insulin-like growth factor I in a patient with Mendenhall's syndrome. N Engl J Med 323:1425-1426, 1990.

49. Yamamoto T, Sato T, Mori T, et al. Clinical efficacy of insulin like growth factor 1 in a patient with auto-antibodies to insulin receptors: A case report. Diabetes Res Clin Pract 49:65-69, 2000.

50. Torres RA, Unger KW, Cadman JA, et al. Recombinant human growth hormone improves truncal adiposity and buffalo humps in HIV positive patients on HAART. AIDS 13:2479-2481, 1999.

51. Kramer N, Rosenstein ED, Schneider G. Refractory hyperglycemia complicating an evolving connective tissue disease: response to cyclosporin. J Rheumatol 25:816-818, 1998.

52. Gavrilova O, Marcus-Samuels B, Graham D, et al. Surgical implantation of adipose tissue reverses diabetes in lipotrophic mice. J Clin Invest 105:271-278, 2000.

53. Shimomura I, Hammer RE, Ikemoto S, et al. Leptin reverses insulin resistance and diabetes mellitus in mice with congenital lipodystrophy. Nature 401:73-76, 1999.

54. Reitman ML, Gavrilova O. A-ZIP/F-1 mice lacking white fat: a model for understanding lipoatrophic diabetes. Int J Obes Relat Metab Disord 24(Suppl 4):S11-S14, 2000.

55. Zhang B. Salituro G, Szalkowski D, et al. Discovery of a small molecule insulin mimetic with antidiabetic activity in mice. Science 284:974-977, 1999.

56. Eriksson JW, Bremell T, Eliasson B, et al. Successful treatment with plasmapheresis, cyclophosphamide, and cyclosporin A in type B syndrome of insulin resistance. Case report. Diabetes Care 21:1217-1220, 1998.

Helpful internet sources for additional information on insulin resistance:

www.diabetes.org

www.acponline.org

www.asim.org

www.endo-society.org

VI. Complications of Diabetes

Chapter 1. Acute Hyperglycemic Syndromes: Diabetic Ketoacidosis and the Hyperosmolar State

Adrienne M. Fleckman

DIABETIC KETOACIDOSIS: CLINICAL PRESENTATION

A typical patient in diabetic ketoacidosis (DKA) becomes severely ill over one to several days and represents a medical emergency.

After increasing urination and thirst, come nausea, vomiting and abdominal pain. Dehydration, weakness and dizziness follow. The patient is confused and slips into coma. The respiratory compensation that accompanies acidemia causes rapid breathing. The sweet smell of the volatile ketone body acetone signals the possibility of ketoacidosis.

The majority of patients in DKA have type 1 diabetes (Figure 1). Consistent with this predominance of type 1 diabetes, the patient is likely to be young, slender, Caucasian (type 1 diabetes is 2-7 times more common in whites than blacks[1]), and lack a family history of diabetes. The DKA patient is often a "repeat offender" who sometimes simply stops taking insulin.

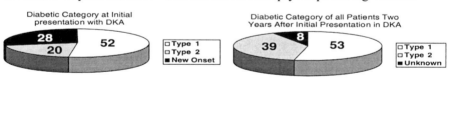

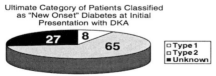

Figure 1. Categories of diabetes in patients with DKA. Diabetic ketoacidosis is predominantly, but not exclusively, a complication of type 1 diabetes[2]. In addition to patients with type 2 diabetes, Black, Japanese and Chinese patients with Atypical Diabetes Mellitus (see text) present with DKA and often do not require insulin after the episode.[3]

The differential diagnosis.

Stupor and coma have many potential causes (Table 1). A decision must be made about which diagnoses to pursue. Alcoholic intoxication or encephalopathy causing coma can be assessed by a history of alcohol intake and blood alcohol levels. Depression of consciousness without focal findings suggests encephalopathy (unilateral weakness on examination suggests a stroke). Emotional instability may suggest that the patient is feigning illness or has taken an overdose; toxicology "screen" is helpful to exclude drugs that can cause coma and acidosis. Kidney failure causing uremic encephalopathy is excluded with blood urea nitrogen (BUN) and creatinine measurements. A "history" or physical evidence of trauma should be sought. Confusion with fever may indicate central nervous system infection. Witnesses can be questioned about seizure activity, which is often followed by a decreased level of alertness. The pneumonic given in Table 1 is not comprehensive; for example, the electrocardiogram may show cardiac arrhythmia or a myocardial infarction that can cause a drop in blood pressure and change in mental state. While reviewing this differential diagnosis, the physician simultaneously obtains the finger stick (capillary) glucose measurement to exclude hypoglycemia (low blood sugar) or hyperglycemia as a cause of coma. An elevated glucose supports a diagnosis of diabetic ketoacidosis or hyperglycemic hyperosmolar coma.

Table 1. Differential diagnosis of diabetic coma

A-E-I-O-U	TIPSI
Alcohol	Trauma
Encephalopathy	Infection
Infectious	Meningitis
Neurologic	Sepsis
Insulin	Psychosis
Hypoglycemia, DKA, hyperosmolar, alcoholic ketoacidosis	Seizure
Opiates, Overdose	post-Ictal state
Uremia	

DEFINITION

Diabetic ketoacidosis (DKA) is a state of metabolic decompensation, caused by a relative or absolute lack of the pancreatic hormone insulin, in which hyperglycemia is associated with excess production of ketoacids resulting in metabolic acidosis.

DKA, the first manifestation of diabetes in a minority of patients, most often occurs in known diabetics who are not taking sufficient insulin. A patient may run out of insulin and not renew a prescription. Adolescents sometimes discontinue insulin as an act of rebellion. Some patients have little understanding of insulin therapy and don't accept the necessity for insulin. When patients are ill and not eating well, they may reduce or omit insulin doses because they do not realize that times of stress may be accompanied by elevation of "counter-regulatory" hormones and require more insulin than usual.

Uncontrolled diabetes leading to DKA is not a definable event like going over a waterfall, but rather is more akin to being caught in a fast-moving stream. The point at which the patient cannot swim against the current is diabetic ketoacidosis. This point is different for each individual[4], requiring agreement on a somewhat arbitrary set of numbers. The customary definition is a glucose level > 250 mg/dl (13.9 mmol/L), acidemia reflected by a pH lower than 7.35, a serum bicarbonate less than 20 meq/L, and positive test for serum ketones.[5] Reasons for some exceptions to this definition are discussed below.

PATHOPHYSIOLOGY

Introduction

Cellular work requires massive amounts of energy. Intermediary metabolism (named for the intermediate compounds that are generated prior to the final metabolic products), largely through the production of ATP (adenosine tri-phosphate), provides this energy and the energy for synthesizing macromolecules.[6, 7, 8]

The fed state is an insulin sufficient state. Insulin affects the internal machinery of cells in the liver, fat (adipose tissue) and muscle to promote energy production and storage.

Glucose, the major cellular nutrient, is transported into cells where it is metabolized in the glycolytic pathway. Enzymes in this pathway are regulated by insulin (whose action is antagonized by glucagon). At the end of this pathway, the three-carbon glucose metabolite pyruvate is further broken down into small molecules used to produce complex cellular components, or can be converted into chemical energy (the nucleotide ATP) when transported into the energy generator of the cell (the mitochondria).

When insulin levels are adequate, energy is stored in small quantities as glycogen for immediate use, or in large quantities as triglycerides for long-term use.

Inside the hepatocyte glucose molecules can be linked in a tightly packed branching structure to form glycogen, the polysaccharide that stores glucose for between meal and overnight "snacks". Alternatively, the two-carbon compound acetyl coenzyme A (acetyl Co-A), which is formed from glucose breakdown, can be used for the manufacture of larger molecules, including fatty acids for energy storage in a large fat depot (adipose tissue). Insulin acts to stimulate and maintain these storage processes.

In DKA, inadequate insulin action does not provide for the excess glucose present in the blood stream to enter cells. The decreased flux of glucose into cells simulates fasting.

With the fall in intracellular glucose, intermediary metabolism of carbohydrates and lipids shifts away from glucose breakdown and storage to an exaggerated imitation of the fasting state. Metabolism shifts away from the utilization of glucose toward gluconeogenesis, which is the production of glucose from pyruvate (Figure 2). Precursors for gluconeogenesis are obtained from fat, which is melted down into fatty acids and glycerol, and from proteins following breakdown into constituent amino acids. Glycerol, amino acids (particularly alanine), and lactate (derived from red cell metabolism) are converted into glucose.

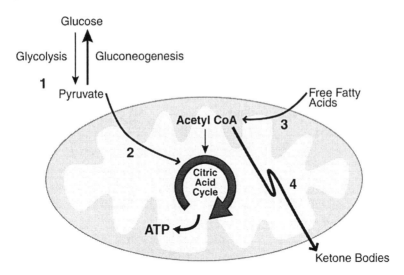

Figure 2. Increased gluconeogenesis, fall in pyruvate levels and formation of ketone bodies.
1 When insulin levels drop, the rate of glycolysis falls and of gluconeogenesis increases, reducing levels of pyruvate. 2 Pyruvate is not available for conversion into oxaloacetate.
3 Without oxaloacetate to be "condensed with", free fatty acids converted into Acetyl-CoA cannot enter the TCA cycle. 4 Acetyl-CoA is therefore diverted to mitochondrial ketone body formation.

The counter-regulatory hormones glucagon and epinephrine, along with growth hormone and cortisol, stimulated by fasting and by stress, antagonize the effects of insulin.

Counter-regulatory hormones antagonize the glucose lowering action of insulin, and act to raise the blood glucose level. Glucagon, a potent counter-regulatory hormone inhibited by insulin, is secreted from pancreatic alpha cells when cells perceive low glucose. In diabetes, pancreatic insulin levels are reduced and glucagon is chronically elevated. In DKA, in addition to low insulin action, there is the cellular perception of low glucose, which further stimulates glucagon secretion. The excessive glucagon levels of DKA dominate hepatic metabolism, promoting breakdown of glycogen to glucose, stimulating gluconeogenesis, inhibiting fatty acid synthesis, and directing long chain fatty acids into the mitochondria where they are dedicated to ketoacid formation (Figure 3).

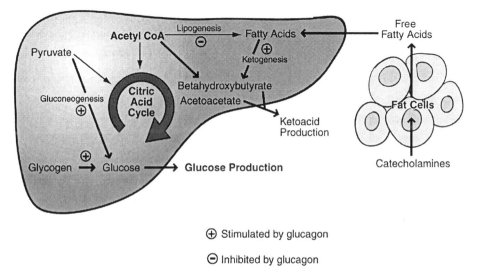

⊕ Stimulated by glucagon

⊖ Inhibited by glucagon

Figure 3. The central role of glucagon in DKA.
Glucagon stimulates glucose production through gluconeogenesis and glycogen breakdown. Lipogenesis is inhibited by glucagon. Free fatty acids derived from lipolysis in fat cells are transported into the mitochondria. Acetyl CoA from fatty acid breakdown is diverted to ketoacid production.

Catecholamines, acting on beta-adrenergic receptors, are the most potent stimulators of lipolysis (breakdown of adipose tissue triglycerides with release of free fatty acids and glycerol). Growth hormone also stimulates lipolysis and liberates free fatty acids.[9] Cortisol contributes to elevations of blood glucose by increasing lipolysis in certain fat depots, increasing the transcription of genes that increase protein catabolism (providing precursors for gluconeogenesis), and up-regulating the expression of the rate-limiting enzyme for gluconeogenesis, phosphoenolpyruvate carboxykinase (PEPCK).[10]

THE CENTRAL ROLE OF FREE FATTY ACIDS (FFAs) IN DKA

Free fatty acids leave the fat cell and are transported to the liver.
Without fatty acids there can't be any ketoacids; without ketoacids there is no diabetic ketoacidosis.[11] Under the influence of insulin, free fatty acids are transported to and imprisoned inside a fat cell (adipocyte) bound as three chains to a glycerol molecule (tri-glyceride). The catecholamines are ready to "spring" FFAs out of "jail", but they are unable to do so while there is adequate insulin. During starvation, when insulin levels drop, lipids stored in adipose tissue as triglycerides (three fatty acids linked to a glycerol molecule) are released from the fat cell as the hydrocarbon long chain fatty acids. These fatty acids are transported to the liver bound to albumin. From the viewpoint of the FFA, the scene in the liver is chaotic. The liver is missing adequate insulin levels. Glycolysis, the most ancient metabolic pathway, is at a standstill. FFAs further inhibit insulin action and stimulate gluconeogenesis and hepatic production of lipoproteins, contributing to hyperglycemia and to the marked elevation of triglycerides seen in some patients. Under the controlled conditions of fasting, this process (coupled with the release of glycerol) provides sufficient calories to serve as the glucose and energy "grocery store" for a month-long trek through the desert. In DKA, this process leads to uncontrolled glucose elevations.

Malonyl Coenzyme A (Co A) levels control free fatty acid transport into the mitochondria, thereby acting as the key control of the rate of hepatic ketoacid production.
Malonyl CoA is a precursor molecule whose levels rise during fatty acid synthesis (an insulin-stimulated process). It functions to inhibit carnitine palmitoyltransferase 1 (CPT1), the transporter of fatty acids into mitochondria. During DKA, since fatty acid synthesis does not occur, malonyl CoA levels decline, permitting a rise in fatty acid transport into mitochondria (Figure 4).

The fate of free fatty acids in the hepatic mitochondria is determined by the activity of the glycolytic pathway, because pyruvate is required for FFA derivatives to enter the TCA cycle (Figure 2).
Pyruvate formed during glycolysis is the glucose-derived metabolite that enters the TCA (tricarboxylic acid, also called the Krebs' or citric acid) cycle. This pathway is oxygen requiring (oxidative) and generates large amounts of ATP. In DKA, pyruvate is diverted to gluconeogenesis, less is available to enter the TCA cycle, and the rate of oxidative metabolism of glucose declines. In addition, the fall in pyruvate alters fat metabolism in the liver. Under normal conditions of energy generation, fatty acid metabolites can enter the TCA cycle in a process that requires pyruvate. Since pyruvate is necessary for fat to enter the TCA pathway, it is said that fat burns in the flame of carbohydrate. In DKA, this energy-generating "flame" is extinguished (Figure 2).

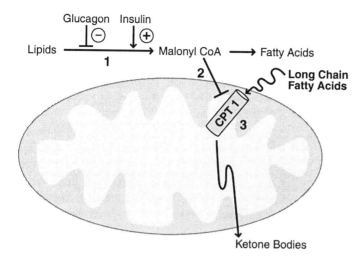

Figure 4. The pivotal role of Malonyl CoA in regulation of ketogenesis.
1 In DKA, the <u>high</u> glucagon and <u>low</u> insulin cause malonyl CoA levels to fall.
2 The fall in malonyl CoA releases the inhibition of the transport protein (CPT 1) that shuttles long chain fatty acids (LCFA) into the mitochondria.
3 Increased LCFA are available for ketone body formation.

Some pyruvate is converted to lactate in a process that restores cytoplasmic NAD+, necessary for minimal cellular metabolism. This can cause a superimposed lactic acidosis on top of ketoacidosis (Figure 5).

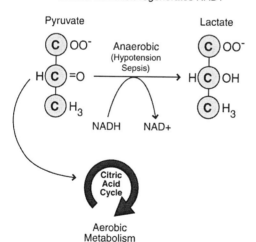

Figure 5. Lactate formed from pyruvate can contribute to acidosis.

When fatty acids cannot enter the TCA cycle in hepatic mitochondria, they are diverted to ketone body (ketoacid) formation.

Fatty acids are broken down in the mitochondrial matrix into the two carbon compound acetyl-CoA. Unable to enter the TCA cycle during intracellular glucose privation, acetyl-CoA in hepatic mitochondria is diverted to the production of the ketoacids beta-hydroxy-butyrate and acetoacetate.[12]

The "redox" (reduction-oxidation) status of the mitochondria, set by the NADH/NAD⁺ ratio, determines the predominant species of ketoacid.

Co-enzymes co-operate with enzymes to catalyze reactions. In these reactions, the co-enzymes are reversibly altered, and can be cycled back and forth between two forms, creating a "pair". The co-enzyme pair NAD^+ (nicotinamide adenine dinucleotide) and NADH functions to carry electrons in oxidation-reduction reactions. An increased NADH/NAD+ ratio develops in DKA during beta-oxidation of fatty acids, and in states of low tissue oxygenation (such as occur if the patient has severe fluid loss and is hypotensive from dehydration or sepsis). NADH <u>reduces</u> the ketoacid acetoacetate to beta-hydroxybutyrate. As will be discussed later, laboratories use the nitroprusside reaction for ketones, which does not measure beta-hydroxybutyrate. When beta-hydroxybutyrate levels greatly exceed acetoacetate, a misleadingly low nitroprusside test can sway the unsuspecting physician away from the correct diagnosis.

Since glucose is not available in DKA, alternative energy-releasing compounds must be utilized. The ketoacids function as an alternate fuel.

Tissues are not able to utilize glucose because of inadequate insulin action. Without insulin, or without <u>enough</u> insulin, cells are left without nutrients. The ketone bodies, or ketoacids, do not require insulin for uptake into cells. If glucose is the electric power line that drives the body, ketone bodies are the battery of the brain and heart. When the electricity fails, hepatic mitochondria produce and export this alternate power. In the heart, skeletal muscle, brain and kidney, ketone bodies can be converted back to acetyl-CoA, which enters the TCA cycle and provides metabolic energy through generation of ATP (Figure 6).

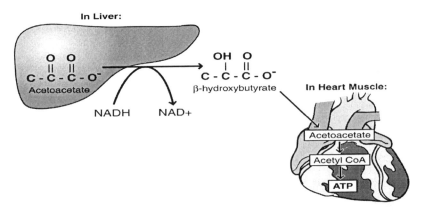

Figure 6. Ketone bodies formed in the liver provide an alternate fuel for the heart, skeletal muscle and brain.

ASSESSMENT OF A PATIENT WITH DKA

Among the long list of potential precipitating factors for DKA are serious conditions that require diagnosis and specific treatment.
Although diabetic ketoacidosis often occurs in repeat offenders who neglect their health, run out of insulin, or stop taking insulin, there is frequently an inciting event that must be discovered. The physician's challenge is to find what went wrong, reverse the process, return the patient to health, and prevent the next episode. In considering the possibilities, it is important to remember that common things occur commonly. The patient may have stopped taking insulin or the pancreas may have gradually lost insulin secretory capacity. Counter-regulatory mechanisms may be activated during any stress and may render antecedent insulin levels insufficient. Particular attention must be given to infections (with elevations of the counter regulatory hormones cortisol and catecholamines), stroke or heart attacks (extremely high epinephrine), or pregnancy (placental lactogen or cortisol). Dehydration during gastrointestinal illness accompanied by vomiting or diarrhea may hasten the development of DKA. An alcohol binge may cause rapid "decompensation" in the patient with limited insulin reserve.

Very unusual causes of counter-regulatory hormone elevation precipitating DKA are growth hormone elevations from acromegaly, glucocorticoid excess in Cushings' syndrome, and glucagon in the rare glucagonoma syndrome. Obscure causes of DKA, such as changing to more active pancreatic enzymes to treat chronic pancreatitis with increased absorption of nutrients, or somatostatin inhibition of insulin secretion in a somatostatinoma, have been described. In teenagers eating disorders are a consideration, especially in recurrent DKA. Medications – the anti-psychotic drugs clozapine and olanzapine - are described to cause DKA. Rare cases of DKA have occurred following pancreatic destruction by a virus.

Infection is the most common precipitating cause of diabetic ketoacidosis; sites that hide infections should be examined carefully.
Elevated glucose levels impair the ability to fight infection, potentially leading to aggressive tissue destruction. Thus it is critical to control the blood glucose and to discover and treat all infections. The physician must be particularly suspicious in patients who are more likely to harbor infections. Infection is twice as likely in women as in men, three times as likely in patients who present with neurologic abnormalities, and two to nine times as likely in patients who fail to clear ketonuria within 12 hours. Hidden sites of infection include the teeth, sinuses, gallbladder, abscesses in the peri-rectal area, and pelvis (in women), and must be examined and re-examined. The nose should be carefully inspected for the eschar (black necrotic tissue) that might indicate the fungus mucormycosis, classically but rarely seen in DKA.

281

Measurements, tests and calculations are used to determine the severity of acidosis, magnitude of ketonemia, and fluid and electrolyte balance.

In order to treat DKA, the physician must measure the degree of acidosis (pH), the ability of the patient to compensate by lowering pCO2, the elevation of the blood glucose level, and the serum potassium (K^+). Initially, an arterial sample is taken for measuring the pH, pO_2, and pCO_2 in order to know if the patient has low oxygenation (hypoxemia), a primary respiratory acidosis (indicating pulmonary disease or central hypo-ventilation), or primary respiratory alkalosis (suggestive of sepsis). After the baseline arterial measurement, the calculated anion gap from serum chemistries (using sodium, chloride and bicarbonate), and the venous pH can be used to evaluate the acid base status (Table 2).[13] To document or follow ketoacid production, serum ketones are typically measured. They are cleared rapidly and may be detected with greater sensitivity in the urine, even when low or absent in the serum. Although it is the dominant "ketoacid" in DKA with a ratio as high as 20:1 compared to acetoacetate, beta-hydroxybutyrate is not measured in the nitroprusside test for ketoacids because beta-hydroxybutyrate is really an acid-alcohol. In the "redox" environment of DKA, an excess ratio of beta-hydroxybutyrate over acetoacetate may result in spuriously low ketone body measurements. The astute clinician knows that DKA may occur without a markedly elevated nitroprusside reaction and is guided by the clinical presentation, pH, anion gap and bicarbonate level.[14]

Table 2. Measurements useful in assessing a patient with DKA

♦ Corrected serum $[Na^+]$ ~ measured serum $[Na^+]$ + 2 x (glucose in mg/dl - 100) ÷ 100

♦ The anion gap = $[Na^+]$ - ($[Cl^-]$ + $[HCO_3^-]$)
  The normal anion gap ~ 8-12

♦ In pure metabolic acidosis the last two digits of the pH = pCO_2
  e.g. if the pH = 7.32, then the pCO_2 should = 32

♦ In pure metabolic acidosis the blood gas pCO_2 ~ (serum HCO_3^- x 1.5) + 8

♦ The calculated effective serum osmolality = 2 (Na^+ + K^+) + (glucose in mg/dl ÷ 18)

♦ Normal total body water (TBW) = lean body mass in kg x 60%
  Current TBW = (normal serum osmolality x normal TBW) ÷ current osmolality
  Water deficit = normal TBW - current TBW

TREATMENT OF DIABETIC KETOACIDOSIS

Introduction

The treating physician seeks to re-establish normal physiology and restore the patient to normal function. Treatment is remarkably straightforward and involves intravenous fluid, insulin, potassium, and vigilance.

The osmotic diuresis of hyperglycemia causes dehydration, which exacerbates the metabolic acidosis.[8] The severity of dehydration determines initial rates of fluid administration.

In the hypotensive patient, fluid resuscitation takes precedence over other concerns. A fluid "challenge" is performed with isotonic fluid given in short blocks of time (in adults, at a rate of 10 cc per minute; in children at a rate of 10-20 ml/kg over 30-60 minutes[15]) – checking the patient every 10 minutes. If intravascular fluid depletion is the cause of hypotension, the blood pressure responds rapidly. Failure to respond to a fluid challenge within 30 minutes suggests another cause for low blood pressure such as cardiac pump failure or peripheral vasodilatation in sepsis. In adults with severe dehydration, initial fluid rates of 1-2 liters/hour may be required. If the patient is not hypotensive, or once blood pressure is restored, a more balanced approach to fluid administration using 250-500 cc per hour is desirable. These slower rates of administration avoid fluid overload with potential for pulmonary edema and hypoxemia, or diuresis of potassium with resultant hypokalemia.[16] Hydration per se decreases counter-regulatory hormone levels, enhances renal perfusion and establishes a glucose diuresis, lowering the blood sugar toward the renal threshold of 300 mg/dl. It is customary to choose isotonic fluid in the hypotensive, dehydrated patient, ½ normal saline as the patient recovers, and dextrose containing fluid as the blood glucose drops below 300 mg/dl.

Fluid administration should be slower in pediatric patients than adults.[15,17]

In children, the physician must be concerned about cerebral edema, which occurs in 1% of DKA episodes in children[18] and is responsible for 70% of diabetic deaths occurring before twelve years of age.[19] The assumption that cerebral edema is caused by organic osmoles that accumulate in the brain to balance the cellular dehydrating effect of the hyperosmolar extracellular fluid, and then cause excess fluid movement into cells with hydration, is unproven.[18] The risk factors recently identified for cerebral edema are more severe acidemia (lower pCO_2), greater dehydration (higher blood urea nitrogen) and the use of bicarbonate.[20] The ketone bodies themselves may increase brain microvascular permeability.[21] Even though the role of rapid fluid administration (greater than 50 ml/kg during the first four hours of therapy) in causing brain herniation[22] is debated, fluid overload is avoided.

Insulin is administered by continuous infusion in doses that range from 0.5 to 4.0 units of regular or lispro insulin per hour.[23]

Insulin doses are adjusted against two parameters – restoring a near normal blood glucose and reversing ketoacidosis. A loading bolus of 10 units regular insulin is commonly administered intravenously while simultaneously beginning continuous infusion at 0.1 units/kg per hour. The glucose should fall by 50-75 mg/dl each hour. If the glucose does not fall as expected, the insulin infusion rate should be doubled. Since prevention of ketoacidosis requires less insulin action than prevention of hyperglycemia, it is a paradox in the therapy of DKA that it is more difficult to stop ketone body generation than to lower serum glucose. Therefore, it is essential that the physician maintain constant insulin infusion, if only at physiologic levels of 0.5 to 1 unit per hour, to restrain lipolysis (release of FFA from adipose tissue). The continued administration of insulin without causing hypoglycemia often requires concomitant administration of glucose containing infusions (usually 5% or, if necessary, 10% dextrose in water at approximately 100cc per hour), which should be started when the serum glucose has fallen to 200-250 mg/dl (11-14 mmol/L).

Potassium repletion is necessary because K^+ is lost during the osmotic diuresis of DKA as the K^+ salt of ketoacids.

The serum potassium level reflects both total body stores, and the distribution between the intracellular (98% of total body K^+) and extracellular spaces. The osmotic diuresis of DKA causes huge urinary K^+ losses. Yet, the serum K^+ can be low, normal or high at the time of presentation. Redistribution of K^+ out of the intracellular compartment and into the intravascular space causes a normal or high serum K^+ in the face of total body depletion.

Physiologic insulin levels drive K^+ into cells[24]. With the decreased insulin action of DKA, potassium moves out of cells into the serum. This redistribution may raise serum K^+. Further elevation of serum K^+ may occur because of redistribution related to acidosis (K^+ moving out of cells in exchange for H^+ moving in). Insulin administration during treatment moves potassium back into the cells, halts the generation of ketoacids and reverses acidosis. Dangerous degrees of hypokalemia may then occur, and are postulated to be the cause of the 30-50% DKA mortality in the 1950's[25]. The treating physician must anticipate and prevent this hypokalemia. Typically, 20-40 meq of K^+ is administered with each liter of fluid. If the fluid is administered more rapidly, the patient will (appropriately) receive more K^+ per unit time. Two caveats against K^+ administration are renal impairment, which prevents normal excretion of excess K^+, and dangerous hyperkalemia at the time of presentation. The physician may administer potassium as soon as urine flow is established. In addition, the physician must order an electrocardiogram (EKG). If signs of hyperkalemia are present (tall peaked T waves, followed by low amplitude P wave and widening QRS complex) (Figure 7), no potassium is given until the "stat" K^+ levels are back from the laboratory. In the absence of signs of hypokalemia on the EKG (low amplitude T waves with rising amplitude U waves), some physicians do not administer K^+ until the laboratory measurement is available.

Figure 7. The electrocardiogram in hyperkalemia progressively shows tall peaked T waves followed by low amplitude "P" wave (not even discernible in this example), and widening of the QRS.

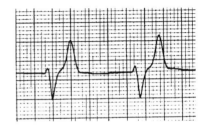

It is increasingly certain that bicarbonate administration plays no role in the therapy of DKA.
When insulin therapy reverses ketoacid formation, bicarbonate is rapidly regenerated from retained ketone body anions. To the extent that these anions were lost in the urine, the kidney takes several days to fully reclaim bicarbonate. In the past, bicarbonate was administered out of concern that severe acidosis would impair cardiac function and precipitate congestive heart failure or vascular collapse. On the other hand, administration of bicarbonate may cause fluid retention, brain edema and unfavorable pH shifts. Current data suggest that bicarbonate administration does not favorably influence patient outcome down to a pH of 6.90.[26] Below this level there would be a consensus to administer bicarbonate even if its value is unproven.

Complications of DKA include death, brain edema, pancreatitis, hyperlipidemia, hypophosphatemia, and pulmonary edema.
Mortality in DKA is 2-10%, striking mostly the very young and the elderly. Almost 2 out of 1000 episodes of DKA in children will result in death from cerebral edema, the major cause of death and disability for children with diabetic ketoacidosis. Multiple organ failure (cardiac, renal, hepatic, and pulmonary) portends a high mortality in adult patients. Elevated pancreatic enzymes, such as amylase and lipase, are correlated with the degree of hyperglycemia, acidemia and dehydration. Although not usually clinically important,[27] dehydration with hypoperfusion of the pancreas and elevations of triglycerides may precipitate acute pancreatitis.[28,29] Elevated triglycerides occur because insulin stimulation of endothelial lipoprotein lipase is necessary to remove lipids from the circulation, and insulin inhibition of adipose tissue lipase prevents mobilization of lipids out of the fat cell. Hypertriglyceridemia resolves following DKA unless there is an underlying defect, but may contribute to pancreatitis.[30] Mild hypophosphatemia commonly occurs in DKA; there is evidence that treatment is not required.[31] Pulmonary symptoms may indicate pneumonia, but may also occur with a "capillary leak" or interstitial edema associated with DKA.[32]

DKA costs lives and dollars; the epidemiology of DKA targets educational and preventive solutions.

In developing countries, mortality rates for type 1 diabetic patients are high, with DKA as the leading cause of death.[33] In U.S. children and young adults with type 1 diabetes mellitus, DKA is also the most common cause of mortality, and appears to affect non-whites with greatly increased frequency compared to whites.[34] DKA, with 100,000 admissions annually in the United States[35], is estimated to represent ~ 25% of the direct medical care dollars of treating type 1 diabetes mellitus.[36]

Educational programs may decrease the incidence of DKA,[37] although the emotional and psychological factors that stimulate knowledgeable patients to discontinue insulin are not easily addressed. Studies have shown that patients can be safely discharged following care in the emergency room if DKA is mild (pH > 7.20, HCO3 > 10)[38]. Admission to a general hospital bed rather than a more expensive intensive care unit bed is also possible for less severely ill patients.[39] Specialty care may provide significant cost savings: endocrinologists treat and discharge their patients with DKA more rapidly, with fewer tests and fewer readmissions than general internists.[35]

Patients may present in DKA with exceptions to the definition including a lower glucose, higher pH and negative nitroprusside test for ketones.

The glucose at presentation in DKA varies widely from less than 180 mg/dl to 1000 mg/dl. If a patient is not eating well prior to the onset of DKA, the glucose may be lower than with a prior good food intake. Young people with good kidney function or pregnant patients with increased glomerular filtration rate (GFR) and lowered glucose threshold can develop DKA with normal blood sugars. Patients who treat their finger stick glucose elevations with small doses of insulin may develop diabetic ketoacidosis with normal glucose levels if the stress hormones during illness stimulate sufficient lipolysis. DKA may develop unusually rapidly during fasting or dehydration because these conditions increase the counter-regulatory hormone glucagon, and increase the pace at which acidosis occurs when insulin is withdrawn. Patients on the insulin pump do not have long acting insulin on board when the pump malfunctions and may go into DKA within hours.

Patients who have excessive vomiting and develop DKA may have pH levels above the definition for DKA (pH < 7.35) because H^+ lost in emesis fluid superimposes metabolic alkalosis on the metabolic acidosis of DKA. Other states that cause metabolic alkalosis can have the same effect, such as DKA with Cushing's syndrome.

Patients with low tissue oxygenation, sepsis and hypotension can present with a large predominance of β-hydroxybutyrate over acetoacetate. The test for ketoacids in these patients may be negative at presentation and become positive as the patient improves and converts β-hydroxybutyrate to acetoacetate.

The patient with atypical diabetes mellitus is exceptional in the ability to recover normal pancreatic function.[3, 40, 41]

In the United States, perhaps 10% of black Americans who present with DKA will have a subsequent course characterized by long-term remission of diabetes mellitus. This course has been labeled "atypical diabetes mellitus", "type 1.5" diabetes, and "Flatbush" diabetes for the area of Brooklyn, New York, where it has been best characterized. Relapses occurred over a time period of months to longer than five years; 20% of patients were in remission beyond six years. Patients may have a family history of similar remissions of diabetes mellitus. This pattern is seen in younger, less obese and more insulin sensitive patients than the typical patient with type 2 diabetes. Unlike in type 1 diabetes, antibodies against glutamic acid decarboxylase (GAD) and islet cell antibodies are negative.[40]

HYPEROSMOLAR HYPERGLYCEMIC SYNDROME (HHS)

Hyperosmolar hyperglycemic syndrome differs from DKA in the more dramatic degree of dehydration, higher serum glucose, lack of acidosis, advanced patient age, and much higher mortality (Figure 8).[42]

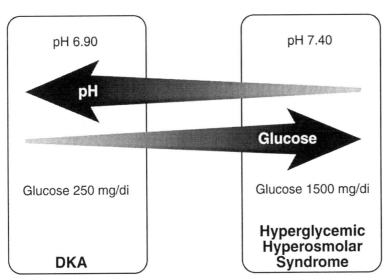

Figure 8. DKA and hyperglycemic hyperosmolar syndrome.
There is no clear separation of DKA and HHS. The less extreme glucose elevations and more extreme acidosis can be labeled DKA. The more extreme glucose elevations with no or minimal acidosis can be labeled HHS. In between, there is overlap and the clinician tailors therapy accordingly.

Hyperosmolar hyperglycemic syndrome (HHS) connotes severe hyperglycemia without (or with mild) acidemia or ketoacidosis. The pathophysiologic assumption is that patients with HHS have a greater insulin reserve and, unlike patients in DKA, are able to inhibit lipolysis and avoid ketoacid formation. Typically, serum glucose is higher than in diabetic ketoacidosis, patients are remarkably more dehydrated, older and with more prominent underlying illnesses. The severe dehydration and hyperglycemia often results in effective serum osmolality (Table 2) greater than 320 mosm/liter, a level at which depression of consciousness or coma can be attributed to the hyperosmolar state.[43,44] Patients commonly have type 2 diabetes mellitus, with poor antecedent glucose control. Thrombotic complications, which may occur in DKA[45], are a feared complication of HHS. Coronary arteries may clot, and arterial clots may propagate from the periphery to include the large central vessels. Presumably, the severe dehydration results in hemoconcentration and a hypercoagulable state. Because of the advanced patient age, and the hypercoagulability and decreased perfusion accompanying severe dehydration, myocardial infarction must be specifically excluded as a precipitating or complicating event (small doses of intravenous heparin [500-1000 units/hour] are appropriate unless contraindicated). Abdominal pain in HHS should be evaluated as a medical emergency, with consideration of perforated viscus, acute cholecystitis and ischemic bowel.

Patients should be treated in an intensive care setting. Fluid management with aggressive rehydration is the critical aspect of treatment of hyperosmolar syndrome. An immediate fluid challenge should be given to guarantee continued renal perfusion and urine output. One or two liters of fluid in the first hour of therapy followed by one liter/hour for the next four hours are commonly recommended. The water deficit can be calculated from the serum osmolality (the serum sodium can be substituted for osmolality in the equation). Half the water deficit should be replaced in the first eight to twelve hours. Exceptions include patients in renal or congestive heart failure, who require highly individualized fluid management.

The "corrected" serum sodium (Table 2) indicates the degree of free water loss - the higher the corrected sodium, the greater the water loss. In spite of marked free water loss, initial fluid replacement is with isotonic solutions, usually normal saline (NS), to establish blood pressure and perfusion. Hypotonic fluids (1/2 NS) are then administered, followed again by isotonic fluids when the glucose falls significantly (for example, to levels of 300-500 mg/dl). The rationale is that hypotonic fluids distribute more evenly between the intravascular and the extravascular space, whereas isotonic fluids remain in the intravascular space. As hyperglycemia resolves, fluid leaves the intravascular space and moves intracellularly. The movement of fluid out of the intravascular space in a severely dehydrated patient may result in vascular "collapse" (hypotension and irreversible shock).

Insulin plays only a minor role in the treatment of HHS, since these patients are not "ketosis-prone", are not acidotic and do not require restraint of free fatty acid release. The glucose osmotic diuresis that occurs with fluid administration is the most important factor in lowering the blood glucose to the renal threshold of 300 mg/dl. Small doses of insulin may be useful, but rapid blood lowering of the serum glucose with insulin is not desirable, because the osmotic pull of glucose helps to maintain intravascular volume, and to prevent cerebral edema. **When it's over, the physician must educate the patient not to omit insulin at times of stress.**

Patients with type 1 diabetes must always take insulin; and patients with type 2 diabetes must understand when insulin doses need to be increased. Common misconceptions have to be corrected. The patient must take insulin even when not able to eat. Ordinarily, the diabetic patient will have long-acting depot insulin or continued pump therapy between meals and during overnight fasting. Patients get confused, however, when they are not eating because of illness, such as gastrointestinal "upset". At these times, counter-regulatory hormones may rise and the patient must know that he or she needs to treat both the fingerstick glucose and urine ketone elevations measured by "ketostik" or other convenient methods.

CONCLUSIONS

The next patient will be different...but the witnesses - glucose, free fatty acids, serum electrolytes and pH, ketoacids - will always tell their stories. The fingerprint of relative insulin deficiency permitting substrates (free fatty acids, amino acids and glycerol) to reach the liver, and counter-regulatory excesses driving hepatic gluconeogenesis and ketogenesis will be clear to your experienced eye. The reversal of controlled storage and synthetic processes resulting in hyperglycemia, systemic acidosis, osmotic diuresis and dehydration will be familiar. Therapy is straightforward, requiring insulin, fluid and electrolyte administration. Key to a successful clinical outcome is careful monitoring of the patient, anticipation of responses, and investigation of potential precipitating factors.

REFERENCES

1. Umpierrez GE, Woo W, Hagopian WA, Isaacs SD, Palmer JP, Lakshmi K, Nepom GT, Clark WS, Mixon PS, Kitabchi AE. Immunogenetic analysis suggests different pathogenesis for obese and lean African-Americans with diabetic ketoacidosis. Diabetes Care 22:1517-1523, 1999.
2. Balasubramanyam A, Zern JW, Hyman DJ, Pavlik V. New profiles of diabetic ketoacidosis: type 1 vs type 2 diabetes and the effect of ethnicity. Arch Intern Med 159:2317-2322, 1999.

3. Winter WE, Maclaren NK, Riley WJ, Clarke DW, Kappy MS, Spillar RP. Maturity-onset diabetes of youth in black Americans. N Engl J Med 316:285-291, 1987.

4. Lebovitz HE. Diabetic ketoacidosis. Lancet 345:767-772, 1995.

5. Fleckman AM. Diabetic ketoacidosis. Endocrinol Metab Clin N Amer 22:181-207, 1993.

6. The cell: a molecular approach. 1st Edition. Cooper GM. ASM Press, Washington, D.C., 39-85, 389-403, 1997.

7. Lehninger Principles of Biochemistry. Nelson DL, Cox MM, Eds; Worth Publishers, New York, 598-622, 869-903, 2000.

8. DeFronzo RA, Matsuda M, Barrett EJ. Diabetic ketoacidosis. Diabetes Rev 2:209-238, 1994.

9. Ottosson M, Lönnroth P, Björntorp P, Edén S. Effects of cortisol and growth hormone on lipolysis in human adipose tissue. J Clin Endocrinol Metab 85:799-803, 2000.

10. Seckl JR, Walker BR. Minireview: 11beta-hydroxysteroid dehydrogenase type 1 - a tissue-specific amplifier of glucocorticoid action. Endocrinol 142:1371-1376, 2001.

11. Zammit VA. Regulation of ketone body metabolism. Diabetes Rev 2:132-155, 1994.

12. Laffel L. Ketone bodies: a review of physiology, pathophysiology and application of monitoring to diabetes. Diabetes/Metab Rev 15:412-426, 1999.

13. Brandenburg MA, Dire DJ. Comparison of arterial and venous blood bas values in the initial emergency department evaluation of patients with diabetic ketoacidosis. Ann Emerg Med 31:459-465, 1998.

14. Fulop M, Murthy V, Michili A, Nalamati J, Qian Q, Saitowitz A. Serum beta-hydroxybutyrate measurement in patients with uncontrolled diabetes mellitus. Arch Intern Med 159:381-384, 1999.

15. White NH. Diabetic ketoacidosis in children. Endocrinol Metab Clin 29:657-682, 2000.

16. Adrogue' HJ, Barrero J, Eknoyan G: Salutary effects of modest fluid replacement in the treatment of adults with diabetic ketoacidosis. JAMA 262:2108-2113, 1989.

17. Kaufman FR. Diabetes in children and adolescents: areas of controversy. Med Clin No Amer 82:721-738 1998.

18. Muir A. Cerebral edema in diabetic ketoacidosis: a look beyond rehydration. J Clin Endocrinol Metab 85:509-513, 2000.

19. Edge JA, Ford-Adams ME, Dunger DB. Causes of death in children with insulin dependent diabetes 1990-96. Arch Disease Child 81:318-323, 1999.

20. Glaser N, Barnett P, McCaslin I, Nelson D, Trainor J, Louie J, Kaufman F, Quayle K, Roback M, Malley R, Kuppermann N. Risk factors for cerebral edema in children with diabetic ketoacidosis. N Engl J Med 344:264-269, 2001.

21. Isales CM, Min L, Hoffman WH. Acetoacetate and beta-hydroxybutyrate differentially regulate endothelin-1 and vascular endothelial growth factor in mouse brain microvascular endothelial cells. J Diabetes & Complic 13:91-97, 1999.

22. Mahoney CP, Vlcek BW, DelAguila M. Risk factors for developing brain herniation during diabetic ketoacidosis. Pediatr Neurol 21:721-727, 1999.

23. Wagner A, Risse A, Brill HL, Wienhausen-Wilke V, Rottman M, Sondern K, Angelkort B. Therapy of severe diabetic ketoacidosis: zero-mortality under very-low-dose insulin application. Diabetes Care 22:674-677, 1999.

24. Weiner ID, Wingo CS. Hypokalemia – consequences, causes, and correction. J Amer Soc Neph 8:1179-1188, 1997.

25. Tattersall RB. A paper which changed clinical practice (slowly). Jacob Holler on potassium deficiency in diabetic acidosis (1946). Diabetic Med 16:978-984, 1999.

26. Viallon A, Zeni F, Lafond P, Venet C, Tardy B, Page Y, Bertrand J. Does bicarbonate therapy improve the management of severe diabetic ketoacidosis? Crit Care Med 27:2690-2693, 1999.

27. Vantyghem MC, Haye S, Balduyck M, Hober C, Degand PM, Lefebvre J. Changes in serum amylase, lipase and leukocyte elastase during diabetic ketoacidosis and poorly controlled diabetes. Acta Diabetol 36:39-44, 1999.

28. Nair S, Pitchumoni CS. Diabetic ketoacidosis, hyperlipidemia, and acute pancreatitis: the enigmatic triangle. Amer J Gastro 92:1560-1561, 1997

29. Nair S, Yadav D, Pitchumoni CS. Association of diabetic ketoacidosis and acute pancreatitis: observations in 100 consecutive episodes of DKA. Amer J Gastro 95:2795-2800, 2000.

30. Fulop M, Eder H. Severe hypertriglyceridemia in diabetic ketosis. Amer J Med Sci 300:361-365, 1990.

31. Fisher JN, Kitabchi AE. A randomized study of phosphate therapy in the treatment of diabetic ketoacidosis. J Clin Endocrinol Metab 57:177-180, 1983.

32. Hoffman WH, Locksmith JP, Burton EM, Hobbs E, Passmore GG, Pearson-Shaver AL, Deane DA, Beaudreau M, Bassali RW. Interstitial pulmonary edema in children and adolescents with diabetic ketoacidosis. J Diabetes & Comp 12:314-320, 1998.

33. Podar T, Solntsev A, Reunanen A, Urbonaite B, Zalinkevicius R, Karvonen M, LaPorte RE, Tuomilehto J. Mortality in patients with childhood-onset type 1 diabetes in Finland, Estonia, and Lithuania: Follow-up of nationwide cohorts. Diabetes Care 23:290-294, 2000.

34. Lipton R, Good G, Mikhailov T, Freels S, Donoghue E. Ethnic differences in mortality from insulin-dependent diabetes mellitus among people less than 25 years of age. Pediatrics 103:952-956, 1999.

35. Levetan CS, Passaro MD, Jablonski KA, Ratner RE. Effect of physician specialty on outcomes in diabetic ketoacidosis. Diabetes Care 22:1790-1795, 1999.

36. Javor KA, Kotsanos JG, McDonald RC, et al: Diabetic ketoacidosis charges relative to medical charges of adult patients with type 1 diabetes. Diabetes Care 20:349-354, 1997.

37. Vanelli M, Chiari G, Ghizzoni L, Costi G, Giacalone T, Chiarelli F. Effectiveness of a prevention program for diabetic ketoacidosis in children: an 8-year study in schools and private practices. Diabetes Care 22:7-9, 1999.

38. Bonadio WA, Gutzeit MF, Losek JD, et al. Outpatient management of diabetic ketoacidosis. Amer J Dis Child 142:448-450, 1988.

39. Marinac JS, Jesa L. Using a severity of illness scoring system to assess intensive care unit admissions for diabetic ketoacidosis. Crit Care Med 28:2238-2241, 2000.

40. Banerji MA, Chaiken RL, Huey H, Tuomi T, Norin AJ, Mackay IR, Rowley JM, Zimmet PZ, Lebovitz HE. GAD antibody negatives NIDDM in adult black subjects with diabetic ketoacidosis and increased frequency of human leukocyte antigen DR3 and DR4. Flatbush diabetes. Diabetes 43:741-745, 1994.

41. Banerji MA, Chaiken RL, Lebovitz HE. Long-term normoglycemic remission in black newly diagnosed NIDDM subjects. Diabetes 45:337-341, 1996.

42. Matz R. Management of the hyperosmolar hyperglycemic syndrome. Am Fam Physician 60:1468-1476, 1999.

43. Fulop M, Tannenbaum H, Dreyer N: Ketotic hyperosmolar coma. Lancet 2:635-639, 1973.

44. Daugirdas JT, Kronfol NO, Tzamaloukas AH, et al: Hyperosmolar coma: cellular dehydration and the serum sodium concentration. Ann Intern Med 110:855-857, 1989.

45. Ileri NS, Buyukasik Y, Karaahmetoglu S, Ozatli D, Sayinalp N, Ozcebe OI, Kirazli S, Muftuoglu O, Dundar SV. Evaluation of the haemostatic system during ketoacidotic deterioration of diabetes mellitus. Haemostasis 29:318-325, 1999.

Chapter 2. Hypoglycemia

Christian Meyer, Steven D. Wittlin, and John E. Gerich

GENERAL CONSIDERATIONS

As indicated earlier in the chapter on Normal Glucose Homeostasis, human plasma glucose concentrations are maintained within a relatively narrow range throughout the day (usually between 55 and 165 mg/dl, ~3.0 and 9.0 mM) despite wide fluctuations in the delivery (e.g. meals) and removal (e.g. exercise) of glucose from the circulation. This is accomplished by a tightly linked balance between glucose production and glucose utilization regulated by complex mechanisms.

Hypoglycemia is to be avoided to protect the brain and prevent cognitive dysfunction. Because of limited availability of ketone bodies and amino acids and the limited transport of free fatty acids across the blood brain barrier, glucose can be considered to be the sole source of energy for the brain except under conditions of prolonged fasting. In the latter situation ketone bodies increase several fold so that these may be used as an alternative fuel.[1]

Since the brain cannot store or produce glucose, it requires a continuous supply of glucose from the circulation. At physiological plasma glucose levels, phosphorylation of glucose is rate-limiting for its utilization. However, because of the kinetics of glucose transfer across the blood brain barrier, uptake becomes rate limiting as plasma glucose concentrations decrease below the normal range. Consequently maintenance of the plasma glucose concentration above some critical level is essential to the survival of the brain and thus the organism. It is therefore not surprising that a complex physiological mechanism has evolved to prevent or correct hypoglycemia (vide infra). Nevertheless for many patients with type 1 or type 2 diabetes hypoglycemia is a frequent complication. Because of its possible detrimental effects on the central nervous system, hypoglycemia is considered to be the main limiting factor for achieving near normal glycemic control.[2]

EPIDEMIOLOGY OF HYPOGLYCEMIA

Type 1 Diabetes

The reported incidence of hypoglycemia varies considerably among studies. In general, patients with type 1 diabetes practicing conventional insulin therapy have an average of ~1 episode of symptomatic hypoglycemia per week, whereas those practicing intensive insulin therapy have ~2 such episodes per week.[3] Thus, over 40 years of type 1 diabetes, the average patient can be projected to experience 2000-4000 episodes of symptomatic hypoglycemia. Since the complete detection of chemical hypoglycemia (commonly defined as a capillary blood glucose concentration < 50 mg/dl)[4] would require continuous blood glucose measurements over prolonged periods, its true frequency is unknown but is undoubtedly much greater than symptomatic hypoglycemia.

The incidence of severe hypoglycemia has been determined more precisely since it is defined as that associated with unconsciousness or requiring external assistance. It occurs more often in intensified insulin therapy than in conventional insulin therapy. For example during the 6.5 year follow-up in the Diabetes Control and Complication Trial (DCCT),[5] 35 % of patients in the conventional treatment group and 65 % of patients in the intensive treatment group had at least one episode of severe hypoglycemia. This corresponds to about 60 episodes per 100 patient years in patients being managed to achieve optimal glycemic control by intensive insulin therapy and to about 20 episodes per 100 patient-years in conventionally treated patients.[5] In a recent meta-analysis of 14 studies, which included 1028 patients on intensified insulin therapy and 1039 patients on conventional insulin therapy, the median incidence of severe hypoglycemia was 7.9 and 4.6 episodes per 100 patient-years in the two treatment groups respectively; the combined odds ratio was 2.99 (p < 0.0001).[6] However the increased incidence of severe hypoglycemia in the intensified treatment group was no longer evident as soon as glycosylated haemoglobin was included in a multivariate regression analysis.[6]

Type 2 Diabetes

Patients with type 2 diabetes generally experience less frequent severe hypoglycemia than those with type 1 diabetes. Both the UKPDS[7] and the Kumamoto study[8] demonstrated a much lower incidence of severe hypoglycemia in insulin treated patients with type 2 diabetes than what was reported in the DCCT study[5] for patients with type 1 diabetes despite similar glycemic control. In the UKPDS study, in which 676 patients with type 2 diabetes were followed for three years on insulin therapy, the incidence was 0.83 episodes per 100 patient-years. In the Kumamoto study, in which 52 type 2 diabetic patients were followed over 6 years on intensive insulin therapy, no severe hypoglycemic episode was reported. However, one retrospective study, which directly compared the incidence of severe hypoglycemia in 104 insulin treated patients with type 2 diabetes with that in 104 equally well controlled type 1 diabetic patients, found a similar incidence of severe hypoglycemia.[9]

In patients with type 2 diabetes treated with sulfonylureas the incidence of severe hypoglycemia has been reported to be approximately 1.5 episodes per 100 patient-years.[10] Its frequency increases with the potency and duration of action of the sulfonylurea, being greatest for second generation sulfonylureas, glimepiride, glyburide and glipizide averaging ~4-6%.[11]

RISK FACTORS FOR HYPOGLYCEMIA

Conventional risk factors for hypoglycemia are those that focus on absolute or relative insulin excess. These include insulin doses that are excessive or ill-timed, missed meals or snacks, lack of compensation for increased exercise, alcohol ingestion or mistaken insulin administration. However, a thorough analysis of a large number of episodes of severe hypoglycemia in the DCCT study has indicated that such conventional risk factors only explained a minority of the episodes;[12,13] indeed, mathematical models incorporating many of these factors were found to have little predictive power.[12] Instead it is now well established that impaired glucose counterregulation and hypoglycemia unawareness (vide infra) are the major risk factors for severe hypoglycemia in type 1 diabetes.[2,14] These defects are particularly common in patients with a long diabetes duration,[15,16] tight glycemic control,[15,17,18] antecedent hypoglycemia,[19,20] and autonomic neuropathy.[21-23] Hypoglycemia awareness may also be compromised by the use of ß-blockers.[24] The risk of severe hypoglycemia is increased 25-fold in patients with impaired hypoglycemia counterregulation[25] and increased 6-fold in those with hypoglycemia unawareness.[26] Other risk factors for severe hypoglycemia due to diabetes complications include renal insufficiency, gastroparesis which causes unpredictable and delayed food absorption, poor vision and rarely insulin antibodies. In the latter hypoglycemia occurs via dissociation of insulin from antibodies causing prolonged hyperinsulinemia.[16]

Despite the fact that most episodes of severe hypoglycemia in type 1 diabetes are related to impaired glucose counterregulation and hypoglycemia unawareness, one should also keep in mind that hypoglycemia can be multifactorial and be the result of several unrelated diseases. These include liver disease, malnutrition, sepsis, burns, total parenteral nutrition, malignancy and administration of certain medications known to reduce plasma glucose concentrations (Table 1).[27]

In principle, the same risk factors for hypoglycemia apply to patients with type 2 diabetes as they do to patients with type 1 diabetes although the importance of each has been less well defined.

Table 1: Drug-Induced Hypoglycemia

Drugs capable of causing hypoglycemia by themselves		Drugs probably causing hypoglycemia only in combination with insulin / sulfonylurea / benzoic acid derivatives
Antidiabetes Drugs	Other	
Insulin	Alcohol	Biguanides
Sulfonylureas	Salicylates	Ace-inhibitors
Benzoic acid	Propranolol	Phenylbutazone
derivatives		
(meglitinide,	Pentamidine	Lidocaine
nataglinide)		
	Sulfonanides	Coumadin
	Vacor	Ranitidine, Cimetidine
	Quinine	Doxipin
	Propoxyphene	Danazol
	Paraamino-	Azopropazone
	benzoic acid	
	Perhexiline	Oxytetracycline
		Clofibrate, Benzofibrate
		Colchicine
		Ketoconozole
		Chloramphenicol
		Haloperidol
		Monoamine oxidase inhibitors
		Thalidomide
		Orphenadrine
		Selegiline

HYPOGLYCEMIA COUNTERREGULATION

Normal Hypoglycemia Counterregulation and Hypoglycemia Awareness

Because of the importance of intact hypoglycemia counterregulation and awareness for the prevention or correction of hypoglycemia this shall be briefly reviewed. Glucose counterregulation refers to the sum of the body's defense mechanisms which prevent hypoglycemia from occurring and which restore euglycemia. Hypoglycemia awareness refers to the symptomatic responses of hypoglycemia which alert the patient of declining blood glucose levels. Our knowledge of counterregulation has accumulated over the past 25 years from studies in which pharmacologic blockade of the secretion or action of individual counterregulatory hormones has been produced during standardized insulin-induced hypoglycemia.[28]

Counterregulatory mechanisms in acute hypoglycemia, i.e. induced by an intravenous insulin injection, differ markedly from those in prolonged hypoglycemia. Clinical hypoglycemia that occurs in patients with diabetes after subcutaneous insulin injection usually develops gradually and is more prolonged.[29] Therefore, in the following discussion mainly counterregulation of prolonged hypoglycemia will be considered.

In normal postabsorptive humans, i.e. after an overnight fast, the sum of glucose release by liver and kidney equals systemic glucose utilization so that plasma glucose concentrations remain unchanged. Since insulin suppresses both hepatic and renal glucose release,[30,31] and stimulates glucose uptake exogenous insulin administration causes systemic glucose utilization to exceed systemic glucose release so that plasma glucose concentrations decrease.

As the plasma glucose levels decrease there is a characteristic hierarchy of responses (Figure 1). Reduction of insulin secretion, the first in the cascade of hypoglycemia counterregulation,[2] derepresses glucose production and reduces glucose utilization. When plasma glucose levels decline to approximately 70 mg/dl, there is an increase in the secretion of counterregulatory hormones (glucagon, epinephrine, growth hormone, cortisol) (21,32-34). Glucagon and epinephrine have immediate effects on glucose kinetics whereas the effects of growth hormone and cortisol are delayed by several hours.[35,36]

Glucagon exclusively increases hepatic glucose release, initially via glycogenolysis, later mainly via gluconeogenesis[37] and does not affect renal glucose release or glucose utilization.[38] In contrast, catecholamines have multiorgan effects, including stimulation of hepatic and renal glucose production,[39,40] inhibition of glucose utilization,[41,42] stimulation of gluconeogenic substrate supply,[39,40,43] suppression of endogenous insulin secretion,[44] and stimulation of lipolysis.[44] Growth hormone and cortisol suppress insulin-mediated tissue glucose uptake and augment glucose release into the circulation.[45,46]

Under normal physiologic conditions, these responses prevent a further decrease in plasma glucose concentrations and restore normoglycemia. Decreases to ~60 mg/dl (3.4 mM) usually evoke the so-called autonomic warning symptoms[47,48] (hunger, anxiety, palpitations, sweating, warmth, nausea) which if interpreted correctly, lead a person to eat and prevent more serious hypoglycemia. However, clues of hypoglycemia may vary considerably from person to person.[49] If, for some reason, plasma glucose levels decrease to about 55 mg/dl (~3.0 mM), this results in so-called neuroglycopenic signs/symptoms of brain dysfunction (blurred vision, slurred speech, glassy-eyed appearance, confusion, difficulty in concentrating).[47,48] Further decreases can produce coma and values below 30 mg/dl (~1.6 mM) if prolonged can cause seizures, permanent neurologic deficits and death. However, it should be pointed out that in otherwise healthy, young (<45 years) individuals, glucose levels averaging 35 mg/dl (~2.0 mM) have been maintained for as long as eight hours without any longterm adverse effects[50] and chronic levels as 24 mg/dl (1.3 mM) in insulinoma patients have been observed in association with apparently normal cerebral function.[51]

Regarding the importance of each of these responses, the exact role of insulin dissipation for hypoglycemia counterregulation is controversial. Heller et al.[52] reported that dissipation of insulin is important but not critical for recovery from hypoglycemia. In contrast, De Feo et al.[53] and Sacca et al.[54] observed that no recovery from hypoglycemia occurs despite increases in counterregulatory hormones when hypoglycemia is induced by continuous low-dose insulin infusion resulting in insulin levels lower (~25 µU/ml)[53] or similar (~40 µU/ml) (54) to those observed postprandially. On the other hand, plasma glucose concentrations stabilized and did not decrease further.

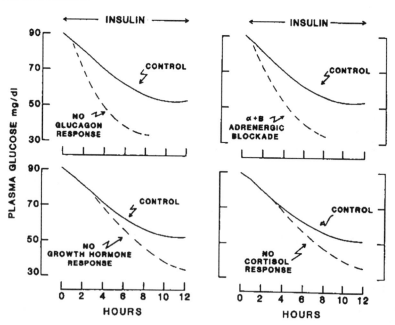

Figure 1. Effect of lack of glucagon, catecholamine (α- and ß-adrenergic blockade), growth hormone, and cortisol responses on insulin-induced hypoglycemia in nondiabetic volunteers studied with pituitary-adrenal-pancreatic clamp.

Roles of individual counterregulatory hormone responses have been delineated using the pituitary-adrenal-pancreatic (PAP) clamp technique.[55] With this technique the spontaneous responses of counterregulatory hormones are simulated by infusions of the hormones during blockade of their secretion so that an isolated lack of response of each hormone can be examined. Studies using this technique have demonstrated that glucagon and epinephrine are the predominant counterregulatory hormones and that cortisol and growth hormone have also major participation in glucose counterregulation (Figure 1).[35,36,56] The consequences of lack of glucagon and epinephrine were quantitatively similar.[28]

These studies have also delineated the time course of action and the relative effects of each hormone on glucose production and glucose utilization.[28] As shown in Figure 2. counterregulation initially involves only changes in glucose production predominantly due to glucagon and, to a lesser extent, catecholamines. Later on, changes in glucose utilization become as important as those of glucose production. At this time, cortisol and growth hormone, through their delayed effects on glucose production and glucose utilization become major hormonal factors and may be more important than catecholamines and glucagon.

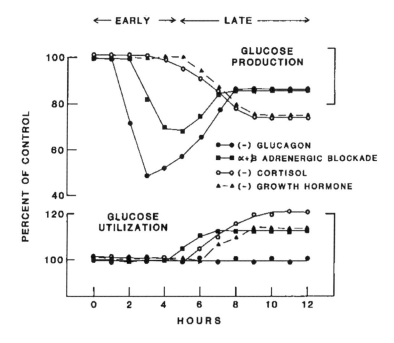

Figure 2. Effect of lack of glucagon, catecholamine (α- and ß-adrenergic blockade), growth hormone, and cortisol responses on counterregulatory changes in glucose production and glucose utilization in nondiabetic volunteers studied with pituitary-adrenal-pancreatic clamp.

299

Hypoglycemia Counterregulation and Hypoglycemia Awareness in Type 1 Diabetes

In type 1 diabetes, the physiology of the defense against hypoglycemia is seriously deranged (Figure 3). First, as endogenous insulin secretion becomes totally deficient over the first few years of type 1 diabetes, the appearance of insulin in the circulation becomes unregulated since it relies on absorption from subcutaneous injection sites. Consequently, as plasma glucose levels are falling insulin levels do not decrease. Second, glucagon responses to hypoglycemia are lost early in the course of type 1 diabetes.[16,57] This defect coincides with the loss of insulin secretion and is therefore the rule in people with type 1 diabetes.[58] Nonetheless, glucose counterregulation appears to be adequate in such patients probably due to compensatory counterregulation by epinephrine.[59] After a few more years epinephrine responses to hypoglycemia are also commonly reduced.[16,60,61] When compared to patients with a defective glucagon response but normal epinephrine responses, patients with a combined defect in glucagon and epinephrine responses have at least a 25-fold increased risk for severe iatrogenic hypoglycemia.[25,62] The combined defect in glucagon and epinephrine responses is therefore considered as the syndrome of impaired hypoglycemia counterregulation.[2] Recently this has been shown to be associated with impaired glucose production in both liver and kidney.[63] This might be different when only glucagon responses are impaired and epinephrine responses are intact. Since glucagon affects exclusively the liver whereas epinephrine has a temporary effect on the liver but a sustained effect on the kidney, only hepatic glucose production might be decreased under these conditions.

In addition to impaired glucose counterregulation people with type 1 diabetes often suffer from hypoglycemia unawareness. These patients no longer have autonomic warning symptoms of developing hypoglycemia which previously prompted them to take appropriate action, i.e. food intake before severe hypoglycemia with neuroglycopenia occurs. Hypoglycemia unawareness has been reported to occur in about 50 % of patients with long-standing diabetes and estimated to affect 25% overall.[14,26,64,65] Hypoglycemia unawareness is associated with six-fold increased risk for severe hypoglycemia.[26]

The mechanisms of impaired hypoglycemia counterregulation and hypoglycemia unawareness are not entirely clear but several factors have been proposed. These include altered intra-islet structure and altered cell-cell interaction (reduced glucagon responses),[66] autonomic neuropathy (reduced catecholamine responses),[21-23] up-regulation of glucose transporters in the central nervous system by antecedent hypoglycemia which prevents central hypoglycemia during subsequent hypoglycemia (reduced hormone and symptom responses),[67] and impaired beta-adrenergic sensitivity to catecholamines which reduces autonomic warning symptoms of hypoglycemia.[68]

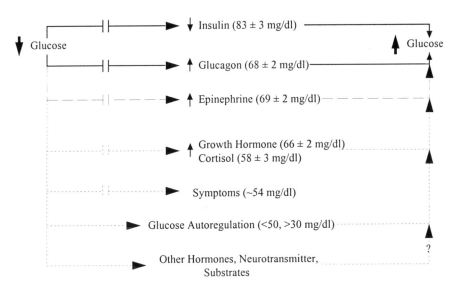

Figure 3. Schematic representation of physiology of glucose counterregulation in normal humans (arrows) and defects in type 1 diabetes (interrupted lines). Mean ± SE arterialized venous glycemic thresholds for the various responses to falling blood glucose concentrations in normal humans are from Schwartz et al.[32] and Mitrakou et al.[33]

Hypoglycemia Counterregulation and Hypoglycemia Awareness in Type 2 Diabetes

In type 2 diabetes the hormonal glucose counterregulation is usually less impaired than in type 1 diabetes.[69-71] Nevertheless defects can be seen when patients become markedly insulin deficient.[72] One important factor for the nearly intact hormonal glucose counterregulation in type 2 diabetes may be that these patients still have some, albeit abnormal, insulin secretion. Normally insulin directly suppresses glucagon secretion. There is now experimental evidence to suggest that the glucagon response to hypoglycemia may depend on the decrease in insulin secretion because the latter would derepress glucagon secretion.[66] Since insulin secretion is absent in type 1 diabetes, no decrease in insulin secretion occurs during hypoglycemia. However, in patients with type 2 diabetes insulin secretion is usually present and decreases appropriately during hypoglycemia which may explain these patients' intact glucagon response to hypoglycemia until they become markedly insulin deficient. Since antecedent hypoglycemia is one of the main factors for impaired epinephrine responses to hypoglycemia and since hypoglycemia rarely occurs in people with type 2 diabetes because of their intact glucagon response, epinephrine responses usually also remain intact.

Once patients with type 2 diabetes become markedly insulin deficient, glucagon responses are commonly impaired. However, in contrast to patients with type 1 diabetes, their epinephrine responses usually remain intact and in fact may partially compensate for the reduced glucagon responses to hypoglycemia[71,73] which may explain their reduced risk for severe hypoglycemia compared to patients with type 1 diabetes. Nevertheless, some studies reported that despite their increased catecholamine responses, patients with type 2 diabetes have impaired endogenous glucose production during hypoglycemia.[73,74] Recently this has been shown to be due to diminished glucose release by the liver which is partially compensated for by an increased glucose release by the kidney.[74] Factors involved in the reduced hepatic glucose release in type 2 diabetes may be diminished hepatic glycogen stores[75] and reduced glucagon activation of hepatic membrane adenylate cyclase.[76] These changes would be expected to impair hepatic glycogenolytic and gluconeogenic responses to glucagon.

COMPLICATIONS OF HYPOGLYCEMIA

Organ Complications

As mentioned above, an episode of severe hypoglycemia can be detrimental or even fatal mostly due to its effects on the central nervous system. At a plasma glucose concentration of ~55 mg/dl (~3 mM) cognitive impairment and EEG changes are demonstrable. Decreases below 40 mg/dl (~2.5 mM) result in sleepiness and gross behavioral (e.g. combativeness) abnormalities. Further decreases can produce coma and values below 30 mg/dl (~1.6 mM) if prolonged can cause seizures, permanent neurologic deficits and death.

In individuals with underlying cardiovascular disease, life-threatening arrhythmias, myocardial infarction and strokes may be precipitated.[77-85] Moreover, in patients with underlying eye disease hypoglycemia has been shown to trigger retinal hemorrhages.[86] It has been suggested that repeated episodes of severe hypoglycemia may lead to subtle permanent cognitive dysfunction.[87] In addition to its physical morbidity and mortality, recurrent hypoglycemia may be also associated with psychosocial morbidity.[64] In fact many patients with diabetes are as much afraid of severe hypoglycemia as they are of blindness or renal failure.[64]

Severe hypoglycemia has been reported to be at least a contributing factor to the cause of death in 3 to 13 % of patients with type 1 diabetes which include motor vehicle accidents, injuries at work etc.[88,89] Severe hypoglycemia due to sulfonylureas has been shown to have a mortality between 4-7 %.[11,90,91]

Somogyi Phenomenon

More than 60 years ago, Somogyi postulated that secretion of counterregulatory hormones provoked by insulin-induced hypoglycemia could lead to hyperglycemia. This sequence has become known as rebound hyperglycemia or the Somogyi phenomenon. It is the result of persistent catecholamine actions initially and growth hormone and cortisol actions later despite return of the plasma glucose concentration to normal. These post-hypoglycemia counterregulatory effects, coupled with the dissipation of insulin injected earlier to produce hypoglycemia, result in posthypoglycemia hyperglycemia in patients with type 1 diabetes. In support of this concept Mintz et al.,[92] and Frier et al.,[93] have shown that hypoglycemia, even in nondiabetic individuals, could cause subsequent glucose intolerance, and several studies demonstrated that prolonged insulin resistance lasting 4-8 hours occurs after hypoglycemia in type 1 diabetes.[94-96]

Despite the evidence cited above, the literature is confounded with studies that have been interpreted to question the mechanism,[97] frequency[98] and even the existence[99] of the Somogyi phenomenon. However, to a large extent study design and selection of patients (inclusion of those with impaired counterregulation[99] for type 2 diabetes)[98] can explain this controversy. It is nevertheless possible that the magnitude of the Somogyi phenomenon has been overestimated in the past. Furthermore, it is of note that the posthypoglycemia hyperglycemia in most patients is probably due to the combination of overtreatment of hypoglycemia with carbohydrate ingestion and the increase in counterregulatory hormones.

MANAGEMENT OF HYPOGLYCEMIA

Treatment

Treatment is aimed at restoring euglycemia, preventing recurrences and, if possible, alleviating the underlying cause. In an insulin-taking diabetic patient with mild hypoglycemia due to a skipped meal, this can simply entail 12-18 gm oral carbohydrate every 30 min until the blood glucose is above 80 mg/dl.[100,101] In the case of more severe hypoglycemia resulting in obtundation where oral administration of carbohydrate might result in aspiration, 1 mg of glucagon subcutaneously or intramuscularly might be sufficient to raise the blood glucose and revive the patient so that oral carbohydrate may be given. Comatose patients should receive intravenous glucose (25 gm bolus, followed by an infusion at an initial rate of 2 mg/kg/min, roughly 10 gm/hr) for as long as necessary for the insulin or sulfonylurea to wear off. Sulfonylurea overdose can result in prolonged hypoglycemia requiring sustained intravenous glucose infusion aimed at keeping the blood glucose at ~4.5 mM (~80 mg/dl) to avoid hyperglycemia causing further stimulation of insulin secretion and setting in motion a vicious cycle. Blood glucose levels should be monitored initially every 30 min and subsequently at 1-2 hour intervals. Rarely diazoxide or a somatostatin analog may be needed to inhibit insulin secretion.[102] Where other drugs may be involved, they should be discontinued if possible (i.e. sulfonamides in a patient with renal insufficiency). In other conditions, the underlying disorder should be treated (e.g. sepsis, heart failure, endocrine deficiency) and the blood glucose supported.

Prevention of Recurrences

Conventional Measures

For prevention of recurrences, it is important to determine whether a particular episode of hypoglycemia was an isolated event or whether it has occurred before. If so, how frequently? Is there any pattern to occurrences, i.e. always at night? For how long have these episodes been occurring? Are they associated with hypoglycemic warning symptoms? If so, usually at what glycemia is hypoglycemia recognized? Are there any precipitating factors, i.e. exercise, skipped meal, erroneous insulin injection, alcohol ingestion, recent weight loss or other precipitating factors (see above). Did the patient spontaneously recover? What did the patient do to prevent recurrences or relieve symptoms? What is the patient's occupation?

Obviously, if these questions reveal precipitating factors for hypoglycemia these factors should be eliminated. However if they do not reveal any apparent precipitating factors but hypoglycemia unawareness, chances are relatively high that there is also impaired hypoglycemia counterregulation especially in a patient with frequent hypoglycemic episodes. Consequently the question arises how to treat these affected patients.

The principles of intensive therapy – patient education, blood glucose self-monitoring, and an insulin regimen that provides basal insulin levels with prandial increments – still apply to the majority of patients who require insulin to control their diabetes. However, glycemic goals must be individualized according to the frequency of hypoglycemia. Since the prevention or correction of hypoglycemia normally involves dissipation of insulin and activation of counterregulatory hormones as discussed above, it follows that patients with impaired glucose counterregulation are extremely sensitive to very little insulin in excess of its requirement resulting in hypoglycemia. It is therefore generally accepted that normoglycemia is not a reasonable goal for such affected patients.[103,104]

Although therapy of type 1 and type 2 diabetes is discussed in detail in other chapters, several suggestions for prevention of hypoglycemia may be useful:

In patients treated with insulin hypoglycemia can be most successfully prevented by continuous subcutaneous insulin infusion (CSII) by means of a minipump. This has been reported to reduce the frequency of severe hypoglycemia by 50 to 75 %[105,106] despite the fact that glycemic control actually improved. If CSII is not feasible, substitution of prepandial rapid insulin (e.g. lispro or aspart) for short-acting (regular) insulin may reduce the frequency of hypoglycemic episodes by reducing prolonged postprandial hyperinsulinemia. In a recent meta-analysis of eight studies comparing 2327 patients treated with insulin lispro with 2339 patients treated with regular insulin, the frequency was approximately 20 % less in those who received lispro despite virtually identical glycemic control.[107] Furthermore, substitution of long acting insulin analogue (glargine) for intermediate-acting insulin (NPH) has recently been shown to reduce the frequency of nocturnal hypoglycemia by about 30 % in patients with type 1 diabetes.[108]

In patients with type 2 diabetes on oral hypoglycemic agents substitution of a long acting sulfonylurea for a short acting sulfonylurea or a benzoic acid derivative (nateglinide, repaglinide) may be useful, especially in patients with chronic renal insufficiency since most of these agents are cleared by the kidney.

If these measures result in strict avoidance of hypoglycemia, hypoglycemia awareness may be restored.[109] A recent report indicates that this might be due to an improvement in beta-adrenergic sensitivity.[110] Although strict avoidance of hypoglycemia does not improve glucagon responses to hypoglycemia in type 1 diabetes,[109,111,114] it does increase epinephrine responses.[113,114] This however seems to be limited to patients with a diabetes duration of less than ~15 years. In patients with type 1 diabetes of more than 15 years epinephrine responses may remain markedly impaired.[109,111] Thus there is unfortunately no conventional therapy available to reverse impaired hypoglycemia counterregulation in such patients. Although the effects of avoidance of hypoglycemia have not been studied in patients with type 2 diabetes it seems likely that these are similar to those in type 1 diabetes.

Pancreas / Islet Transplantation

Because of the irreversibly impaired hypoglycemia counterregulation in long-standing type 1 diabetes, pancreas or islet transplantation have been proposed as a possible treatment in patients who suffer from recurrent severe hypoglycemia despite all conventional measures.[115-117] Pancreas transplantation has been found to improve glucagon responses to hypoglycemia in most studies[118-124] and to improve or normalize epinephrine responses.[120-122,124-126] Furthermore, it has been reported to improve hypoglycemia awareness in type 1 diabetes.[124]

Experience in the effects of islet transplantation on hypoglycemia counterregulation and awareness is very limited.[115,116] It seems that glucagon responses remain impaired after islet transplantation[115,116] possibly because of the transplantation site.[127] However, epinephrine responses and hypoglycemia awareness have been reported to improve in long-standing type 1 diabetes in one small study.[116]

Although pancreas transplantation and islet transplantation may be promising alternatives for some patients with recurrent severe hypoglycemia, risk benefits ratios should be extremely carefully analyzed because of the invasive nature of these forms of therapy and the necessity for immunosuppression.

SUMMARY AND CONCLUSIONS

In summary severe hypoglycemia is a relatively common, potentially life-threatening complication of diabetic treatment more often affecting patients with type 1 than those with type 2 diabetes. Major risk factors for severe hypoglycemia are impaired hypoglycemia counterregulation and hypoglycemia unawareness whereas conventional risk factors explain only a minority of the hypoglycemic episodes. Treatment is to be aimed at acute restoration of normoglycemia and prevention of recurrences. The latter can be accomplished by temporary loosening of glycemic control and changes in types and administration of insulin in addition to education, frequent blood glucose monitoring and ongoing professional guidance. This may restore hypoglycemia counterregulation and hypoglycemia awareness which subsequently may allow tightening of glycemic control.

REFERENCES

1. Owen O, Morgan A, Kemp H, Sullivan J, Herrera M, Cahill G. Brain metabolism during fasting. J Clin Invest 46:1589-1595, 1967.
2. Cryer P. Banting Lecture: Hypoglycemia, the limiting factor in the management of IDDM. Diabetes 43:1378-1389, 1994.
3. Cryer P, Binder C, Bolli G, Cherrington A, Gale E, Gerich J, Sherwin R. Hypoglycemia in IDDM. Diabetes 38:1193-1199, 1989.
4. Foster D, Rubenstein A. Hypoglycemia. In: Wilson J , Braunwald E, Isselbacher K: Harrison's Principles of internal medicine, New York McGraw-Hill, 1759, 1991.
5. DCCT Research Group. The effect of intensive treatment of diabetes on the development and progression of long-term complications in insulin dependent diabetes mellitus. N Engl J Med 329:977-986, 1993.

6. Egger M, Smith GD, Stettler C, Diem P. Risk of adverse effects of intensified treatment in insulin-dependent diabetes mellitus: ameta-analysis. Diabet Med 14:919-928, 1997.

7. UK Prospective Diabetes Study (UKPDS) Group. Intensive blood-glucose control with sulphonylureas or insulin compared with conventional treatment and risk of complications in patients with type 2 diabetes (UKPDS 33). Lancet 352:837-853, 1998.

8. Ohkubo Y, Kishikawa H, Araki E, Miyata T, Isami S, Motoyoshi S, Kojima Y, Furugoshi N, Shichiri M. Intensive insulin therapy prevents the progression of diabetic microvascular complications in Japanese patients with non-insulin- dependent diabetes mellitus: a randomized prospective 6-year study. Diabetes Res Clin Pract 28:103-117, 1995.

9. Hepburn D, MacLeod K, Pell A, Scougal I, Frier B. Frequency and Symptoms of hypoglycemia experienced by patients with type 2 diabetes treated with insulin. Diab Med 10:231-237, 1993.

10. Van Staa T, Abenhaim L, Monette J. Rates of hypoglycemia in users of sulfonylureas. J Clin Epidemiol 50:735-741, 1997.

11. Gerich J. Sulfonylureas in the treatment of diabetes mellitus. Mayo Clin Proc 60:439-443, 1985.

12. DCCT Research Group. Epidemiology of severe hypoglycemia in the diabetes control and complications trial. Am J Med 90:450-459, 1991.

13. Nilsson A, Tideholm B, Kalen J, Katzman P. Incidence of severe hypoglycemia and its causes in insulin-treated diabetics. Acta Med Scand 224:257-262, 1988.

14. Amiel S. R.D. Lawrence Lecture 1994. Limits of normality: the mechanisms of hypoglycemia unawareness. Diabetic Med 11:918-924, 1994.

15. Mokan M, Mitrakou M, Veneman T, Ryan C, Korytkowski M, Cryer P, Gerich J. Hypoglycemia unawareness in IDDM. Diabetes Care 17:1397-1403, 1994.

16. Bolli G, DeFeo P, Compagnucci P, Cartechini M, Angeletti G, Santeusanio F, Brunetti P, Gerich J. Abnormal glucose counterregulation in insulin-dependent diabetes mellitus: interaction of anti-insulin antibodies and impaired glucagon and epinephrine secretion. Diabetes 32:134-141, 1983.

17. Amiel S, Tamborlane W, Simonson D, Sherwin R. Defective glucose counterregulation after strict control of insulin-dependent diabetes mellitus. N Engl J Med 316:1376-1383, 1987.

18. Simonson D, Tamborlane W, DeFronzo R, Sherwin R. Intensive insulin therapy reduces counterregulatory responses to hypoglycemia in type I diabetes. Ann Int Med 103:184-188, 1985.

307

19. Davis M, Mellman M, Shamoon H. Further defects in counterregulatory responses induced by recurrent hypoglycemia in IDDM. Diabetes 41:1335-1340, 1992.
20. Lingenfelser T, Renn W, Sommerwerck U, Buettner U , Zaiser-Kaschel H, Kaschel R, Eggstein M, Jakober B. Compromised hormonal counterregulation, symptom awareness, and neurophysiologic function after recurrent short-term episodes of insulin-induced hypoglycemia in IDDM patients. Diabetes 42:610-618, 1993.
21. Meyer C, Großmann R, Mitrakou A, Mahler R, Veneman T, Gerich J, Bretzel R. Effects of autonomic neuropathy on counterregulation and awareness of hypoglycemia in type 1 diabetic patients. Diabetes Care 21:1960-1966, 1998.
22. Horie H, Hanafusa T, Matsuyama T, Namba M, Nonaka K, Tarui S, Yamatodani A, Wada H. Decreased response of epinephrine and norepinephrine to insulin- induced hypoglycemia in diabetic autonomic neuropathy. Horm Metab Res 16:398-401, 1984.
23. Hoeldtke R, Boden G, Shuman C, Owen C. Reduced epinephrine secretion and hypoglycemic unawareness in diabetic autonomic neuropathy. Ann Int Med 96:459-462, 1982.
24. Hirsch I, Boyle P, Craft S, Cryer P. Higher glycemic thresholds for symptoms during b-adrenergic blockade in IDDM. Diabetes 40:1177-1186, 1991.
25. White N, Skor D, Cryer P, Bier D, Levandoski L, Santiago J. Identification of type I diabetic patients at increased risk for hypoglycemia during intensive therapy. N Engl J Med 308:485-491, 1983.
26. Gold A, MacLeod K, Frier B. Frequency of severe hypoglycemia in patients with type 1 diabetes with impaired awareness of hypoglycemia. Diabetes Care 17:697-703, 1994.
27. Gerich J. Hypoglycemia. In: DeGroot L. Endocrinology, 4 edn., Philadelphia, W. B. Saunders, 2001, 921.
28. Gerich J. Glucose counterregulation and its impact on diabetes mellitus. Diabetes 37:1608-1617, 1988.
29. Bolli G, Dimitriadis G, Pehling G, Baker B, Haymond M, Cryer P, Gerich J. Abnormal glucose counterregulation after subcutaneous insulin in insulin-dependent diabetes mellitus. N Engl J Med 310:1706-1711, 1984.
30. Cersosimo E, Garlick P, Ferretti J. Renal glucose production during insulin-induced hypoglycemia in humans. Diabetes 48:261-266, 1999.
31. Meyer C, Dostou J, Gerich J. Role of the human kidney in glucose counterregulation. Diabetes 48:943-948, 1999.

32. Schwartz N, Clutter W, Shah S, Cryer P. The glycemic thresholds for activation of glucose counterregulatory systems are higher than the threshold for symptoms. J Clin Invest 79:777-781, 1987.

33. Mitrakou A, Ryan C, Veneman T, Mokan M, Jenssen T, Kiss I, Durrant J, Cryer P, Gerich J. Hierarchy of glycemic thresholds for counterregulatory hormone secretion, symptoms, and cerebral dysfunction. Am J Physiol 260:E67-E74, 1991.

34. Fanelli C, Pampanelli S, Epifano L, Rambotti A, Ciofetta M, Modarelli F, DiVincenzo A, Annibale B, Lepore M, Lalli C, DelSindaco P, Brunetti P, Bolli G. Relative roles of insulin and hypoglycemia on induction of neuroendocrine responses to, symptoms of, and deterioration of cognitive function in hypoglycemia in male and female humans. Diabetologia 37:797-807, 1994.

35. DeFeo P, Perriello G, Torlone E, Ventura M, Santeusanio F, Brunetti P, Gerich J, Bolli G. Demonstration of a role of growth hormone in glucose counterregulation. Am J Physiol 256:E835-E843, 1989.

36. DeFeo P, Perriello G, Torlone E, Ventura M, Fanelli C, Santeusanio F, Brunetti P, Gerich J, Bolli G. Contribution of cortisol to glucose counterregulation in man. Am J Physiol 257:E35-E42, 1989.

37. Lecavalier L, Bolli G, Cryer P, Gerich J. Contributions of gluconeogenesis and glycogenolysis during glucose counterregulation in normal humans. Am J Physiol 256:E844-E851, 1989.

38. Stumvoll M, Meyer C, Kreider M, Perriello G, Gerich J. Effects of glucagon on renal and hepatic glutamine gluconeogenesis in normal postabsorptive humans. Metabolism 47:1227-1232, 1998.

39. Stumvoll M, Meyer C, Perriello G, Kreider M, Welle S, Gerich J. Human kidney and liver gluconeogenesis: evidence for organ substrate selectivity. Am J Physiol 274:E817-E826, 1998.

40. Meyer C, Stumvoll M, Welle S, Nair S, Haymond M, Gerich J. Sites, substrates and mechanisms of epinephrine stimulated glucose production in humans. Diabetes 47(Suppl 1):A305, 1998(Abstract).

41. Rizza R, Haymond M, Cryer P, Gerich J. Differential effects of physiologic concentrations of epinephrine on glucose production and disposal in man. Am J Physiol 237:356-362, 1979.

42. Sacca L, Morrone G, Cicala M, Corso G, Ungaro B. Influence of epinephrine, norepinephrine and isoproterenol on glucose homeostasis in normal man. J Clin Endocrinol Metab 50:680-684, 1980.

43. Sacca L, Vigorito C, Cicala M, Corso G, Sherwin R. Role of gluconeogenesis in epinephrine-stimulated hepatic glucose production in humans. Am J Physiol 245:E294-E302, 1983.

44. Clutter W, Bier D, Shah S, Cryer P. Epinephrine plasma metabolic clearance rates and physiologic thresholds for metabolic and hemodynamic actions in man. J Clin Invest 66:94-101, 1980.
45. Gerich J, Campbell P. Overview of counterregulation and its abnormalities in diabetes mellitus and other conditions. Diabetes Metab Rev 4:93-111, 1988.
46. McMahon M, Gerich J, Rizza R. Effects of glucocorticoids on carbohydrate metabolism. Diabetes Metab Rev 4:17-30, 1988.
47. Hepburn D, Deary I, Frier B, Patrick A, Quinn J, Fisher B. Symptoms of acute insulin-induced hypoglycemia in humans with and without IDDM. Factor-analysis approach. Diabetes Care 14:949-957, 1991.
48. Towler D, Havlin C, Craft S, Cryer P. Mechanism of awareness of hypoglycemia: perception of neurogenic (predominantly cholinergic) rather than neuroglycopenic symptoms. Diabetes 42:1791-1798, 1993.
49. Cox D, Gonder-Frederick L, Antoun B, Cryer P, Clarke W. Perceived symptoms in the recognition of hypoglycemia. Diabetes Care 16:519-527, 1993.
50. Bolli G, DeFeo P, Perriello G, DeCosmo S, Ventura M, Campbell P, Brunetti P, Gerich J. Role of hepatic autoregulation in defense against hypoglycemia in humans. J Clin Invest 75:1623-1631, 1985.
51. Mitrakou A, Fanelli C, Veneman T, Perriello G, Calderone S, Plantanisiotis D, Rambotti A, Raptis S, Brunetti P, Cryer P, Gerich J, Bolli G. Reversibility of unawareness of hypoglycemia in patients with insulinomas. N Engl J Med 329:834-839, 1993.
52. Heller S, Cryer P. Hypoinsulinemia is not critical to glucose recovery from hypoglycemia in humans. Am J Physiol 261:E41-E48, 1991.
53. DeFeo P, Perriello G, DeCosmo S, Ventura M, Campbell P, Brunetti P, Gerich J, Bolli G. Comparison of glucose counterregulation during short-term and prolonged hypoglycemia in normal humans. Diabetes 35:563-569, 1986.
54. Sacca L, Sherwin R, Hendler R, Felig P. Influence of continuous physiologic hyperinsulinemia on glucose kinetics and counterregulatory hormones in normal and diabetic humans. J Clin Invest 63:849-857, 1979.
55. DeFeo P, Perriello G, Ventura M, Brunetti P, Santeusanio F, Gerich J, Bolli G. The pancreatic-adrenocortical-pituitary clamp technique for study of counterregulation in humans. Am J Physiol 252:E565-E570, 1987.
56. DeFeo P, Perriello G, Torlone E, Fanelli C, Ventura M, Santeussanio F, Brunetti P, Gerich J, Bolli G. Contribution of adrenergic mechanisms to glucose counterregulation in humans. Am J Physiol 261:E725-E736, 1991.

57. Gerich J, Langlois M, Noacco C, Karam J, Forsham P. Lack of glucagon response to hypoglycemia in diabetes: evidence for an intrinsic pancreatic alpha-cell defect. Science 182:171-173, 1973.

58. Fukuda M, Tanaka A, Tahara Y, Ikegami H, Yamamoto Y, Kumahara Y, Shima K. Correlation between minimal secretory capacity of pancreatic ß-cells and stability of diabetic control. Diabetes 37:81-88, 1988.

59. Rizza R, Cryer P, Gerich J. Role of glucagon, epinephrine and growth hormone in glucose counterregulation. J Clin Invest 64:62-71, 1979.

60. Hirsch B, Shamoon H. Defective epinephrine and growth hormone responses in type I diabetes are stimulus specific. Diabetes 36:20-26, 1987.

61. Dagogo-Jack S, Craft S, Cryer P. Hypoglycemia-associated autonomic failure in insulin dependent diabetes mellitus. J Clin Invest 91:819-828, 1993.

62. Bolli G, DeFeo P, DeCosmo S, Perriello G, Ventura M, Benedetti M, Santeusanio F, Gerich J, Brunetti P. A reliable and reproducible test for adequate glucose counterregulation in Type I diabetes mellitus. Diabetes 33:732-737, 1984.

63. Cersosimo E, Ferretti J, Sasvary D, Garlick P. Adrenergic stimulation of renal glucose release is impaired in type 1 diabetes. Diabetes 50(Suppl 2):A54, 2001.

64. Pramming S, Thorsteinsson B, Bendtson I, Binder C. Symptomatic hypoglycemia in 411 type I diabetic patients. Diabetic Med 8:217-222, 1991.

65. Hepburn D, Patrick A, Eadington D, Ewing D, Frier B. Unawareness of hypoglycemia in insulin-treated diabetic patients: prevalence and relationship to autonomic neuropathy. Diabetic Med 7:711-717, 1990.

66. Unger R. Insulin-glucagon relationships in the defense against hypoglycemia. Diabetes 32:575-583, 1983.

67. Boyle P, Kempers S, O'Connor A, Nagy R. Brain glucose uptake and unawareness of hypoglycemia in patients with insulin-dependent diabetes mellitus. N Engl J Med 333:1726-1731, 1995.

68. Fritsche A, Stumvoll M, Grüb M, Sieslack S, Renn W, Schmülling R-M, Häring H-U, Gerich J. Effect of hypoglycemia on b-adrenergic sensitivity in normal and type 1 diabetic subjects. Diabetes Care 21:1505-1510, 1998.

69. Heller S, MacDonald I, Tattersall R. Counterregulation in type 2 (noninsulin-dependent) diabetes mellitus: normal endocrine and glycemic responses, up to 10 years after diagnosis. Diabetologia 30:924-929, 1987.
70. Levy C, Kinsley B, Bajaj M, Simonson D. Effect of glycemic control on glucose counterregulation during hypoglycemia in NIDDM. Diabetes Care 21:1330-1338, 1998.
71. Shamoon H, Friedman S, Canton C, Zacharowicz L, Hu M, Rossetti L. Increased epinephrine and skeletal muscle responses to hypoglycemia in non-insulin-dependent diabetes mellitus. J Clin Invest 93:2562-2571, 1994.
72. Segel S, Paramore D, Cryer P. Defective glucose counterregulation in type 2 diabetes. Diabetes 49(Suppl 1):A131, 2000 (Abstract).
73. Bolli G, Tsalikian E, Haymond M, Cryer P, Gerich J. Defective glucose counterregulation after subcutaneous insulin in noninsulin-dependent diabetes mellitus. J Clin Invest 73:1532-1541, 1984.
74. Woerle HJ, Meyer C, Popa E, Cryer P, Gerich J. Renal compensation for impaired hepatic glucose release during hypoglycemia in type 2 diabetes. Diabetologia (In Press).
75. Magnusson I, Rothman D, Katz L, Shulman R, Shulman G. Increased rate of gluconeogenesis in type II diabetes. A 13C nuclear magnetic resonance study. J Clin Invest 90:1323-1327, 1992.
76. Arner P, Einarsson K, Ewerth S, Livingston J. Altered action of glucagon on human liver in Type 2 (noninsulin- dependent) diabetes mellitus. Diabetologia 30:323-326, 1987.
77. Krahn D, Mackenzie T. Organic personality syndrome caused by insulin-related nocturnal hypoglycemia. Psychosomatics 25:711-712, 1984.
78. Silas J, Grant D, Maddocks J. Transient hemiparetic attacks due to unrecognised nocturnal hypoglycaemia. Brit Med J 282:132-133, 1981.
79. Chalmers J, Risk M, Kean D, Grant R, Ashworth B, Campbell I. Severe amnesia after hypoglycemia. Clinical, psychometric, and magnetic resonance imaging correlations. Diabetes Care 14:922-925, 1991.
80. Fisher B, Quin J, Rumley A, Lennie S, Small M, MacCuish A, Lowe G. Effects of acute insulin-induced hypoglycaemia on haemostasis, fibrinolysis and haemorheology in insulin-dependent diabetic patients and control subjects. Clinical Science 80:525-531, 1991.
81. Wredling R, Levander S, Adamson U, Lins P. Permanent neuropsychological impairment after recurrent episodes of severe hypoglycaemia in man. Diabetologia 33:152-157, 1990.

82. Patrick A, Campbell I. Fatal hypoglycaemia in insulin-treated diabetes mellitus: clinical features and neuropathological changes. Diabetic Med 7:349-354, 1990.

83. Pladziewicz D, Nesto R. Hypoglycemia-induced silent myocardial ischemia . Am J Cardiol 63:1531-1532, 1989.

84. Duh E, Feinglos M. Hypoglycemia-induced angina pectoris in a patient with diabetes mellitus. Ann Intern Med 121:945-946, 1994.

85. Perros P, Frier B. The long-term sequelae of severe hypoglycemia on the brain in insulin-dependent diabetes mellitus. Horm Metab Res 29:197-202, 1997.

86. Kohner E, McLeod D, Marshall J. Complications of Diabetes, London, Edward Arnold, 1982.

87. Deary I, Crawford J, Hepburn D, Langan S, Blackmore L, Frier B. Severe hypoglycemia and intelligence in adult patients with insulin-treated diabetes. Diabetes 341-344, 1993.

88. Paz-Guevara A, Hsu T-H, White P. Juvenile diabetes mellitus after forty years. Diabetes 24:559-565, 1975.

89. Nabarro J, Mustaffa B, Morris D, Walport M, Kurtz A. Insulin deficient diabetes. Contrasts with other endocrine deficiencies. Diabetologia 16:5-12, 1979.

90. Seltzer H. Severe drug-induced hypoglycemia: a review. Comprehensive Therapy 5:21-29, 1979.

91. Berger W, Caduff F, Pasquel M, Rump A. Die relative haufigkeit der schweren Sulfonylharnstoff- hypoglykamie in den letzten 25 Jahren in der Schweiz. Schwerz.Med.Wschr. 116:145-151, 1986.

92. Mintz D, Finster J, Taylor A, Fefea A. Hormonal genesis of glucose intolerance following hypoglycemia. Am J Med 45:187-197, 1968.

93. Frier B, Corrall R, Ashby J, Baird J. Attenuation of the pancreatic beta-cell response to a meal following hypoglycemia in man. Diabetologia 18:297-300, 1980.

94. Attvall S, Fowelin J, von Schenck H, Smith U. Insulin resistance in type I (insulin-dependent) diabetes following hypoglycemia-evidence for the importance of B- adrenergic stimulation. Diabetologia 30:691-697, 1987.

95. Kollind M, Adamson U, Lins P. Insulin resistance following nocturnal hypoglycemia in insulin- dependent diabetes mellitus. Acta Endocrinol 116:314-320, 1987.

96. Clore J, Brennan J, Gebhart S, Newsome H, Nestler J, Blackard W. Prolonged insulin resistance following insulin-induced hypoglycemia. Diabetologia 30:851-858, 1987.

97. Gale E, Kurtz A, Tattersall R. In search of the Somogyi effect. Lancet 2:279-282, 1980.

98. Havlin C, Cryer P. Nocturnal hypoglycemia does not commonly result in major morning hyperglycemia in patients with diabetes mellitus. Diabetes Care 10:141-147, 1987.

99. Tordjman K, Havlin C, Levandoski L, White N, Santiago J, Cryer P. Failure of nocturnal hypoglycemia to cause fasting hyperglycemia in patients with insulin-dependent diabetes mellitus. N Engl J Med 31:1552-1559, 1987.

100. Gaston S. Outcomes of hypoglycemia treated by standardized protocol in a community hospital. Diabetes Educ 18:491-494, 1992.

101. Slama G, Traynard P, Desplanque N, Pudar H, Dhunputh I, Letanoux M, Bornet F, Tchobroutsky G. The search for an optimized treatment of hypoglycemia. Carbohydrates in tablets, solution, or gel for the correction of insulin reactions. Arch Intern Med 150:589-593, 1990.

102. Palatnick W, Meatherall R, Tenenbein M. Clinical spectrum of sulfonylurea overdose and experience with diazoxide therapy. Arch Intern Med 151:1859-1862, 1991.

103. Cryer P, Gerich J. Glucose counterregulation, hypoglycemia, and intensive insulin therapy in diabetes mellitus. N Engl J Med 313:232-241, 1985.

104. Bolli G. How to ameliorate the problem of hypoglycemia in intensive as well as nonintensive treatment of type 1 diabetes. Diabetes Care 22(Suppl 2):B43-B52, 1999.

105. Boland E, Grey M, Oesterle A, Fredrickson L, Tamborlane W. Continuous subcutaneous insulin infusion. A new way to lower risk of severe hypoglycemia, improve metabolic control, and enhance coping in adolescents with type 1 diabetes. Diabetes Care 22:1779-1784, 1999.

106. Bode B, Steed RD, Davidson P. Reduction in severe hypoglycemia with long-term continuous subcutaneous insulin infusion in type 1 diabetes. Diabetes Care 19:324-327, 1996.

107. Brunelle R, Llewelyn J, Anderson J, Gale E, Koivisto V. Meta-analysis of the effect of insulin lispro on severe hypoglycemia in patients with type 1 diabetes. Diabetes Care 21:1726-1731, 1998.

108. Pieber T, Eugene-Jolchine I, Derobert E, The European Study Group of HOE 901 in Type 1 Diabetes. Efficacy and safety of HOE 901 versus NPH insulin in patients with type 1 diabetes. Diabetes Care 23:157-162, 2000.

109. Dagogo-Jack S, Rattarason C, Cryer P. Reversal of hypoglycemia unawareness, but not defective glucose counterregulation in IDDM. Diabetes 43:1426-1434, 1994.

110. Fritsche A, Stumvoll M, Haring H, Gerich J. Reversal of hypoglycemia unawareness in a long-term type 1 diabetic patient by improvement of beta-adrenergic sensitivity after prevention of hypoglycemia. J Clin Endocrinol Metab 85:523-525, 2000.

111. Fanelli C, Pampanelli S, Epifano L, Rambotti A, Vincenzo A, Modarelli F, Ciofetta M, Lepore M, Annibale B, Torlone E, Perriello G, DeFeo P, Santeusano F, Brunetti P, Bolli G. Long-term recovery from unawareness, deficient counterregulation and lack of cognitive dysfunction during hypoglycemia, following institution of rational, intensive insulin therapy in IDDM. Diabetologia 37:1265-1276, 1994.

112. Cranston I, Lomas J, Maran A, MacDonald I, Amiel S. Restoration of hypoglycemia unawareness in patients with long- duration insulin-dependent diabetes. Lancet 344:283-287, 1994.

113. Davis M, Mellman M, Friedman S, Chang C, Shamoon H. Recovery of epinephrire response but not hypoglycemic symptom threshold after intensive therapy in type 1 diabetes. Am J Med 97:535-542, 1994.

114. Fanelli C, Epifano L, Rambotti A, Pampanelli S, Di Vincenzo A, Modarelli F, Lepore M, Annibale B, Ciofetta M, Bottini P, Porcellati F, Scionti L, Santeusanio F, Brunetti P, Bolli G. Meticulous prevention of hypoglycemia normalizes the glycemic thresholds and magnitude of most of neuroendocrine responses to, symptoms of, and cognitive function during hypoglycemia in intensively treated patients with short-term IDDM. Diabetes 42:1683-1689, 1993.

115. Kendall D, Teuscher A, Robertson R. Defective glucagon secretion during sustained hypoglycemia following successful islet allo- and autotransplantation in humans. Diabetes 46:23-27, 1997.

116. Meyer C, Hering B, Großmann R, Brandhorst H, Brandhorst D, Gerich J, Federlin K, Bretzel R. Improved glucose counterregulation and autonomic symptoms after intraportal islet transplants alone in patients with long-standing type I diabetes mellitus. Transplantation 66:233-240, 1998.

117. Federlin K, Pozza G. Indications for clinical islet transplantation today and in the foreseeable future--The diabetologist's point of view. J Mol Med 77:148-152, 1999.

118. Bosi E, Piatti P, Secchi A, Monti L, Traeger J, Dubernard J, Pozza G. Response of glucagon and insulin secretion to insulin-induced hypoglycemia in diabetic patients after pancreatic transplantation. Diab Nutr Metab 1:21-27, 1988.

119. Diem P, Redman J, Abid M, Moran A, Sutherland D, Halter J, Robertson R. Glucagon, catecholamine, and pancreatic polypeptide secretion in type I diabetic recipients of pancreas allografts. J Clin Invest 86:2008-2013, 1990.

120. Bolinder J, Wahrenberg H, Persson A, Linde B, Tyden G, Groth C, Ostman J. Effect of pancreas transplantation on glucose counterregulation in insulin-dependent diabetic patients prone to severe hypoglycaemia. J Int Med 230:527-533, 1991.

121. Bolinder J, Wahrenberg H, Linde B, Tyden G, Groth C, Ostman J. Improved glucose counterregulation after pancreas transplantation in diabetic patients with unawareness of hypoglycemia. Transplant Proc 23:1667-1669, 1991.

122. Landgraf R, Nusser J, Riepl R, Fiedler F, Illner W, Abendroth D, Land W. Metabolic and hormonal studies of Type 1 (insulin-dependent) diabetic patients after successful pancreas and kidney transplantation. Diabetologia 34(Suppl 1):S61-S67, 1991.

123. Barrou Z, Seaquist E, Robertson R. Pancreas transplantation in diabetic humans normalizes hepatic glucose production during hypoglycemia. Diabetes 43:661-666, 1994.

124. Kendall D, Rooney D, Smets Y, Bolding L, Robertson R. Pancreas transplantation restores epinephrine response and symptom recognition during hypoglycemia in patients with long-standing type 1 diabetes and autonomic neuropathy. Diabetes 46:249-257, 1997.

125. Luzi L, Battezzati A, Perseghin G, Bianchi E, Vergani S, Secchi A, La Rocca E, Staudacher C, Spotti D, Ferrari G, Di Carlo V, Pozza G. Lack of feedback inhibition of insulin secretion in denervated human pancreas. Diabetes 41:1632-1639, 1992.

126. Battezzati A, Luzi L, Perseghin G, Bianchi E, Spotti D, Secchi A, Vergani S, Di Carlo V, Pozza G. Persistence of counter-regulatory abnormalities in insulin-dependent diabetes mellitus after pancreas transplantation. Eur J Clin Invest 24:751-758, 1994.

127. Gupta V, Wahoff D, Rooney D, Poitout V, Sutherland D, Kendall D, Robertson R. The defective glucagon response from transplanted intrahepatic pancreatic islets during hypoglycemia is transplantation site-determined. Diabetes 46:28-33, 1997.

Chapter 3. Microvascular Complications of Diabetes Mellitus

Vincent Yen

INTRODUCTION

The common feature underlying the diverse complications of diabetes is vasculopathy, both "micro" and "macro", characterized by progressive narrowing of lumen as well as abnormal permeability to proteins. Diabetes and its complications have been used as a model for accelerated aging.[1] In this model of aging, the ongoing biochemical process of non-enzymatic cross-linking of several types of macromolecules, including proteins and nucleic acids, leads to modification and then decline in structure and function of these molecules, as the cross-links accumulate both extracellularly and intracellularly over time. A prime example would be the crosslinking of collagen, which is thought to lead to typical phenomena observed in aging, such as increased susceptibility to atherosclerosis, osteoporosis, decreased joint elasticity, the formation of cataracts, and cardiac enlargement. Crosslinked collagen, found in increased levels in aged animal aorta and cartilage[2] as well as in aged human collagen of tendon and skin,[3] has been considered a biological marker for aging. Cross-linking of nucleic acids similarly might lead to increased errors in information transfer.

The cross-linking process is enhanced by a number of types of small reactive molecules (the most important being glucose and other reducing sugars) and their Amadori products, which act as a type of molecular glue by instigating the eventually irreversible glycosylation of proteins and other macromolecules, the so-called Maillard reaction (Figure 1).[2] Examples of the Maillard reaction can be observed in the kitchen, where an apple cut in half, or a turkey in the oven, turn yellow and then brown; yellowing of teeth is another example. In diabetes, while the exact mechanisms by which hyperglycemia causes vascular damage have not been fully elucidated, it can be demonstrated that matrix proteins, such as collagen, both within and outside the vessel walls, once glycosylated, can physically cross link with each other, with extravasated plasma proteins, such as albumin and immunoglobulins, and with lipoproteins.[4] Over time, these tight sugar-protein bonds cause alterations in structure and function, causing conformational changes, impairing fluxes of both nutrient and waste material and leading to vascular hypertrophy and stiffening of collagen with subsequent reduction of arterial compliance. These are processes that are associated with aging but seem to be accelerated by hyperglycemia. These cross-linked macromolecules, called advanced glycosylation end products (AGEs), are implicated in the pathogenesis of vascular complications. Once

AGEs are taken up by specific AGE receptors (RAGE), cytokines, growth factors, and adhesion factors are released, leading to further cellular changes. AGEs also can impair endothelial function and vascular reactivity, such as in response to nitric oxide. Modification of LDL as a result of glycation may contribute to foam cell formation.[4] Thus, AGEs appear to be main players not only in the development of diabetic complications and atherosclerosis, but in some ways may even be considered the final common pathway for pathologic processes associated with aging. One might speculate that this role of glucose in the formation of AGEs underlies the well described phenomenon in animals whereby caloric restriction prolongs lifespan in animals.[5]

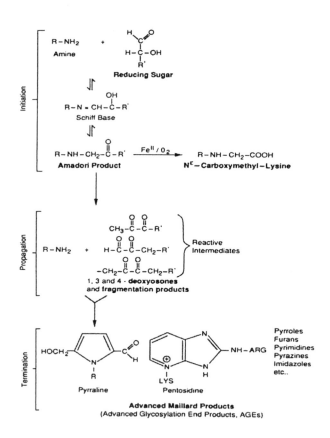

Figure 1. General scheme of the Maillard reaction. The initial step is generally referred to as nonenzymatic glycosylation or glycation. (From Monnier VM. Nonenzymatic glycosylation, the Maillard reaction and aging process. J Gerontol Biol Sci 45:B105-111, 1990, with permission).

318

Chemically, the following sequence of events unfolds:[2]

1) The process begins with the nucleophilic addition of glucose to free amino groups on proteins, typically on lysine residues, resulting in the reversible formation of a Schiff base. The rate of this process is proportional to the glucose concentration.

2) Over weeks, the Schiff base is transformed to a stable sugar-protein adduct, a ketoamine, the so-called Amadori type early glycosylation product. Importantly, hemoglobin A1c, or glycosylated hemoglobin, widely used clinically as a measure of ambient glucose exposure, is an example of an Amadori product. This covalently bound product is still slowly reversible. Schiff base and Amadori product are in equilibrium with glucose.

3) Over months to years the Amadori product rearranges to produce a now irreversibly bound glucose-protein compound, collectively called AGE's, or advanced glycosylation end products. The type of sugar, the sugar concentration, duration of macromolecule exposure, and rate of oxidative degradation determine the amount of Amadori product available to form AGEs. These irreversibly bound moities persist for the lifetime of the protein or substrate and will therefore accumulate continuously, for example on long lived proteins of vessel walls. These AGEs are measured by characteristic fluorescence and absorbance properties, as well as with anti AGE antibodies, and can be isolated from both tissue samples and from serum. Note that the precise chemical identities of individual AGEs at this point are for the most part unclear; at present, AGEs are mostly designated by their various immunochemical classes. Two defined AGE compounds include carboxy methyl lysine (CML) and pentosidine.

Once formed, AGEs continue to cross-react with neighboring amino groups to form a tightly interwoven matrix of intramolecular and intermolecular crosslinks. Since prolonged exposure to hyperglycemia has the clearest correlation for development of microvascular complications in both type 1 and type 2 diabetes, (two otherwise very different conditions), the standard, especially since the Diabetes Control and Complications Trial (DCCT)[6] and United Kingdom Prospective Diabetes Study (UKPDS)[7] data have been available, has been to try to decrease the risk for vascular complications by controlling hyperglycemia. On the other hand, since maintenance of euglycemia, especially over time, is imperfect at best and impossible at worst, there is a rationale to try to arrest or interfere with the glycosylation process in an attempt to prevent complications, independently of glycemic control (interestingly, aminoguanidine, an agent that has been examined as a possible blocker of the glycosylation process, is a popular player on "fountain of youth" internet websites). Notably, as AGEs accumulate as a function of area under the glucose exposure curve, they eventually continue to form on long lived glucose modified proteins and macromolecules even in the absence of hyperglycemia. This phenomenon is illustrated by patients whose proliferative retinopathy progresses despite pancreatic transplant.[8]

Clinically, there are some as yet uncharacterized genetic components to susceptibility of the micro- and macrovasculature to the development of the changes in response to the chronic exposure to hyperglycemia and AGE. These components might involve genetically determined differences in monokine secretory response or end organ response to the monokines.[9]

Some shared pathophysiologic processes are seen across the spectrum of the otherwise very diverse complications of diabetes. These include (Table 1):[9]

1) Accumulation of periodic acid Schiff (PAS) positive deposits of CHO-containing plasma proteins that have extravasated because of increased vascular permeability and leakage; these deposits are demonstrated in glomerular, retinal, and endoneural microvessels as well as in arterial media and subintima. These serum proteins, such as albumin, globulin, and lipoprotein, appear to be tightly crosslinked and immobilized into vessel wall matrix components by collagen linked AGEs, which act as foci for these deposits. The increased vascular permeability may be related to AGE crosslinked vessel wall changes.

2) expanded extracellular matrix production, such as by glomerular mesangial cells or retinal basement membrane. The term "extracellular matrix" refers to the polymer substances occupying the spaces between cells in a tissue. Notably, AGE-protein can be recognized, taken up, and degraded by various cell surface macrophage receptors. In vitro, it has been demonstrated that, once AGEs are taken up, cytokines, such as tumor necrosis factor (TNF), and interleukin (IL-1), are secreted.[10] Additional endothelial growth factors such as platelet-derived growth factor (PDGF),[11] an inducer of angiogenesis, and insulin-like growth factor-1 (IGF-1)[4] as well as transforming growth factor (TGF-β)[12] and vascular endothelial growth factor (VEGF)[13] contribute to this expanded vessel wall matrix and mesenchymal cell proliferation. VEGF is also known to be a main cytokine involved in retinopathy and neovascularlization. Elevated levels of both VEGF and AGE have been measured in diabetic ocular fluid;[13] in vitro AGEs promote VEGF expression, while in vivo, rats injected with AGE showed increased VEGF immunoreactivity in retinal vessels, with increased permeability.[14] Rat aortic smooth muscle cells, cultured with AGEs, demonstrated stimulated growth promoting signal transduction pathways, such as MAP-kinase.[15] AGE receptor activity also increases the transcription factor Nf-kB, which may be involved in the development of atherosclerosis and apoptosis.[16] Normally, monocyte derived macrophages, activated through adhesion molecules, play a central role in the maintenance of vascular wall homeostasis and tissue remodeling in terms of proteolysis,

degradation, removal, and replacement; the presence of accumulated AGEs, however, may interfere with this balance in favor of expansion.[9] Additionally, endothelial cells demonstrate elaboration of downregulated cell surface heparin binding as well as altered transmembrane signaling that result in altered matrix interactions with platelets and vascular wall cells and increased synthesis of procoagulant tissue factors.[4,17] Thus, AGE-modified vessel matrix can contribute to the clinically observed vasoconstriction and focal thrombi seen in diabetic vasculopathy.

3) cellular hypertrophy and hyperplasia, such as that seen in retinal endothelial cells and in arterial smooth muscle cells in atherosclerotic plaques. AGE modified matrix proteins have been shown to block the antiproliferative effect of nitric oxide on vascular smooth muscle and renal mesangial cells.[18] AGE-collagen inactivates nitric oxide as well as other vascular smooth muscle relaxing factors.[4] Of note, inhibition of the cross-linking process by aminoguanidine has been shown to slow this loss of vascular reactivity.

Table 1. AGE-related processes

1. Accumulation of periodic acid Schiff (PAS) deposits.
2. Expanded extracellular matrix production.
3. Cellular hypertrophy and hyperplasia

Thus, AGE-formation on diabetic vessel wall matrix proteins involves the cross-linking of extravasated plasma proteins to the matrix components, as well as cross linking of matrix components with each other. In diabetic nephropathy, the hallmark of disease is thickening of the glomerular and tubular basement membranes. Anti AGE-antibodies can be used to localize AGEs within kidney specimens from both diabetic and nondiabetic patients. This approach demonstrates high levels of accumulation of AGEs in both diabetic and aged vascular intima, particularly the inner elastic layer of arteries.[18] There is also positive staining within nodular and severe diffuse glomerular lesions as well as in hyaline deposits of arterioles. AGE-modified glomerular basement membrane is seen to be more resistant to physiologic digestion and thus, when combined with the enhanced synthesis of mesangial matrix, will over time display thickening, decreased elasticity, and an altered ability of the basement membrane molecules to interact with laminin, heparan sulfate proteoglycan, and type IV collagen and to form ordered complexes.[9,17] The postulate is that there would then be a conformational change in intermolecular spacing and thus even pore size. When injected into normal rats, AGEs cause glomerular lesions, proteinuria, and renal dysfunction.[20] As mentioned previously, there is early and continuous accumulation of extravasated plasma proteins in the arterial wall. In the arterial subintima, extravasated LDL that has been immobilized by cross-linked AGEs can be demonstrated in vitro; AGE formation also occurs on the lipoprotein components of LDL. AGE-immobilized LDL, in the environment of other AGE-crosslinked matrix complexes that interfere with scavenging macrophages, could presumably become the focus for foam cell and plaque formation;[9] thus, perhaps measurement of AGE-LDL might be the true indicator for vasculature at risk for oxidative modification. AGE-LDL incubated with human aortic endothelial cells demonstrated increased surface expression of adhesion molecules, such as vascular cell adhesion molecule (VCAM-1), which promote monocyte adherence.[21] Platelet activation in vitro has been demonstrated by addition of food derived AGE (e.g., cola; cocoa); there is speculation that this postprandial increase in thrombogenicity, especially given the high AGE content of the western diet, might underlie the high incidence of post-prandial ischemic events.[22] The accumulation of proteins themselves contributes to progressive luminal wall narrowing, and, as mentioned earlier, the long lived proteoglycan components of the vascular matrix, themselves altered by AGE accumulation, demonstrate decreased binding of heparins, altered transmembrane signaling, altered interactions with platelets/cell wall components, and a decreased vasodilatory response to nitric oxide. The overall effect of AGE on vasculature is thus luminal narrowing, microthrombus formation, vasoconstriction, oxidative tissue injury, cytokine mediated tissue remodeling, and plaque formation.[23,24]

At the organism level, elevated serum concentrations of AGEs have been shown in patients with type 2 diabetes mellitus compared to non-diabetic controls; additionally, among those with diabetes, the patients who had coronary heart (CHD) disease had significantly higher AGE levels than those that did not have CHD.[25] The circulating serum AGEs seem to be comprised of serum proteins, themselves modified by AGEs (including AGE-LDL), as well as catabolized tissue-bound AGEs. These levels are seen to accumulate dramatically in end stage renal disease and are felt to contribute to the morbidity associated with uremia.[23] Using enzyme linked immunoassays, similarly significant increases in serum AGEs have been found in diabetic patients as compared to controls, with significant correlation with level of nephropathy and retinopathy.[26] Skin AGE levels are also correlated with complication rates; levels have been correlated over a three year period with Hgb A1C, with the suggestion that AGE levels might be useful to describe even longer term glycemic control, as well as the presence of complications.[27] AGE-collagen levels also yield similar correlations.[30]

Regarding the role of other known risk factors for the development of atherosclerosis and a possible role of AGE in this process, the postulate is that hypertension and increased intra-vascular pressure would lead to an increased rate of protein extravasation through the endothelial barrier; as described earlier this could lead to increased AGE linked protein deposits in the vascular matrix as well as increased stimulation of cells having AGE receptors, with subsequent increase in PDGF and thrombomodulin leading to hypercoagulability and platelet aggregation at the site.[31] Additionally, AGE may contribute to the hypertension itself by their inactivation of nitric oxide. One study did not find a correlation of serum AGE levels with smoking.[25] Diabetic mice on folate deficient diet and subsequent increase in the levels of homocysteine demonstrated increased levels of RAGE in renal vasculature; additionally, bovine aortic endothelial cells exposed to homocysteine showed an increase in mRNA for RAGE as well as an increase in activation of an oxidant sensitive Nuclear factor kappa B (NF-kB), suggesting that homocysteine may enhance RAGE, especially in diabetes, by mechanisms linked to oxidative stress. [32]

Many theories regarding pathogenesis of neuropathy exist.[33] A widely held partial hypothesis is that of the polyol pathway, whereby hyperglycemia, via mass action, increases the concentration of sorbitol and other polyols. Aldose reductase is the rate-limiting enzyme in the polyol pathway. The accumulation of sorbitol causes the intracellular depletion of myo-inositol and consequently, phosphatidylinositol, a key intracellular signal transducer which is required for the activation of protein kinase C. Myo-inositol depletion impairs Na/K-ATPase activity, which is seen to be correlated with decreased nerve conduction velocity in diabetic rodents. Note that the pathways that might integrate polyol pathway induced abnormalities in nerve myoinositol metabolism , Na/K-ATPase activity and the observed clinical findings in peripheral nerve are still obscure and that aldose reductase inhibitors have had mixed clinical results in treating neuropathy.

AGE involvement in neuropathic changes could include protein glycation of the endoneural vascular supply in ways already described; glycation of the extracellular matrix, with subsequent interference with neurotrophic functions; or glycation of the cells themselves. It this respect, sorbitol can be converted to fructose, which can then serve as a substrate for crosslinking. When cultured cerebro cortical neurons were incubated with various AGE classes cellular death was demonstrated; this cytopathic effect was prevented by anti-AGE antibodies.[34] As an interesting aside, the authors of this study postulated a contribution of AGE to Alzheimer's disease.

The formation of DNA-linked AGEs, on amino groups of DNA nucleotides and likely on histones as well, has been shown to lead to complex DNA rearrangements and mutations in prokaryotic cells. Expression by human coronary artery plaque cells of transforming genes involved in apoptosis may be an example.[35,31,9] DNA-AGE may also play some role in the increased incidence of congenital malformations seen in fetuses of diabetic mothers. This concept of DNA linked AGEs may thus partially explain the phenomenon of the need for preconception glycemic control to reduce risk.[35,4]

Given the compelling evidence for an association of AGEs with diabetic vascular complications, there have been efforts to use aminoguanidine, a nucleophilic hydrazine compound, to block reactive carbonyl groups on AGE precursors, such as 3-deoxyglucose, in an attempt to block the crosslinking process and thereby forestall the onset of microvascular disease.[36] Notably, aminoguanidine does not interfere with formation of normal enzymatic collagen cross-links. In vitro, aminoguanidine, via preferential binding, inhibits AGE formation, AGE cross linking of soluble proteins to matrix, AGE cross-linking of collagen, and prevents cross linked induced defects of heparin binding to collagen/fibronectin and cross linked induced defects of heparin sulfate proteoglycan binding to basement membrane.[37]

In animal studies, there are effects of decreased AGE's seen in the retina, kidney, nerve, and artery of diabetic rats. The retina shows highly significant decrease in proliferation of capillaries and microaneurysms.[37] In a 5 year study of experimental diabetes in dogs during which the treatment with aminoguanidine was initiated at the onset of diabetes, aminoguandine prevented the development of retinal microaneurysms, acellular capillaries, and pericyte ghosts.[38] It also prevented some gene expression changes related to neuronal apoptosis and neuroglial activity in diabetic rat retina.[39] The kidneys showed decreased albuminuria and prevention of increase in mesangial volume.[40,41] In rats nerve conduction is normalized and myelin is preserved, in relation to decreased AGE levels seen in the neural tissue.[42]

Aminoguanidine has been shown to inhibit coronary atherosclerosis in rabbits[43] and rats.[44] It prevents decreases in myocardial compliance and prevents age related arterial stiffening and cardiac hypertrophy.[45]

Clinical data in patients with both type 1 and type 2 diabetes using doses of 150-300 mg bid of pimagedine (aminoguanidine) are in progress; as might be expected, long trials might be required to see results. Aminoguanidine itself appears to be well tolerated with few side effects, except for vitamin B6 deficiency, via aminoguanidine's reactivity with pyridoxal compounds.[46] Patients treated with aminoguanidine have demonstrated decreased levels of serum Hgb-AGE.[27]

Additional agents under investigation include n-phenacyl-4,5-dimethylthiazolium, or ALT-711 (Alteon Corporation), a so-called cross-link breaker, rather than cross link inhibitor. Rats with streptozotocin induced diabetes, with higher levels of AGEs in skin collagen, who were treated with ALT-711 did not show decreased crosslinks as measured by half-time for solubilization of collagen[47] but demonstrated a suggestion of improved systemic arterial compliance and distensibility.

SUMMARY[9]

AGEs accumulate on macromolecules (such as protein) as a function of exposure to glucose and nonenzymatic glycosylation. These accumulations may be involved in the pathogenesis of chronic diabetic complications by causing dysfunctional changes in:
- extracellular matrix
- endothelium
- vessel wall

Pathophysiology includes:
- abnormal receptor mediated production of cytokines, such as TNF, IL-1, IGF-1;
- altered function of intracellular proteins and DNA;
- vessels show enhanced subintimal protein and lipoprotein deposition;
- increased vascular permeability, e.g. to albumin;
- inactivation of nitric oxide;
- activation of endothelial receptors, leading to vasoconstriction and thrombosis;
- altered proteoglycan milleu;
- altered basement membrane cellular structure;
- proliferation of matrix.

Strategies directed at the prevention of formation or the disruption of AGE cross-links may be promising.

REFERENCES:

1. Monnier VM, Kohn RR, Cerami A Accelerated age-related browning of human collagen in diabetes mellitus. Proc Natl Acad Sci USA 81:583-587, 1984.
2. Monnier VM. Nonenzymatic glycosylation, the Maillard reaction and the aging process. J Gerontol 45:B105 – B111, 1990.
3. Dyer DG, Dunn JA, Thorpe SR, Bailie KE, Lyons TJ, McCance DR, Baynes JW. Accumulation of Maillard reaction products in skin collagen in diabetes and aging. J Clin Invest 91:2463-2469, 1993.
4. Bucala R, Cerami A, Vlassara H. Advanced glycosylation end products in diabetic complications. Diabetes Reviews 3:258-26, 1995.
5. Holehan A, Merry BJ The experimental manipulation of aging by diet. Biol Rev 61:329-68, 1986.
6. Diabetes Control and Complications Trial Research Group. The effect of intensive therapy of diabetes mellitus in the development and progression of long term complications of IDDM. N Engl J Med 329:977-986. 1993.
7. UKPDS study. Lancet 352:837-53, 1998.

8. Ramsay RC, Goetz FC, Sutherland DE. Progression of diabetic retinopathy after pancreatic transplant for IDDM. N Engl J Med 318:208-214, 1988.
9. Brownlee M, Cerami A, Vlassora H. Advanced glycation end products in tissue and the biochemical basis of diabetic complications. N Engl J Med 318:1315–1321, 1988.
10. Vlassara H, Brownlee M, Manogue KR, Dinarella CA, Pasagian A. Cachectin/TNF and IL-1 induced glucose-modified proteins: role in normal tissue remodelling. Science 240:1546–1548, 1988.
11. Kirstein M, Brett J, Radoff S, Ogawa S, Stern D, Vlassara H. Advanced protein glycosylation induces transendothelial human monocyte chemotaxis and secretion of platelet derived growth factor: role in vascular disease and aging. Proc Natl Acad Sci USA 93:3902-3907, 1996.
12. Reeves WB, Andreoli TE. Transforming growth factor beta contributes to progressive diabetic nephropathy. Proc Natl Acad Sci USA 97:7667-7669, 2000.
13. Endo M, TuchidaK, Sone M, Obara S, Miyoshi H, Makita Z, Korike T. Increased vascular endothelial growth factor (VGEF) and AGEs in the aqueous humor in diabetic retinopathy. Diabetes 48 (Suppl 1): A66, 0281, 1999
14. Stitt A, Simpson D, Bhaduri T, Gardiner T, Archer D Coinduction of retinal vasopermeability and VEGF expression by AGEs in vitro and in vivo. Diabetes 48 (Suppl 1): A155, 0672, 1999.
15. Ihm SH, Yoo HJ, Park SW, Ihm J. Effect of AGE on rat aortic vascular smooth muscle cells. Diabetes 49 (Suppl II): A14, :572-P, 2000.
16. Yeh CH, Sturgis L, Haidacher J, Zheng XN, Sherwood S, Bjerche RJ, Juhasz O, Crow MT, Tilton RG, Denner L. Requirements for p38 and p44/p42 mitogen-activated protein kinases and RAGE-mediated Nuclear Factor kappa-B transcriptional activation and cytokine secretion. Diabetes 50:1495-1504, 2001.
17. Tarsio JF, RegerLA, Furcht LT. Molecular mechanisms on basement Membrane complications of diabetes alterations in heparin, laminin, and Type IV collagen association. Diabetes 37:532-540, 1988.
18. Rumble JR, Cooper ME, Soulis T, Cox A, Yousef S, Jasik M, Jerums G, Gilbert RE. Vascular hypertrophy in experimental diabetes: role of advanced glycation end products. J Clin Invest 99:1016-1027, 1997.
19. Nishino T, Horii Y, Shiiki H, Yamamoto H, Makita Z, Bucala R, Dohi K. Immunohistochemical detection of AGE products within the vascular lesions and Glomeruli in diabetic nephropathy. Human Pathol 26:308-313, 1999.
20. Vlassara H, Striker LJ, Teichberg S, Fuh H, Li YM, Steffes M. Advanced glycation end products induce glomerular sclerosis and albuminuria in normal rats. Proc Natl Acad Sci USA 91(24):11704-8, 1994.

21. Lopes-Virella M, Takei A, Crawford A, Huang Y. AGE-LDL stimulates adhesion molecule expression in human aortic endothelial cells Diabetes 48 (Suppl 1): A31, 0134, 1999.

22. Koschinsky T, Schwippert B, Ruetter R, Buenting C, Vlassara H, Tschoepe D. Food AGE induce expression of P-selectin in platelets from diabetic and non diabetic subjects. Diabetes 49 (Suppl II): A142, 581-P, 2000.

23. Makita Z, Yanagisawa K, Kuwajima S, Bucala R, Vlassara H, Koike T. The role of AGE products in the pathogenesis of atherosclerosis. Nephrol Dialysis Transplantation 11 (Suppl 5):31-3, 1996.

24. Sims TJ, Rasmussen LM, Oxlund H, Bailey AJ. The role of glycation cross links in diabetic vascular stiffening. Diabetologia 39:951-964, 1996.

25. Kilhovd B, Berg TJ, Birkeland KI, Thorsby P, Hanien KF. Serum levels of advanced glycation end products are increased in patients with type 2 diabetes and coronary heart disease. Diabetes Care 22:1543–1548, 1999.

26. Ono Y, Aoki S, Ohnishi K, Yasuda T, Kawano K, Tsukada Y. Increased serum levels of AGE in NIDDM patients with diabetic complications (letter). Diabetes Care 21:1027, 1998.

27. Beisswenger PJ, Makita Z, Curphey TJ, Moore LL, Jean S, Brinck-Johnsen T, Bucala R, Vlassara H. Formation of immunohistochemical AGE products precedes and correlates with early manifestations of renal and retinal disease in diabetes. Diabetes 44: 824-9, 1995.

28. Makita Z, Vlassara H, Rayfield E, Cartwright K, Friedman E, Rodby R, Cerami A, Bucala R. Hemoglobin-AGE: a circulating marker advanced glycosylation. Science 258:651-653, 1992.

29. Makita Z, Takeuchi M, Tschchida KI, Obara S, Miyoshi H, Koike T. Circulating AGEs as an indicator of long term glycemic control. Diabetes 48 (Suppl 1): A351, 1537, 1999.

30. Monnier VM, Vishwanath V, Frank KE, Elmets CA, Dauchot P, Kohn RR. Relation between complications of Type I diabetes mellitus and collagen-linked fluorescence. N Engl J Med 314:403-408, 1986.

31. Brownlee M. Advanced products of nonenzymatic glycosylation and the pathogenesis of diabetic complications. In Ellenberg & Rifkins Diabetes Mellitus. Stamford,CT, Appleton & Lange 229-245, 1997

32. Hofmann M, Lu Y, Schermer C, Ferran L, Kohl B, Lalla E, Schmidt AM. Modulation of expression of receptor for advanced glycosylated endproducts (RAGE) by homocysteine in cultured endothelium of diabetic mice. Diabetes 48, (Suppl 1):A31, 0132, 1999.

33. Greene DA, Feldman EL, Stevens MJ, Albers JW, Sima AAF, Pfeifer MA. Diabetic Neuropathy. In Ellenberg & Rifkin's Diabetes Mellitus. Stamford, CT, Appleton & Lange 1009-1078, 1997.

34. Takeuchi M, Bucala P, Suzuki T, Ohkubo T, Yamazaki M, Koike T, Kamada Y, Makita Z. Neurotoxicity of advanced glycosylation end products for cultured cortical neurons. J Neuropath & Exp Neurol 59:1094-1105, 2000.

35. Dandona P, Thusu K, Cook S, Snyder B, Makowski J, Armstrong D, Nicotera T. Oxidative changes to DNA in diabetes mellitus. Lancet 347:444-445, 1996.

36. Brownlee M, Vlassara H, Kooneg A, Ulrich P, Cerami A. Aminoguanidine prevents diabetes induced arterial wall protein cross-linking. Science 232:1629-1632, 1986.

37. Hammes HP, Martin S, Federlin K, Geisen R, Brownlee M. Aminoguanidine treatment inhibits the development of experimental diabetic retinopathy. Proc Natl Acad Sci USA 88:11555-11558, 1991.

38. Kern TS, Engerman RL. Pharmacological inhibition of diabetic retinopathy. Aminoguanidine and aspirin. Diabetes 50:1636-1642, 2001.

39. Gerherdinger C, Zanello S, Zhang J, O'Neill B, Lorenzi M. Gene expression profiling of early experimental diabetic retinopathy and effects of aminoguanidine. Diabetes 50 (Suppl 2): A18, 73-OR, 2001.

40. Soulis T, Cooper ME, Vranes D, Bucala R, Jerums G. Effects of aminoguanidine in preventing experimental diabetic nephropathy are related to duration of treatment. Kidney Intl 50:627-634, 1996.

41. Ellis E, Good BH Prevention of glomerular basement membrane thickening by aminoguanidine in experimental diabetes mellitus. Metabolism 40:1016-1019, 1991.

42. Yagihashi S, Kamijo M, Baba M, Yagihashi N, Nagai K. Effect of aminoguanidine on functional and structural abnormalities in peripheral nerve of STZ-induced diabetic rats. Diabetes 41:47-52, 1992.

43. Li YM, Steffes M, Donelly T, Liu C, Fuh H, Basgen J, Bucala R, Vlassara H: Prevention of cardiovascular and renal pathology of aging by the advanced glycation inhibitor aminoguanidine. Proc Natl Acad Sci USA 93:3902–3907, 1996.

44. Panagiotpolous S, O'Brien RC, Bucala R ,Cooper ME, Jerums G. Aminoguanidine has an anti-atherogenic effect in the cholesterol-fed rabbit. Atherosclerosis 136:125 – 131, 1998.

45. Norton GR, Candy G, Woodiwiss AJ. Aminoguanidine prevents the decreased myocardial compliance produced by streptozoticin-induced diabetes in rats. Circulation 93:1905 – 1912, 1998.

46. Miyashi M, Taguchi T, Yanagisawa K, Tsuchida KI, Korke T, Miwa I, Makita Z. Aminoguanidine-pyridoxal adduct is superior to aminoguanidine in preventing experimental diabetic retinopathy.Diabetes 49, Suppl II: A158, 647-P, 2000.

47. Yang S, Thorpe SR, Baynes JW. AGE-breakers fail to break cross linksin skin collagen of diabetic rats. Diabetes 49, Suppl II, A130, 527P, 2000.

Chapter 4. Diabetic Retinopathy

Joseph A. Murphy and Firas M. Rahhal

INTRODUCTION

Diabetic retinopathy (DR) is the leading cause of blindness in working-age Americans.[1] It accounts for 12% of cases of new blindness in the United States each year.[2] Of the 12 to 16 million Americans who have diabetes mellitus (DM), it is estimated that 700,000 have proliferative diabetic retinopathy (PDR) and 325,000 have macular edema[3]—the most significant forms of sight – threatening DR. Patients who have diabetic retinopathy are 29 times more likely to be blind than non diabetic persons.[3] Each year, 25,000 Americans are blinded by DR. In 90% of these cases, early detection and timely management might have prevented visual loss from DR.[4] Given these facts, it is obvious that the public health impact of DR is tremendous, and our efforts to better understand this potentially devastating complication of diabetes must continue and, indeed, increase so that improved treatments and preventive measures can be developed.

The prevalence of DR increased significantly after the development of life-saving insulin treatment in 1921.[5] The resultant prolonged life expectancy of diabetic patients allowed more time for the development of diabetic retinopathy. Since the landmark discovery of "light photocoagulation" by Meyer – Schwickerath in the 1950's, treatment of DR has steadily improved using various laser surgical techniques.[6] Subsequently the development of vitreous and retinal microsurgical techniques in the 1970's and 1980's improved our ability to help even the most advanced cases of DR. Today our understanding of the pathogenesis and biochemical basis of DR grows rapidly, and pharmacological, hormonal, and additional surgical treatments are on the horizon which may even prevent the development of the more serious forms of DR. This chapter will introduce you to the prevalence, pathogenesis, clinical findings, differential diagnosis, natural history, and treatment of diabetic retinopathy. We hope that familiarity with these basic topics will help the student of DM and the practitioner rendering care to diabetic patients better understand this serious complication of the disease, and remove some of the mystery often associated with this portion of the patients' overall care.

EPIDEMIOLOGY

A variety of types of epidemiological studies investigate the incidence and prevalence of DR. Prevalence studies are generally not highly accurate because their findings are usually based on the reporting of blindness caused by DR to various public agencies. These numbers are then presented as a percentage of total population from a given geographical region. These data will most likely underestimate the true incidence or prevalence of DR because of under-reporting by patients and/or health care workers. Population based studies, such as the Wisconsin Epidemiologic Study of Diabetic Retinopathy, which identified a population of diabetic patients through their primary care physicians and then studied a random sampling of these patients, are more likely to be accurate.[7-11] These studies, like many others, have proven that the major risk factor for development of DR is duration of DM.[12-17] This is true for both type 1 DM,[7,10,14,15] and for type 2 DM.[8,18] DR does not appear to occur prior to three years from the onset of DM.[7,8,15] It appears that the median time of onset of DR is approximately 5–10 years after the diagnosis of DM for both type 1 and type 2, although one study showed it to be somewhat later in type 2.[18] There are definite differences, however, in the clinical development and prevalence of DR between type 1 and type 2 DM. For example, the prevalence of DR after 15 years in type 1 patients exceeds 95% and appears to be less than 70% in patients with type 2 DM.[7,8,18] One study by Yanko et al., found the prevalence of DR to be only 60% after 16 years with type 2 DM. Naturally, the time of diagnosis of DM in type 2 can be difficult to ascertain exactly, and many patients may have had hyperglycemia long prior to the actual diagnosis of DM. This could confound epidemiological data and have the effect of artificially shortening duration to diagnosis of DR in these patients.

The differences in disease prevalence between type 1 and type 2 DM are more profound when the severity and subtype of DR are considered. After 15 years, type 1 DM patients have as high as a 50% prevalence[7] of proliferative diabetic retinopathy (PDR), whereas that number is less than 10% in type 2 DM.[8,18] When the other major sight threatening complication of DR is considered, macular edema, the reverse may be true. One investigator[19] found the prevalence of diabetic macular edema (DME) related proportionally to the age of the patient and hence, was more common in type 2 DM. The Wisconsin study did not confirm this, reporting that the prevalence rates of DME were similar between type 1 and type 2 DM, and were, again, directly related to duration of DM.[9] Clinically, many ophthalmologists specializing in the treatment of DR recognize that the proportion of patients developing PDR is much higher with type 1 DM and, at least early in the course of DR, the proportion developing DME is higher in type 2 DM.

ASSOCIATED SYSTEMIC CONDITIONS

Systemic Hypertension and Nephropathy

The role of hypertension in DR receives a great deal of attention from both clinical ophthalmologists and investigators. Most clinicians believe that poorly controlled hypertension can exacerbate and promote progression of non proliferative (NPDR) and proliferative diabetic retinopathy (PDR), and in particular, make DME difficult to manage. Several scientific studies have supported this position[20-23] but some have drawn into question this conclusion. They report that blood pressure alone is not a significant factor when nephropathy is removed as a confounding variable.

The United Kingdom Prospective Diabetes Study (UKPDS) reported the results of a randomized controlled trial comparing tight blood pressure control, average 144/82, with less tight control, average 154/87.[24] Nephropathy and glucose control were similar in both groups. UKPDS showed that over 9 years tight blood pressure control also reduced the risk of 3 lines of visual loss by 47%. Tight blood pressure control reduced the risk of progression of retinopathy by 34%. Tight blood pressure control also reduced the risk of photocoagulation by 37%. These results were independent of the patients randomization to treatment with an angiotensin converting enzyme inhibitor or beta-blocker. This study emphasises the importance of blood pressure control for preservation of vision in patients with DR.

Clearly, hypertension and nephropathy can be related and it is difficult to assess purely the role of one or the other in promoting or exacerbating DR.[25-27] Nephropathy itself is a predictor of DR (using serum BUN, creatinine, and/or proteinuria as evidence of nephropathy).[7,28-32] The opposite is also true: patients with symptomatic retinopathy have a higher rate of nephropathy.[33]

Puberty

The role of puberty in the development and progression of DR is not well understood but several studies suggest a significant causal relationship.[10,14,15] When looking at duration of DM, and its relationship to the development of DR in young patients, it appears that the number of years of DM prior to puberty are not as important[12,14,15,34] as the number after puberty.

Pregnancy

The role of pregnancy in DR development and progression has been more controversial. The risk of developing DR, in patients who enter pregnancy with no evidence of DR, has been reported as approximately 10%.[35] Progression of DR has also been reported with subsequent partial

331

regression after delivery.[36-38] It is difficult to assess pregnancy's effect on DR independent of the natural history of DM or DR. In 1990, Klein, et al performed a well controlled study and concluded that current pregnancy was unquestionably an independent risk factor for retinopathy progression.[21] The etiology of this causal relationship may simply relate to hyperglycemia suddenly changing from poorly controlled prior to pregnancy to tightly controlled during pregnancy.[37,39,40] As noted these changes may be partially reversible after delivery. Fortunately, there is good evidence that laser photocoagulation for DR prior to or during pregnancy has beneficial effects, and may prevent or limit progression during pregnancy.[35]

CLINICAL FINDINGS & PATHOGENESIS

The clinical definitions of diabetic retinopathy focus on vascular lesions. Other tissues are also damaged but there is practical clinical value in using vessel disease for classification. The vessels are easily seen and categorized and the condition of the vessels is of great use prognostically. The vascular changes progress along a recognized spectrum of disease which is directly related to risk of vision loss.

Non-Proliferative Diabetic Retinopathy (NPDR)

NPDR is characterized clinically by the presence of microaneurysms, nerve fiber layer infarcts (cotton wool spots), intraretinal hemorrhages, intraretinal microvascular abnormalities (IRMA), venous beading, vascular dilation and macular edema (Figure 1).

The initial lesion of diabetic retinopathy is a microangiopathy involving the small arterioles, capillaries and venules. Microaneurysms, capillary closure, basement membrane thickening, loss of pericytes and IRMA are histopathologically documented in the small vessels of diabetics.[41-43]

Microaneurysms are the first lesions seen by ophthalmoscopy. They appear as small red dots in the substance of the retina which represent small outpouchings of the capillary wall. If they rupture in the deep layers of the inner retina they produce a dot hemorrhage. If they rupture in the nerve fiber layer the blood forms a flame-shaped hemorrhage. They have an incompetent blood-retinal barrier and leak plasma components. This contributes to macular edema and lipid deposition. Fluorescein angiography demonstrates leakage of dye from patent microaneurysms.

Capillary closure is a feature of NPDR which increases as the disease progresses. It leaves increasing portions of inner retina unperfused. This is not directly visible on clinical exam but is readily apparent on fluorescein angiography (Figure 1, right). The mechanism of the closure is unknown. Capillary non-perfusion provides a stimulus for neovascularization. Capillary non-perfusion usually affects the peripheral retina before the macula. Capillary closure in the macula may erode the capillaries at the edge of the foveal avascular zone (FAZ) producing an undersirable enlargement of the FAZ. If it affects a large portion of the macula it produces an ischemic macula and severe loss of vision. There is no known way of restoring capillary patency.

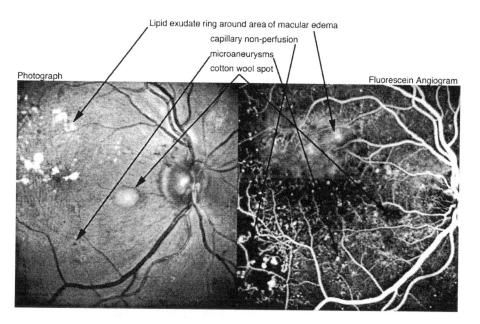

Figure 1. Non-proliferative diabetic retinopathy.

Nerve fiber layer infarcts are also known as soft exudates or cotton-wool spots. They appear as white fluffy areas in the nerve fiber layer. They are accumulations of stalled axoplasmic flow in the retinal ganglion cell axons and usually occur in areas of ischemic damage.[44]

IRMA appear as dilated retinal capillaries and can be difficult to differentiate from surface retinal neovascularization on clinical exam. They serve as shunt vessels adjacent to areas of non-perfusion. Fluorescein dye does not leak from IRMA while it leaks profusely from neovascularization.

Venous beading refers to a beaded or bumpy look of the large veins. The normal uniform diameter may become highly variable in advanced NPDR. The veins may also form loops. This is a sign of sluggish retinal circulation and an indicator of the presence of capillary nonperfusion. Early in NPDR the vasculature shows dilation.

Macular Edema is one of the most important causes of visual loss in DR. It appears as retinal thickening on stereoscopic biomicroscopy using a

+90, +78, or +60 diopter lens or contact lens. If the thickening is great enough cysts form in the retina, known as cystoid macular edema (CME). The thickening is due to fluid accumulation. Increased capillary permeability and decreased vascular resistance upstream of capillaries produce changes in oncotic and hydrostatic pressures respectively which foster fluid collection.[45] Microaneurysms leak plasma components. The water and protein transudate components lead to edema. Lipids in the transudate may deposit in the retina as hard exudates.

Proliferative Diabetic Retinopathy (PDR)
PDR is characterized by new vessel growth from retinal vessels. Neovascularization appears as fine red vessels over the optic disk or elsewhere growing on the surface of the retina or into the vitreous (Figure 2). These vessels usually appear at the borders of non-perfused retina but do not help relieve the non-perfusion problem. Fluorescein angiography is very useful for revealing the pronounced capillary non-perfusion and neovascular leakage characteristic of PDR.

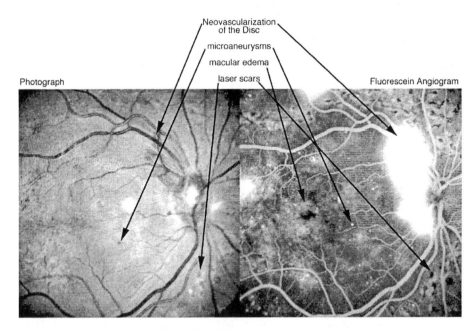

Figure 2. Proliferative diabetic retinopathy.

Patients with PDR are at risk for severe visual loss for several reasons. The neovascularization is fragile and prone to bleed producing vitreous hemorrhage. As new vessels proliferate there is a fibrous contractile response in the vitreous. This places traction on the retina which can produce

334

macular edema, macular drag (heterotopia) or a tractional retinal detachment. If the traction is great enough a hole may develop producing a rhegamatogenous retinal detachment. The neovascular stimulus may produce neovascularization of the iris (NVI), subsequent neovascularization of the drainage angle (NVA) and finally neovascular glaucoma (NVG). The degree of visual impairment varies depending on the type and extent of pathology. It may be minimal or produce no light perception.

Molecular Mechanisms of Diabetic Retinopathy

The cellular and biochemical events involved in DR have received increasing attention in recent years. Experimental evidence has amassed for the involvement of several metabolic and cell signaling pathways in the pathophysiologic changes of DR.

The occurrence of retinal neovascularization in disorders which produce ischemic retina such as DR, sickle cell anemia, central retinal vein occlusion and others suggests a common mechanism. The hypothesis of growth factor involvment is attributed to Michaelson.[3] Some of the requirements for a growth factor which could induce retinopathy are the following: the growth factor must be induced by ischemia, produced by retinal cells, able to induce endothelial cell growth, diffusable in the eye, elevated before or as neovascularizatin occurs and reduced with regression of neovascularization.

Miller et al reviewed the substantial evidence which implicates vascular endothelial growth factor (VEGF) in retinal neovascularization (46). VEGF is produced by retinal cells in response to hypoxia.[47] It is a potent mediator of vascular permeability[48] and vascular endothelial proliferation.[49] These changes characterize macular edema and new vessel growth respectively. It has high affinity receptors present on endothelial cells[50] and has freely soluble and bound isoforms.[51] These different forms may account for the neovasculariztion commonly found immediately adjacent to ischemic retina and iris neovascularization which is distant to ischemic areas. VEGF is increased in the ocular fluid of patients with PDR when compared to NPDR, and the intraocular concentration of VEGF falls after successful scatter laser photocoagulation.[52] Intravitreal injections of VEGF are sufficient to produce NVI in non human primates[53] Experiments have shown that VEGF is necessary for ischemia induced neovascularization. Antagonism of VEGF activity using various techniques inhibits neovascularization in animal models of ischemia-induced intraocular neovascularization.[54,55]

A number of theories exist to explain the changes of non proliferative DR. The roles of protein kinase C, advanced glycosylation end products and the sorbitol pathway are briefly described below.

335

The protein kinase C (PKC) family of enzymes functions in intracellular signaling and is implicated along with VEGF in the pathogenesis of diabetes.[56] PKC has several isoforms most of which modulate their phosphorylating activitiy in proportion to diacylglycerol (DAG) and Ca^{+2} levels. Diabetes produces several metabolic changes which increase the activity of PKC. Hyperglycemia increases DAG concentrations and leads to activation of PKC beta in the retina.[57] PKC activation regulates hypoxia and hyperglycemia induced VEGF expression.[58,59] Additionally VEGF induces a dose-dependent increase in PKC activity.[60] A PKC beta inhibitor (LY333531)[61] has been used to provide compelling experimental evidence for the role of PKC in diabetic disease. Oral LY333531 reverses the increases in retinal mean circulation time seen in diabetic rats.[62] Oral or intravitreal LY333531 prevents the increased retinal permeability normally caused by intravitreal injection of VEGF.[63] In vitro, LY333531 inhibits VEGF induced endothelial cell proliferation.[60] Oral LY333531 suppresses neovascularization in a porcine central retinal vein occlusion model of neovascularization.[64] PKC is involved in the pathways for expression of VEGF and for production of effects of VEGF. These findings and the lack of clinical side effects have led to a multicenter randomized controlled clinical trial of LY333531 for DR. The results of the trial are eagerly awaited.

The involvement of advanced glycosylation end products (AGE) is postulated in DR. AGE are the result of non-enzymatic condensation reactions of reducing sugars with amine groups on proteins, lipids and nucleic acids.[65] The Maillard reaction is the name given to this complex series of reactions which through the production of reactive intermediates over weeks to months can cross-link long-lived macromolecules.[66] The Maillard reaction is responsible for the "browning" of foods. The hemoglobin A_{1c} (HgbA$_{1c}$) assay measures glycated hemoglobin which is an Amadori product, not an AGE but the first step on the path to AGE. AGE are implicated in various diverse diseases by their co-localization with pathologic findings. AGE accumulates in retinal vessels of diabetic and AGE exposed rats.[67] Basement membrane thickening and an accumulation of basement membrane material seen in the retina of diabetic mice is reduced with antibodies that specifically recognize Amadori-modified glycated albumin.[68] Administration of AGE-modified albumin to non diabetic rats leads to increased vascular permeability and increased expression of VEGF mRNA.[69] Incubation of retinal microvascular endothelial cells in high ambient glucose or glycated albumin produces a dose-dependent reduction of nitric oxide (NO) synthesis.[70] PKC inhibitors partially restore NO synthesis. This study implicates glycated proteins and PKC in the vascular dysfunction of DR. Aminoguanadine (pimagedine) inhibits AGE formation. In Phase III clinical trials over 1 year pimagedine reduced progression of retinopathy in type 1 diabetics by 50%.[65] Its usefulness however may be limited by side effects.

The polyol pathway is another suspect in the pathogenesis of DR. High glucose concentrations lead to saturation of hexokinase and with subsequent increased glucose flux through the alternate sorbitol (polyol) pathway.[71] The accumulation of sorbitol and fructose is hypothesized to generate osmotic and oxidative stress. Aldose reductase inhibitors reduce glucose flux through the sorbitol pathway. They reduce the accumulation of the pathway metabolites, sorbitol and fructose, reduce osmotic stress and impact on pathway cofactors. An inhibitor of aldose reductase normalizes sorbitol, fructose, and other metabolite concentrations in a in vitro model of rat retina.[72] The aldose reductase inhibitor ponalrestat ameliorates capillary basement membrane thickening in diabetic rats.[73] The Sorbinol Retinopathy Trial Research Group examined the effect of sorbinil, an aldose reductase inhibitor, on the progression of DR in humans. A 3 year trial of sorbinil failed to show a reduction of DR progression.[74]

A recent preliminary report ties PKC, AGE and sorbitol observations together.[75] Elevated glucose concentrations produce reactive oxygen species in bovine aortic endothelial cells. In vitro inhibition of superoxide production succeeded in abolishing the elevations of PKC activity, AGE formation and sorbitol formation usually induced by incubation in high concentrations of glucose. This suggests that elevated superoxide production from the mitochondrial electron transport chain is a causal link between elevated glucose levels and pathogenic changes in PKC, AGE and sorbitol.

DIFFERENTIAL DIAGNOSIS

Any retinal vascular disease causing retinal edema, hemorrhages, lipid exudates, cotton wool spots, retinal ischemia, and/or retinal or optic disc neovascularization can mimic DR. There are many clinical situations where other conditions can result in these physical findings and be considered in the differential diagnosis of DR.

Hypertensive retinopathy, in its more advanced or severe stages, can resemble DR. In a patient with both severe hypertension and diabetes, it can be difficult to assess the proportionate role of either in the development of retinopathy. Conversely, mild hypertensive retinopathy would rarely be confused with DR. Many patients with even mild hypertension, however, develop retinal vein occlusions, which can closely mimic DR (Figure 3). Fortunately, the hemorrhages and other retinal changes in vein occlusions usually have a geographic distribution within the retina (outlining an area drained by a single vein) rendering the diagnosis more clear. DR tends to be more diffuse in its presentation. Additionally, vein occlusions are almost always more abrupt in onset and cause sudden visual symptoms whereas DR can be more chronic and insidious.

Radiation retinopathy can be identical to DR but there is usually an obvious antecedent history of ocular radiation exposure (usually a few months to a few years prior to clinical signs and symptoms). Sickle cell disease tends to create retinopathy more anteriorly in the retina than DR and can easily be screened with a sickle prep or hemoglobin electrophoresis. Carotid insufficiency retinopathy is relatively uncommon and is usually unilateral whereas DR tends to be bilateral.

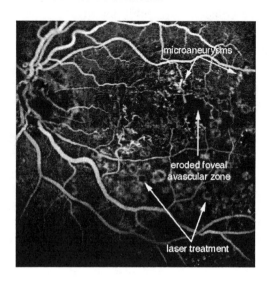

Figure 3. Branch vein occlusion.

NATURAL COURSE

There is evidence that visual function is affected early in diabetes before there is clinical evidence of vascular changes. The electroretinogram shows depressed oscillatory B wave function.[76] Color and contrast sensitivity testing may show subtle defects.[77] Although most patients perceive no change in vision, some, particularly those who work in graphic arts complain of loss of color and contrast discrimination despite a normal retinal exam.

There are several diabetes related causes of visual loss in addition to those directly due to retinopathy. These include problems of the ocular media: corneal epithelial erosions, cataracts, and transient lens swelling. Wide fluctuations in blood sugar can lead to osmotic lens swelling and blurred vision correctable with a change in spectacle refraction. The knowledgeable eye professional refers these patients to an internist to confirm the suspicion of diabetes. Optic nerve papillopathy and diabetic cranial neuropathies can reduce vision.

The causes of vision loss attributable to diabetic retinopathy include macular ischemia, macular edema, and hemorrhage. Fibrotic contraction (cicatrization) of the neovascular tissue characteristic of proliferative diabetic retinopathy produces retina traction. Traction can induce macular distortion (macular heterotopia), edema, and tractional or rhegomatogenous retinal detachments.

Patients are often not symptomatic until they have advanced PDR. Regular dilated fundus exams by an eye professional are needed to detect DR before it becomes advanced.[78] Advanced disease is much harder to stabilize and the risk of vision loss in this case is greater than if DR is managed on a regular basis. The natural history and effects of therapeutic trials were examined in several large national clinical trials summarized below. Implementing the conclusions of these trials can reduce visual loss by over 90%.[4]

EXAMINATION TECHNIQUE

Direct or indirect ophthalmoscopy can be used to visualize the fundus. Direct ophthalmoscopy is readily available and provides a magnified image. It suffers from its limited (5°) field of view and lack of stereopsis. Welch Allyn's new PanOptic (TM) Ophthalmoscope, introduced in March 2001, offers the ease of use of a handheld direct, a magnified image and a 25° field of view.[79] Slit lamp biomicroscope ophthalmoscopy using a contact, +90D, or +78D lens generates the best view of the retina posterior to the equator of the eye. Magnification, light intensity and stereopsis are excellent. Head mounted indirect ophthalmoscopy with a +20D or +28D lens offers the best view of the peripheral retina which lies anterior to the equator. Both the slit lamp biomicroscope and head mounted indirect are technically challenging and of limited availability.

Fluorescein angiography (FA) is a valuable tool in diagnosing causes of visual loss in diabetics (Figure 2). Sodium fluorescein is loosely bound to albumin and normally does not cross the tight junctions of the retinal pigment epithelial cells or the retinal vascular endothelial cells. This intact blood-retinal barrier normally prevents leakage of fluorescein into the retina. When normal barrier function is lost, leakage of fluorescein pinpoints areas of diabetic macular edema, traction, ischemia and neovascularization. Lack of hyperfluorescence demonstrates areas of nonperfusion. Despite the sensitivity of FA for these lesions it is not used to screen for DR. FA is used to guide treatment of macular edema, look for neovascularization and evaluate unexplained visual loss.

TREATMENT

Impact of clinical trials.
Ophthalmology's entry into the modern era of NIH funded large-scale multi-center clinical trials was heralded by the Diabetic Retinopathy Study.[80] The national trials have set the standard of care for many aspects of DR as well as other ophthalmic diseases. Kertes and Conway have provided a very useful summary of clinical trials in ophthalmology.[81]

Diabetic Retinopathy Study (DRS)
Laser photocoagulation is currently the most common modality employed in the surgical treatment of diabetic retinopathy. Treatment of the neovascular lesions of diabetic retinopathy with light dates to the 1950's with Meyer-Schwickerath's Xenon photocoagulator. Photocoagulation technique evolved over the decades from the direct treatment of neovascular lesions or their feeder vessels to treatment in a standard panretinal "scatter" pattern.

The DRS tested and proved the value of extensive "scatter" photocoagulation (panretinal photocoagulaton, PRP) in reducing the risk of severe visual loss in patients with proliferative diabetic retinopathy.[80,82] Additionally the natural history of disease was examined with attention paid to identifying "high-risk characteristics" for visual loss.

1758 patients were enrolled from 1972 to 1975. Eligible patients had a confirmed diagnosis of diabetes (type 1 or type 2), vision better than 20/100 in each eye, media clear enough to undergo photocoagulation and PDR in one eye or severe NDPR in both eyes. One eye of each participant was randomized to "scatter" photocoagulation while the other was followed without treatment. The primary outcome measured in the DRS was the development of severe visual loss, defined as visual acuity less than 5/200.

Analysis of the data showed a 50% reduction in severe vision loss in treated eyes (Figure 4). Although the percentage of patients with severe visual loss increases with time for both treated and untreated groups, the risk for the treated group is significantly lower at all times after treatment.

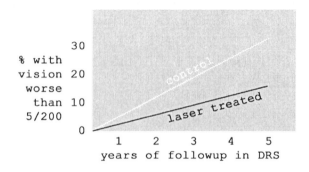

Figure 4. Results of Diabetic Retinopathy Study (DRS).

340

Examination of the characteristics of the proliferative disease in patients who progressed to severe visual loss revealed features associated with increased risk. These features are: 1) vitreous hemorrhage in the presence of any neovascularization or 2) moderate neovascularization of the disc regardless of vitreous hemorrhage. Practically speaking ophthalmolscopically obvious NVD is at least moderate in extent. The presence of high-risk characteristics bestowed the untreated eyes with a 2 year risk for severe visual loss of 25% to 37%. Scatter treatment reduced that risk by 50%.

Early Treatment Diabetic Retinopathy Study (ETDRS)
While the DRS proved the benefit of PRP in reducing severe visual loss in PDR with high risk characteristics it did not provide clear direction in cases of less advanced retinopathy. The question remained as to whether prompt treatment or deferral of treatment until reaching high risk characteristics provided better preservation of vision.[83]

The ETDRS addressed three questions:[84]
1) When in the course of diabetic retinopathy is it most effective to initiate photocoagulation?
2) Is photocoagulation effective for the treatment of macular edema?
3) Does aspirin alter the course of diabetic retinopathy?

Eligible patients had mild NPDR to early PDR with visual acuity better than 20/200 in each eye. 3711 patients were enrolled from 1980 to 1985. The patients were 50% male, 76% white and 70% type 2 diabetics. The primary outcome measure was the development of severe visual loss defined as vision worse than 5/200.

One eye of each patient was assigned to either early photocoagulation or to deferral of photocoagulaton. Five year rates of severe visual loss were 2.6% in the early treatment group and 3.7% in the deferral group.[85] The small benefit of early treatment was offset by adverse affects of scatter photocoagulation on visual acuity and visual fields. As a result scatter photocoagulation is not recommended for mild to moderate nonproliferative diabetic retinopathy. Scatter photocoagulation should be considered for advanced NPDR and PDR. It should not be deferred in eyes with high risk characteristics for visual loss.

The ETDRS also examined the benefit of focal and grid photocoagulation for diabetic macular edema. They defined clinically significant macular edema (CSME) as:
1) retinal thickening within 500μm of the fovea;
2) exudate within 500μm of the fovea contiguous with retinal thickening
3) retinal thickening greater than 1 disc area in size within one disc diameter of the fovea.

Focal and grid photocoagulation were found to reduce the risk of moderate visual loss, defined as loss of 3 lines on the vision chart, by about 50%.

The use of aspirin to medically treat DR was based on clinical observations and the reasoning that the anti-platelet function of aspirin may be able to help prevent capillary closure seen in DR and thus forestall DR progression.[84] The ETDRS showed no effect of 650 mg of aspirin daily on the progression of retinopathy or visual loss. Additionally this dose of aspirin did not increase the frequency of vitreous hemorrhage.[86] Aspirin did however reduce the risk of cardiac events by 17% compared to the non-aspirin taking group.[87] The ETDRS showed that aspirin should be used in diabetics not to influence DR but to reduce increased risk for cardiac morbidity. PDR is not a contraindication to aspirin use.

Diabetic Retinopathy Vitrectomy Study (DRVS)

Vitreous hemorrhage from PDR can produce media opacity sufficient for severe visual loss. This occurs when the disease advances to severe proliferation of vessels and fibrous tissue before photocoagulation can be offered or when it progresses despite photocoagulation. The development of a vitreous cutter by Machemer permitted the removal of the vitreous gel.[88] Vitrectomy allows the removal of media obscuring blood. It is also used to relieve detachment producing retinal traction caused by cicatrized fibrovascular tissue and vitreous.

Controversy existed over the role of vitrectomy for severe PDR. At the time of the study vitrectomy was not offered unless VH persisted beyond a year. The DRVS examined the value of vitrectomy soon after VH and in cases prior to VH. It asked two questions in addition to examining the natural history of eyes with severe PDR. Is early vitrectomy advantageous in cases of:

1) very severe PDR?
2) severe vitreous hemorrhage from PDR?

For the first question 370 eyes with severe PDR, no hemorrhage and acuity of 20/400 or better were randomly assigned to either early vitrectomy or conventional management. After 4 years of follow-up, the percentage of eyes with a visual acuity of 20/40 or better was 44% in the early vitrectomy group and 28% in the conventional management group. The proportion with very poor visual outcome was similar in the two groups. The advantage of early vitrectomy tended to increase with increasing severity of new vessels. In the group with the least severe new vessels, no advantage of early vitrectomy was apparent.[89]

For the second question 616 eyes with recent severe diabetic VH were randomly assigned to either early vitrectomy or deferral of vitrectomy for 1 year. Early vitrectomy produced a higher proportion of eyes seeing 20/40 or better throughout the 4 year follow-up. Early vitrectomy increased the chances of good vision most in eyes with more severe PDR. The advantage of early vitectomy was not found in those patients who were older and tended to have less severe retinopathy.

The findings support early vitrectomy in eyes with very severe PDR for improving the chances of restoring or maintaining good vision.[90]

Diabetes Control and Complications Trial (DCCT)

It is sensible to postulate that the complications of diabetes including DR will be fewer when blood glucose is under better control. Circumstantial evidence for this was provided in a population based observational study, the Wisconsin Epidemiologic Study of Diabetic Retinopathy.[91] Conclusive evidence for this was provided in a multicenter, randomized clinical trial, The Diabetes Control and Complications Trial (DCCT). The DCCT sought to answer two questions:

1) Does intensive treatment of blood glucose reduce the incidence of diabetic retinopathy in those who do not yet have it? The patients recruited for this arm of the study (primary-prevention) had a diagnoisis of type 1 DM but no DR on clinical examination.

2) The second question was: does tight control of blood glucose reduce the progression of diabetic retinopathy? The patients recruited for this arm of the study (secondary-intervention) had type 1 DM and mild to moderate non proliferative DR (NPDR).

The study enrolled 1441 type 1 diabetics aged 13 to 39 with good vision and no hypertension, hypercholesterolemia or severe complications of diabetes. In the entire study population the patients assigned to intensive treatment maintained a $HgbA_{1c}$ (~7%) about 2 percentage points lower than those assigned to conventional treatment group (~9%).

The results showed that intensive treatment reduced the risk for both onset and progression of DR. Those in the primary-prevention arm receiving intensive treatment had a 76% reduction of their risk for development of DR. Likewise patients in the secondary-intervention arm receiving intensive treatment reduced their risk of DR progression by 54%.

In summary, the DCCT showed that tight control of blood glucose reduced the incidence and progression of DR. The amount of risk reduction was proportional to the degree of $HgbA_{1c}$ decrease. The treatment benefit was not apparent until after three years. An unexpected finding was that some patients in the tight control group experienced a worsening of DR soon after the initiation of tight control. However, the long-term benefits of tight control on vision outweighed the early worsening.

Can the conclusions of the DCCT be applied to all type 1 diabetics? Comparison of DCCT patient characteristics with those of the population-based WESDR study type 1 patients show demographic and clinical similarities.[92] This suggests that the conclusions can be applied to the general population of type 1 diabetics.

United Kingdom Prospective Diabetes Study Group (UKPDS)

The UKPDS was a randomized clinical trial performed in 23 centers in Britain over 20 years. It sought to determine the effect of intensive blood glucose control on predetermined clinical end points. More than 5000 patients with type 2 diabetes were recruited. The UKPDS demonstrated a 28% reduction in the retinal photocoagulation of type 2 patients with intensive therapy ($HgbA_{1c}$ = 7%) compared to type 2 patients under conventional therapy ($HgbA_{1c}$ = 7.9%).[93] This finding confirms the benefit of reduced blood glucose for type 2 diabetics.

Clinical Treatment Recommendations

The trials reviewed above provide solid evidence upon which to base treatment of DR. Clinical practice still requires good clinical judgement in deciding when and how to treat each patient. General guidelines are provided below.

CSME is treated as per the recommendations of the ETDRS with focal or grid photocoagulation. Using a plano contact lens and 100μm spot size enough power (typically 80-100mW) of a green or yellow laser is applied for 0.1 seconds to just whiten the outer retina. Leaking microanuerysms may be treated directly or they may be ignored in favor of a grid of treatment spots across the macula. Most retina specialists combine a grid treatment with focal treatment of some particularly leaky microanuerysms.

NPDR is treated with copious advice and encouragement about the benefits of good blood glucose control and value of regular follow up with physicians. Laser treatment is usually not offered.

PDR is treated with scatter laser photocoagulation (panretinal photocoagulation, PRP) when high risk characteristics (HRC) are reached as per the recommendations of the DRS and ETDRS. PRP may be given before HRC are reached for several reasons: poor patient compliance, impending cataract surgery, aggressive disease in this eye or the other, comorbidities, and pregnancy. Treatment is with visible or infrared laser light, 200mW, 0.2 seconds, and 400μm diameter spot for a total of 1200 to 1500 solid white spots. When ME exists with NPDR or PDR treatment with scatter photocoagulation may exacerbate the ME. Splitting the treatments over 2 or 3 sittings reduces this risk. Advanced PDR may require 4000 to 6000 spots. This essentially ablates the retina peripheral to the vascular arcades.

VH is given a variable amount of time to clear before vitrectomy is offered, typically 3 months. Uniocular patients or those with bilateral hemorrhages are offered surgery when they can no longer live their lives with the visual impairment. Consistent with findings in the DRVS those with active severe PDR benefit more from earlier intervention.

Tractional retinal detachments (TRD) are generally not treated with vitrectomy until they threaten or actually detach the macula.

Macular ischemia and other areas of capillary non perfusion have no treatment at this time.

EXAMINATION GUIDELINES

Type 1 diabetics are seen yearly by ophthalmologists or others knowledgeable about DR with a dilated funduscopic examination starting 5 years after diagnosis. Type 2 diabetics are seen yearly upon diagnosis. Yearly follow-up is acceptable as long as there is no DR or only mild NPDR. Moderate NPDR should be evaluated twice a year, severe NPDR every 4 months, and early PDR and PDR with HRC every 2 to 3 months.[78]

SUMMARY

It is well known that one of the most potentially devastating complications of diabetes mellitus is diabetic retinopathy. Although it is not well understood how chronic hyperglycemia results in this very specific and (in some ways) unique microvascular retinal disease, it is proven that excellent control of the hyperglycemia reduces the incidence and severity of disease. We also know that the most important risk factor for the development of retinopathy is duration of diabetes. Until about 30 years ago, there was little that ophthalmologists could offer as specific treatment for retinopathy. As has been reviewed in this chapter, the last three decades have seen tremendous advances in the specific treatment of proliferative diabetic retinopathy, macular edema, vitreous hemorrhage, and retinal detachment, the most sight-threatening complications of diabetic retinopathy. The development of laser and vitrectomy techniques, and their appropriate testing with randomized controlled clinical trials, has improved our management of these problems and, therefore, the quality of our patients' lives. Clearly, none of these treatments are cures for the overall disease process. Much attention is now directed toward understanding the pathogenesis and molecular biology underlying diabetic retinopathy. There have been many studies in the last decade analyzing the role of vascular endothelial growth factor and other mediators in the pathogenesis of retinopathy. It is our hope that important discoveries in this area will lead directly to a cure or prevention of diabetic retinopathy in the near future.

REFERENCES

1. Kahn HA and Hiller R. Blindness caused by diabetic retinopathy. Am J Ophthalmol 78(1):58-67, 1974.
2. Vision Problems in the US: A Statistical Analysis. New York, National Society to Prevent Blindness, 1980.
3. Flynn HW, Smiddy WE, ed. Diabetes and ocular disease : past, present, and future therapies. Ophthalmology Monographs. Vol. 14, Am Acad Ophthal 334, 2000.
4. Ferris FL 3rd. How effective are treatments for diabetic retinopathy? Jama 269(10):1290-1, 1993.
5. Banting FG, Best CH. The internal secretion of the pancreas. J Lab Clin Med 7:251-266, 1922.
6. Meyer-Schwickerath G. Light coagulation. St. Louis: Mosby - Yearbook, Inc., 1960.
7. Klein R et al. The Wisconsin epidemiologic study of diabetic retinopathy. II. Prevalence and risk of diabetic retinopathy when age at diagnosis is less than 30 years. Arch Ophthalmol 102(4):520-6, 1984.
8. Klein R et al. The Wisconsin epidemiologic study of diabetic retinopathy. III. Prevalence and risk of diabetic retinopathy when age at diagnosis is 30 or more years. Arch Ophthalmol 102(4):527-32, 1984.
9. Klein R et al. The Wisconsin epidemiologic study of diabetic retinopathy. IV. Diabetic macular edema. Ophthalmology 91(12):1464-74, 1984.
10. Klein R et al. Retinopathy in young-onset diabetic patients. Diabetes Care 8(4):311-5, 1985.
11. Klein R et al. Glycosylated hemoglobin predicts the incidence and progression of diabetic retinopathy. JAMA 260(19):2864-71, 1988.
12. Kostraba JN et al. Contribution of diabetes duration before puberty to development of microvascular complications in IDDM subjects. Diabetes Care 12(10):686-93, 1989.
13. Sjolie AK. Ocular complications in insulin treated diabetes mellitus. An epidemiological study. Acta Ophthalmol Suppl 172:1-77, 1985.
14. Palmberg P et al. The natural history of retinopathy in insulin-dependent juvenile-onset diabetes. Ophthalmology 88(7):613-8, 1981.
15. Frank RN et al. Retinopathy in juvenile-onset type I diabetes of short duration. Diabetes 31(10):874-82, 1982.
16. Frank RN et al. Retinopathy in juvenile-onset diabetes of short duration. Ophthalmology 87(1):1-9, 1980.
17. Dwyer MS et al. Incidence of diabetic retinopathy and blindness: a population-based study in Rochester, Minnesota. Diabetes Care 8(4):316-22, 1985.

18. Yanko L et al. Prevalence and 15-year incidence of retinopathy and associated characteristics in middle-aged and elderly diabetic men. Brit J Ophthalmol 67(11): p. 759-65, 1983.
19. Aiello LM et al. Diabetic retinopathy in Joslin Clinic patients with adult-onset diabetes. Ophthalmology 88(7):619-23, 1981.
20. Klein R et al. Is blood pressure a predictor of the incidence or progression of diabetic retinopathy? Arch Intern Med 149(11):2427-32, 1989.
21. Klein BE, SE Moss, and Klein R. Effect of pregnancy on progression of diabetic retinopathy. Diabetes Care 13(1): p. 34-40, 1990.
22. Knowler WC, Bennett PH, and Ballintine EJ. Increased incidence of retinopathy in diabetics with elevated blood pressure. A six-year follow-up study in Pima Indians. N Engl J Med 302(12):645-50, 1980.
23. Kornerup T. Studies in diabetic retinopathy. Acta Med Scand 153:81-101, 1955.
24. Anonymous. Tight blood pressure control and risk of macrovascular and microvascular complications in type 2 diabetes: UKPDS 38. UK Prospective Diabetes Study Group. Brit Med J 317 (7160):703-13, 1998.
25. Janka HU et al. Risk factors for progression of background retinopathy in long-standing IDDM. Diabetes 38(4): 460-4, 1989.
26. Dornan T, JI Mann, and R Turner. Factors protective against retinopathy in insulin-dependent diabetics free of retinopathy for 30 years. Brit Med J (Clin Res Ed) 285(6348):1073-7, 1982.
27. Gray RS et al. HLA antigens and other risk factors in the development of retinopathy in type 1 diabetes. Brit J Ophthalmol 66(5):280-5, 1982.
28. Jerneld B and P Algvere. Proteinuria and blood glucose levels in a population with diabetic retinopathy. Am J Ophthalmol 104(3): p. 283-9, 1987.
29. Young RJ et al. Alcohol: another risk factor for diabetic retinopathy? Brit Med J (Clin Res Ed) 288(6423):1035-7, 1984.
30. Barnett AH et al. Microalbuminuria and diabetic retinopathy. Lancet 1(8419):53-4, 1985.
31. Microalbuminuria predicts proliferative diabetic retinopathy. Lancet 1(8444): p. 1512-3, 1985.
32. Nelson RG et al. Proliferative retinopathy in NIDDM. Incidence and risk factors in Pima Indians. Diabetes 38(4):435-40, 1989.
33. Feldman JN, Beyer MM, et al. Prevalence of diabetic nephropathy at time of treatment for diabetic retinopathy. In : Diabetic Renal – Retinal Syndrome, ed. L.E.F. Firedman EA. Vol 2., New York: Grune & Stratton. 9, 1982.
34. Becker B. Diabetes and glaucoma. Vascular complications of diabetes mellitus, ed. K.S.a.K. WM. St Louis: Mosby – Yearbook, Inc., 1967.

35. Dibble CM et al. Effect of pregnancy on diabetic retinopathy. Obstet Gynecol 59(6):699-704, 1982.
36. Ohrt V. The influence of pregnancy on diabetic retinopathy with special regard to the reversible changes shown in 100 pregnancies. Acta Ophthalmol (Copenh) 62(4):603-16, 1984.
37. Moloney JB, Drury MI. The effect of pregnancy on the natural course of diabetic retinopathy. Am J Ophthalmol 93(6):745-56, 1982.
38. Laatikainen L et al. Occurrence and prognostic significance of retinopathy in diabetic pregnancy. Metab Pediatr Ophthalmol 4(4):191-5, 1980.
39. Sinclair SH et al. Macular edema and pregnancy in insulin-dependent diabetes. Am J Ophthalmol 97(2):154-67, 1984.
40. Phelps RL et al. Changes in diabetic retinopathy during pregnancy. Correlations with regulation of hyperglycemia. Arch Ophthalmol 104(12):1806-10, 1986.
41. Bloodworth J. Diabetic microangiopathy. Diabetes 12:99, 1963.
42. Toussaint D, Dustin P. Electron micorscopy of normal and diabetic retinal capillaries. Arch Ophthalm 70:96, 1963.
43. Ashton N. Vascular basement membrane changes in diabetic retinopathy. Br J Ophthal 58:344, 1974.
44. Apple DJ, Rabb MF. Ocular Pathology. Third ed. St Louis: C.V. Mosby. 560, 1985.
45. Kristinsson JK, Gottfredsdottir MS, Stefansson E. Retinal vessel dilatation and elongation precedes diabetic macular oedema. Br J Ophthalmol 81(4): p. 274-8, 1997.
46. Miller JW, Adamis AP, Aiello LP. Vascular endothelial growth factor in ocular neovascularization and proliferative diabetic retinopathy. Diabetes-Metabolism Reviews 13(1):37-50, 1997.
47. Pierce EA et al. Vascular endothelial growth factor/vascular permeability factor expression in a mouse model of retinal neovascularization. Proc Natl Acad of Sci 92(3):905-9, 1995.
48. Senger DR et al. Purification and NH2-terminal amino acid sequence of guinea pig tumor-secreted vascular permeability factor. Cancer Research 50(6):1774-8, 1990.
49. Plate KH et al. Vascular endothelial growth factor is a potential tumour angiogenesis factor in human gliomas in vivo. Nature 359(6398):845-8, 1992.
50. Olander JV, Connolly DT, DeLarco JE. Specific binding of vascular permeability factor to endothelial cells. Biochem Biophysic Res Com 175(1):68-76, 1991.
51. Houck KA et al. Dual regulation of vascular endothelial growth factor bioavailability by genetic and proteolytic mechanisms. J Biol Chem 267(36): 26031-7, 1992.

52. Aiello LP et al. Vascular endothelial growth factor in ocular fluid of patients with diabetic retinopathy and other retinal disorders. N Engl J Med 331(22):1480-7, 1994.

53. Tolentino MJ et al. Intravitreous injections of vascular endothelial growth factor produce retinal ischemia and microangiopathy in an adult primate. Ophthal 103(11):1820-8, 1996.

54. Adamis AP et al. Inhibition of vascular endothelial growth factor prevents retinal ischemia-associated iris neovascularization in a nonhuman primate. Arch Ophthal 114(1):66-71, 1996.

55. Robinson GS et al. Oligodeoxynucleotides inhibit retinal neovascularization in a murine model of proliferative retinopathy. Proc Natl Acad Sci 93(10):4851-6, 1996.

56. Ways DK and MJ Sheetz. The role of protein kinase C in the development of the complications of diabetes. Vitamins & Hormones 60:149-93, 2000.

57. Xia P et al. Characterization of the mechanism for the chronic activation of diacylglycerol-protein kinase C pathway in diabetes and hypergalactosemia. Diabetes 43(9):1122-9, 1994.

58. Mazure NM et al. Induction of vascular endothelial growth factor by hypoxia is modulated by a phosphatidylinositol 3-kinase/Akt signaling pathway in Ha-ras-transformed cells through a hypoxia inducible factor-1 transcriptional element. Blood 90(9):3322-31, 1997.

59. Williams B et al. Glucose-induced protein kinase C activation regulates vascular permeability factor mRNA expression and peptide production by human vascular smooth muscle cells in vitro. Diabetes 46(9):1497-503, 1997.

60. Xia P et al. Characterization of vascular endothelial growth factor's effect on the activation of protein kinase C, its isoforms, and endothelial cell growth. J Clin Investigation 98(9):2018-26, 1996.

61. Jirousek MR et al. (S)-13-[(dimethylamino)methyl]-10,11,14,15-tetrahydro-4,9:16, 21-dimetheno-1H, 13H-dibenzo[e,k]pyrrolo[3,4-h][1,4,13]oxadiazacyclohexadecene-1,3(2H)-d ione (LY333531) and related analogues: isozyme selective inhibitors of protein kinase C beta. J Med Chem 39(14):2664-71, 1996.

62. Ishii H et al. Amelioration of vascular dysfunctions in diabetic rats by an oral PKC beta inhibitor. [see comments]. Science 272(5262):728-31, 1996.

63. Aiello LP et al. Vascular endothelial growth factor-induced retinal permeability is mediated by protein kinase C in vivo and suppressed by an orally effective beta-isoform-selective inhibitor. Diabetes 46(9):1473-80, 1997.

64. Danis RP et al. Inhibition of intraocular neovascularization caused by retinal ischemia in pigs by PKCbeta inhibition with LY333531. Investigative Ophthalmology & Visual Science 39(1):171-9, 1998.

65. Singh R et al. Advanced glycation end-products: a review. Diabetologia 44(2): 129-46, 2001.
66. Maillard LC. Action des acides amines sur les sucres: formation des melanoides par voie methodique. CR Acad Sci 154: 66-68, 1912.
67. Stitt AW et al. Advanced glycation end products (AGEs) co-localize with AGE receptors in the retinal vasculature of diabetic and of AGE-infused rats. Am J Pathol, 150(2):523-31, 1997.
68. Clements RS Jr, Robison WG Jr, and Cohen MP. Anti-glycated albumin therapy ameliorates early retinal microvascular pathology in db/db mice. J Diab Compl 12(1):28-33, 1998.
69. Stitt AW et al. Advanced glycation end products induce blood-retinal barrier dysfunction in normoglycemic rats. Molecular Cell Biology Research Communications 3(6):380-8, 2000.
70. Chakravarthy U et al. Constitutive nitric oxide synthase expression in retinal vascular endothelial cells is suppressed by high glucose and advanced glycation end products. Diabetes 47(6): p. 945-52, 1998.
71. Gonzalez RG et al. Direct measurement of polyol pathway activity in the ocular lens. Diabetes 33(2):196-9, 1984.
72. Van den Enden MK et al. Elevated glucose levels increase retinal glycolysis and sorbitol pathway metabolism. Implications for diabetic retinopathy. [see comments]. Investigative Ophthalmology & Visual Science 36(8):1675-85, 1995.
73. Chakrabarti S and Sima AA. Effect of aldose reductase inhibition and insulin treatment on retinal capillary basement membrane thickening in BB rats. Diabetes 38(9):1181-6, 1989.
74. Anonymous. A randomized trial of sorbinil, an aldose reductase inhibitor, in diabetic retinopathy. Sorbinil Retinopathy Trial Research Group. Arch Ophthal 108(9):1234-44, 1990.
75. Nishikawa T et al. Normalizing mitochondrial superoxide production blocks three pathways of hyperglycaemic damage. Nature 404(6779): 787-90, 2000.
76. Coupland SG. A comparison of oscillatory potential and pattern electroretinogram measures in diabetic retinopathy. Doc Ophthalmol 66(3):207-18, 1987.
77. Sokol S et al. Contrast sensitivity in diabetics with and without background retinopathy. Arch Ophthalmol 103(1):51-4, 1985.
78. Preferred Practice Pattern, Diabetic Retinopathy. American Academy of Ophthalmology: San Francisco. p. 36., 1998.
79. Panoptic ophthalmoscope. Welch Allyn, 2001.
80. Anonymous. Preliminary report on effects of photocoagulation therapy. The Diabetic retinopathy study research group. Am J Ophthal 81(4): 383-96, 1976.
81. Kertes PJ, Conway MD, ed. Clinical trials in ophthalmology: a summary and practice guide. Williams and Wilkins: Baltimore, 1998.

82. Anonymous. Diabetic retinopathy study research group: Design, methods, and baseline results. DRS report Number 6. Invest Ophthalmol Vis Sci 21:149-201, 1981.

83. Anonymous. Photocoagulation treatment of proliferative diabetic retinopathy. Clinical application of diabetic retinopathy study (DRS) findings, DRS Report Number 8. The Diabetic Retinopathy Study Research Group. Ophthalmology 88(7):583-600, 1981.

84. Anonymous. Early treatment diabetic retinopathy study design and baseline patient characteristics. ETDRS report number 7. Ophthalmology 98(Suppl 5):741-56, 1991.

85. Anonymous. Early photocoagulation for diabetic retinopathy. ETDRS report number 9. Early treatment diabetic retinopathy study research group. Ophthalmology 98(Suppl 5):766-85, 1991.

86. Anonymous. Effects of aspirin treatment on diabetic retinopathy. ETDRS report number 8. Early treatment diabetic retinopathy study research group. Ophthalmology 98(Suppl 5):757-65, 1991.

87. Anonymous. Aspirin effects on mortality and morbidity in patients with diabetes mellitus. Early treatment diabetic retinopathy study report 14. ETDRS Investigators. JAMA 268(10):1292-300, 1992.

88. Machemer R et al. Vitrectomy: a pars plana approach. Transactions - American Academy of Ophthalmology & Otolaryngology 75(4):813-20, 1971.

89. Anonymous. Early vitrectomy for severe proliferative diabetic retinopathy in eyes with useful vision. Results of a randomized trial-- Diabetic retinopathy vitrectomy study report 3. The Diabetic Retinopathy vitrectomy study research group. Ophthalmology 95(10):1307-20, 1998.

90. Anonymous. Early vitrectomy for severe vitreous hemorrhage in diabetic retinopathy. Four-year results of a randomized trial: Diabetic retinopathy vitrectomy study report 5. [erratum appears in Arch Ophthalmol Oct; 108(10):1452]. Arch Ophthal 108(7): 958-64, 1990.

91. Klein R et al. Relationship of hyperglycemia to the long-term incidence and progression of diabetic retinopathy. Arch Intern Med 154(19):2169-78, 1994.

92. Klein R and Moss S. A comparison of the study populations in the Diabetes Control and Complications Trial and the Wisconsin Epidemiologic Study of Diabetic Retinopathy. Arch Intern Med 155(7): 745-54, 1995.

93. Anonymous. Intensive blood-glucose control with sulphonylureas or insulin compared with conventional treatment and risk of complications in patients with type 2 diabetes (UKPDS 33). UK Prospective Diabetes Study (UKPDS) Group. [erratum appears in Lancet 1999 Aug 14;354(9178):602]. Lancet 352(9131):837-53, 1998.

ON-LINE RESOURCES:

Diabetic Retinopathy: Epidemiology, Diagnosis and Management,
http://www.aao.org/aaoweb1/OEC/405.cfm

Diabetes in America, http://diabetes-in-america.s-3.com/ Diabetes in
America, 2nd Edition, is a 733-page compilation and assessment
of epidemiologic, public health, and clinical data on diabetes and
its complications in the United States.

Chapter 5. Diabetic Nephropathy

Jordan L. Rosenstock and Gerald B. Appel

PREVALENCE AND COSTS OF DIABETIC RENAL DISEASE

Diabetes is the most important cause of end stage renal disease (ESRD) in the United States. Over 50% of all new patients entering ESRD programs are now diabetics and over one-third of the entire ESRD population of over 300,000 persons has diabetes mellitus as a cause of renal failure.[1] The increase in diabetics as a percentage of all patients developing ESRD has been about 2% annually with no indication of a future decline. The ESRD program cost now exceeds 16 billion dollars annually. The exact percentage of patients with type 1 and type 2 diabetes who will progress to ESRD has been debated. From 25-40% of type 1 patients will develop nephropathy and most will progress to ESRD.[2] If a type 1 diabetic has not developed proteinuria at 20-25 years, the risk of renal disease decreases to only a few percent. Of type 2 diabetes patients a smaller percentage will progress to ESRD. Nevertheless, since type 2 diabetics make up a far greater percentage of the overall diabetic population, the total number of diabetics who progress to ESRD is weighted towards type 2 rather than type 1 patients. Moreover, with improved treatment of hypertension and coronary heart disease, more type 2 diabetics are surviving long enough to develop ESRD. White patients have a lower risk of developing ESRD than do Blacks, Hispanics, or native Americans with type 2 diabetes. Almost 50% of diabetic Pima Indians develop nephropathy by 20 years of diabetes and 15% will have progressed by this time to ESRD.

CLINICAL MANIFESTATIONS AND COURSE OF DIABETIC NEPHROPATHY

At the earliest stage of diabetic glomerulopathy, before there is any elevation of the BUN, creatinine, or clinical proteinuria on routine dipstick, most patients who are destined to progress to clinical nephropathy have been shown to have an increased glomerular filtration rate. This is associated with an increased renal blood flow and an increase in renal size when measured by ultrasound. In animal models this hyperfiltration and increased renal plasma flow have been shown to correlate with increased transcapillary glomerular pressures, or intraglomerular hypertension.[2] In these models intraglomerular hypertension is associated with the development of proteinuria and glomerulosclerosis. Mechanisms which decrease the intraglomerular pressures (low protein diet and use of angiotensin converting enzyme [ACE] inhibitors or angiotensin II receptor antagonists) are associated with a decrease in both proteinuria and glomerulosclerosis.

In this early stage of diabetic renal disease, low but abnormal levels of albumin are present in the urine. The routine dipstick and standard laboratory assays for albumin will not detect albuminuria at this level, so called "microalbuminuria." One can check for microalbuminuria on a 24 hour urinary specimen, on a timed specimen, or with a spot urine albumin-to-creatinine ratio. The National Kidney Foundation (NKF) has declared all methods to be of comparable efficacy and predictive value when performed accurately. Normal values for urinary albumin excretion are <30 mg/dl (<20 mcg/min or a spot urine albumin/creatinine ratio <0.3). Microalbuminuria is defined as 30-300 mg albuminuria/day (20-200 mcg/min) and overt proteinuria as >300 mg/day (>200 mcg/min).

Several factors can cause transient increases in urinary protein excretion and thus lead to a positive test for microalbuminuria which might not necessarily imply incipient diabetic nephropathy. These include uncontrolled hyperglycemia, exercise, urinary infections, severe hypertension, congestive heart failure, and acute febrile illnesses.

In patients without clinically detectable dipstick positive proteinuria, screening for microalbuminuria should be performed annually in type 1 diabetics after five years of diabetes or at puberty, and in all type 2 diabetics.[3,4] Although at least two of three collections done in a 3-6 month period are recommended by the American Diabetes Association (ADA) and NKF to establish the presence of fixed microalbuminuria, many clinicians feel a single abnormal value in a setting excluding the above interfering influences is adequate to treat the patient vigorously.

Microalbuminuria predicts the progression to clinical proteinuria in the majority of type 1 diabetics. Almost 80% of patients with microalbuminuria will progress to overt nephropathy in a 10-15 year time period.Given the presence of clinical proteinuria (>300 mg/day) most patients with type 1 diabetes will progress to ESRD but at a variable rate (with a loss of GFR from 2- 20 cc/min/year). After 10 years of clinical proteinuria 50% of type 1 diabetics develop ESRD, and by 20 years the number rises to over 75%. The percentage of type 2 diabetics found initially with microalbuminuria will be greater than in type 1 diabetes but only about 20% will progress to ESRD over 20 years after they develop clinically overt proteinuria. In several studies in Caucasian populations, the rate of decline of renal function has been identical in type 1 and type 2 diabetics once there is a reduced GFR with clinical nephropathy.

As the GFR declines, proteinuria increases and eventually reaches over 3-3.5 g/day. At this point of nephrotic range proteinuria, many patients develop the other manifestations of the nephrotic syndrome: hypoalbuminemia, edema, hyperlipidemia, and a coagulation tendency. Diabetes is by far the most common cause of the nephrotic syndrome in the United States. During this period most of the patients will also develop hypertension. It is extremely unusual for a diabetic patient to develop significant clinical nephropathy without becoming hypertensive along the way. In type 1 diabetes approximately 5% of patients are hypertensive at 10 years, 33% at 20 years, and 70% at 40 years of diabetes. In type 2 diabetes, over one third are hypertensive at diagnosis and 50% have hypertension before the onset of microalbuminuria. Moreover, retinopathy detectable on ophthalmologic examination is almost always present in the type 1 diabetic with clinical renal disease, and it is often present in the type 2 diabetic as well.

As the renal function worsens, insulin requirements may decrease because the kidney is responsible for 30-40% of the catabolism of insulin and patients may also lose their appetite with the onset of uremia. Diabetic patients may develop uremic signs and symptoms and require dialysis at higher GFR levels (10-15 cc/min) than non-diabetics.[2] Risk factors for progressive renal disease in patients with diabetes are summarized in Table 1.

Table 1. Risk factors for progressive renal disease in diabetes

1. Hypertension
2. Hyperglycemia
3. Smoking
4. High dietary protein intake
5. ?Hyperlipidemia

DIALYSIS AND TRANSPLANTATION

Once a patient with nephropathy has reached ESRD, options for treatment are hemodialysis, peritoneal dialysis, or transplantation. In terms of dialysis modalities, there is probably no significant difference in outcomes whether a patient is treated with peritoneal dialysis or hemodialysis; however, currently only 12% of diabetics with ESRD are treated with peritoneal dialysis. The mortality rate of diabetics on dialysis is very high and approximately 40-50% of diabetic ESRD patients in the U.S. die within two years of initiating hemodialysis.[1] The most common cause of death is cardiovascular disease. It must be noted though that the mortality rate has been improving annually over the past decade.

Transplantation is a viable option for diabetic patients with ESRD. Patient survival at one and two years is equivalent in diabetic and non-diabetic patients and graft survival is probably only marginally decreased in diabetic patients. A study published in 1999[5] found that diabetics who underwent renal transplantation had a 73% reduction in mortality when compared with those who remained on dialysis still waiting for a transplant. This was projected to mean a likely gain of 11 years of life in a diabetic patient who received a transplant, a larger increase than in all other groups of patients. This added benefit in diabetics existed in all age groups analyzed, including the group of patients 60-74 years old. For type 1 diabetics, simultaneously transplanting a pancreas together with a kidney is now an option. Candidates for this surgery remain a highly select group: type 1 diabetics usually younger than 50 years old without any obvious cardiovascular disease. There is growing evidence that combining the two transplants will decrease patient mortality and help preserve kidney graft function in the long term.

PATHOLOGY OF DIABETIC NEPHROPATHY

Diabetes may lead to multiple renal problems including obstruction due to bladder atonic disease, renal arterial lesions, renal vein thrombosis, and tubulo-interstitial damage from reflux, infections, and vascular problems. However, glomerulosclerosis is the most common finding associated with proteinuria in the diabetic. Thickening of the glomerular capillary basement membrane is an early and sensitive indicator of renal involvement with diabetes. Progressive expansion of the extracellular matrix in the mesangial areas of the diabetic glomerulus correlates most closely with years of diabetes, degree of proteinuria, and renal dysfunction. Hyperglycemia and intraglomerular hypertension appear to contribute to both abnormalities. Kimmelstiel Wilson (KW) nodules—acellular nodular glomerulosclerosis—is only one of many later findings in the glomerulus with well-developed diabetic changes. Other lesions include arteriolar sclerosis of the afferent and efferent arterioles, microaneurysm formation of the glomerular capillaries and capsular drop lesions. In late stages, the degree of interstitial fibrosis correlates well with the progressive loss of renal function. It is virtually impossible to distinguish the appearance of a kidney biopsy specimen of a patient with type 1 diabetes from that of a patient with type 2 diabetes. Both types of patients with significant nephropathy may have nodules of intercapillary glomerulosclerosis (Kimmelstiel-Wilson nodules), mesangial sclerosis, arteriolar sclerosis of the afferent and efferent arterioles, and thickening of the glomerular capillary walls.[2]

PREVENTION AND AMELIORATION OF NEPHROPATHY— ESTABLISHED FACTORS

Glycemic Control

Several studies published within the last few years clearly show that good glycemic control is associated with a reduction of the complications of diabetes in certain populations. The Diabetes Control and Complications Trial[6] followed over 1400 type 1 diabetics for seven years. In the half randomized to "tight" control with either three insulin injections daily or an insulin pump, there was a significantly better control of both capillary glucose measurements at several points during daily measurement (breakfast, lunch, etc.) and a better control of the HgbA1C levels. In the patients without retinopathy, a group with presumably less fixed damage, there was a significant reduction in microalbuminuria, but not in clinical proteinuria. In the group with retinopathy already present, "tight" glucose control led to less microalbuminuria and to significantly less clinical proteinuria as well. There was also a reduction in retinopathy and neuropathy in the well-controlled group. A study in Japanese type 2 diabetics has shown similar results with a marked reduction in the development of microalbuminuria and in the progression of nephropathy.[7] The United Kingdom Prospective Diabetes Study (UKPDS) trial showed that strict glycemic control with a number of hypoglycemic agents led to fewer micro and macrovascular complications including a 34% decrease in albuminuria.[8] Thus, although there is somewhat less data in the type 2 patient, good glycemic control should be a part of every diabetic's care. This may be a major factor in the prevention of nephropathy and slowing its rate of progression. The exact method of control and to what level is left for the clinician to decide. Although many clinicians would recommend a HgbA1C value < 6-6.5%, others would argue that <7% is adequate.

Control of Hypertension

Many recent studies have focused on the choice of anti-hypertensive agent in patients with diabetes. It is important to realize that control of hypertension itself, regardless of the method, is crucial in slowing the progression of nephropathy. In type 1 diabetics, hypertension develops along with microalbuminuria, and over one-third of type 2 diabetics have hypertension at the time of diagnosis of diabetes. Both systolic and diastolic hypertension have been correlated with the progression of diabetic nephropathy. In classic studies by Parving,[9] control of blood pressure was shown to decrease the rate of GFR decline and proteinuria over years. Since these studies were conducted before the advent of ACE inhibitors, calcium channel blockers, or angiotensin II receptor antagonists, it is clearly the effect of blood pressure control itself that makes a clinical difference. The UKPDS trial has confirmed the benefits of strict blood pressure control in preventing cardiovascular and all cause mortality in adult onset diabetics.[10] In 1148 type 2 diabetics there was a 24% decrease in mortality with tight blood pressure control (<150/85 vs. <180/105 mm Hg). Blood pressure control has been shown to lead to a reduced mortality and the need for dialysis and transplantation.

The ideal blood pressure for the diabetic patient has been the concern of many investigators and clinicians. Some guidelines recommend a blood pressure < 120-130 / 80-85 mm Hg for non-pregnant diabetics over the age of 18 years (ADA), while others recommend < 130/85 as a goal.[11,12] The recommendations are more modest for isolated systolic hypertension and hypertension in older individuals. Other measures to reduce blood pressure and cardiovascular risk, such as weight reduction, limiting sodium intake, limiting alcohol use, and exercise should also be instituted. Despite the evidence for beneficial effect of individual types of medications, the overwhelming importance of just controlling the blood pressure elevation in diabetics cannot be over-emphasized.

ACE Inhibitors

Angiotensin II (AII) has been shown in animal models to have several detrimental effects upon the glomerulus.[13] It may increase efferent arteriolar vasoconstriction leading to associated intra-glomerular hypertension, proteinuria, and glomerulosclerosis. It may promote mesangial proliferation and sclerosis and act as a co-growth factor on various glomerular cells as well. These effects have been ameliorated or reversed in cell culture and animal studies. In diabetic animals, the use of either ACE inhibitors or AII receptor antagonists has led to decreased proteinuria and glomerulosclerosis. In cell culture, AII receptor antagonists prevent mesangial cell proliferation and production of matrix proteins.

In humans, several recent studies have clearly shown benefit from the use of ACE inhibitors in diabetic populations. In a classic study in type 1 diabetics,[14] over 400 patients were randomized to receive either captopril three times daily or other antihypertensive medications. After four years of follow-up there was a 48% risk reduction in patients in the ACE inhibitor group doubling their creatinine and a 50% risk reduction in rate of death, dialysis, or transplantation (This effect was present despite the fact that blood pressure control was similar in both groups, 140/90 mm Hg). This study clearly showed the benefits of ACE inhibition in type 1 diabetics.

A long-term randomized trial in 100 normotensive type 2 diabetics with microalbuminuria found that the ACE inhibitor enalapril prevented the progression to clinical proteinuria at 5 years of follow-up, with a 66% risk reduction over the control group.[15] At 7 years of follow-up, patients maintained on an ACE inhibitor did even better than control populations and still had no clinical proteinuria.[16] These and other studies in microalbuminuric hypertensive patients suggest that ACE inhibitors have, by their unique intrarenal effects, an advantage over other classes of medications in preventing the progression to renal failure in diabetics. Two large recent European trials with benazepril and ramipril likewise found reductions of proteinuria and renal disease progression in patients with glomerular diseases (AIPRI Study[17] and REIN Trial[18]). Although there were few diabetics in these studies and almost no African-Americans, these studies confirmed the role of ACE inhibition in glomerular diseases. Most recently, the HOPE trial[19] found that the addition of ACE inhibition to high risk cardiovascular patients, including diabetics, led to major reductions in cardiovascular events and mortality.

Angiotensin II Receptor Blockers (ARBs)

Six angiotensin II receptor antagonists are now clinically available and becoming widely used. Since, unlike ACE inhibitors, they do not lead to a blockade of kininase, they are much less likely to cause cough and angioedema, two significant side effects of ACE inhibitors.[20,21] In patients with reduced renal function ARBs are also associated with less hyperkalemia than ACE inhibitors. In a controlled blinded comparison this advantage of ARBs over the ACE inhibitors was shown to be due to the less pronounced inhibition of aldosterone secretion.[22] ACE inhibitors and ARBs do have an equal incidence of increasing the serum creatinine in patients with marginal renal blood flow by dilating the efferent arterioles of the glomeruli and decreasing intraglomerular pressures. In diabetic animals, ARBs reduce proteinuria and prevent glomerulosclerosis just like ACE inhibitors.[13] Several studies have documented reduction in microalbuminuria with use of ARBs in type 2 diabetics. In a one year study, one hundred type 2 diabetics with microalbuminuria were randomized to losartan or enalapril. Hypertension was equally controlled and microalbuminuria was equally decreased in both groups.[23] Two recent studies of microalbuminuria have confirmed the beneficial effect of ARBs. IRMA 2 (Irbesartan Reduction of Microalbumininuria)[24] studied type 2 diabetics and found that high dose irbesartan therapy (300 mg/day) reduced the progression to overt nephropathy from 14.9% to 5.2% over placebo, a 70% reduction (p=0.004). MARVAL (Microalbuminuric Reduction with Valsartan) studied 332 normotensive or hypertensive type 2 diabetics for 24 weeks to receive eighteen ARB or the calcium channel blocker amlodipine. Reduction of urinary albumin was greater with the ARB and urinary albumin was normalized in a greater percentage of patients despite equivalent lowering of blood pressure (data unpublished at the time of this writing).

In two large long term randomized studies in type 2 diabetes, ARBs have now been shown to slow the progression of diabetic glomerulopathy in humans. In the RENAAL Trial (Reduction of Endpoints in NIDDM with AII Antagonist)[25] 1513 patients with type 2 diabetes were treated with either the ARB losartan plus other antihypertensives versus the other antihypertensive agents alone. The mean age was 60 years, 2/3 were males, and 94% hypertensive. Subjects had a mean blood pressure of 153/82 mm Hg. Mean protein excretion was approximately 3 g/day and mean serum creatinine level 1.9 mg/dl. At 3.5 years of follow-up, there was a 28% reduction in ESRD (p=0.002) and a 25% reduction in doubling of serum creatinine (p=0.006). Although mortality was equivalent for the losartan and control (other antihypertensive) groups, the reduction in ESRD or death was 20% (p= 0.01). Proteinuria was reduced markedly, by 35%, in the losartan group (p=0.001). Although this study was not powered to show reduced cardiovascular mortality (1500 patients studied for 3.5 years as opposed to 9,000 in the HOPE trial followed for 4 years), hospitalizations for congestive heart failure were reduced by 32%. Discontinuations for adverse events were also less frequent in the losartan group. In a second trial, IDNT (Irbesartan Diabetic Nephropathy Trial)[26], 1715 type 2 diabetics with proteinuria and hypertension were randomized to the ARB irbesartan, the calcium channel blocker amlodipine or placebo with other antihypertensives. The ARB reduced doubling of plasma creatinine by 33% over the placebo group (p=0.003) and 37% over the amlodipine group (p<0.001) while reducing proteinuria significantly. ARB also reduced the risk of ESRD by 23% compared with other group but this did not reach statistical significance (p=0.07). These studies document for the first time that blockade of the renin angiotensin system in type 2 diabetics can prevent the progression of diabetic nephropathy to end stage renal failure.

Two studies have found comparable over-all and cardiovascular mortality when losartan was compared to captopril in elderly patients with severe congestive heart failure (CHF).[20,21] Side effects leading to study withdrawal were less frequent with the ARB in both studies. Studies are currently ongoing comparing ARBs to ACE inhibitors in other CHF populations as well as studies comparing ARBs in addition to ACE inhibitors versus ACE inhibitors alone in a number of different populations.[27]

Calcium Channel Blockers

Although many groups recommend ACE inhibitors as the treatment of choice at present for diabetic patients with hypertension or microalbuminuria, there is data to suggest that some calcium channel blocking medications (CCB's) can slow the progression of diabetic nephropathy. These studies have shown both reduction of proteinuria and slowing of the decline in GFR over time. The best data comes from comparative studies using non-dihydropyridine CCB's which appeared in some trials as effective as ACE inhibitors in preventing the progression of diabetic nephropathy.[28] However, the studies have been performed in small numbers of patients and it is unclear whether the data can be extrapolated to other diabetic populations and to other newer medications of this class of agents. Thus, further studies are warranted. Of interest, in recent large, blinded, randomized trials using the AII receptor antagonists, calcium channel blockers are often used in the "control" arms of the study,[24,25,26] and these and other studies seem to indicate that ARBs or ACE inhibitors are more effective than calcium channel blockers in reducing microalbuminuria and the progression to renal failure in type 2 diabetics. Although some studies have suggested an increase in mortality due to cardiovascular disease in type 2 diabetics from the dihydropyridine CCBs versus ACE inhibitors, recent studies, such as the Syst-Eur[29] trial and the HOT trial,[30] show that dihydropyridines are effective and decrease mortality especially when added to an ACE inhibitor in diabetics with hypertension. It is more likely that it was the protective effect of ACE inhibition that caused mortality to be lower in the ACE inhibitor group rather than any toxicity of the CCB. Ongoing studies should clarify the picture in the future, and also show which calcium channel blockers are effective and safe in the diabetic population.

Dietary Protein Restriction and Lipid Control

Dietary protein restriction in diabetic animals leads to reduction of intraglomerular capillary hypertension and reduced rates of proteinuria and glomerulosclerosis. In humans, several small studies in diabetics showed that protein restriction did lead to reduced progression of renal disease.[31] In the largest trail of dietary protein restriction, the Modified Diet in Renal Disease (MDRD), dietary protein restriction led to equivocal results in renal protection.[32] It should be noted that only 3 % of the MDRD patients had type 2 diabetes. Protein restriction may be particularly difficult in diabetic patients many of whom are already calorie-restricted, saturated fat and cholesterol restricted, sodium restricted, and potassium restricted. Nutritional deficiency with protein restriction has not been studied long-term in this population with other dietary restrictions. Thus, some recommend dietary protein restriction to 0.8 g/kg/day in diabetics and further restriction to 0.6 g/kg/day in those with a reduced GFR. Many would not recommend dietary protein restriction at this time since 1) it is the least proven method to delay progression of nephropathy; 2) its long-term consequences need to be studied; and 3) inhibitors of the renin-angiotensin system may accomplish the same outcome in these patients (as they do in animal models).

There is little doubt that control of hyperlipidemia can ameliorate macrovascular disease in the diabetic. Indeed, the ideal goals for diabetics are more stringent than for the general population with the goals of LDL <100 mg/dl desirable even in diabetics without other risk factors. However the relationship between lipid control and diabetic nephropathy is less clear. While some studies suggest that hyperlipidemic patients have a poor renal prognosis, they are confounded by the strong correlation between hypercholesterolemia and proteinuria. Thus, while control of lipids should be a goal in every diabetic patient, its effects on progression of renal disease need more study.

Blockers of Advanced Glycation End-products (AGEs)

Methods to prevent damage produced by advanced glycation end products (AGEs) are currently being evaluated. In diabetic animal models AGEs are associated with retinopathy and nephropathy. An experimental medication, aminoguanidine, prevents formation and cross-linking of AGEs, resulting in less retinopathy and nephropathy.[33,34] Human studies have recently been completed in type 1 diabetics. The results have been equivocal. The medication reduced retinopathy and proteinuria significantly, but did not significantly reduce progression to renal failure (doubling of serum creatinine in 26% of the placebo group versus 20% of the aminoguanidine group).[35] However, this was confounded by the fact that 94% of all patients were taking an ACE inhibitor or ARB throughout the four years of the study thus slowing the progression to renal failure of the placebo group significantly over what had been originally predicted. It is clear that in all current trials, attempting to show any benefit from newer medications will be more difficult since all patients will be treated to achieve close monitoring of their blood pressure and glycemic control, and blockade of the renin angiotensin system. Current studies in laboratory animals focus on a new generation of AGE blockers and blockers of the AGE receptor (RAGE). The promise in the future for slowing the progression of diabetic nephropathy and perhaps preventing it is exciting. Strategies to prevent progressive nephropathy in diabetes are summarized in Table 2.

Table 2. Preventing progressive nephropathy in diabetes

1). Maintain blood pressure at optimal level*
2). Use ACE inhibitor or ARB to control BP and proteinuria
3). Achieve glycemic control
4). Discontinue smoking
5). Avoid high protein intake
6). Control lipids (*<120/80 for most type 1 and type 2 diabetics. <140/85 for older type 2 diabetics)

SUMMARY

Diabetes is the most important cause of ESRD in this country. The natural history of diabetic nephropathy begins with hyperfiltration, progresses from microalbuminuria to proteinuria, followed by renal insufficiency, and finally to renal failure. The overall pattern is similar for type 1 and type 2 diabetes and 20-40% of diabetics ultimately develop ESRD. Dialysis or transplantation are options for management of diabetics with ESRD. Interventions that have been shown to prevent or slow renal complications of diabetes include tight glucose control, blood pressure control, use of ACE inhibitors and angiotensin II receptor blockers, and, to a lesser extent, dietary protein restriction, smoking cessation and lipid control. Newer agents which interfere with the formation and cross-linking of advanced glycation end products (AGEs) are being investigated as another potential therapy for the prevention of diabetic nephropathy.

REFERENCES

1. United States Renal Data System, USRDS 2000 Annual Data Report. The National Institutes of Health, National Institute of Diabetes and Digestive and Kidney Diseases. Bethesda, MD, June 2000.
2. Breyer J. Diabetic Nephropathy. In: Greenberg A ed: Primer on kidney diseases 2nd ed. Academic Press, New York, 215- 220, 1998.
3. Mogenson CE, Keane WF, Bennett PH, et al. Prevention of diabetic renal disease with special reference to microalbuminuria. Lancet 346:1080-1084, 1995.
4. Bennett PH, Haffner S, Kasiske BL, Keane W, Mogensen CE, Parving HH, Steffes MW, Striker GE. Screening and management of microalbuminuria in patients with diabetes. Amer J Kidney disease 25: 107-112, 1995.
5. Wolf RA, Ashby VB, Milford EL, Ojo AO, Ettenger RA, Agodoa L, Held PJ, Port FK. Comparison of mortality in all patients on dialysis, patients on dialysis awaiting transplant, and recipients of a first cadaveric transplant. N Engl J Med 341: 1725-1730 ,1999.
6. Diabetes Control and Complication Trial Research Group. The effect of intensive treatment of diabetes on the development and progression of long-term complications in insulin-dependent diabetes mellitus. N Eng J Med 329:977-986, 1993.
7. Okhubo Y, Kishikawa H, Araki E, et al. Intensive insulin therapy prevents progression of microvascular complications in Japanese patients with NIDDM: a randomized prospective six year study. Diab Res Clin Pract 28: 103-117, 1995.
8. UK Prospective Diabetes Study (UKPDS) Group. Intensive blood glucose control with sulphonylureas or insulin compared with conventional treatment and risk of complications with type 2 diabetes. Lancet 352: 837-853, 1998.
9. Parving HH, Anderson AR, Smidt UM, Svendsen PA. Early aggressive antihypertensive treatment reduced rate of decline in renal function in diabetic nephropathy. Lancet 1 (8335): 1175-1179, 1983.
10. UK Prospective Diabetes Study (UKPDS) Group. Tight blood pressure control and risk of macrovascular and microvascular complications in type 2 diabetes. Brit Med J 317: 703-713,1998.
11. American Diabetes Association Treatment of Hypertension in Diabetes (Consensus Statement). Diabetes Care 19 (Suppl 1):S107-S113, 1996.
12. The Sixth Report of the Joint national Committee on Prevention, Detection, Evaluation, and Treatment of High Blood Pressure. Arch Int Med 157: 2413-2446, 1997.

13. Remuzzi A, Perico N, Amuchastegui CS, Malanchini B, Mazerska M, Battaglia C, Bertani T, Remuzzi G. Short and long-term effect of angiotensin II receptor blockade in rats with experimental diabetes. J Amer Soc Nephr 4: 40-49,1993.

14. Lewis EJ, Hunsicker L, Bain RP, et al. The effect of angiotensin-converting enzyme inhibition on diabetic nephropathy. N Eng J Med 329:1456-1462,1993.

15. Ravid M, Savin H, Jutrin I, Bental T, Kats B, Lishner M. Long-term stabilizing effect of ACE inhibition on plasma creatinine and on proteinuria in type 2 diabetic patients. Ann Int Med 118:577-581, 1993.

16. Ravid M, Lang R, Rachmani R, Lishner M. Long-term renoprotective effect of ACE inhibition in NIDDM: A 7 year follow-up study. Arch Int Med 156:286-289, 1996.

17. Maschio G, Alberti D, Janin J, Locatelli F, Mann JF, Motolese M, Ponticelli C, Ritz E, Janin G, Zucchelli P, Angiotensin-Converting Enzyme Inhibition in Progressive Renal Insufficiency Study Group. Effect of the angiotensin-converting enzyme inhibitor benazepril on the progression of chronic renal insufficiency. N Engl J Med 334: 939-945, 1996.

18. The GISEN Group (Gruppo Italiano di Studi Epidemiologici in Nefrologia). Randomized placebo controlled trial of effect of ramipril on decline in glomerular filtration rate and risk of terminal renal failure in proteinuric, non-diabetic nephropathy. Lancet 349: 1857-1863, 1997.

19. HOPE Investigators. Effects Of ACE inhibitor ramipril on cardiovascular events in high risk patients. N Engl J Med 342:145-153, 2000.

20. Pitt B, Segal R, Martinez FA, et al. Randomized trial of losartan versus captopril in patients over sixty five with heart failure (Evaluation of Losartan in the Elderly Study, ELITE). Lancet 349: 747-752, 1997.

21. Pitt B, Poole-Wilson PA, Segal R, et al. Effect of losartan compared with captopril on mortality in patients with symptomatic heart failure- ELITE II. The Lancet 355:1582-1587, 2000.

22. Bakris GL, Siomos M, Richardson D, et al. ACE inhibition or angiotensin receptor blockade: impact on potassium in renal failure. VAL-K Study Group. Kid Int 58:2084-2092, 2000.

23. LaCourciere Y, Belanger A, Godin C et al. Long-term comparison of losartan and enalapril on kidney function in hypertensive type 2 diabetics with early nephropathy. Kid Int 58:762-769, 2000.

24. Parving HH, Lehnert H, Brochner-Mortensen J, et al, with the Irbesartan in Patients with Type 2 Diabetes and Microalbuminuria Study Group. The effect of irbesartan on the development of diabetic nephropathy in patients with type 2 diabetes. N Engl J Med 345: 870-878, 2001.

25. Brenner BM, Cooper ME, de Zeeuw D, Keane WF, Mitch WE, Parving H, Remuzzi G, Snapinn SM, Zhang Z, Shahinfar S and the RENAAL Study Investigators. Effect of losartan on renal and cardiovascular outcomes in patients with Type 2 diabetes and nephropathy. N Engl J Med 345: 861-869, 2001.

26. Lewis EJ, Hunsicker LG, Clarke WR, Berl T, Pohl MA, Lewis JB, Ritz E, Atkins RC, Rohde R, Raz I with the Collaborative Study Group. Renoprotective effect of the angiotensin-receptor antagonist irbesartan in patients with nephropathy due to Type 2 diabetes. N Engl J Med 345: 851-860, 2001.

27. Russo D, Pisano A, Belleta MM, et al. Additive antiproteinuric effect of ACE inhibitor and losartan in normotensive patients with IgA Nephropathy. Amer J of Kid Dis 33: 851-856, 1999.

28. Bakris GL, Copley JB, Vicknair N, et al. Calcium channel blockers versus other antihypertensive therapies on progression of NIDDM associated nephropathy. Kidney Int 50:1641-1650, 1996.

29. Tuomilehto J, Ratenyte D, Birknhager WH, et al. for the Systolic Hypertension in Europe Trial Investigators. Effects of calcium channel blockade in older patients with diabetes and systolic hypertension. N Engl J Med 340:677-684, 1999.

30. Hansson L, Zanchetti A, Carruther SG, et al. Effect of intensive blood pressure lowering and low-dose aspirin in patients with hypertension: principal results of the Hypertension Optimal Treatment (HOT) randomized trial. The Lancet 351:1755-1762,1997.

31. Zeller K, Whittaker E, Sullivan L, et al. Effect of dietary protein on the progression of renal failure in patients with insulin-dependent diabetes mellitus. N Eng J Med 324:78-84, 1991.

32. Klahr S, et al. The Effects of dietary protein restriction and BP control on the progression of chronic renal disease. Modification of Diet in Renal Disease Study Group. N Eng J Med 330:877, 1994.

33. Brownlee M. Advanced protein glycosylation in diabetes and aging. Ann Rev Med 46:223-234, 1995.

34. Soulis T, Cooper ME, Vranes D, Bucala R, Jerums G. Effects of aminoguanidine in preventing experimental diabetic nephropathy are related to the duration of treatment. Kidney Int 50:627-634, 1996.

35. Appel GB, Bolton K, Freedman B, Wuerth JP, Cartwright K, for the ACTION 1 Investigator Group. Pimagedine lowers total urinary protein and slows progression of overt diabetic nephropathy in patients with type 2 diabetes mellitus (abstract). J Am Soc Neph 10: 153A, 1999.

Chapter 6. Diabetic Neuropathy

Russell Chin, and Michael Rubin

INTRODUCTION

Diabetes mellitus (DM) is the most common cause of peripheral neuropathy in the United States. Approximately 16 million Americans suffer from diabetes and as many as 100% may have neuropathy. Evidence suggests that the incidence of neuropathy increases with the duration and severity of disease, and that strict glycemic control delays its development and progression.[1,2]

Neuropathies in DM are a heterogeneous group of disorders with different mechanisms accounting for the various forms of neuropathy.[3] A causal relationship with DM has been demonstrated only for diabetic polyneuropathy (DPN) and perhaps for lumbosacral plexus neuropathies and carpal tunnel syndrome. The remaining neuropathies found with DM may have only a chance association.

Data on the exact incidence and natural history of neuropathic complications are limited. The most reliable statistics come from Rochester, Minnesota, where Dyck *et al* found a 1.3 % prevalence of diabetes in a population of 64,573.[4] Most had non-insulin dependent DM (NIDDM). Sixty six percent of the insulin dependent diabetics and 59% of NIDDM patients had some form of neuropathy but only 20% were symptomatic.[4]

Neuropathy is the most common late complication of DM and may lead to a significant burden of disability for the patient including painful foot ulceration, Charcot neuroarthropathy, and symptomatic autonomic dysfunction.[5] In this chapter we will focus on the clinical characteristics of the most common neuropathies resulting from diabetes, their hypothesized etiopathogenesis, and the various avenues of therapy available for their treatment.[6,7]

DEFINITIONS

Neuropathy is a nonspecific term implying an abnormality of nerve. It is often used synonymously and imprecisely with *polyneuropathy* or *peripheral neuropathy*, the latter two being equivalent.

Polyneuropathy or *peripheral neuropathy* identifies a predominantly distal, bilaterally symmetric abnormality of nerves which usually begins in the feet and ascends proximally. *Mononeuropathy* indicates the presence of an abnormality of a single nerve. *Multiple mononeuropathy* or *mononeuropathy multiplex* indicates the presence of an abnormality of more than one nerve. Multiple nerves are involved, usually in a random, asymmetric manner. Note that these terms imply nothing regarding the underlying etiology.

CLASSIFICATION

Numerous classifications have been proposed for the various neuropathies which occur in DM, some based on clinical subtype, others on pathophysiological mechanism. Classification provides a framework with which to develop a differential diagnosis, while offering important information regarding prognosis. For example, the natural history of distal polyneuropathy is indolently progressive over many years, whereas, patients with diabetic lumbosacral radiculoplexus neuropathy (DLSRPN) have an acute or subacute monophasic illness followed by slow, but spontaneous, resolution. Identifying the type of neuropathy thus allows for more precise prognostication.

For this review we offer the following classification (Table 1).

Table 1. Classification of Diabetic Neuropathies

Symmetrical Length-Dependent Neuropathy
1. Diabetic polyneuropathy (DPN) - mixed sensory, motor, autonomic
2. Predominantly sensory neuropathy
   Predominantly large fiber (ataxic or pseudotabetic)
   Mixed large and small fiber
   Predominantly small fiber (painful or anesthetic)
3. Predominantly motor neuropathy
4. Predominantly autonomic neuropathy

Asymmetrical Neuropathies (Non-Length-Dependent)
1. Diabetic lumbosacral radiculoplexus neuropathy (DLSRPN)
2. Diabetic thoracolumbar radiculoneuropathy (DTLRN)
3. Cranial neuropathy
4. Entrapment neuropathy

(Modified from Dyck PJ, Thomas PK, et al. *Diabetic Neuropathy*, 2nd Edition. WB Saunders, Philadelphia, 1999)

CLINICAL CHARACTERISTICS

Given the variety of neurologic symptoms a diabetic patient may have at presentation, it is important to develop a directed line of questioning that will thoroughly investigate the extent of the patient's neurologic problem(s). Table 2 offers guidance for questions to be asked, as well as answers one might expect from the patient.

Table 2. Neuropathic Symptoms and Signs in Diabetes Mellitus

Sensory
Negative symptoms: numbness, deadness, "cotton wool feeling", "thick", "less sensitive", loss of dexterity, painless injuries, ulcers
Positive symptoms: burning, prickling, pain, hypersensitivity to light touch, stabbing, electric shock-like, tearing, tight, band-like
Motor
Proximal weakness: difficulty rising from a seated position, difficulty climbing stairs, falls secondary to knees "giving out", difficulty raising arms above the shoulders (as in combing or shampooing hair)
Distal weakness: difficulty turning keys or opening jars, impaired fine hand coordination, toe scuffing, tripping, foot slapping

---

(Adapted from Windebank AJ and Feldman EL. Diabetes and the Nervous System, in Aminoff M (ed): *Neurology and General Medicine*, 3rd Ed. Churchill Livingstone, Philadelphia, 2001).

Diabetic Polyneuropathy (DPN)

This is by far the most common neuropathy associated with DM, with an estimated incidence ranging from 10 to 100%.[4] The wide variability results from canvassing patients at different intervals during the course of their disease. Basically, the longer a patient has had DM, the more likely he is to have neuropathy. Pirart found clinical evidence of neuropathy in 8% of patients at the time of diagnosis, which increased to 50% after 25 years of follow-up.[5]

Most cases of DPN involve a combination of sensory, motor, and autonomic nerve abnormalities. Clinically, the first signs are a reduction or loss of ankle reflexes, accompanied by decreased or lost vibratory sensation in the toes. This may progress to sensory loss of multiple modalities including pain, temperature, position and vibration, with positive or negative symptomatology. Negative symptoms, thought to be related to neural hypofunction, include numbness, deadness, or a "cotton wool" or "walking on pebbles" feeling. Positive symptoms, perhaps secondary to neural hyperfunction, include lancinating, burning, or electric shock-like pain. Weakness and atrophy of the small foot muscles and ankle dorsiflexors, with varying degrees of autonomic dysfunction, follow. The predominantly distal "stocking and glove" pattern of involvement develops because the distal portions of the longest nerves, being furthest from the nucleus in the dorsal root ganglion or anterior horn cell, are affected first.

The electrodiagnostic findings of DPN (see below: Electrodiagnostic Features) include slowed nerve conduction velocities and diminished amplitudes, findings which correlate well with clinical abnormalities.[8] Most patients also have an absent sympathetic skin response and many demonstrate a decreased heart rate response to deep breathing and Valsalva maneuver.[4,9]

The clinical course of DPN is characterized by an insidious onset and slow course. There tends to be a higher association with total hyperglycemic exposure and type 1 DM. DPN has also been found to be strongly associated with concurrent retinopathy and nephropathy. These points may be useful in differentiating DPN from other diabetic neuropathies.

An acute, painful, small fiber polyneuropathy with weight loss may be a variant of DPN with similar etiopathogenesis.[10] Alternatively, it may be a distinct entity, given its particular clinical hallmarks: a monophasic course, a lack of association with the duration or severity of diabetes, and the increased incidence in men with non-insulin dependent diabetes mellitus. This, however, remains controversial and warrants further study.[11]

Table 3. Diagnostic Criteria for Diabetic Polyneuropathy

Presence of diabetes mellitus
Sufficient chronic hyperglycemic exposure
A characteristic pattern of neuropathy consisting of a symmetrical distal lower limb sensorimotor polyneuropathy
An association with diabetic retinopathy or nephropathy
Exclusion of other neurologic diseases or neuropathies
Exclusion of other varieties of diabetic neuropathy (e.g. diabetic lumbosacral radiculoplexus neuropathy)

It is important to remember that there may be little to distinguish diabetic-related distal sensorimotor polyneuropathy with variable autonomic involvement from other causes of polyneuropathy. Remain alert to the possibility of other pathologic processes (Table 4).

Diabetic Autonomic Neuropathy (DAN)

Diabetic autonomic neuropathy (DAN) is associated with increased mortality among diabetics.[12] Although more commonly associated with long-standing diabetes, it may evolve early in the course of disease. DAN presents mainly in the form of cardiac autonomic neuropathy, but also affects the gastrointestinal, genitourinary, thermoregulatory, and pupillary

Table 4. Differential Diagnosis of Diabetic Polyneuropathy

Hereditary neuropathies
Hereditary motor and sensory neuropathy (e.g. Charcot-Marie Tooth syndrome)
Hereditary sensory and autonomic neuropathy (e.g. familial dysautonomia)
Acquired neuropathies
Autoimmune processes (e.g. Sjogren's, vasculitis)
Infectious (e.g. Lyme, HIV, syphilis, leprosy)
Demyelinating (e.g. chronic inflammatory demyelinating polyneuropathy)
Toxic (e.g. medication-related)
Nutritional disorders (e.g. alcohol, B12 deficiency)
Idiopathic

(Modified from Dyck PJ, Thomas PK, et al; Diabetic Neuropathy, 2nd Edition. WB Saunders, Philadelphia, 1999)

systems. The cardiovascular hallmark is reduced heart rate variability with clinical manifestations including lightheadedness, orthostatic hypotension, and syncope.[13] Patients with DAN may have complement-fixing autoantibodies to sympathetic and parasympathetic ganglia, but the significance and pathogenic role of those antibodies have yet to be determined. They do not appear to be associated with cardiac dysautonomia.[14]

Presenting symptoms vary with the organ system involved (Table 5). Impotence may be an early manifestation of autonomic dysfunction, occurring in 30-60% of male diabetics. The incidence of gastrointestinal symptoms is reportedly as high as 75% and symptoms of either increased or decreased gastric motility may coexist.[15]

Table 5. Autonomic Symptoms by Organ System

Sudomotor: loss of sweating or excessive sweating in defined areas, gustatory sweating, dry skin
Cardiovascular: postural light-headedness, fainting, micturition syncope, cough syncope, exertional syncope
Pupillary: usually asymptomatic, poor dark adaptation, poor tolerance of bright lights
Sexual: impotence, loss of ejaculation, retrograde ejaculation, inability to reach sexual climax
Urinary: urgency, incontinence, dribbling, hesitancy
Gastrointestinal: nausea, vomiting, early satiety, nocturnal diarrhea

A careful history is crucial. Additionally, bedside testing for dry skin, pupillary reactivity, and heart rate and blood pressure variability in the lying and upright position are simple screening methods for autonomic dysfunction. Sophisticated quantifiable tests for dysautonomia, including skin sympathetic response, quantitative sudomotor axon reflex test (QSART), thermoregulatory sweat test, sweat imprints, and pupil edge light cycle testing, are beyond the scope of primary care practices. Management of the more common manifestations of DAN is outlined in Table 6.[15]

Table 6. Management of DAN-Related Disorders

Impotence:	Meds: α2-adrenergic receptor blockers (e.g. yohimbine), sildenafil citrate
	Vacuum devices, penile injections or implants
Neurogenic bladder	Intermittent self-catheterization
Gastroparesis:	Reduce meal size, limit fats and high calorie foods
	Meds: cisapride, domperidone, erythromycin, Metoclopramide
Orthostatic hypotension:	Head elevation at night (prevents Na and water loss and supine hypertension)
	Compression stockings
	Increase salt intake to 10-20 grams
	Meds: fludrocortisone, midodrine, phenylpropanolamine, NSAID's (inhibit prostaglandins)

Diabetic Lumbosacral Radiculoplexus Neuropathy

This syndrome of subacutely evolving, painful, usually asymmetric, proximal weakness was originally described in 1890. Through the years this syndrome has been given a confusing array of names, including diabetic amyotrophy, femoral neuropathy, proximal motor neuropathy, and subacute proximal diabetic neuropathy.[16] Proximal diabetic neuropathy is the most commonly accepted term but Dyck advocates the more precise, though cumbersome, diabetic lumbosacral radiculoplexus neuropathy (DLSRPN).

This uncommon complication usually occurs in males in their seventh decade with a mean duration of about 11 years of type 2 DM. The patient initially complains of pain, often described as deep, aching and localized to the anterior thigh, occasionally involving the buttock and lumbar musculature. Typically worse at night, the pain is not increased with straight leg raising, mechanical movement, coughing or sneezing. This is followed by weakness and atrophy of the pelvic girdle and thigh musculature, resulting in weakness of hip flexion and knee stabilization, and depressed or absent knee reflexes. There is little sensory loss. It may be unilateral or bilateral, and distal sensory polyneuropathy may coexist. An associated weight loss of 4.5 kg or more has also been reported.[17]

Recovery is spontaneous but slow, usually beginning within 1 to 12 months, with pain resolving first, followed by motor improvement. Most cases resolve without residual disability or relapse. Pathologic findings of inflammatory changes in the intermediate cutaneous nerve of the thigh raise the possibility that a vasculitic etiology may be involved.[18]

Glycemic control, physiotherapy, and pain control are recommended. Intravenous immunoglobulin or corticosteroids have occasionally been beneficial but are generally reserved for patients who have severe, bilateral, progressive deficits.[17]

Diabetic Thoracolumbar Radiculoneuropathy

Also known as truncal radiculopathy, diabetic thoracolumbar radiculoneuropathy (DTLRN) is characterized by the acute onset of aching or burning pain that usually occurs unilaterally in a band-like distribution around the lower thoracic or abdominal wall. Older men are more commonly affected and both type 1 and type 2 diabetics are susceptible. DTLRN is not related to the duration or severity of diabetes and an association with retinopathy and nephropathy has not been noted as it has been with DPN.

The pain is worse at night and may be associated with hypersensitivity to touch. Focal motor weakness, though rare, may occur and result in localized bulging of the abdominal wall resembling a hernia.[19] Profound weight loss may accompany this neuropathy.[20]

The first priority for patients with subacute onset of unilateral truncal pain is to rule out visceral pathology including myocardial infarction and dissecting abdominal aortic aneurysm. A history of trauma may suggest rib fracture or chest wall muscle strain. Thoracic intervertebral disc herniation is uncommon but must be considered, as must herpes zoster (shingles), especially in elderly and immunosuppressed patients.

Electrophysiologic findings include the presence of denervation potentials in the intercostal, anterior abdominal, and paraspinal muscles at the affected level. Coexisting polyneuropathy is also common.

As with diabetic DLSRPN, DTLRN is associated with a relatively acute onset of pain followed by remission over 6 to 18 months. The acute nature of DTLRN favors an ischemic etiology.[19] Management of these patients usually involves only supportive care. Steroids or immunosuppressive treatments have not proven effective.

Cranial Neuropathy

Isolated cranial neuropathies are a well-known consequence of DM in older patients. Most commonly affected are the oculomotor, abducens and trochlear nerves. Facial neuropathy may have an increased association, whereas an association with trigeminal neuralgia is less clear.

Oculomotor neuropathy occurs acutely, over several hours, and is marked by pain and ipsilateral headache associated with diplopia and ptosis. The exam is noteworthy for ophthalmoparesis, usually with pupillary sparing, because the pupillomotor fibers travel circumferentially along the surface of the optic nerve and retain their vascular supply in this micro-infarctive process.[21,22] The pupil may be involved in up to 18% but this should prompt a search for a compressive lesion, such as an aneurysm or tumor.

Prognosis is generally excellent with recovery within days to a few months.[23]

Entrapment and Compression Neuropathy

Diabetics are at greater risk for compression or entrapment neuropathy, particularly of the median, ulnar and peroneal nerves. The reasons for this, however, are not clear.[24]

The most commonly associated mononeuropathy is carpal tunnel syndrome (CTS). More frequent in women than men, CTS presents initially with sensory changes in a median nerve distribution (particularly digits I-III) or even all five fingers. The patient may develop a pins and needles sensation or a deep aching pain in the forearm. This may be followed by weakness and wasting of the thenar muscles. Treatment includes wrist splints, anti-inflammatory medication, and steroid injections, with carpal tunnel surgical release reserved for severe cases.

Ulnar neuropathy at the elbow is the second most common mononeuropathy associated with DM. Symptoms include pain and paresthesiae in the fourth and fifth fingers, often accompanied by pain or tenderness along the medial aspect of the elbow. Weakness and atrophy of ulnar innervated muscles, particularly the interossei, are common. Nerve conduction studies can confirm the diagnosis. Treatment includes anti-inflammatory medication and avoidance of elbow bending. Surgery is offered for progressive cases.

Peroneal neuropathy is the most common compressive neuropathy of the lower extremity. Involvement at the fibular head results in foot drop and foot eversion, but not inversion, weakness. Numbness over the dorsolateral foot and lower leg may also be seen. Most cases improve spontaneously with conservative management and a foot brace.[25]

Sciatic, lateral femoral cutaneous (meralgia paresthetica), radial, and obturator neuropathies have been reported with diabetes; however a causal relationship is difficult to prove.

PATHOGENESIS

Defining a precise cause for diabetic neuropathy has proven difficult. Numerous theories have been offered individually but the overall mechanism may ultimately be multifactorial and complex. A review of these hypotheses is valuable in trying to understand the pathophysiology and different treatment approaches attempted in diabetic neuropathy.

Metabolic Hypothesis. Hyperglycemia is associated with the development of neuropathy. The Diabetes Control and Complications Trial demonstrated that intensive control of blood glucose decreases the occurrence of neuropathy by 60% in those without neuropathy, and slows its progression in those already affected.[1] The stricter the glucose control the better but at a cost of more frequent hypoglycemic reactions. Hyperglycemia thus results in neuropathy but how it does remains unclear.

A popular hypothesis invokes myoinositol depletion. Aldose reductase converts glucose into sorbitol, accumulation of which lowers intracellular myoinositol (Figure 1). Reduced myoinositol impairs sodium-potassium ATPase activity and is associated with slowed nerve conduction velocities. This hypothesis underlies the rationale for using aldose reductase inhibitors to prevent diabetic neuropathy. However, their success has been mediocre at best. Sorbinil resulted in only small increases in nerve conduction velocities and Tolrestat had some clinical benefit but the study involved mild diabetic neuropathy. The poor results are not surprising. Study of sural nerve biopsy specimens show no correlation between sorbitol content and neuropathy[26] and dietary myoinositol replacement resulted in no improvement in neuropathy. Nevertheless, clinical trials using more powerful aldose reductase inhibitors continue.[27]

Vascular Hypothesis. Nerve ischemia due to small vessel disease is another hypothetical cause for diabetic neuropathy. Work in several areas supports this hypothesis. Blood flow is reduced in diabetic neuropathy and endoneurial hypoxia has been demonstrated.[28,29] Oxygen supplementation prevents, and hyperbaric oxygenation reverses, electrophysiologic and biochemical abnormalities in experimental diabetic neuropathy.[30,31] Pathological study of sural nerve has shown blood vessel thickening with hyalinization of the vessel walls, reduplication of the basal lamina, and occlusion with platelet aggregates, further supporting a vascular pathogenesis. Focal neuropathy with sudden onset in diabetics is certainly consistent with this hypothesis but DPN and autonomic neuropathy may also have a vascular basis.

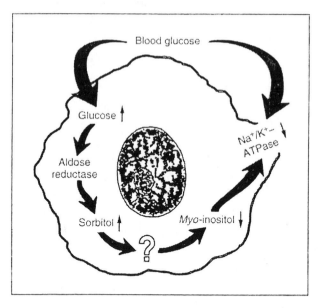

Figure 1. The Aldose Reductase Pathway of Glucose Metabolism.

The aldose reductase pathway is activated by intracellular hyperglycemia, resulting in increased sorbitol formation. This, in turn (through an unknown mechanism, indicated by the question mark), results in decreased *myo*-inositol formation and ultimately in decreased cellular activity of Na⁺K⁺–ATPase. Hyperglycemia also directly inhibits ATPase activity. The vertical arrows indicate increases (↑) and decreases (↓) in the substances in question.

(From: Clark CM, Lee DA. Prevention and treatment of complications of diabetes mellitus. N Engl J Med 332:1210-1217, 1995. Reprinted with permission.)

Ischemia *per se* may directly contribute to the development of neuropathy and explains the benefit of vasodilators in improving nerve conduction velocities. Ischemia also increases oxidative stress and, thus, antioxidants are another avenue of investigation for neuropathy treatment.

Immune Hypothesis: Evidence supporting an immune pathogenesis is strongest for diabetic autonomic neuropathy. Autonomic ganglia heavily infiltrated by lymphocytes, plasma cells, and macrophages were found at autopsy in five type 1 diabetics with symptomatic autonomic neuropathy. Striking cervical sympathetic ganglia atrophy was reported in another with severe sensory and autonomic neuropathy.[32]

Autoimmune pathogenesis may be involved in proximal diabetic neuropathy as well. Pathologic study among 15 such patients revealed, in four, polymorphonuclear small vessel vasculitis affecting epineurial vessels with polymorphonuclear transmural infiltration of postcapillary venules.

IgM deposits were found in affected vessel walls and endoneurium, and activated complement was seen along small vessel endothelium. Perivasculitis was seen in another six and demonstrated findings suggestive of healed vasculitis.[33]

Evidence for an autoimmune basis for the common symmetrical DPN remains scanty.

Altered Protein Synthesis and Axonal Transport: Pathologic findings in human diabetic neuropathy support a distal axonopathy of the dying back variety. Such distal degeneration may result from impaired protein synthesis combined with abnormal axonal transport, both of which have been demonstrated in the experimental diabetic rat model (the streptozocin-treated rat).

Nerve Growth Factor: Nerve growth factor (NGF) is an endogenous protein necessary for small diameter nerve fiber development and survival. Levels of NGF are decreased in animal models of diabetic neuropathy and NGF was felt to play a role particularly in the development of small fiber painful diabetic neuropathy. Unfortunately multicenter Phase III clinical trials showed no significant benefit of NGF in the treatment of diabetic neuropathy and this avenue of investigation has been halted.

ELECTRODIAGNOSTIC FEATURES

Standard nerve conduction studies (NCS) allow the physician to directly measure *large* fiber motor and sensory nerve function. These fibers are involved in position and vibration sensation, deep tendon reflex function, and muscle strength. *Small* diameter fibers, which convey pain and temperature sensation and autonomic function, are not routinely studied. Thus, in diabetes where large fiber nerve function is often impaired, NCS are ideally suited to define the extent and severity of disease.

Motor and sensory nerves are tested individually with NCS but the underlying principle for each is similar. A nerve is stimulated at one or more sites along its course and a recording is made at a second site. If a motor nerve is being studied, the recording is made over a muscle which the nerve supplies. If a sensory nerve is studied, both the recording and stimulating electrodes are placed over the nerve at some distance apart, and the nerve is stimulated. Recording of the sensory response is made over the *nerve* for sensory NCS, rather than over an end organ, as it is for motor NCS where the recording electrode is over the muscle and not the nerve. This is because, unlike motor nerves, sensory nerves have no end organ from which a recording can easily be made.

Electromyography (EMG) complements NCS in the study of peripheral nerve function. Indeed, NCS and EMG are often performed in tandem and referred to, together, as "an EMG". Specifically, EMG is the study of the electrical activity of muscle, performed by means of a needle electrode inserted directly into the muscle. Together with NCS, EMG can distinguish neuropathy from myopathy, localize neuropathic disorders, and quantify and provide prognostic information for nerve and muscle disorders.

Electrophysiologic findings in diabetes are well described. When large diameter nerve fibers are affected in diabetic polyneuropathy, NCS reveal decreased evoked response amplitudes of both motor and sensory nerve fibers with mild slowing of sensory and motor nerve conduction velocities. If the polyneuropathy is purely small fiber in nature (e.g. painful diabetic polyneuropathy) standard NCS are often normal. This is because the potentials produced by these smaller fibers are not measured by routine NCS. Computers (CASE IV systems) have been designed which can evaluate small diameter nerve fiber function and when warranted, patients may be referred to centers where this is available. In most instances, however, this will not be necessary.

As a general rule, electrophysiological deficits, when present, should be symmetrical in the context of a polyneuropathy. If the clinical problem is asymmetrical, the NCS will reflect this as well. For example, NCS in peroneal neuropathy at the fibular head causing unilateral foot drop, will show abnormalities limited to the peroneal branch of the sciatic nerve, sparing of the tibial nerve, and slowing of peroneal conduction velocity across the fibular head but not in the distal calf. Similarly, ulnar neuropathy at the elbow or median neuropathy at the wrist (carpal tunnel syndrome) will demonstrate slowing localized to the elbow or wrist, respectively. EMG textbooks should be consulted for details in any specific case.[34]

TREATMENT

The twin goals of treatment are to manage the clinical symptoms and halt or slow down progression of disease by targeting the underlying pathophysiological mechanisms.[35,20] Of the strategies aimed at the underlying pathophysiology (Table 7), strict glycemic control has proven to have the most scientific support and clinical applicability. The DCCT showed a 50% reduction in the prevalence rates for clinical or electrophysiologic evidence of neuropathy in patients treated with intensive insulin therapy.

Advances in basic pain research have contributed to strategies for diabetic neuropathy. Current medical management of neuropathic pain includes: 1) anti-epileptic medications, 2) anti-depressants, 3) Na and Ca channel antagonists, 4) centrally-acting analgesics, and 5) miscellaneous medications (e.g. capsaicin, clonidine). These treatment modalities are summarized in Table 8.

Table 7. **Management Aimed at Underlying Pathogenic Mechanisms**

Glycemic control—Found to reduce clinical and electrophysiologic evidence of neuropathy

Aldose reductase inhibitors—Found to diminish the reduction in motor nerve conduction velocity. Clinical benefits unclear at this time.

Alpha-lipoic acid—Possible effect in reducing somatic and autonomic neuropathies. Currently under investigation.

Gamma-linoleic acid—an important constituent of membrane phospholipids. Under investigation.

Aminoguanidine—Inhibits formation of advanced glycosylation end products. Human trials discontinued secondary to toxicity.

Human intravenous immunoglobulin—Possible benefit in forms of diabetic neuropathy associated with autoimmunity, e.g. diabetic lumbosacral radiculoplexus neuropathy

Neurotrophic therapy—Initial positive effects of recombinant human nerve growth factor in sensory neuropathy not borne out in two large multicenter studies.

Strict glycemic control remains the hallmark for managing diabetic neuropathy. Careful drug selection for symptom management should take into account the patient's age and comorbidities. Currently gabapentin is a well-tolerated first-line treatment. Tricyclic antidepressants are less well-tolerated but have been proven effective in selected populations.

CONCLUSIONS

The neuropathic complications of diabetes are varied in nature. The most frequent complication is a mixed sensory-motor polyneuropathy which is usually chronic and progressive. Tight glycemic control slows progression[1,45] and the options for symptomatic treatment have widened with the arrival of new anti-convulsants[46]. Other neuropathies tend to affect individual nerves (e.g. cranial neuropathies, intercostal or entrapment neuropathies) or groups of nerves in close proximity to each other (asymmetrical proximal motor neuropathy). These tend to have a monophasic course with spontaneous resolution.

The future of diabetic neuropathy research lies in finding new and tolerable ways to halt the progression of the disease and discovering novel ways of treating symptoms, which range from numbness to severe pain.

Table 8. Medications for Pain of Peripheral Neuropathy

Medication	Dosage	Side effects/Comments
Anti-depressants[36,37]		Inhibits re-uptake of NE or
Amitriptyline	Titrate up from 25 mg/day to average of 50-150 mg qhs	5HT. Accentuates effects of these NT's in activation of pain-inhibitory systems.
Nortriptyline		SE's: cognitive impairment
Desipramine	50-150 mg/day	orthostatic hypotension
Paroxetine	100 mg qd	increased intraocular pressure
	40 mg qd	urinary retention
Antiepileptics[38,39]		Effective for lancinating pain
Carbamazepine	300-600 mg/day	SE's: somnolence, dizziness gait disturbance
Phenytoin	300 mg/day 15 mg/kg IV infusion	Moderately effective in one study; IV infusion resulted in significant reduction in hyperalgesia.
Gabapentin[40]	Titrate from 300 mg/day up to 3600 mg/day	Improved pain in small study SE's: dizziness, nausea, & somnolence were tolerable MOA unclear; no direct effect on GABA receptors. Target dose unclear;
Lamotrigine[41]	Titrate up from 25 mg to 400 mg/day	SE: Rash; titrate slowly Improvement in pain, sleep
Pregabalin	300 mg or greater/day	and global impression of change scores SE's: dizziness, somnolence peripheral edema
Mexilitine[42]	75-225 mg tid, slow titration.	Class 1B-antiarrhythmic agent; Cardiology clearance required. SE: GI upset
Clonidine	Oral or topical	Acts as a sympathetic blocking agent
Capsaicin cream[43]	0.075% cream qid	Inhibits substance P uptake at sensory endings.
Tramadol[44]	50 mg qd, 100 mg qid max	Inhibits uptake of monoamines; has low-affinity binding to mu-opioid receptors

NE=norepinephrine; 5-HT=serotonin; NT=neurotransmitters; SE=side effects; MOA=mechanism of action

REFERENCES

1. Diabetes Control and Complications Trial (DCCT) Research Group. The effect of intensive treatment of diabetes on the development and progression of long-term complications in insulin-dependent diabetes mellitus. N Engl J Med 329:977-986, 1993.
2. Melton LJ III, Dyck PJ. Epidemiology, 239-252. in Dyck PJ, Thomas PK, et al (eds): Diabetic Neuropathy. WB Saunders, Philadelphia, 1999.
3. Thomas PK, Tomlinson DR: Diabetic and hypoglycemic neuropathy. p. 1219-1250. in Dyck PJ, Thomas PK, et al (eds). Peripheral Neuropathy. W.B. Saunders, Philadelphia, 1993.
4. Dyck PJ, Karnes JL, O'Brien PC, et al. The Rochester Diabetic Neuropathy Study: reassessment of tests and criteria for diagnosis and staged severity. Neurology 42:1164-70, 1992.
5. Pirart J. Diabetes Mellitus and its degenerative complications: a prospective study of 4,400 patients observed between 1947 and 1973. Diabetes Care 1:168-188, 1978.
6. Boulton Andrew JM, Malik RA. Diabetic Neuropathy. Medical Clinics of North America 82:909-929, 1998.
7. Vinik AL, Park TS, et al. Diabetic neuropathies. Diabetologia 43:957-973, 2000.
8. Halar EM, Graf RJ, Halter JB, Brozovich FV, Soine TL. Diabetic neuropathy: a clinical, laboratory, and electrodiagnostic study. Arch Phys Med Rehabil 63:298-303, 1982.
9. Niakan E, Harati Y. Sympathetic skin response in diabetic peripheral neuropathy. Muscle Nerve 11:261-4, 1988.
10. Blau, RH. Diabetic Neuropathic Cachexia: Report of a Woman with this syndrome and review of the literature. Arch Intern Med 143:2011-2012, 1983.
11. Archer AG, Watkins PJ, Thomas PK, et al. The natural history of acute painful neuropathy in diabetes mellitus. J Neurol Neurosurg Psychiatry 46:491, 1983.
12. Ewing DJ, Campbell IW, Clarke BF. The natural history of diabetic autonomic neuropathy. Q J Med 49:95-108, 1980.
13. Aronson D. Pharmacologic modulation of autonomic tone: implications for the diabetic patient. Diabetologia 40:476-481, 1997.
14. Schnell O, Schwarz A, Becker DM, Standl E. Autoantibodies against autonomic nervous tissues in type 2 diabetes. Exp Clin Endocrinol Diabetes (Germany) 108:181-6, 2000.
15. Wein TH, Albers JW. Diabetic neuropathies. Phys Med and Rehab Clinics of North America 12(2):307-320, 2001.

16. Barohn RJ, Sahenk Z, Warmolts JR, Mendell JR. The Bruns-Garland Syndrome (Diabetic Amyotrophy): Revisited 100 Years Later. Arch Neurol 48:1130-1135, 1991.

17. Pascoe MK, Low PA, Windebank AJ, Litchy WJ. Subacute diabetic proximal neuropathy. Mayo Clin Proc 72:1123-1132, 1997.

18. Said G, Goulon-Goeau C, Lacroix C, Moulonguet A. Nerve biopsy findings in different patterns of proximal diabetic neuropathy. Ann Neurol 35:559-569, 1994.

19. Stewart JD. Diabetic truncal neuropathy: Topography of the sensory deficit. Ann Neurol 25:233-238, 1989.

20. Sun SF, Streib EW. Diabetic thoracoabdominal neuropathy: Clinical and electrodiagnostic features. Ann Neurol 9:75-79, 1981.

21. Goldstein JE, Cogan DG. Diabetic ophthalmoplegia with special reference to the pupil. Arch Ophthalmol 64:592, 1960.

22. Jacobson DM. Pupil involvement in patients with diabetes-associated oculomotor nerve palsy. Arch Ophthalmol 116:723-727, 1998.

23. Richards BW, Jones FR, Younge BR. Causes and prognosis in 4,278 cases of paralysis of the oculomotor, trochlear, and abducens cranial nerves. Am J Ophthalmol 113:489-496, 1992.

24. Dahlin LB, Meiri KF, McLean WG, et al. Effects of nerve compression on fast axonal transport in streptozotocin-induced diabetes mellitus. Diabetologica 29:181-185, 1986.

25. Shahani B, Spalding JMK. Diabetes mellitus presenting with bilateral foot-drop. Lancet 2:930-931, 1969.

26. Dyck PJ, Sherman WR, Hallcher LM et al. Human diabetic endoneurial sorbitol, fructose, and myoinositol related to sural nerve morphometry. Ann Neurol. 8:590-6, 1980.

27. Airey M, Bennet C, Nicolucci A, Williams R. Aldose reductase inhibitors for the prevention and treatment of diabetic peripheral neuropathy. Cochrane Database Syst Rev 285 (2):CD002182, 2000.

28. Newrick PG, Wilson AJ, Jakubowski J, et al. Sural nerve oxygen tension in diabetes. Brit Med J 293:1053-1054, 1986.

29. Tuck RR, Schmelzer JD, Low PA. Endoneurial blood flow and oxygen tension in the sciatic nerves of rats with experimental diabetic neuropathy. Brain 107:935-950, 1984.

30. Low PA, Tuck RR, Dyck PJ, et al. Prevention of some electrophysiologic and biochemical abnormalities with oxygen supplementation in experimental diabetic neuropathy. Proc Natl Acad Sci USA 81:6894-6898, 1984.

31. Low PA, Schmelzer JD, Ward KK, et al. Effect of hyperbaric oxygenation on normal and chronic streptozotocin diabetic peripheral nerves. Exp Neurol 99:201-212, 1988.

32. Watkins PJ, Gayle C, Alsanjari N, et al. Severe sensory autonomic neuropathy and endocrinopathy in insulin dependent diabetes. Q J Med 88:795-804, 1999.
33. Kelkar P, Masood M, Parry GJ. Distinctive pathologic findings in proximal diabetic neuropathy (diabetic amyotrophy). Neurology 55:83-88, 2000.
34. Kimura J. Electrodiagnosis in diseases of nerve and muscle: principles and practice, 3rd Ed. Oxford University Press, New York. 2001.
35. Low PA, Dotson RM. Symptomatic Treatment of Painful Neuropathy. JAMA 280:1863-1864, 1998.
36. Max MB, Lynch SA, Muir J et al. Effects of desipramine, amitriptyline, and fluoxetine on pain in diabetic neuropathy. N Engl J Med 326 (19):1250-1256, 1992.
37. Sindrup SH, Jensen TS. Pharmacologic treatment of pain in polyneuropathy. Neurology 55:915-920, 2000.
38. Bennet GJ, Dworkin RH, Nicholson B. Anticonvulsant Therapy in the Treatment of Neuropathic Pain. Neurology Treatment Updates. Medscape. www.medscape.com. Accessed May 9, 2001
39. Tremont-Lukats IW, Megeff C, Backonja M-M. Anticonvulsants for Neuropathic Pain Syndromes: Mechanisms of action and place in therapy. Drugs 60(5):1029-1052, 2000.
40. Gorson KC, Schott C, Herman R, et al. Gabapentin in the treatment of painful diabetic neuropathy: a placebo controlled, double blind, crossover trial. J Neurol Neurosurg Psychiatry 66:251-252, 1999.
41. McCleane G. Two hundred mg daily of lamotrigine has no analgesic effect in neuropathic pain: a randomized, double-blind, placebo controlled trial. Pain 83:105-107, 1999.
42. Jarvis B, Coukell AJ. Mexiletine: a review of its therapeutic use in painful diabetic neuropathy. Drugs 56(4):691-707, 1998.
43. Rains C, Bryson HM. Topical capsaicin. A review of its pharmacological properties and therapeutic potential in post-herpetic neuralgia, diabetic neuropathy and osteoarthritis. Drugs Aging 7(4):317-328, 1995.
44. Harati Y, Gooch C, Swenson M, et al. Double-blind randomized trial of tramadol for the treatment of the pain of diabetic neuropathy. Neurology 50(6):1842-1846, 1998.
45. Diabetes Control and Complications Trial (DCCT) Research Group. Effect of intensive diabetes treatment on nerve conduction in the diabetes control and complications trial. Ann Neurol 38:869-880, 1995.
46. Feldman EL, Stevens MJ, Greene DA. Clinical management of diabetic neuropathy: an overview. In Veves A (ed): Clinical Management of Diabetic Neuropathy. Humana Press, Totowa, NJ, 1998.

INTERNET RESOURCES

www.aan.com - Homepage of the American Academy of Neurology; features helpful practice advisories for the treatment of most neurological conditions

www.mayohealth.org - Of interest to your patients for general health advice and reviews of neurological conditions

www.neuroland.com - A good page from Baylor College of Medicine for review of neurological diseases; also has a site for patients with links to patient help sources and foundations.

www.neuroguide.com - A helpful guide to general neuroscience with numerous links to neurology sites

www.ninds.nih.gov/healinfo/nindspub.htm - NINDS site, brief disease description, synopsis and information about NINDS research.

www.neuropathy.org - Homepage of the American Neuropathy Association

www.theacpa.org - Homepage of the American Chronic Pain Association

Chapter 7. Peripheral Vascular Disease in Diabetes

Jennifer K. Svahn

INTRODUCTION

Diabetes mellitus is a ubiquitous disease which affects millions of Americans, incurs significant comorbidities and costs billions annually in healthcare dollars. The morbidities associated with diabetes mellitus include a substantial increase in both small vessel (microvascular) and large vessel (macrovascular) disease. The macrovascular effects of diabetes, causing serious morbidity and mortality, are found in the coronary, cerebral (extra and intracranial) and peripheral vascular circulation. The focus of this chapter's discussion will be on the lower extremity peripheral vascular complications of diabetes.

The atherosclerotic nature of peripheral vascular disease (PVD) in diabetics is similar histologically to that found in non-diabetics but tends to be more virulent and aggressive in its behavior and natural history. The early notion of "small vessel disease" unique to diabetics has been disproved. Initially proposed in 1959[1], it led to the misguided conclusion that diabetics have untreatable micro-occlusive arteriolar disease. This tenet, although subsequently disproved[2-4], is still espoused by many practitioners today. The very nature of modern vascular surgery and the concept of limb salvage that is so vital to the treatment of the diabetic patient is premised on the knowledge that diabetics do not suffer from untreatable occlusive microvascular disease of the lower extremities. These patients are almost always amenable to infrainguinal and tibial reconstruction for limb salvage, even in the most seemingly dismal circumstances.

There are approximately 16 million diabetics currently in the United States. As many as 25% will require medical attention at some point in the course of their disease for diabetes related foot problems. An astounding 60,000 major amputations are performed annually for these problems.[5]

PATHOPHYSIOLOGY OF PERIPHERAL VASCULAR DISEASE IN DIABETES

Exact factors responsible for the development of peripheral vascular disease in diabetics are poorly and incompletely understood (Table 1).

Table 1. Factors Predisposing Patient with Diabetes to PVD

Thickening of capillary basement membrane
Impaired white blood cell migration
Impaired vasodilatation response to injury
Maldistribution of dermal capillaries
Altered endothelium-derived nitric oxide release
Increased oxygen free-radical production
Alteration in function of Na^+-K^+ ATPase

The recognition that the vascular endothelium plays a major role in impaired endothelial cell function and the development of diabetic vascular disease is pivotal.[6] The change that does characterize the vascular disease in diabetics is most notably a thickening of the capillary basement membrane. This change does not result in capillary narrowing or diminished arteriolar blood flow, however.[7] Nevertheless, white blood cell migration and response in the setting of injury to the diabetic foot may be impeded by this thickening of the basement membrane and thus leave the diabetic foot more susceptible to severe infection.[8,9] Diabetics also suffer from an impaired ability to vasodilate in response to injury, with a maldistribution of skin capillaries which results in local skin ischemia, and impaired neurogenic vasodilatory response.[10] All of these changes lead to an increased susceptibility to trauma and subsequently increased risk of infection.

Prolonged and persistent exposure to elevated glucose levels may alter the production, release and action of endothelium-derived nitric oxide (EDNO) and result in abnormal relaxation of the vascular smooth muscle and impaired vasodilation.[6] EDNO, previously known as endothelium-derived relaxing factor (EDRF), is produced by the normal endothelium and is responsible for mediating arterial smooth muscle relaxation and vasodilatation.[11,12] In diabetics, the synthesis, release, and response to EDNO is decreased which may play a significant role in the atherosclerotic process in this patient population.[13] The generation of oxygen-derived free radicals may also be increased in diabetics with a concomitant decrease in free radical scavenger systems and this may further impair the activity of EDNO.[14,15] In addition, elevated levels of vasoconstrictive prostanoids have been proposed to be produced by endothelium that is chronically exposed to elevated glucose levels. The increase in deleterious free radicals may exaggerate both the effect of hyperglycemia on impaired endothelial relaxation as well as the vasoconstrictive properties of circulating prostanoids. Finally, reduction in the activity of Na+, K+-ATPase in the vascular smooth muscle of diabetics may be yet another factor contributing to the impaired vessel response seen in the diabetic patient.[6]

Additional mechanisms by which hyperglycemia may result in diabetic PVD include the following (Table 2): glycation of proteins resulting in dysfunctional or toxic endproducts; interference with the fluid, vascular

386

and platelet phases of coagulation; abnormal lipid metabolism; abnormal insulin/proinsulin levels; and an impairment in the immune system lymphokine production and polymorphonuclear leukocyte function.[16]

Table 2. Mechanisms by which hyperglycemia increases the risk of PVD

Glycation of serum proteins (toxic products)
Alteration in coagulation pathways
Abnormal lipid metabolism
Alteration in insulin/proinsulin levels
Impairment in polymorphonuclear leukocyte function/cytokine production

A clear understanding of the exact factors involved in this "glucose toxicity" and the method by which they interact to culminate in the vascular pathophysiology unique to diabetics remains elusive. Ultimately, therapy aimed at reversing these abnormalities could result in minimizing or eliminating the negative effects of hyperglycemia on the vascular system of the diabetic patient.

THE DIABETIC FOOT

Nearly half of all diabetics in the United States will develop some degree of PVD and significant lower extremity ischemia beginning approximately one decade after the onset of their disease. As noted previously, the atherosclerosis in patients with diabetes begins at an earlier age and is more severe than in non-diabetics. 25% of diabetics will need evaluation at some time for foot lesions. The latter carry a 0.6% risk of major amputation per year, resulting in 60,000 major amputations annually in this country.[17] The likelihood of major amputation is an event that is 40 times more likely in the diabetic population and parallels the risk for vascular disease in general.

More hospitalizations in diabetics are for care of foot lesions than for anything else. Diabetic foot ulcers are the result of a combination of peripheral neurotrophic changes, chronic ischemic changes, and infection in the lower extremity and foot. Peripheral neuropathy is a significant problem in diabetics which contributes to and exacerbates the complications of PVD and is discussed in great detail in Chapter VI.6.

Careful attention to and fastidious care of the diabetic foot is of utmost importance in an attempt to avoid ulceration, infection, gangrene, and limb-loss. Ischemic ulcers are typically located on the digits or heel of the foot and are usually painful. Ischemic pain, however, may be blunted by neuropathic changes prevalent among diabetics. Neurotrophic ulcers are typically found beneath the metatarsal heads on the plantar aspect of the foot and are present often in the setting of a well-perfused foot.[5] Table 3 represents a comparison between characteristics of diabetic and ischemic ulcers.

Table 3. Comparison of neuropathic vs. ischemic ulcers

Diabetic	Ischemic
Metatarsal head	Tips of toes/heel
Painless	Painful
Pulses present (frequently)	Absent pulses

Even extensive infection in the diabetic foot often presents without the classic signs of fever and elevated white blood cell count. A thorough exam and a high degree of suspicion on the part of the physician evaluating the diabetic foot are mandatory to avoid underestimating the extent of infection and the grave consequences of delay in appropriate, aggressive therapy.[18] When patients with diabetes mellitus present with foot lesions, early control of the spreading infection and surgical drainage of established infection remain the cornerstone of initial care.[19] Even a seemingly well-perfused diabetic foot with a normal pedal pulse exam may harbor a severe polymicrobial infection and abscess. The most common organisms involved in diabetic foot infections include staphylococcus aureus, staphylococcus epidermidis, and streptococcus. Early complete debridement of infected and devitalized tisssue and drainage of abscess cavities in the operating room are required. Immobilization and non weight-bearing on the affected extremity are also necessary. Wound and bone cultures and appropriate antimicrobial therapy in concert with frequent dressing changes, return trips to the operating room for further debridement, and wound care are required to treat the infection, promote tissue healing, and avoid major amputation and limb loss. When indicated, early revascularization should follow initial control of active infection.

ISCHEMIA IN THE DIABETIC EXTREMITY: ASSESSMENT AND TREATMENT

Assessment of the degree of peripheral vascular disease present in the diabetic patient is important (table 4). It is not uncommon that the chronically ischemic diabetic foot will require revascularization in order to heal ulcers, control local sepsis, prevent progressive gangrene, and avoid digit, foot or leg amputation. When physical exam and clinical judgement indicate that ischemia is present in the affected extremity and foot, complete evaluation of the arterial tree is required to plan appropriate intervention and revascularization.

Table 4. Assessment of Ischemia

History
Physical Exam
Noninvasive vascular studies (pulse/volume recordings; ankle brachial index)
Magnetic Resonance Angiography
Angiography
Clinical Judgement

A thorough history is required when assessing the diabetic patient for evidence of PVD. Patients may describe intermittent claudication as calf pain or heaviness, aching, or fatigue that is reproducible and consistent with ambulation and which is relieved with rest. This pattern of symptoms is present because the gastrocnemius muscle has the highest oxygen consumption of any leg muscle and develops ischemic pain earliest during exercise. More advanced ischemia may be manifested as rest pain when perfusion even in the non-exercising muscle is inadequate. Minimum nutritional requirements of resting skin, muscle, bone, and nerve are not met and lead to rest pain, ulceration, and eventual gangrene. Rest pain in the foot is worse at night with leg elevation in the recumbent position and is improved with standing. Patients with severe rest pain often sleep with the leg and foot left dangling over the side of the bed. It is important to keep in mind that neuropathic foot pain may often be confused with ischemic rest pain. Moreover, the insensate diabetic foot may mask the rest pain that is the hallmark typical of severe atherosclerosis in nondiabetics.

Physical exam of the diabetic extremity must also be thorough. The examiner should look for signs of trophic changes that are consistent with chronic ischemia. These changes include thin, shiny skin, subcutaneous atrophy, brittle toenails, diminished muscle mass and poor hair growth. The feet are often pale and cool with sluggish capillary refill, dependent rubor and weak or absent pedal pulses. In severe ischemia, there is loss of sweating resulting from sympathetic denervation, signs of neuropathy, and signs of tissue loss with ulceration and gangrene. Ulcers are most often located on the tips of toes or on the heel of the foot, with irregular borders and a pale base.[20] Accuracy and success of different examiners in locating the site of arterial obstruction varies considerably with experience. In a study by Baker and String[21], medical students, resident physicians and attending surgeons all determined the location of arterial disease based on physical examination. These assessments were then compared to vascular lab and arteriographic findings. Residents and students were partially correct 35% of the time and totally correct only 65% of the time, while attending surgeons were accurate 98% of the time. Thus, for most vascular specialists, physical exam is nearly as accurate as the vascular lab and angiography in identifying the level of occlusive disease.

When indicated, noninvasive vascular lab studies and angiography supplement the findings on physical exam and are important tools in establishing whether or not PVD and ischemia are critical factors in the foot ulcer or infection. The ankle-brachial index (ABI) compares the systolic blood pressure at the ankle with that of the brachial artery. A normal ABI is 1.0 to 1.1. Progressively diminishing ABI's are found in patients with worsening degrees of PVD – claudication is typically found with ABI's in the range of 0.5 – 0.9. Rest pain is usually experienced with results less than 0.5 and tissue loss is common below 0.3. Pulse volume recordings (PVR) are wave tracings that reflect volume changes in the lower extremity with blood flow. Normally triphasic, the PVR tracing becomes biphasic, monophasic and eventually flat with progressively more severe vascular disease. When interpreting the results of noninvasive studies in diabetic patients, it is important to keep in mind that medial calcification of tibial vessels may artifactually elevate segmental limb pressures and ABI readings as a result of poorly compressible vessels. Absolute ankle pressures of less than 30-40 mm Hg are reliable predictors of nonhealing in the diabetic. Because digital vessels, unlike tibial vessels, are rarely calcified even in diabetics, digital pressure readings may be even more accurate predictors of successful healing.[5] Toe pressures less than 20 mm Hg correlate consistently with no healing while toe pressures greater than 40 mm Hg predict successful healing.[17]

When the diabetic patient requires revascularization to treat rest pain and/or to heal tissue loss and infection, angiography is indicated. Additionally it is recognized that distal arterial reconstruction and the reversal of hypoxia halt the progression of diabetic neuropathy which is a significant factor in diabetic foot lesions and ulceration. This represents, therefore, another possible indication for angiography.[22] When performing lower extremity angiography, the use of selective digital subtraction angiography with attention to careful pre and post-angiography hydration to minimize the risk of renal toxicity, has proven invaluable. The angiogram must demonstrate not only the more proximal extremity vessels but must also define the tibial and pedal vessels to adequately assess the outflow. Only with this complete information can the appropriate intervention to revascularize the diabetic extremity be planned (19).

REVASCULARIZING THE DIABETIC EXTREMITY

As noted earlier, lower extremity peripheral vascular disease in the diabetic is a result of atherosclerosis which is grossly similar to the atherosclerotic process seen in nondiabetics. However, the distribution of vessels involved and the virulence of the atherosclerotic process in diabetic patients are unique. Patients with diabetes classically have atherosclerosis involving the tibial and peroneal arteries with sparing of the relatively normal suprageniculate and foot vessels. Frequently though the diabetic patient also has other risk factors for atherosclerosis (most notably, tobacco smoking) and suffers from atherosclerosis of the more proximal arterial tree in addition to the classic vascular disease below the knee.

When physical exam and clinical judgement indicate that ischemia is present in the affected extremity and foot, complete evaluation of the arterial tree is required to plan appropriate intervention and revascularization (table 5).

Table 5. Principles of Lower Extremity Revascularization

Demonstrate necessity for improvement in blood supply
Define vascular anatomy (contrast or magnetic angiography)
Potential interventional therapy (angioplasty +/- stent) as adjunct to surgery
Appropriate choice of conduit (vein, PolyTetraFluoroEthylene)
Careful choice of surgical bypass

While occlusive disease of the proximal, large arteries can often be successfully treated nonoperatively with a combination of percutaneous balloon angioplasty and stent placement, smaller vessel disease below the popliteal artery requires surgical bypass to patent distal tibial, peroneal, or foot vessels. Often, a combined cooperative approach between the disciplines affords the patient the best result. Occlusive iliac vessels, for example, can be successfully opened with angioplasty and stent placement by the interventional radiologists thereby providing adequate inflow to the femoral vessels so that the vascular surgeon can perform the lower extremity femoral-to-distal vessel bypass.

Accurate and detailed preoperative information regarding the status of the affected extremity's arterial tree is vital to planning a successful operation. This typically requires contrast angiography or magnetic resonance angiography of the entire inflow and outflow tract, including foot vessels. The classic dictum is that the goal in healing ischemic tissue in the lower extremity or foot is to bring normal, pulsatile arterial flow to the level of tissue loss. In the foot, this means attempting to restore palpable pedal pulses. There are certainly cases where tissue healing is achieved without restoring pedal pulses, limiting the operation to more proximal bypasses or simply improving the arterial inflow to the extremity without a distal bypass. These cases, however, are the exception and every attempt should be made to restore palpable distal flow when an acceptable patent outflow vessel exists in a medically suitable patient.

Autogenous greater saphenous vein (left in-situ with valvulotomy or reversed ex-situ and tunneled) is clearly the conduit of choice in below-the-knee distal bypasses with superior long-term patency and decreased risk of infection as compared to synthetic conduits (PolyTetraFluoroEthylene or

PTFE). When the greater saphenous vein is not available for use, autogenous arm vein may also be used as the bypass conduit with good long-term results. However, many surgeons have achieved and described successful operations using a composite graft of autogenous vein and PTFE or PTFE alone (18). LoGerfo et al (19) described the successful decrease in major amputation rates with the application of an increasing rate of dorsalis pedis artery bypass. Bypass to patent dorsalis pedis vessels resulted in a 3-year patency rate of 87% and a limb salvage rate of 92%. Additionally, despite the increased rate of distal bypass surgery, the authors did not experience an increase in mortality in this patient population. Diabetics with reconstructible lesions demonstrated on angiography do just as well as nondiabetics in terms of long-term graft patency and limb salvage. Pedal bypass is safe, effective, and durable and should be considered even in "high-risk" patients with critical ischemia before major amputation (23). That noted, however, there can be a recurrence of diabetic foot ulcers despite patent distal bypasses and adequate blood supply.

SUMMARY

"Understanding the pattern of atherosclerotic occlusive disease in patients with diabetes mellitus is the foundation for a successful clinical management plan (19)." Recognizing that the infra-geniculate vessels are involved with atherosclerosis while the pedal vessels, particularly the dorsalis pedis artery, are often spared and are thus amenable to extreme distal revascularization is the cornerstone of successful management. Rejection of the concept of microvascular occlusive disease is stressed. There is no evidence to support the notion of diminished blood flow in the microcirculation as a result of basement membrane thickening – so called "small-vessel disease" or microangiopathy (5).

General maintenance and preventive care of the diabetic patient with peripheral vascular disease is mandatory and includes the following: control of hyperglycemia and hyperlipidemia and strict avoidance of smoking, a reasonable exercise regimen, close attention to and care of the feet, nails and skin with avoidance of local trauma, antifungal care when indicated, control of hypertension and body weight reduction. Additionally, various drugs may be useful adjunctive therapy. Medications which afford the diabetic patient with PVD only varying and inconsistently positive results include hemorrheologic agents (pentoxifylline), antithrombotic therapy, anticoagulants, platelet-inhibitors, and thrombolytic drugs.

Together, improved metabolic control, an appreciation of the nature of peripheral vascular disease typical of the diabetic patient and the success of distal bypasses in this population will lead to decreases in lower extremity amputation and an increase in limb salvage in this patient population.

REFERENCES

1. Goldenberg SG, Alex M, Joshi RA, Blumenthal HT. Nonatheromatous peripheral vascular disease of the lower extremity in diabetes mellitus. Diabetes 8:261-73, 1959.
2. Strandness DE Jr, Priest RE, Gibbons GE. Combined clinical and pathologic study of diabetic and nondiabetic peripheral arterial disease. Diabetes 13:366-72, 1964.
3. Conrad MC. Large and small artery occlusion in diabetics and nondiabetics with severe vascular disease. Circulation 36:83-91, 1967.
4. Bamer HB, Kaiser GC, Willman VL. Blood flow in the diabetic leg. Circulation 43:391-4, 1971.
5. Current therapy in vascular surgery. Ernst-Stanley, Ed, 3rd edition, 1995.
6. Cohen RA. Dysfunction of vascular endothelium in diabetes mellitus. Circulation 87:67–76, 1993.
7. Parving HH, Viberti GC, Keen H, Christiansen JS, Lassen NA. Hemodynamic factors in the genesis of diabetic microangiopathy. Metabolism 32:943-9, 1983.
8. Flynn MD, Tooke JE. Aetiology of diabetic foot ulceration: a role for the microcirculation? Diabetes Med 8:320-9, 1992.
9. Rayman G, Williams SA, Spencer PD, et al. Impaired microvascularhyperaemic response to minor skin trauma in type 1 diabetes. Br Med J 292:1295-8, 1986.
10. Parkhouse N, LeQueen PM. Impaired neurogenic vascular response in patients with diabetes and neuropathic foot lesions. N Engl J Med 318:1306-9, 1988.
11. Furchgott RF, Zawadzki JV. The obligatory role of endothelial cells in the relaxation of arterial smooth muscle by acetylcholine. Nature 288:373-6, 1980.
12. Palmer RM, Ferrige AG, Moncada S. Nitric oxide release accounts for the biologic activity of endothelium-derived relaxing factor. Nature 327:524-6, 1987.
13. Baron AD. The coupling of glucose metabolism and perfusion in humanskeletal muscle. The potential role of endothelium-derived nitric oxide. Diabetes 45:S105-9, 1996.
14. Wolff SP, Dean RT. Glucose autoxidation and protein modification: the role of oxidative glycosylation in diabetes. Biochem J 245:234-50, 1987.
15. Timimi FK, Ting HH, Haley EA, Roddy M, Ganz P, Creager MA. Vitamin C improves endothelium-dependent vasodilation in patients with insulin-dependent diabetes mellitus. J Am Coll Cardiol 31:552-7, 1998.
16. Vascular Surgery: A comprehensive review. Wesley S. Moore, Ed., 5th ed., W.B. Saunders Co., Philadelphia, PA.

17. Vascular disease: a multi-specialty approach to diagnosis and management Darwin Eton, Fred Weaver, Ed. Landes Bioscience, 1998.
18. Akbari CM, LoGerfo FW. Diabetes and peripheral vascular disease. J Vasc Surg 30:373-84, 1999.
19. LoGerfo FW, Gibbons GW, Pomposelli FB, et al. Trends in the care of the diabetic foot. Arch Surg 127:617-21, 1992.
20. Vascular, Medicine: A textbook of vascular biology and diseases Loscalzo J, Creager MA, Dzau VJ, Eds; 2nd ed., Little, Brown, 1996.
21. Baker WH, String ST, Hayes AC, Turner D. Diagnosis of peripheral occlusive disease: comparison of clinical evaluation and noninvasive laboratory. Arch Surg 113(11):138-10, 1978.
22. Akbari CM, Gibbons GW, Habershaw GM, et al. The effect of arterial reconstruction on the natural history of diabetic neuropathy. Arch Surg 132:148-52, 1997.
23. Gloviczki P, Bower TC, Toomey BJ, et al. Microscope-aided pedal bypass is an effective and low-risk operation to salvage the ischemic foot. Am J Surg 168(2):76-84, 1994.

Chapter 8. The Diabetic Foot

Dennis Shavelson

INTRODUCTION

The importance of the physician's role in examining and assessing the diabetic foot is hard to overstate.[1] Fifteen percent of the 16 million diabetic patients in the United States will develop foot ulcers.[2] The diabetic foot is responsible for more than half of the 67,000 annual non-traumatic lower extremity amputations in the developed world.[3] Complications of the diabetic foot account for 25% of all diabetic hospital admissions in the USA.[3] Lower extremity amputation is 15 times more likely to occur in a patient with diabetes and 50% of diabetic patients with an amputation have contralateral amputation within five years. The annual cost of amputations is $600 million and lost wages and morbidity are estimated at $1 billion, annually. Finally, studies have shown that primary care physicians are rarely performing foot examinations on their diabetic patients during routine visits.[4,5]

Physicians treating diabetic individuals must obtain a foot history and perform a foot examination in the course of office visits. Using advice and instruction during routine visits, primary care physicians can assist diabetic patients in developing good foot care habits. They must also know when to refer the patient to the appropriate specialist for preventive and curative care or to the emergency room for admission. The United States National Diabetes Advisory Board stated that "the early detection, monitoring and treatment of the risk factors will lead to an 85 percent reduction in lower extremity amputation."[2] The foot history and exam will enable the physician to classify each patient according to the Relative Risk Factor (RRF) for Lower Extremity Amputation Scale (this scale will be explained later in the chapter). If the RRF rating is high, a consultation with a podiatrist is in order. It has been found that the preventive care, diagnosis and treatment of the existing risk factors by a podiatrist are important in determining the health and longevity of diabetic patients' feet and that podiatry is an integral part of the team approach to diabetes.[6]

The Lower Extremity Amputation Prevention (LEAP) project provides a resource for diabetic patients for information and self care. LEAP was developed in 1992 and is now maintained by the U.S. Bureau of Primary Health Care in Washington, DC. LEAP reported that we can dramatically reduce lower extremity amputations in individuals with diabetes mellitus, Hansen's disease, or any condition that results in loss of protective sensation in the feet.[7]

The LEAP program consists of five relatively simple activities: annual foot screening, patient education, daily self-inspection of the foot, appropriate footwear selection and management of simple foot problems (Table 1).

Table 1. Lower Extremity Amputation (LEAP) Project

1. Annual foot screening
2. Patient education
3. Daily self-inspection of the foot
4. Appropriate footwear selection
5. Management of simple foot problems

In addition, it is becoming more appropriate to be aggressive in reducing or removing risk factors in order to prevent future ulcers and amputations. For example, if there is an extremely prominent metatarsal bone that would serve as the site of an eventual malum perforans neurotrophic ulcer, a foot insert (orthotic) or even a surgical elevation or removal of the metatarsal head should be considered before the ulcer or a recurrence develops.[8]

BIOMECHANICS OF THE FOOT

Understanding the biomechanics of the foot is an important component in the evaluation of the diabetic foot. Functional Lower Extremity Biomechanics (FLEB) is the field of knowledge which focuses on the human body from the low back down, when in *closed chain kinetics* (standing [stance] or active [gait] and weighted upon the ground). Classical medicine studies subjects in *open chain kinetics* (on an examining table or not weighted).

The etiological forces that must be overcome in managing a patient biomechanically are the hard unyielding ground, hard unyielding shoeboxes and the deforming force of the earth's gravity. Secondary etiological forces that compound biomechanical pathology are obesity, inactivity or hyperactivity and the presence of diabetes or other metabolic diseases.

Removing pathological forces from the weightbearing surface of the foot, balancing the posture and providing functional and safe footwear for the diabetic foot are the biomechanical keys to preventing and treating foot ulcers, gait and balance problems and painful foot syndromes. The use of straps, pads, foot orthotics and therapeutic footwear reduces foot ulcers, foot infections, amputation and hospitalizations in a diabetic population while allowing the patient to maintain and improve walking and active functioning.

Biomechanical Anatomy of the Foot. Biomechanically, the foot is divided into two functional segments, the medial arch and the lateral arch (Figure 1).

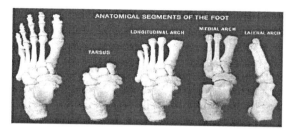

Figure 1. Functional anatomy of the foot. (Adapted from Glick JB. Dynamics of the foot in locomotion. Pod Management 4:136, 2001, with permission).

The medial arch is composed of the calcaneus, talus, navicular, the three cuneiforms and the three medial metatarsals. The lateral arch is composed of the calcaneus, the cuboid and the two lateral metatarsals.[9]

The Gait Cycle

The gait cycle defines a complete step from heel contact to heel contact using one limb, either left or right. The gait cycle is first divided into a stance phase (60%), when the foot is in contact with the ground, and a swing phase (40%), when the foot is free floating. The stance phase is further divided into heel contact (20%), flat foot (40%), heel rise (20%), push off (10%) and toe off (10%). Since pathology usually develops when the foot is touching the ground, FLEB concentrates on the stance phase of gait.

Because the tendo Achilles is medially inserted, it places the foot in an inverted position when the stance phase of gait begins and so the heel strikes the ground on the lateral arch. As the foot descends rapidly, the heel everts (pronation) in order to place the medial surface of the foot upon the ground. Because of pronation, the ball of the foot contacts the ground (flat foot) with the metatarsals hitting in order of 5,4,3,2 and 1 as the medial arch supports weight. Then, as the leg continues to move forward, the heel comes off the ground (heel rise) and when muscular power increases to the point where it is stronger than the ground reactive forces and the metatarsal heads are firmly planted, the foot pushes off the ground (push off) (figure 2).

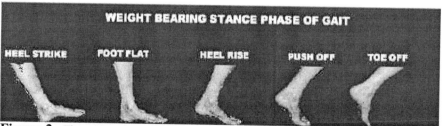

Figure 2. The stance phase of gait. (Adapted from Glick JB. Dynamics of the foot in locomotion. Pod Management 4:138, 2001, with permission).

Since heel strike places the foot on the lateral arch which is naturally strong and stable, there is no need for the ligaments or muscles to assist at this moment in order to have weightbearing. Unlike in the case of the lateral arch, ligamentous and muscular integrity and power must be available to offer assistance in order to strengthen and stabilize the medial arch, since the medial arch collapses when not supported. Therefore, depending on the ability of the ligaments and muscles to lock the bones of the medial arch during the flat foot phase of gait, the foot can be flexible, normal or tight (i.e. flat to high arch).

Foot Types

Groups of feet share similarities with respect to range of motion, functional advantage and weakness and predisposition to pathology. However, a dialogue remains as to how these various groups should be typed.[10,11,12, 13] In a foundational sense, the range of motion and neutral position of two joints, the subtalar joint and the midtarsal joint define how feet compensate and what types of pathology they are prone to. The subtalar joint represents the Rearfoot (RF) and the midtarsal joint, represents the Forefoot (FF). Depending on genetic bony structure and position, each of these joints can be flexible (Flex), normal (Norm) or rigid (Rig). This translates into nine pure foot types (Table 2).

Table 2. The Nine Pure Foot Types

Foot Type	Features/Callus Pattern	Associated Problems
Flexible Rf/flexible Ff	Flat foot, early bunion Callus 2-3 mets, hallux IP,	Early poor posture, fatigue tired feet
Flexible Rf/Normal Ff	flat foot, bunions, Callus 2nd met, IP hallux	poor posture, fatigue, 2nd and 5th toe hammertoes
Flexible Rf/Rigid Ff	flat foot, 1st, 5th callus, hammertoes	
Normal Rf/Flexible Ff	normal arch sitting, flat foot standing	bunions, heel spurs
Normal Rf/Normal Ff	no callus, normal arch	no problems
Normal Rf/Rigid Ff	normal arch, 5th met callus	low back pain, Forefoot pains
Rigid Rf/Flexible Ff Mechanical	high arch sitting, low arch Standing callus 2nd and 5th met, 2 and 5 hammertoes, bunions	heel and arch pain, postural cramps
Rigid Rf/Normal Ff	high arch sitting, normal arch standing 5th met callus	low back pain
Rigid Rf/RigidFf	high arch, callus sub 1st met/ 5th met, 1-5 Hammertoes, met-cun exostosis	low back and shock problems, heel and arch pain

After diagnosing a subject's foot type, a podiatrist can cast and fabricate a semi rigid foot orthotic that will decompensate pathological forces between the ground and the foot, preventing biomechanical sequelae. This means that the location of future ulcerations and pressure problems can be predicted and prevented by using a semi rigid foot orthotic.

The Unequal Limb Syndrome (TULS)
Since 60% or more of all people have one leg at least one quarter of an inch shorter, the balancing of this biomechanical variation is fundamental to treating any unilateral (asymmetrical) foot problem.

By measuring the distance from the anterior superior iliac spine (ASIS) to the center of the medial malleolus on both sides an examiner can determine a short side. Also, the short side foot well be held down and in equinovarus position when compared to its mate.[14]

The use of heel lifts or platforms placed on the inside or outside of the short side shoe or incorporated into the short side orthotic biomechanically compensates TULS.

Corn, callus and poroma formation
Biomechanical pathology causes pressure and friction to develop in areas of the foot that are not meant to tolerate such loads. As a result, compensatory protective hyperkeratoses in the form of corns, callus and porokeratotic (poroma) lesions can develop. Continued pressure can cause a breakdown of these protective lesions in the form of pressure ulcers and wounds. Monitoring and controlling compensatory hyperkeratoses is a vital part of diabetic foot care.

THE PHYSICIAN FOOT EVALUATION

The Diabetic Foot History and Physical must include a history of the patient's feet, a physical examination focusing on the foot and the development of a preventive medical foot treatment plan. The treatment plan may involve annual examination (if there are no abnormal findings) or more rapid follow-up and consultation if there are abnormalities.

History and Chief Complaint
The patient should be questioned regarding all foot problems, including the location and severity of corns, calluses, thick or ingrown toenails, infection and ulceration. Existing deformities, such as bunions and hammertoes, should be listed. Problems with mechanics and posture, such as flat feet or high arches, should be noted, as should a family history of foot and postural problems. Shoe sizing and fit problems must be discussed along with a discussion of lifestyle and activity level. Existing metabolic and systemic conditions should be determined, as well as a surgical history. The patient should be asked if he or she is a "slow wound healer" or has poor circulation, pedal numbness, burning, tingling or anesthesia.

The Diabetic Foot Examination

All tests should be performed bilaterally, with asymmetry noted. **Neurological.** Sharp, cold and vibratory sense, as well as joint position sense must be tested and the deep tendon reflexes recorded for Achilles and patela. The Semmes-Weinstein monofilament test (Fig 3) should be taken at ten sites to determine insensitivity (refer to section on loss of protective sensation or LOPS).[15]

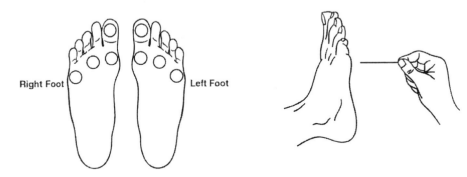

Figure 3. The monofilament sensation test and common test sites. Adapted from LEAP project website www.bphc.hrsa.dhhs.gov/leap/def.htm, with permission.

Vascular. Dorsalis pedis and posterior tibial pulses should be recorded. Pedal hair growth, temperature and skin texture should be examined. Capillary return time and venous filling tests should be performed. The lower extremity should be checked for varicosity and edema. Cuts, abrasions and wounds should be checked for healing.

Dermatological. The toenails should be checked for deformity, fungus infection and ingrowing. Skin texture, dryness and fissures should be appreciated. Skin rashes, such as tinea pedis, should be noted. Location and severity of corns and callus should be noted. The location of ulcers, wounds and infections should be determined.

Orthopedic. Pedal and digital deformities, such as bunions, hammer toes and prominent metatarsal heads, should be located and graded. The foot should be examined for small (intrinsic) muscle wasting. The biomechanical foot type should be determined. Shoes should be checked for wear and fit. Gait and postural abnormalities should be noted.

The Diabetic Foot Ulceration Prevention Plan

The physician must list the risk factors for each patient and, utilizing a classification system, develop a plan of preventive foot care[16]. Classification systems for determining ulceration risk in diabetics, when properly used, are capable of preventing not only ulceration, but also infection, hospitalization and amputation. These systems utilize various risk factors to classify the level of problem and level of care necessary to prevent ulceration. The risk factors include the degree of loss of protective sensation (LOPS), the degree of foot deformity, of limited joint mobility and the existence of current or previous ulceration, infection, peripheral vascular disease or Charcot foot. The University of Texas or UT Risk Classification System (Fig 4) which utilizes all of these risk factors to classify Diabetic Foot Risk is rapidly becoming the "gold standard". Once the relative risk factors are determined, a patient can be followed according to the flowchart since every risk level gives the corresponding level of foot care needed in order to prevent lower extremity amputation. For example, if a patient has a loss of protective sensation and a previous history of ulceration of the foot,

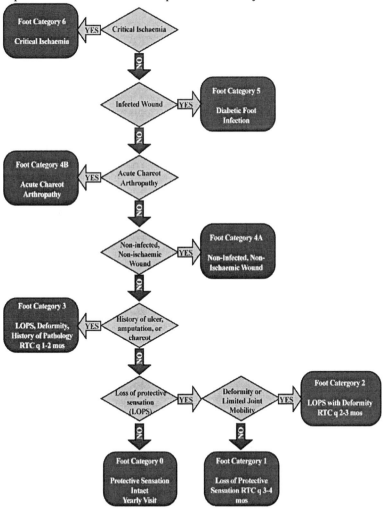

Figure 4. The UT risk classification flowchart. (Adapted from Armstrong DG et al. Who is at risk for diabetic foot ulceration? Clin Pod Med Surg 15(1): 11-19, 1998, with permission).

he or she would be rated as belonging to the UT foot category 3 and require foot care every 1-2 months. In this manner, an appropriate plan of prevention can be established for each patient to monitor and care for his/her feet.

THE TEAM APPROACH TO DIABETIC FOOT CARE

Successful management of the diabetic foot involves a concept of "The Team Approach". The team consists of medical specialists, each focusing on specific risk factors, and commonly includes an endocrinologist, vascular surgeon, neurologist, podiatrist, diabetic nurse educator and nutritionist[18].
In successful models, the "captains" of the team could include an endocrinologist, vascular surgeon or podiatrist. New patients undergo a diabetic foot history and physical examination and have an initial consultation with the each of the team members. Each specialist provides a baseline report including diagnosis, recommended immediate care and long term follow-up.
Relative risk factors (RRF) are determined and the patient is classified according to the UT Diabetic Foot Risk Classification. The patient is then referred to the primary care physician for treatment and monitoring according to this classification, see above.

RISK FACTORS FOR AMPUTATION
The risk factors for lower extremity amputation are classified into primary and secondary (Table 3).

Table 3. Risk factors for Diabetic Foot Ulceration and Amputation

Primary risk factors
1. Loss of protective sensation (LOPS)
2. Autonomic neuropathy (dryness and fissuring of the skin)
3. Peripheral vascular disease
4. Structural and biomechanical deformities
5. Prior infection
6. Prior ulceration

Secondary Risk Factors
1. Obesity
2. Impaired vision and retinopathy
3. Nephropathy
4. Poor control of diabetes
5. Poor footwear selection
6. At home non-compliance
7. Lack of adequate home support system

The *primary risk factors* include peripheral neuropathy, peripheral vascular disease, structural and functional foot deformities, infection, and ulceration. The *secondary risk factors* include obesity, impaired vision, improper footwear, lack of a home based support system and apparent non compliance on the patients' part.

Primary Risk Factors

Peripheral neuropathy
   Loss of protection sensation (LOPS). Insensitivity coexists with diabetic foot wounds more than 80% of the time.[19] The combination of structural foot deformities, biomechanical abnormalities and poor fitting shoes with a lack of protective sensation in diabetic feet dictate the need for frequent foot examination. Repetitive friction or trauma that would ordinarily cause no more than a painful blister can fester into a lower extremity amputation when LOPS is concomitant.[20]
   When a 5.07mm nylon monofilament (a 10-gram force) is pressed against the skin to the point of buckling (fig 3), patients who cannot feel the filament are at risk for ulceration and require special care. A test with the monofilament is as effective as more time consuming tests of vibration and thermal sensation for identifying patients prone to ulceration.[21] All patients with diabetes should be tested frequently with this inexpensive, rapidly performed test.
   Autonomic neuropathy. The autonomic component of the diabetic neuropathy produces reduced sweating and fissuring of the skin of the heels and toe web spaces in the diabetic foot making it prone to infection and ulceration. In addition, there is a potential for osseous hyperemia that can be involved in the development of a Charcot foot (see below).
Peripheral vascular disease (PVD)
   Occlusive arterial disease of the posterior tibial and common perioneal arteries is four times more prevalent in diabetic patients.[22] Reduced pedal pulses, pedal hair loss, claudication, rest and night pain in the arch and calf, cool feet, indurated or shiny skin, dependent rubor, clubbed digits and thickened toenails, as well as poor healing of cuts and wounds, indicate the existence of PVD.[23]
Structural and biomechanical deformities
   Structural deformities, such as bunions and rigid hammertoes, as well as normal anatomical prominences, such as the fifth metatarsal head and the base of the fifth metatarsal, serve as predictable locations for ulceration in the diabetic. It is important to document where these deformities exist for each patient and to instruct the patient to observe these areas carefully for change.
   Biomechanical deformities involve pathology that reduces weightbearing under one anatomical site thereby producing a compensatory

increase in weightbearing under another specific pedal location. This increased weightbearing creates repetitive injury, callus formation and ulceration. This is the common mechanism in the creation of plantar metatarsal ulcers (malum perforans) in the diabetic patients with LOPS.

Infection

Diabetic patients tend to have slow healing cuts, contusions and superficial tineal infections. These otherwise minor injuries tend to get infected and, because of concomitant risk factors (such as PVD), multiple aerobic bacteria, yeast and anaerobic organisms are frequent pathogens in these wounds, making them difficult to control and cure. In addition, because the deep structures in the foot (such as the bone) are actually quite close to the surface, deep infections, such as osteomyelitis, are more common in diabetic feet.[24]

Ulceration

Repetitive microtrauma, repetitive friction and continuous pressure in the insensitive foot lead to corn and callus formation which, if left unattended, leads to a sublesional hemorrhage (intracorneal exsanguination) within the keratoses, with subsequent ulceration.

Ulceration usually occurs in areas of bony prominence that are being irritated by shoes or excessive weightbearing plantar pressure.

Secondary Risk Factors

Obesity

It has long been known that obesity plays an important role in initiating and maintaining type 2 diabetes. It also plays a role in lower extremity amputation since, with obesity, weight bearing increases for all foot structures. The presence of obesity magnifies all biomechanical pathology and for this reason, among others, weight reduction must be considered a critical goal in obese diabetics.

Impaired vision

The demographic characteristics for lower extremity amputation are skewed towards senior citizens with an age greater than sixty. This population usually suffers from age-related vision problems such as cataracts and glaucoma. In addition, these patients may suffer from diabetic retinopathy. Impaired vision keeps a patient from self examination and self care of the feet and when added to a lack of sensation in the diabetic foot, may allow problems to escalate.

Improper footwear

Irritation and pressure from poor sizing and selection of footwear in the diabetic plays a critical role in the development of ulcers and infections. Since insensitivity also includes proprioception, patients with diabetes cannot tell if their shoes are well fit or creating irritation. Therefore, diabetic patients need skilled shoe fitters and continual monitoring of their shoes.

Stylish shoes, high heels and improper fitting (either too small or too large) may press or rub on bony prominences and contribute to the formation of ulcers. Shoes must be properly selected and sized with sufficient toe box, width, closing systems and depth in order to accommodate all existing deformities without being too large. Selecting a larger size, if in doubt, should reduce errors but it should be noted that as a shoe becomes too large for a patient's foot, balance and gait problems would ensue.

The Congress has tried to address this issue by initiating The Medicare Therapeutic Shoe Bill in 1996.[25] Under this bill, a physician must certify that a patient is diabetic, is under a treatment plan for diabetes and has a related foot problem. A professional with shoe prescribing knowledge, such as a podiatrist, may then prescribe a pair of shoes with protective insoles. Medicare will pay for one pair of shoes and three protective insoles or a molded shoe annually.

Shoe non-compliance at home

Diabetics with LOPS often do not wear their protective shoes when at home.[26] Since this may be where they spend most of their day, slippers should be dispensed with protective foot inserts (orthotics) and the use of diabetic socks should be considered.

Lack of a home-based support system

The ability to observe and care for a wound and the additional needs of a diabetic patient are enhanced by the support system. Without adequate support from a family member or visiting professional, such as a wound care nurse, wounds that would otherwise heal uneventfully can lead to a lower extremity amputation in a matter of days. The physician must coordinate home support or change the patient environment in order to prevent such tragedies.

Apparent Non Compliance on the Patients Part

When working with diabetic feet, a physician may experience a false sense that the patient is non-compliant. Since the lack of pain sensation can interfere with the patients' compliance, it is the responsibility of the physician to alert all parties involved in the patient's care, including the patient himself, to this problem.

PLANTAR OFFLOADING OF THE DIABETIC FOOT

The feet are the foundation of the posture and must accept a lifetime of weightbearing stress. Biomechanics, body weight and activity level determine the location and timing of areas of potential breakdown. It is necessary to disperse the plantar weightbearing forces away from high stress areas in order to prevent ulceration or to heal an existing wound.

Thermography and computerized pressure scanning can be used to predict sites that will ulcerate on the plantar surface of the diabetic foot. Plantar offloading of the diabetic foot encompasses the use of pads, inserts (foot orthotics), shoe modifications, pressure distributing boots and prophylactic foot surgery to remove or redistribute stress away from areas under extreme pressure.[27]

Principles of padding

The use of ¼ " adhesive felt and sponge pads to relocate pressure proximally to a problematic area is a hallmark of podiatry care. Because we walk heel-toe, pads that are horseshoe or rectangular in shape and placed just proximal to a callus (or ulcer) will reduce pressure under the callused area (or ulceration). This will prevent the breakdown of a callus (or heal the ulcer). These pads can be adhered directly to the foot or incorporated into the footbed of a shoe. It should be noted that pads placed directly on a pressure area would actually add to the pressure.

Foot orthotics

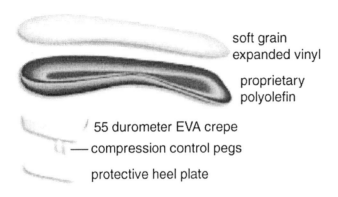

soft grain
expanded vinyl

proprietary
polyolefin

55 durometer EVA crepe

— compression control pegs

protective heel plate

Figure 5. Components of a custom foot orthotic. (Adapted from www.benefoot.com, with permission).

Foot orthotics can be *prefabricated* (over-the-counter), *customized prefabricated* (over-the-counter with custom modifications) or *custom* (taken from a cast of the foot). They are made from materials that vary from soft and accommodating to rigid and supportive. Orthotics may be soft, hard or mixed in nature, depending on their function. A rigid device can support and control the arch of a flat footed youth. An accommodative device can cushion and give comfort and protection to a weak or diabetic foot. A mixed material orthotic, when custom casted, can support the arch while removing pressure from specific overweighted areas.

Since an orthotic can be utilized to improve function and quality of life, as well as to reduce pressure in desired locations, the diabetic foot and especially the insensitive diabetic foot deserves a custom orthotic shoebed (Figure 5) for safe and maximum performance.

Shoe modifications

Because of cosmetics, shoe modifications should be a last resort. Today, there is over-the-counter footwear that fills the need for almost all diabetic patients. Depth inlay shoes, therapeutic shoes, velcro closure shoes, wound healing shoes, walking shoes and comfort shoes have largely replaced the molded shoe from a cast. Modifications, such as rocker bars, lifts, cutouts and heel and sole wedge, can then be added to overcome specific problems.

Pressure distributing boots

Non healing wounds (older than six months) can often be healed with total contact casting (TCC). Weekly application of a pressure distributing cast reduces pressure underneath the wound, yet allows for weightbearing function. This gold standard is slowly being replaced by a new generation of healing boots that reduce pressure under wounds yet, unlike TCC, allow for their removal for inspection, physical therapy and unencumbered bed rest.

Prophylactic foot surgery

Podiatrists and orthopedic surgeons perform osteotomies, corrective digital procedures and bony spur excisions on diabetic feet in order to eliminate the creation or the recurrence of ulcers and infections. Utilizing the information on foot typing, weightbearing x-rays, thermography and pressure mat scanning a surgeon can predict the precise locations that will ulcerate and become infected in the future. In well-selected cases, foot surgeons can prevent a future problem at a time when the vascular system is adequate to allow healing. The same surgical procedures, if performed at a later date, in the face of PVD, may be contraindicated. For example, if a diabetic with an insensate foot but adequate circulation has a plantarflexed second metatarsal that is rapidly forming thick callus, a prophylactic dorsiflectory osteotomy of the second metatarsal will prevent a future malum perforans at this site.

DIABETIC NEUROPATHY AND PODIATRY TREATMENT

Historically, PVD has been considered the most common complication observed in diabetic lower extremities. However, it is now accepted that the distal symmetric sensory, autonomic and motor polyneuropathy occurs in up to 60% of patients with longstanding disease[22].

Furthermore, insensitivity coexists with diabetic foot wounds more than 80% of the time.[20] Peripheral nerve dysfunction is significantly associated with both impaired balance and lower extremity impairments, such as walking speed.

In addition to the sensory and autonomic components of the diabetic neuropathy, there is a motor component. The motor component of this polyneuropathy reveals itself by affecting the intrinsic muscles of the foot. Atrophy within the intermetatarsal spaces, reduced plantarflexion of the digits and hammering of the toes are the most noticeable changes to the examiner. The use of long and short acting local anesthetics and cyanocobalamine as first interspace and posterior tibial nerve "chemical sympathectomies" has been shown to be affective in the treatment of diabetic peripheral neuropathy.[28]

There is evidence that insufficient dietary intake of gamma linoleic acid (GLA) is a possible cause of the diabetic peripheral neuropathy.[29] Normal subjects can convert linoleic acid (LA), which is readily available in our diet, into GLA. However, some diabetics have a reduced capacity for this conversion. Evening Primrose Oil (EPO) seeds, when crushed, are a safe source of GLA. 450mg, given orally, twice a day, may reverse the signs and symptoms of diabetic neuropathy in 10-14 days in a diabetic individual.[30]

Topical capsaicin cream in low concentration (0.025%) applied sparingly to affected areas, may be of some use in subjects that cannot tolerate other treatment.

For the motor portion of the diabetic peripheral neuropathy, home exercises are generally effective in remobilizing the hammered digits. Toe fists (15X), toe pickups (picking up cotton balls or pencils) (15X), extending the toes over the binding of a book (20X) and toe creeping (crawling with the toes on the ground) (2 minutes) should be repeated 1-2 times/day.

CELLULITIS AND OSTEOMYELITIS

Cellulitis and osteomyelitis are no longer major causes for limb loss due to advances in diagnostic techniques, oral and intravenous antibiotics and the team approach to care. The bone scan and MRI studies have replaced x-rays as the standard techniques for early diagnosis and monitoring. Modern antibiotics are more effective and have reduced side effects. In a vascularized limb, with appropriate antibiotic therapy cellulitis resolves in a matter of days[31] and 6-8 week course of antibiotics will heal osteomyelitic bone. If this protocol fails, the insertion of antibiotic beads can be considered.[32] Since early diagnosis is critical, the physician must react quickly and aggressively when the signs and symptoms of cellulitis and osteomyelitis are apparent.[33]

THE BIOMECHANICS OF CHARCOT FOOT

Charcot foot involves a devastating collapse of one of three specific areas of the foot. Since an inherited biomechanical weakness can exist at the midtarsal joint, the tarsometatarsal joint or the first metatarsalphalangeal joint, it is these areas of the foot that are affected. Diabetes is the number one disease associated with Charcot foot with end stage syphilis and leprosy as distant second and third. Once a Charcot foot develops, morbidity of the foot is permanent and progressive.[33] The patient's lifestyle and his/her ability to walk, work and wear normal shoes are reduced.

Biomechanically, Charcot foot is composed of a triad of symptoms:
1) LOPS;
2) a structurally weak foot type;
3) an active lifestyle and personality and/or obesity.

An individual with preserved pain sensation will experience pain and swelling in the area of potential collapse when this area is stressed. The pain forces the patient to reduce activity, lose weight or introduce a biomechanical support, such as a custom foot orthotic, and therefore prevent the potential collapse of the foot. The patient with LOPS in this triad remains pain-free and thus does not adjust his or her active lifestyle.

Eventually, the weakest link in the biomechanical chain collapses, producing a Charcot foot (Figure 6).

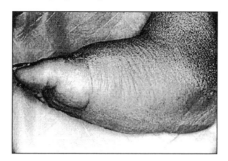

Figure 6. The rocker bottom deformity of a Charcot foot. (Adapted from Sommer, TA. Charcot foot, the diagnostic dilemma. Amer Fam Prac 11: 109, 1995, with permission).

There is no successful way to re-establish a normal lifestyle and biomechanics once a Charcot foot occurs. Therefore, it is essential for the physician to detect the impending signs of this triad and to consider a biomechanical evaluation with a podiatrist for all patients with LOPS.

NON-HEALING WOUND CARE

With the evolution of modern antibiotics, diagnostic tools such as MRI, and home wound care and educational programs that allow the physician to make an earlier diagnosis and provide more effective treatment than in the past, most diabetic foot wounds heal uneventfully.[34] However, wounds that have not significantly healed after three to six months of care can be considered non-healing. They have sparse angiogenesis, reduced growth factor release and are more likely to become infected. These wounds can be converted into fresh, healing wounds with proper management.

After evaluation of the status of the foot and of the wound a clinician can classify a wound according to its depth, size and healing ability. Only then can a multifaceted program of care can be instituted and monitored.

Clinical attention to many factors involved in healing a wound, rather than focus on a single risk factor, can lead a non-healing wound to improve at a time when it seems to be stagnant. If the status of a particular system or risk is uncertain, then immediate consultation with a specialist is in order.

Evaluation of the status of the wound

The wound should be measured and photographed.[35] The wound should be classified according to depth as:

1) Pre or post ulceration, completely epithelialized;
2) Superficial and not involving tendon, capsule or bone;
3) Penetrating to tendon or capsule;
4) Penetrating to bone.

The location of the wound is critical and will determine the importance for offloading. The margins should be examined for redness, heat, swelling. The level of pain should be determined but since insensitivity of wounds in diabetics is the rule, painless wounds should not be considered low risk. The epithelial borders of the wound should be assessed. The quality of the base of the wound should be determined. A fresh, granular base is desirable and necrosis and detritus are to be avoided. The presence of bleeding and/or exudate should be recorded. Microbial culture and sensitivity should be obtained and an antibiotic should be started if the wound is showing even early signs if infection and not healing. It should be noted that even the smallest amount of healing every week will lead to a healed wound but a wound that remains status quo for more than two weeks needs reassessment. Some change in the treatment regimen or consultation is necessary at this critical time.

Evaluation of the status of complications

Wounds should be classified according to the vascular status and the presence of infection:

1) absence of vascular complications and infection;
2) presence of infection;
3) presence of vascular complications;
4) presence of both infection and vascular complications.

A vascular and/or infectious disease consultation becomes critical when these complications are present.

Classification of diabetic foot wounds

Once the clinician determines the status of the wound and the foot, it is necessary to utilize this information to classify the wound and establish a treatment protocol. The UT wound classification[36] gives a wound status number (zero-3) and a foot status letter (A-D) which gives a final description of the wound. For example, a UT wound classification of C-3 wound be a wound penetrating to bone involving an avascular foot. Figure 7 shows the University of Texas Wound Classification Flowchart which incorporates both the status of the wound and complications.

Meticulous debridement

Meticulous debridement is the most important service that a chronic, non-healing wound deserves since wounds that are not aggressively debrided form a callus that masks the clinicians ability to evaluate, treat and monitor a wound. In a poorly healing wound, the epithelial edges seal and stop growing inward, preventing closure of the wound.

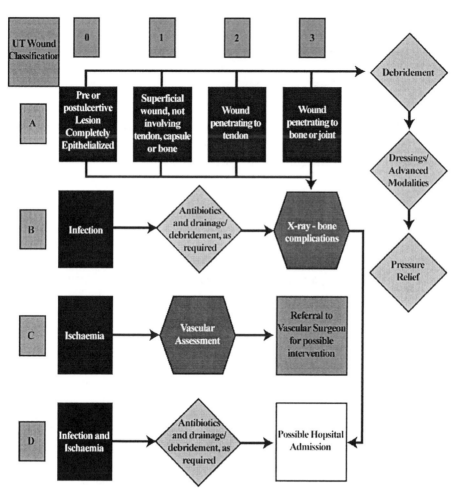

Figure 7. The UT Wound Classification Flowchart. (Adapted from Armstrong, DM et al. Validation of a diabetic wound classification system: the importance of depth, infection and ischaemia. J Amer Pod Med Assoc 79:150, 1998, with permission).

The base of the wound becomes necrotic and infected and growth factors cease to be released (Fig 8). Meticulous debridement utilizes aggressive sterile surgery to remove peripheral callus and make the epithelial edges raw. It eliminates necrotic tissue and detritus as well as free bleeding at the base and periphery of the wound.

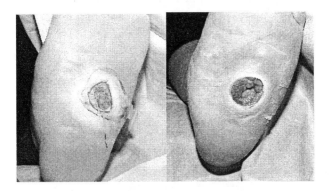

Figure 8. A diabetic ulcer under the cuboid of a Charcot foot, before and after meticulous debridement. (Adapted from Brenner, MA, Ed. Management of the diabetic foot. Williams and Wilkins, Baltimore, MD, 1987, with permission.)

Debridement stimulates the release and production of the multiple growth factors that contribute to wound healing.[37] It denudes circumferential epithelial margins so that the skin margins can continue to close instead of "sealing off" at the wound edge. It stimulates angiogenesis and the vascular cascade. Wounds should be measured weekly and debrided using a sterile field and instruments, as they heal. Surgeons should consider the use of gentian violet to paint non-healing wounds. Since gentian violet is astringent, anti-fungal, anticandida and antiseptic it remains one of the best topical preparations for diabetic wounds. Likewise, since gentian violet is rapidly absorbed by healthy tissue and stains the skin edge, it allows for simple monitoring of new growth and vitality of the wound.

Offloading of the non-healing wound

The use of ¼ inch adhesive sponge horseshoe shaped pads just proximal to non-healing wounds reduces plantar pressure on these wounds dramatically. Wound healing shoes and boots with custom insoles to reduce weightbearing pressure are invaluable. If, in spite of these measures, a wound remains resistant to healing, a wheelchair, contact casting, or bed rest must be considered.

Advances in wound healing

The three most utilized advances in wound care are hyperbaric oxygen treatment,[38] recombinant growth factors[39] and autograft skin substitutes.[40] These modalities are adjunctive to meticulous debridement

412

and off-loading and, although costly, when used in properly selected cases, can reduce the healing time of wounds as well as the overall cost of care.

Hyperbaric oxygen treatment (HBO) uses pressurized 100% oxygen, delivered in a full body chamber. If the PO2 of the wound surface is low, then HBO may be of benefit.

Platelet derived growth factor (PDGF) has been successfully produced in a gel form and, when applied to large and deep non-infected wounds, can accelerate the healing process. Other growth factors are under investigation and additional products are on the horizon.

Autograft skin substitutes are becoming more useful when treating large and deep wounds which are the most resistant to healing. The use of autograft substitutes, such as irradiated allografts and bioengineered human skin equivalents, can produce adequate coverage of these wounds without the additional morbidity of a donor graft site. The most sophisticated product to date is composed of living keratinocytes and dermal fibroblasts derived from neonatal foreskin and propagated in culture.[41] This product is easy to apply and, since it serves as a substrate for the patient's own skin repair, the end result is a plantar wound covered by plantar tissue.

CONCLUSIONS

Diabetes affects the feet, the eyes and the kidneys. These organs must be monitored closely in diabetic patients. Complications of the foot are the number one cause for hospital admission in diabetics today.

By implementing a foot care program that involves risk classification, biomechanical evaluation, the team approach and close monitoring, the physician will be able to keep his/her patients active, functional, ulcer and infection free and will reduce the risk of limb loss.

REFERENCES

1. Brenner MA, Ed. Management of the diabetic foot (chapter 6). Williams and Wilkins, New York, 1987.
2. The American Diabetes Association Advisory Board. Diab Care 17:122-128, 1996.
3. Bulat T, Kosinski M. Diabetic foot: strategies to prevent and treat common problems. Geriatrics 46:55-57, 1995.
4. Mayfield J. Foot examinations reduce the risk of diabetic amputations. J Fam Practice 49:499-504, 1998.
5. American Diabetes Association. Foot care in patients with diabetes mellitus. Diab Care 21:54-58, 1998.
6. Todd WF, Armstrong DG, Liswood PJ. Evaluation and treatment of the infected foot in a community teaching hospital. J Am Podiatr Med Assoc 86:421-426, 1996.
7. LEAPP. Diabetes Care 21: 23-25, 1998.

8. Armstrong DG, Lavery LA, Stern S, et al. Is prophylactic diabetes foot surgery dangerous? J Foot Ankle Surg, 35:585-590, 1996.

9. Glick JB. Dynamics of the foot in locomotion. Pod Management 4: 134-142, 2001.

10. Root ML, Orien WP and Weed JH. Normal and abnormal function of the foot. In *Clinical biomechanics*, Vol 2, Clinical Biomechanics Corp, LA, California, 1977.

11. Inman VT. The joints of the ankle. Mann/Inman, Ed. Williams and Wilkins, New York, 1976.

12. Donatelli R. The biomechanics of the foot and ankle. FA Davis Comp, Phila, PA, 1990.

13. Kevin KA. Biomechanics of the normal and abnormal foot. J Amer Pod Med Assoc 90:88-92, 2000.

14. Shavelson D. The unequal limb syndrome: biomechanical considerations. J Am Acad Pod Sport Med 1:18-23, 1983.

15. Caputo GM. The nylon monofilament test for sensation. New Eng J Med 331:854-859, 1994.

16. Frykberg R, Ed. The high risk foot in diabetes. Churchill Livingstone, New York, 1991.

17. Armstrong DG, Lavery LA, Harkless LB. Who is at risk for diabetic foot ulceration? Clin Podiatr Med Surg 15:11-19, 1998.

18. Frykberg RG. Team approach toward lower extremity amputation prevention in diabetes. J Am Podiatr Med Assoc 87:5-12, 1997.

19. Selby JV, Hang D. Risk factors for lower extremity amputation in persons with diabetes. Diab Care 18:509-516, 1995.

20. Day MR, Harkless LB. Factors associated with pedal ulceration in patients with diabetes mellitus. J Am Podiatr Med Assoc 87:365-369, 1997.

21. Young MJ, Breddy JL, Veves A, et al. The prediction of diabetic neuropathic foot ulceration using vibration perception thresholds. Diab Care 17:557-562, 1994.

22. McNeely MJ, Boyko EJ, Ahroni JH, et al. The independent contributions of diabetic neuropathy and vasculopathy in foot ulceration. Diab Care 18:216-219, 1995.

23. Sykes MT, Godsey JB. Vascular evaluation of the problem diabetic foot. Clin Podiatr Med Surg 15:49-83, 1998.

24. Apelqvist J. Wound healing in diabetes: outcome and costs. Clin Podiatr Med Surg 15:21-39, 1998.

25. The Medicare Therapeutic Shoe Bill. Department of Health and Human Services, Medical Carriers Manual, Section 2134, p2-85.1-2-86. US Gov't Printing Office, Washington, D.C., 1994.

26. Armstrong DG, et al. Continuous activity monitoring in persons at high risk for diabetes-related lower extremity amputation. J Am Pod Med Assoc 91: 451-455, 2001.

27. Lavery LA, Vela SA, Lavery DC, et al. Reducing dynamic foot pressures in high-risk diabetic subjects with foot ulcerations. Diab Care 19:818-821, 1999.

28. Shavelson D. Local anesthetics and injectable cortisone. In T Delauro, Ed. Clinics in Pod Med & Surg, Chapter 8, W.B. Saunders, Phila, 1993.

29. Jamal GA. The use of gamma linoleic acid in the prevention and treatment of diabetic neuropathy. Diab Medicine 11:145-149, 1994.

30. Hounsom L, et al. GLA is effective against multiple indices of experimental diabetic neuropathy. Diabetologia 41:839-843, 1998.

31. Resneck HE, et al. Independent effects of peripheral nerve dysfunction on lower-extremity physical function in old age. Diab Care 23: 132-138, 2000.

32. Marcinko DE. Antibiotic-impregnated polymethyl methacrylate beads. In *Infections of the foot: diagnosis and management*. Habershaw GM Ed. Mosby-Year Book Pub, St Louis, MO, 174-176, 1998.

33. Gibbons GW, Habershaw GM. Diabetic foot infections: anatomy and surgery. Infect Dis Clin North Am 9:131-142, 1995.

34. Sommer TA. Charcot foot: the diagnostic dilemma. J Fam Practice 11:1591-1599, 2001.

35. Frykberg RG. Diabetic foot ulcers: current concepts. J Foot Ankle Surg 37: 440-446, 1998.

36. Sage RA. The management of foot ulcers. In Advances in podiatric medicine and surgery. W Joseph, Ed. Mosby-Year Book Pub, St. Louis, Mo 139-153, 1995.

37. Armstrong DG, Harkless LB, et al. Validation of a diabetic wound classification system: the importance of depth, infection and ischaemia, J Am Pod Med Assoc 79: 144-153, 1998.

38. Faglia E, Favales F, Aldeghi A, et al. Adjunctive systemic hyperbaric oxygen therapy in treatment of severe prevalently ischemic diabetic foot ulcer: a randomized study. Diab Care 19:1338-1342, 1996.

39. Wieman TJ, Smiell JM, Su Y. Efficacy and safety of a topical gel formulation of recombinant human platelet-derived growth factor-BB (becaplermin) in patients with chronic neuropathic diabetic ulcers: a phase III randomized placebo-controlled double-blind study. Diabetes Care 21:822-829, 1998.

40. Snyder RJ, Simonson DA. Cadaveric allograft as adjunct therapy for nonhealing wounds. J Foot Ankle Surg 38:93-101, 1999.

41. Falanga V. How to use Apligraf to treat venous ulcers. Skin and aging 2:30-36, 1999.

Chapter 9. Male Sexual Dysfunction in Diabetes Mellitus

Albert C. Leung and Arnold Melman

INTRODUCTION

Male sexual dysfunction can be classified in the following categories: erectile dysfunction (ED); orgasmic and ejaculatory dysfunction; priapism; and decreased libido. Of these various dysfunctions, more patients with ED are likely to seek medical attention. ED, or impotence, is defined as the inability to achieve or maintain an erection sufficient for satisfactory sexual function[1]. In recent years, there has been an escalated awareness of ED, partly attributed to the advent of Viagra™ and its associated promotion. The impact of ED can be appreciated by the estimation that its prevalence in men 40 to 70 years old is 52%, based on the Massachusetts Male Aging Study.[2] Based on these data and United States population projections for the year 2005 of more than 50 million men 40 to 70 years old, ED will affect more than 25 million men, and millions more over the age of 70. The projected worldwide prevalence of ED for year 2025 will be staggering at 322 million men. Certain patients are found to have a significantly higher prevalence of ED; for example, diabetic men command a more than threefold increase in risk of ED than their nondiabetic counterparts. Indeed, diabetes mellitus is the single most common cause of ED.[2] More than 50% of diabetic patients are afflicted with some degree of ED, and approximately 50% of the patients evaluated at our Center for Male Sexual Dysfunction are diabetic.

Studies have found ED to be an age-dependent disease process that is accelerated in age-matched diabetic men, with the prevalence of ED in diabetics ranging from 35% to 75%,[2] depending on patient age, duration of diabetes, and disease severity. The onset of ED occurs at an earlier age in diabetic men, on average 10 to 15 years earlier than in the general population, regardless of insulin dependency status.

ETIOLOGY

ED can be multifactorial in origin, but for simplicity, it can be described as either organic or psychogenic.[4] Organic ED can be secondary to vasculogenic, neurogenic, hormonal, or cavernosal smooth muscle abnormalities or lesions, whereas psychogenic ED is due to central inhibition of the erectile mechanism and is most prevalent in younger men. The most common cause of the organic component of diabetic ED is the autonomic neuropathy and vascular abnormalities often associated with diabetes, reflecting disease in major arteries, arterial insufficiency, veno-occlusive dysfunction, and microvascular abnormalities.[5-9] Corporal smooth muscle abnormalities, such as dysfunctional corporal muscle tone, are also essential factors in diabetic ED. Endocrine disorders such as hypogonadism, hyperprolactinemia, hypothyroidism and hyperthyroidism, testicular failure, and estrogen excess may also result in ED, although they cause ED in only a small proportion of the general population.[8] Numerous medications and substances of abuse are commonly associated with ED. These drugs include certain antihypertensives, antidepressants, hormones, diuretics, and cardiac medications.[4-8] Cummings et al describe the striking degree of overlap between the risk factors of ED and common comorbidities of diabetes: cardiovascular disease, treated and untreated hypertension, multiple drug therapy, neuropathy, and obesity.[10] Thus, the vulnerability of diabetic men to ED is further compounded by their additional need for multiple medications for other diabetes-associated medical conditions. Finally, trauma, irradiation or surgery involving the pelvic region can also result in iatrogenic ED. Table 1 summarizes the various processes that contribute to ED.

GENERAL PENILE ERECTION PHYSIOLOGY

The presentation of diabetic ED can be described in 1 of 3 ways: 1) chemical diabetes followed years later by impotence, 2) impotence as a first sign of diabetes, and 3) temporary impotence resulting from poorly controlled diabetes, which is more likely caused by associated malnutrition and weakness.[11] The onset of organic ED is usually insidious and gradual, with the presenting symptom being the inability to sustain erection, followed by incomplete rigidity and ultimately complete loss of erectile function. In order to appreciate the penile erectile physiology and dysfunction, knowledge of the penile anatomy and hemodynamics of erection is imperative.

Table 1. Etiology of Erectile Dysfunction

Systemic diseases	Penile
Diabetes mellitus	Peyronie's disease
Atherosclerosis	Epispadias
Arterial hypertension	Priapism
Myocardial infarction	
Scleroderma	**Psychiatric**
Renal failure	Depression
Liver cirrhosis	Widower's syndrome
Idiopathic hemochromatosis	Performance anxiety

Neurogenic	Nutritional
Epilepsy	Protein malnutrition
Cerebrovascular accidents	Zinc deficiency
Multiple sclerosis	
Guillain-Barre	**Hematologic**
Alzheimer's disease	Sickle cell anemia
	Leukemias
Respiratory	
Chronic obstructive pulmonary disease	**Infections**
	Brucellosis
Endocrine	Tuberculosis
Hyperthyroidism	AIDS
Hypothyroidism	Trypanosomiasis
Hypogonadism	

The penis originates as separate, paired structures, the crura, which are attached by dense facial fibers to the periosteum of the ischiopubic rami. As the crura course toward the pubic symphysis, they join to one another and to the corpus spongiosum on the caudal aspect to form a tripartite structure. The corpora cavernosa are enclosed in a thick fibrous sheath, the tunica albuginea, whose fibers unite medially to form a perforated septum that allows the 2 bodies to function as a single unit. Cavernosal tissue contains a meshwork of interconnected cavernosal spaces known as sinusoidal or lacunar spaces, which are lined with vascular endothelium and separated by trabeculae composed of bundles of smooth muscle fibers with an extracellular matrix of collagen, elastin, and fibroblasts. Gap junctions, hexamer protein lined aqueous intercellular channels, connect the smooth muscle cells of the corpora cavernosa into a syncytial network.[8-12]

The arterial inflow to the penis is the end terminal of the internal pudendal artery, a branch of the hypogastric or internal iliac artery. Upon emerging from Alcock's canal, the internal pudendal artery gives rise to the common penile artery, which further subdivides into the bulbo-urethral, cavernosal (deep) and dorsal penile end arteries. The cavernosal arteries of the penis give off multiple helicine branches that are tortuous and contracted in the flaccid state while becoming straight and larger in caliber during erection. While the vascular elements lead to tumescence, it is ultimately the tone of the corporal bodies or the intracavernosal pressure that determines erectile function.

The penis is a complex vascular organ that requires the coordination of vascular, neural, and hormonal factors in order to achieve satisfactory penile erection. Any abnormalities that affect the integrity of the penile vasculature may result in ED. Four physiologic mechanisms must function to effect penile erection: 1) intact neuronal innervation, 2) intact arterial supply, 3) appropriately responsive corporal smooth muscle with normally functional intercellular communication, and 4) intact veno-occlusive mechanism. Nonetheless, penile erection and detumescence are principally vascular events coordinated by the relaxation and contraction of corporal smooth muscle respectively. In the absence of severe arterial insufficiency, relaxation of the corporeal smooth muscle is sufficient to elicit a sustained erection.[13-14] The corporal smooth muscle tone is thus a primary determinant of erectile function. In the flaccid state, the cavernosal arteries are constricted, thereby permitting venous outflow, and only a minimal amount of blood (3-5 mL/min) flows through the cavernous artery into the cavernous spaces. Sexual stimulation leads to a decrease in peripheral resistance secondary to vasodilation and increased blood flow through the cavernous and helicine arteries. The intracavernous pressure increases without any increase in systemic pressure. Relaxation of the trabecular smooth muscle causes increased compliance of the cavernosal spaces, leading to penile engorgement and erection. In the full erectile state, the cavernosal arteries are relaxed, with resultant increased arterial inflow and compression of the trabecular smooth muscle against the fibroelastic tunica albuginea, and thus causing closure of the emissary veins and accumulation of blood in the sinusoidal bodies. Detumescence ensues during contraction of the trabecular smooth muscle, with resumption of arterial blood flow at the prestimulation level and reopening of venous outflow channels. The intracavernosal pressure declines and the veno-occlusive mechanism is inactivated, leading to the flaccid state. Any interruption or interference in this cascade of vascular events may potentially precipitate ED.[8, 15-16]

PATHOPHYSIOLOGY OF DIABETIC ERECTILE DYSFUNCTION

Neurologic/Biochemical Physiology

There has been a concensus that ED in diabetics is primarily caused by neurologic abnormalities.[5, 17, 18] Ellenberg attributed the increased incidence of diabetic impotence to autonomic neuropathy.[5, 6] Penile erection is under the regulation of the autonomic system, and studies demonstrated that erection is controlled by both the sympathetic and parasympathetic nerves, with the sympathetic nervous system inhibiting erections while the parasympathetic system contains excitatory pathways. Sexual stimuli result in neurological impulses via somatic and autonomic motor tracts to the penis, generating tumescence and erection. Recent studies suggest that the motor control of erection is exerted via both sympathetic and parasympathetic nerve fibers, and that neither a cholinergic nor an adrenergic neurotransmitter system is solely responsible for erectile function. Nevertheless, the exact role of cholinergic neurotransmitters remains unclear. For instance, intravenous or intracavernous injection of atropine fails to inhibit penile erection.[19] Moreover, in vitro experiments on human erectile tissue treated with exogenous acetylcholine have demonstrated either contractile responses or relaxation, or even no responses at all. Saenz de Tejado et al suggest that acetylcholine is probably an inhibitory modulator of adrenergic constrictor nerves and a facilitatory modulator of nonadrenergic noncholinergic relaxation.[20] Studies from Blanco et al demonstrated an impaired ability of penile cholinergic nerves from impotent diabetic men to synthesize and release acetylcholine, thereby concluding that these patients have dysfunctional penile cholinergic nerves and that this autonomic neuropathy within the corporal tissue worsens with disease duration.[18]

Studies have also suggested a role for adrenergic neurotransmitters in erectile function. High concentration of norepinephrine has been demonstrated in the blood vessels and corporal smooth muscle, as well as a significant decrease in norepinephrine concentration in impotent diabetic patients.[21] Animal experiments show that the sympathetic noradrenergic fibers innervating the penis appear to demonstrate neuropathic changes in uncontrolled streptozotocin-induced diabetic rats along with a markedly reduced norepinephrine content, thereby providing support for the presence of noradrenergic sympathetic nerve damage in the penis as a complication of diabetes.[22-25] Our studies also demonstrate that alterations in α-adrenoceptor (phenylephrine) responsiveness are positively correlated with age in diabetic human erectile tissues but not the nondiabetic tissues.[26] Nonetheless, it has been observed that the addition of β-adrenergic blockers to isolated corporal tissue strips has no apparent effect on the contractile response to catecholamines, indicating that corporal smooth muscle relaxation cannot be effectively achieved by endogenous catecholamines.[16]

Since neither cholinergic nor adrenergic mechanisms can fully delineate erectile function, the possibility of nonadrenergic and noncholinergic neurotransmitters (NANC) has been explored. One of the peptides being studied as a neurotransmitter in penile physiology is vasoactive intestinal polypeptide (VIP). A potent vasodilator contained in the neurons of the major pelvic ganglion, VIP immunospecific fibers have been demonstrated in the cavernosal tissue.[27] Experiments have demonstrated a dose-dependent relaxation response to VIP,[28] and VIPergic nerves have been found to be depleted in the corpora of diabetic men.[29] Additional data demonstrate a consistent reduction of VIP-like immunoreactivity density in penile tissue from streptozotocin-diabetic rats and human diabetic penile tissue when compared with control subjects.[30] Lincoln et al utilized an immunohistochemical, histochemical, and biochemical investigation of the VIPergic, cholinergic, and adrenergic innervation in penile tissue from impotent patients, and provided evidence that all three types may be affected in diabetes.[31]

Endothelial cell derived modulators, such as endothelin-1 (a potent vasoconstrictor peptide), nitric oxide, and prostanoids, have been identified in the corpus cavernosum.[32, 33] Endothelin-1(ET-1) may serve as a crucial modulator in ED, supported by evidence that cultured endothelial cells from human corpus cavernosum are capable of expressing endothelin mRNA, the presence of specific binding sites for ET-1 on human corporal smooth muscle cells, the effect of ET-1 on intracellular calcium levels, and the long-lasting and potent contractile effects of ET-1 on human corpus cavernosum smooth muscles strips.[34] Elevated ET-1 levels are also observed in peripheral venous blood from diabetic patients.[35] Our studies suggest that the physiological relevance of ET-1 to corporal smooth muscle physiology may be related to its ability to augment the contractile responses of other vasomodulators present in the human corpora. ET-1 potentiates contractile responses to several spasmogens such as norepinephrine, serotonin, and angiotensin II in diverse vasculature, and may affect corporal smooth muscle tone via augmentation of underlying α1-adrenergic activity.[34] Elevated ET-1 levels may reflect local overproduction of peptide from damaged endothelial cells with plasma spillover secondary to disease processes,[35] and cause an increased intracellular calcium levels in diabetic cavernosal tissue.[36] Organic ED may thus be fostered through altered regulation of ET-induced vasoconstriction, and thereby resulting in heightened corporal vascular tone. Data from Francavilla et al also reveal elevated circulating ET-1 levels in diabetic and nondiabetic men with ED compared with normal men, as well as elevated ET-1 levels in diabetic impotent patients when compared with nondiabetic impotent ones, thus suggesting that diffuse endothelial dysfunction contributes to diabetic ED.[35] ET-1 receptor binding has also been shown to increase in the diabetic rat corpora, possibly secondary to upregulation.[37] These data all serve to suggest ET-1 as a putative modulator of ED.

Nitric oxide (NO) is demonstrated to induce vascular smooth muscle relaxation, and is deemed by some to be the putative principal mediator of penile erection. Produced from L-arginine via nitric oxide synthase, NO is identified in corporal smooth muscle cells and there is a consensus that endothelium dependent relaxation in the corpora is achieved by activation of cholinergic receptors on corporal endothelial cells and increased NO production.[32, 38, 39] NO may be released via other mechanisms; for example, it may be related to mechanical deformation or shear-stress of the endothelial cells subsequent to the increased blood flow produced by the helicine arterioles dilalation, or it may be released from nonadrenergic or noncholinergic neurons.[16] Nevertheless, there are several families of the phosphodiesterase enzymes, of which cyclic GMP-specific phosphodiesterase 5 (PDE5) plays a major role in the human corpora. Sildenafil (Viagra™), a potent and selective PDE5 inhibitor that revolutionized the field of oral agents in ED treatment, functions by inhibiting the breakdown of cGMP and thereby promoting smooth muscle relaxation. Moreover, advanced glycosylation end-products, formed from glucose and amino groups of tissue proteins and elevated in diabetic and/or aging patients, may contribute to diabetic ED by binding NO and thereby quenching its supply.[40] The collagen and elastin present in penile smooth muscle and tunica albuginea are suspected to be the target of injury by glycosylated end-products formed in diabetic animals.[41, 42] Deleterious effect on NO formation and diminished nitrergic innervation of the diabetic rat corpora has also been documented.[43-45] While NO mediates corporal smooth muscle relaxation and penile erection, studies demonstrate significantly higher NO synthase activity in diabetic rats when compared with control rats, with a marked increase in plasma NO.[46] Despite the elevated NO levels, its action or pathway may be hindered in the diabetic corpora secondary to impaired receptors or transduction mechanism for second messengers, failed corporal smooth muscles, or increased catabolism.[46, 47] Miller and associates demonstrate a reduction in the hydrolysis of cAMP and cGMP in diabetic rats, and conclude that the increased intracellular cyclic nucleotide levels constitute an adaptive response to counteract the deleterious effects of diabetes.[48] The mechanism leading to the functional blockade of NO in diabetic penile tissues will need to be further elucidated.

As Ellenberg and Kolodny et al proposed autonomic neuropathy to be the primary cause of increased incidence of diabetic impotence, other investigations have also corroborated that conclusion.[5, 6, 20, 49, 50] ED may not be a late complication of diabetes, as ED can present early during the course of the disease, or the diagnosis of ED can lead to the discovery of otherwise unrecognized diabetes.[51] The correlation of bladder neuropathies or dysfunction in diabetic impotent patients, such as decreased bladder sensation, increased residual urine and detrusor instability, is crucial in supporting autonomic neuropathy as cause of diabetic impotence since the bladder and penis receive autonomic innervation from common origins, the hypogastric sympathetic and the pelvic parasympathetic nerves. Ellenberg and Faerman et al both report high incidence of bladder dysfunction in diabetic impotent patients.[6, 52] Neurophysiological, hormonal, and vascular investigations from Bemelmans and associates conclude that diabetic urogenital neuropathy along with poor diabetes regulation plays a crucial role in the etiology of diabetic ED while vasculopathy appears to be of secondary importance.[53] Their studies demonstrate a significantly lower glycosylated hemoglobin values and plasma glucose in the potent diabetic men than the impotent diabetic ones, suggestive of better diabetes control in the former group. Morphologic alterations or abnormalities, consisted of beaded thickenings, vacuolated thickenings, hyperargentophilia and moniliform thickenings, are also revealed in the autonomic nerve fibers of diabetic corporal tissue,[52] although our earlier studies demonstrate that the anatomic integrity of the sympathetic nerves retrieved from the corporal tissue of impotent diabetic men is intact.[54] The host of neurotransmitters implicated in the physiology of penile erection, along with the various neuroeffector systems, also lend support to the notion that diabetic penile neuropathy is the primary origin of diabetic ED. Nevertheless, knowledge gaps remain regarding the exact contribution of diabetic neuropathy to ED and bladder dysfunction at the molecular and cellular level. Is there a secondary response of the corporal tissue per se or changes in the myocytes when the innervation to the tissue is altered? Current efforts at our Urology

Research Laboratory focus on studying the differential control of smooth muscle cell tone in physiologically distinct organ systems such as the excitable bladder detrusor myocytes and nonexcitable corporal smooth muscle, and propose that differential organ function is attributable to quantifiable differences in the way that ionic mechanisms participate in the control of myocyte tone. Our data also support that altered neural and/or myocyte function will differentially contribute to diabetic ED and bladder dysfunction, and can thus lead to novel therapeutic possibilities by better defining the mechanisms involving diabetic neuropathy or myopathy.

Integrative Corporal Smooth Muscle Physiology

Recent clinical data demonstrate the essential role of corporal smooth muscle in modulating penile blood flow during erection, with an emerging concensus that the etiologic basis of organic ED lies in the primary changes of corporal smooth muscle physiology and function.[55] Regardless of the primary defect or abnormality, corporal smooth muscle relaxation is both necessary and sufficient to elicit an erection in many cases.[55]

The modulation of corporal smooth muscle tone is an intricate process necessitating the integration of a host of intracellular events and extracellular signals. Data reveal that the neurotransmitters that participate in erection and detumescence modulate corporal muscle tone largely via their effects on the gap junctions, calcium and potassium channels.[55] Figure 1 depicts the major mechanisms regulating corporal smooth muscle tone. Broadly, events linked to calcium mobilization and muscle contraction favor increases in the level of intercellular communication, whereas events linked to the activation of cAMP and muscle relaxation decrease the level of intercellular communication.[8]

Potassium channels, ubiquitous in myocytes, appear to exhibit a greater diversity than any other ion channels. At least four distinct subtypes have been identified in corporal smooth muscle: calcium-sensitive potassium channel (maxi-K or K_{Ca}); ATP dependent potassium channel (K_{ATP}); inwardly rectifying channel (K_{ir}); and voltage-gated potassium channel (K_v). Of these four subtypes, the K_{ATP} and maxi-K channels are the most thoroughly studied, and are physiologically relevant to the control of corporal smooth muscle tone. The importance of potassium channels to the modulation of corporal smooth muscle tone is related to the intricate interplay between membrane potential, cellular excitability, and contractility.[56,57] In other words, sustained contractions of corporal smooth muscle are dependent on continuous transmembrane calcium flux through voltage-dependent calcium channels, and hyperpolarization of corporal smooth muscle cells via potassium channels may represent an important mechanism for modulating corporal muscle tone.[55] Recent studies report that diabetic corporal tissues from patients are less sensitive to relaxation with potassium modulators.

Gap junction proteins have a vital role in the initiation, maintenance, and modulation of corporal smooth muscle tone,[58-60] since the sparse neuronal innervation of corporal smooth muscles may not explain their synchronized and coordinated relaxation, as well as the rapid and diffuse response of corpora cavernosa to locally released or injected neuromodulators. Our studies demonstrate the diffusion of current carrying ions and second messengers (calcium ions and IP_3) through gap junctions between coupled corporal smooth muscle cells in culture.[58] A significant increase in connexin43 mRNA expression in the rat corpora is reported in STZ-induced diabetic rats,[61] and Giraldi et al reveal a twofold to eightfold variability in connexin43 mRNA in corporal tissue isolated from patients with organic ED,[62] which signifies that the connexin43 mRNA level may be a crucial regulatory point in organic ED. Interestingly, changes in connexin43 mRNA expression are also correlated with physiologically significant alterations in other smooth muscle tissues, such as myometrial smooth muscle.[63,64] Gap junction dysfunction may be accountable for the impaired smooth muscle relaxation and contraction coordination in vascular disease due to the presence of collagen fibers between cellular membranes.[65] Thus, there is strong evidence to support a role for intercellular communication in the integration of corporal smooth tissue responses, and gap junctions play an invaluable role in modulating corporal smooth muscle tone and consequently penile erection.

Streptozotocin (STZ)-Induced Diabetic Erectile Dysfunction in a Rat Model

Our recent studies propose that differential organ function is attributed to quantifiable organ-specific differences in the way that ionic mechanisms participate in the control of myocyte tone. We hypothesize that altered neural functions such as diabetic peripheral neuropathy, impaired myocyte function such as loss or decrease in myocytes, change in myocyte responsiveness to agonist stimulation such as alterations in potassium channels or gap junctions, will differentially contribute to STZ-induced diabetic bladder and erectile dysfunction. These alterations may be related to differences in the severity and duration of diabetes. Isolating the effects of altered myocyte function versus altered neural regulation in our experiments is monumental since a more direct or accurate cause-and-effect relationship can then be elucidated, and development of a more appropriate remedy can thus be targeted. Diabetes or hyperglycemia may induce direct effects on myocyte function. It has been demonstrated that alterations in neural and myocyte function are unequivocally related to the hyperglycemia, and not a nonspecific effect of STZ.[43, 61] The following alterations have been observed in STZ-induced diabetic rats: a significant reduction in penile erectile reflexes, decrease in erectile response to cavernous neurostimulation, loss of erectile rigidity similar to the loss of erection in diabetic men, and loss of efferent neurons as evidenced by altered synaptophysin staining.[43,44,66]

425

Diminished hyperpolarizing ability of the corporal smooth muscle, possibly secondary to decreased potassium channel mRNA expression, may lead to impaired smooth muscle relaxation as hyperpolarization of corporal smooth muscle cells via potassium channels may be vital in modulating corporal smooth muscle tone. Through the aforementioned mechanism, STZ-induced alterations in potassium channel activity can manifest as quantifiable changes in their ability to modulate contractility. Our studies reveal a significant diabetes-related difference in the maximal amplitude of the phenylephrine-(PE, equipotent as endogenous norepinephrine on corporal tissue strips) induced contractile response, and a virtually absent pinacidil-induced relaxation in the corporal tissue strips from STZ-diabetic rats. Moreover, our pharmacological assays measure the ability of purinergic agonists (ATP and UTP) to induce changes in the intracellular calcium levels, and discover a significant reduction in ATP-mediated calcium mobilization in the diabetic corporal tissue and a sevenfold decrease in the sensitivity of the corpora to ATP. This observation may reflect a functional reduction/expression of the P2-receptor, mediator of corporal smooth muscle relaxation induced by stimulation of the penile purinergic innervation. These changes in purinergic signaling may possibly contribute to diabetic ED.

Vascular factors

Vascular abnormalities associated with diabetes mellitus and atherosclerosis is a major cause of organic ED. Atherosclerosis is the cause of approximately 40% of ED in men older than 50 years, and is characterized by the proliferation of smooth muscle and deposition of lipid or collagen in the vessel wall. The presence of arteriogenic ED in men older than 50 years of age is considered by some investigators as an ominous sign for the presence of atherosclerotic disease and microangiopathy in other parts of the body.[67,68] Diabetic retinopathy is often a manifestation of small vessel disease in diabetic patients. Diffuse vascular process such as atherosclerosis can lead to arteriogenic ED by causing vessel obstruction or arterial insufficiency, commonly the internal pudendal artery and sometimes even the collaterals, and consequently reducing arterial inflow. Thickening of the capillary basement membrane and increased vascular permeability with extravasation of lipoproteins into the vessel walls are considered to be the etiologies of small vessel disease in diabetic patients.[69] Jevtich and associates conclude from their studies that stenosis and obliteration of penile arteries is the primary contributor to diabetic ED.[69] Other studies demonstrate that in patients with leg ischemia, there is significant pudendal arterial stenosis in impotent diabetic and nondiabetic men compared to potent men.[70] Diabetes is also associated with increased risk of developing hypercholesterolemia and hypercoagulopathy.[71] Hypercholesterolemia may contribute to ED as well as atherosclerosis via deposition of lipid in vascular lesions;[68] thus, diabetic patients are subject to compounded risk factors and insults when they develop hypercholesterolemia and atherosclerosis

426

independently. The hypercoagulopathic state associated with diabetes, which is induced by increase in coagulation factors such as the von Willebrand factor and tissue plasminogen, can lead to thrombosis and reduced arterial inflow.[72,73] Diabetic impotent patients may also have other vascular risk factors, such as hypertension and cigarette smoking, which can all cause atherosclerotic vessel changes.[2, 74-76] Corporal veno-occlusive dysfunction associated with atherosclerotic alterations is also implicated in the etiology of ED in diabetic men,[77] via structural changes in the fibroelastic components of the corpora.

DIAGNOSTIC MODALITIES

As the first step in the evaluation process, a complete history and physical examination should be performed with primary attention toward sexual and genital development as well as identifying any vascular, endocrine, or neurologic abnormalities. Approximately 20% of men by history and physical examination alone will be overdiagnosed with organic ED.[78] Any patients who describe overt, rigid, straight erections (for example with mistress but not with wife, during masturbation) should be referred for sex therapy without further diagnostic testings. A careful neurologic examination is important in a patient with a history suggestive of peripheral or central neuropathies such as diabetes. The endocrine studies that may be performed for evaluation of impotent men are targeted toward hypothalamic-pituitary-testicular axis. These assays measure serum testosterone, prolactin, thyroid, and luteinizing hormones. A screening glycosylated hemoglobin Alc should also be performed to assess for a diabetic cause of ED.

To diagnose the presence of ED, initial tests such as Rigiscan™ analysis, visual sexual stimulation, and penile plethysmography (pulse volume recording) can be performed as baseline studies. Rigiscan™ analysis monitors nocturnal penile tumescence and rigidity by measuring penile circumference and radial rigidity through loops connected to a microcomputer that is strapped to the patient's thigh. Rigiscan remains the only objective way of monitoring the presence or absence of erectile ability. Intracavernous pharmacotesting can also serve as a treatment trial to assess the quality of erection. If erection is not achieved, the test should be considered as inconclusive and other diagnostic tests should be sought. Penile plethysmography is a good screening test that measures volume changes with each pulsatile expansion of the penis during flaccidity. Duplex sonography is a minimally invasive initial diagnostic test of vascular impairment.[79, 80] The advantages of penile duplex ultrasound are the ability to visualize penile anatomy, measure arterial flow velocity or peak systolic velocity, assess arterial compliance and pharmacologic response, and evaluate venous efflux.

Although autonomic neuropathy is the primary cause of erectile dysfunction there are no direct measure to assess the autonomic nervous

427

system. Penile biothesiometry simply measures the sensory function or vibration perception threshold of the penis, and can be used as an initial screening test. Aging and diabetes accelerate the diminished perception of vibratory sensation.[81] Since first described by Haldeman et al, somatosensory evoked potential testing has evolved into a promising tool in the evaluation of neurogenic impotence.[82]

Although no tests can directly measure the autonomic component of erectile function, testing of the autonomic cardiovascular reflexes suggests that abnormal reflexes are associated with aging and organic impotence, indicating the equal importance of autonomic dysfunction in the etiology of erectile failure.[83] Cystometrography and tests of certain vascular functions regulated by the autonomic nervous system, including blood pressure and pulse response to cold, sympathetic skin responses to electrical stimulation, and orthostatic measurements of blood pressure and pulse, have been suggested as ways of identifying autonomic neuropathy in impotent patients.[84]

THERAPEUTIC OPTIONS

After the diagnosis of ED is established, a treatment plan should be configured. The applicability of the particular therapeutic option is dependent on the underlying pathology, potential reversibility of the dysfunction, and of course, wishes of the patient.

No treatment
Some 25 to 30% of patients are content to be told of the etiology of their dysfunction, and desire no further treatment[81].

Medical Therapy
The drug therapies available to induce penile erection are nonspecific and may promote erection in the presence of psychological, hormonal, neurologic, or vascular pathologies. If the vascular flow obstruction or vessel stenosis, veno-occlusive dysfunction, corporal fibrosis, micro- and macro-angiopathies are too severe, drug treatment will be ineffective and other noninvasive therapies must be sought.

The introduction of oral sildenafil (Viagra[TM]) has contributed to increased public awareness of ED. Sildenafil exerts its effects via prolonging the action of cGMP, thereby increasing calcium efflux and consequent corporal smooth muscle relaxation. Impotent patients with long history of severe poorly-controlled diabetes may not optimally benefit from sildenafil secondary to microangiopathy, altered myocyte function and neural regulation. But Rendell et al report improved erections in 57% of diabetic impotent patients receiving sildenafil versus 10% in the placebo group, which is encouraging despite the pathophysiologic alterations diabetes can impose on penile physiology.[85] However, the study of 268 patients excludes those presenting with more severe diabetic complications such as unstable glucose control and severe autonomic neuropathy. In other words, patients sustaining more severe diabetic complications may not be suited to administration of sildenafil, despite the study's conclusion that oral sildenafil is an effective and well-tolerated treatment for men with diabetic ED.[85] Price et al also report good efficacy of oral sildenafil in treating diabetic impotent, although only 21 men are included in the study and only 6 have evidence of autonomic neuropathy.[86] To reiterate, we believe that oral sildenafil may not be an effective treatment option for impotent men suffering from the more advanced or severe diabetes-induced pathophysiologic alterations secondary to myocyte function and neural regulation impairment, and a possible direct diabetic effect on the cavernous tissue independent from any other alterations. Nevertheless, the advent of such a relatively effective oral agent for ED is encouraging, and since none of its adverse effects exacerbates diabetes, diabetic impotent patients should be given a trial of oral sildenafil. Common minor side effects include headache, flushing, and blurred vision, and an enhanced hypotensive effect may be incurred to patients already receiving nitrates.

Patients with primary hormonal abnormalities such as severe hypotestosteronemia may benefit from testosterone therapy while those with hyperprolactinemia induced by prolactin-secreting tumors can utilize either oral bromocriptine, radiation, or surgical ablation of the pituitary tumor.

Prostaglandins have been identified in human corporal tissue, and are known to modulate autonomic nerve function and the effect of vasoactive hormones that contribute to the myogenic tone of vascular smooth muscle.[87] Intraurethral alprostadil, the synthetic formulation of prostaglandin E1 administered as a pellet in 500-μg quantities, has rapid absorption rates and can induce penile erection in some patients. This "medicated urethral system for erection" or "MUSE" may incur side effects of urethral pain and bleeding, hypotension, or infection.[88]

Intracorporal pharmacotherapy or injection of vasoactive agents is a minimally invasive therapy pioneered by Virag in 1983. The pharmacologic erection can be induced with an intracavernous injection of 0.20 mL of Trimix (papaverine 30 mg/mL, 2.5 mL; phentolamine 5 mg; and prostagladin E1, 25 μg, 1.2 mL saline) or 10 μg of prostagladin E1. Papaverine is another phosphodiesterase inhibitor that prolongs the action of intracellular cyclic AMP and causes vascular smooth muscle relaxation. This form of therapy works best in patients with good or marginal penile blood supply and properly functioning corporal smooth muscle, and may be used alone or in conjunction with other drugs. Diabetic impotent patients who have the complications of atherosclerosis and venous corporal incompetence may not benefit from intracavernous pharmacotherapy. Side effects include priapism, scarring, and bleeding.

Vacuum Devices

The external vacuum device offers a relatively safe and nonsurgical alternative for almost all types of ED. It functions by being placed over the penis in which a vacuum is generated. The vacuum pulls blood into the corpora, thus generating an erection-like state. A tourniquet or tension band is then placed at the penile base in order to trap blood in the shaft, and the band is left in place for a maximum of 30 minutes.

Surgical Treatment

Penile prosthesis is an effective surgical alternative to impotent patients with organic or systemic diseases. The basic choice is between the placement of a semi-rigid and inflatable prostheses. The primary side effect is infection at the time of surgery with a reported incidence of about 3%. Studies report that penile prosthesis is effective in diabetic impotent men with low complication rates.[89, 90]

FUTURE DIRECTIONS IN DIABETIC ERECTILE DYSFUNCTION

ED is commonly associated with diabetes, and each disease process by itself incurs debilitating consequences. Diabetes is now the leading cause of new blindness in adults, the leading cause of end-stage renal disease, the leading cause of lower extremity amputations not related to injury, and one of the major contributing factors to cardiac disease and stroke, and a host of many other comorbidities. The diabetes-related changes observed in ED and bladder dysfunction are permanent and require medical therapy to ameliorate the symptoms.[91] Since hyperglycemia per se appears to be responsible for the complications and glucose management remains to be problematic, there will be a high priority for development of novel therapeutic options to tackle the various complications from diabetes. There is an impressive reduction in the incidence and progression of microangiopathy and neuropathy via tight glycemic control. Since the pathophysiology from diabetic ED is related to the duration and severity of hyperglycemia and its complications,[92] aggressive tight metabolic control from the onset, or possibly even prevention, of the disease is key to avoiding ED and all the other comorbidities associated with diabetes.

SUMMARY

Recognized since antiquity, diabetes mellitus has become ubiquitous in many developing and newly industrialized countries. Dubbed the silent killer, diabetes causes more deaths per year in the United States than AIDS. Although the effect of diabetes on sexual function in men has been known since approximately 200 years ago, their association has become well-recognized only during the last 3 decades. The impact of diabetes on male sexual function can be appreciated by the fact that more than 50% of patients with diabetes have ED. The most common causes of diabetic ED include autonomic neuropathy and vascular abnormalities often associated with diabetes. Numerous neurotransmitters are implicated in the modulation of penile erection, including vasoactive intestinal polypeptide, endothelin-1, and nitric oxide, further strengthening the notion that diabetic neuropathy plays a crucial role in the genesis of diabetic ED. Our current research efforts at the molecular level on gap junctions and potassium channels are invaluable in further deciphering the mechanisms governing penile smooth muscle relaxation and contraction, and thereby suggesting novel therapeutic options.

Several therapeutic options are offered with the diagnosis of ED: medical therapy such as oral sildenafil, intracorporal pharmacotherapy; vacuum devices; or surgical modalities such as penile prosthesis. But despite the advancement and efficacy of such treatments, the biggest hope of patients and physicians alike will be a cure of diabetes and thus the eradication of its associated co-morbidities. The prevention of diabetes can also eliminate the onset of its deleterious effects such as ED. As we strive to search for more answers, a cure for diabetes mellitus may be on the horizon.

REFERENCES

1.   NIH Consensus Development Panel on Impotence. NIH Consensus Conference. JAMA 270: 83, 1993.
2.   Feldman HA, Goldstein I, Hatzichristou DG, Krane RJ, McKinlay JB. Impotence and its medical and psychosocial correlates: results of the Massachusetts Male Aging Study. J Urol 151: 54-61, 1994.
3.   Zonszein J. Diagnosis and management of endocrine disorders of erectile dysfunction. Urol Clin N Am 22: 789-802, 1995.
4.   Benet AE, Melman A. The epidemiology of erectile dysfunction. Urol Clin N Am 22: 699-709, 1995.
5.   Ellenberg M Impotence in diabetes: the neurologic factor. Ann Intern Med 75: 213-219, 1971.
6.   Ellenberg M. Sexual function in diabetic patients. Ann Intern Med 92: 331-333, 1980.
7.   Ryder RE, Close CF, Moriarty KT, Moore KT, Hardisty CA. Impotence in diabetes: aetiology, implications for treatment and preferred vacuum device. Diabetes Med 9: 893-898, 1992.
8.   Melman A, Gingell JC. The epidemiology and pathophysiology of erectile dysfunction. Urol 161: 5-11, 1999.
9.   Buvat J, Lemaire A, Buvat-Herbaut M, et al. Comparative investigations in 26 impotent and 26 nonimpotent diabetic patients. J Urol 133: 34-38, 1985.
10. Cummings MH, Alexander WD. Erectile dysfunction in patients with diabetes. Hosp Med 60: 638-644, 1999.

11. Lehman TP, Jacobs JA. Etiology of diabetic impotence. J Urol 129: 291-294, 1983.
12. Christ GJ, Brink PR, Melman A, Spray DC. The role of gap junctions and ion channels in the modulation of electrical and chemical signals in human corpus cavernosum smooth muscle. Int J of Impotence Res 5: 77, 1993.
13. Goldstein I. Impotence (editorial). J Urol 51:1533, 1994.
14. Lue TF. Erectile dysfunction associated with cavernous and neurological model (editorial). Am J Physiol 260: H1590, 1991.
15. Andersson KE, Wagner G. Physiology of penile erection. Physiol Rev 75: 191, 1995.
16. Lerner SE, Melman A, Christ GJ. A review of erectile dysfunction: new insights and more questions. J Urol 149:1246-1255, 1993.
17. McCulloch DK, Campbell IW, Wu FC, Prescott RJ, Clarke BF. The prevalence of diabetic impotence. Diabetologia 18:279-283, 1980.
18. Blanco R, Saenz de Tejada I, Goldstein I, Krane RJ, Wotiz HH, Cohen RA. Dysfunctional penile cholinergic nerves in diabetic impotent men. J Urol 144:278-280, 1990.
19. Wagner G, Brindley GS. The effect of atropine, alpha and beta blockers on human penile erection: a controlled pilot study. In: Zorgniotti AW, Rossi G, eds. Vasculogenic Impotence. Proceedings of the First International Conference on Corpus Cavernosum Revascularization. Springfield, Illinois: Charles C Thomas Publishers, pp. 77-81, 1980.
20. Saenz de Tejada I, Goldstein I. Diabetic penile neuropathy. Urol Clin N Am 15:17-22, 1988.
21. Melman A, Henry DP. The possible role of the catecholamines of the corpora in penile erection. Urol 121:419-421, 1979.
22. Felten DL, Felten SY, Melman A. Noradrenergic innervation of the penis in control and streptozotocin-diabetic rats: evidence of autonomic neuropathy. Anat Rec 206: 49-59, 1983.
23. Melman A, Henry DP, Felten DL. Catecholamine content of the penile corpora in patients with diabetes associated impotence. Surg Forum 29: 634-636, 1978.
24. Melman A, Henry DP, Felten DL, O'Connor BL. The effect of diabetes mellitus upon the sympathetic nerves of the penile corpora in patients with erectile impotence. South Med J 73:307-309, 1980a.
25. Melman A, Henry DP, Felten DL, O'Connor BL. Alteration of the nerves of the penile corpora in patients with erectile impotence. Invest Urol 17: 474-477, 1980.
26. Christ GJ, Maayani S, Valcic M, Melman A. Pharmacological studies of human erectile tissue: characteristics of spontaneous contractions and alterations in alpha-adrenoceptor responsiveness with age and disease in isolated tissues. Br J Pharmacol 101: 375-381, 1990.

27. Gu J, Polak JM, Probert L, Islam KN, et al. Peptidergic innervation of the human male genital tract. J Urol 130:386-391, 1983.
28. Adaiken PG, Kottegoda SR, Ratnam SS. Is vasoactive intestinal peptide the principal transmitter involved in human penile erection? J Urol 135:638-640, 1986.
29. Gu J, Polak J, Lazarides M, Morgan RJ, et al. Decrease of vasoactive intestinal polypeptide (VIP) in the penises from impotent men. Lancet 2:315-318, 1984.
30. Crowe R, Lincoln J, Blacklay PF, Pryor JP, Lumley JS, Burnstock G. Vasoactive intestinal polypeptide-like immunoreactive nerves in diabetic penis. A comparison between streptozocin-treated rats and man. Diabetes 32: 1075-1077, 1983.
31. Lincoln J, Crowe R, Blacklay PF, Pryor JP, Lumley JS, Burnstock G. Changes in the VIPergic, cholinergic and adrenergic innervation of human penile tissue in daibetic and non-diabetic impotent males. J Urol 137: 1053-1059, 1987.
32. Azadzoi K, Kim N, Brown ML, Goldstein I, Cohen RA, Saenz de Tejada I. Endothelium-derived nitric oxide and cyclooxygenase products modulate corpus cavernosum smooth muscle tone. Urol 147:220-225, 1992.
33. Saenz de Tejada I, Carson MP, de las Morenas A, Goldstein I, Triash AM. Endothelin: localization, synthesis, activity, and receptor types in human penile corpus cavernosum. Am J Physiol 26:H1078-1085, 1991.
34. Christ GJ, Lerner EE, Kim DC, Melman A. Endothelin-1 as a putative modulator of erectile dysfunction: Characteristics of contraction of isolated corporal tissue strips. J Urol 153:1998-2003, 1995.
35. Francavilla S, Properzi G, Bellini C, Marino G, Ferri C, Santucci A. Endothelin-1 in diabetic and nondiabetic men with erectile dysfunction. J Urol 158: 1770-1774, 1997.
36. Sullivan ME, Dashwood MR, Thompson CS, Muddle JR, Mikhailidis DP, Morgan RJ. Alterations in endothelin B receptor sites in cavernosal tissue of daibetic rabbits: potential relevance to the pathogenesis of erectile dysfunction. J Urol 158:1966-1972, 1997.
37. Bell CRW, Sullivan M, Dashwood MR, Muddle JR, Morgan RJ. The density and distribution of endothelin-1 and endothelin receptor subtypes in normal and diabetic rat corpus cavernosum. Br J Urol 76: 203-207, 1995.
38. Kim N, Azadzoi K, Goldstein I, Saenz de Tejada I. A nitric oxide-like factor mediates nonadrenergic-noncholinergic neurogenic relaxation of penile corpus cavernosum smooth muscle. J Clin Invest 88:112-118, 1991.

39. Rajfer J, Aronson WJ, Bush PA, Dorey FJ, Ignarro LJ. Nitric oxide as a mediator of relaxation of the corpus cavernosum in response to nonadrenergic, noncholinergic neurotransmission. N Engl J Med 326: 90-94, 1992.

40. Seftel AD, Vaziri ND, Ni Z, Razmjouei K, Fogarty J, Hampel N, Polak J, Wang RZ, Ferguson K, Block C, Haas C. Advanced glycation end products in human penis: elevation in diabetic tissue, site of deposition, and possible effect through iNOS or eNOS. Urology 50:1016-1026, 1997.

41. Makita Z, Vlassara H, Cercimi, Bucola R. Immunochemical detection of advanced glycosylation products in vivo. J Biol Chem 267: 5133-5138, 1992.

42. Maher E, Bachoo M, Elabbady AA, Polosa C, Begin LR, Collier B, Elhilali MM, Hassouna MM. Vasoactive intestinal peptide and impotence in experimental diabetes mellitus. Br J Urol 77: 271-278, 1996.

43. Cellek S, Rodrigo J, Lobos E, Fernandez P, Serrano J, Moncada S. Selective nitrergic neurodegeneration in diabetes mellitus - a nitric oxide-dependent phenomenon. Br J Pharmacol 128:1804-1812, 1999.

44. el-Sakka AI, Lin CS, Chui RM, Dahiya R, Lue TF. Effects of diabetes on nitric oxide synthase and growth factors genes and protein expression in an animal model. Int J Impotence Res 11:123-132, 1999.

45. Sullivan M, Thompson CS, Mikhailidis DP, Morgan RJ, Angelini GD, Jeremy JY. Differential alterations of prostacyclin, cyclic AMP and cyclic GMP formation in the corpus cavernosum of the diabetic rabbit. Br J Urol 82:578-584, 1998.

46. Elabbady AA, Gagnon C, Hassouna MM, Begin LR, Elhilali MM. Diabetes mellitus increases nitric oxide synthase in penises but not in major pelvic ganglia of rats. Bri J Urol 76: 196-202, 1995.

47. Basar MM, Yildiz M, Soylemezoglu F, et al. Histopathological changes and nitric oxide synthase activity in corpus cavernosum from rats with neurogenic erectile dysfunction. Br J Urol Int 83: 101-107, 1999.

48. Miller MA, Morgan RJ, Thompson CS, Mikhailidis DP, Jeremy JY. Hydrolysis of cyclic guanosine monophosphate and cyclic adenosine monophosphate by the penis and aorta of the diabetic rat. Br J Urol 78:252-256, 1996.

49. Kolodny RC, Kahn CB, Goldstein HH, Barnett DM. Sexual dysfunction in diabetic men. Diabetes 23: 306-309, 1974.

50. Jensen SB. Sexual dysfunction in insulin-treated diabetes: a six year follow-up study of 101 patients. Arch Sex Behav 15: 271, 1986.

51. Deutsch S, Sherman L. Previously unrecognized diabetes mellitus in sexually impotent men. JAMA 244: 2430-2432, 1980.

52. Faerman I, Glocer L, Fox D, Jadzinsky MN, Rapaport M. Impotence and diabetes. Histological studies of the autonomic nervous fibers of the corpora cavernosa in impotent diabetic males. Diabetes 23: 971-976, 1974.

53. Bemelmans BL, Meuleman EJ, Doesburg WH, Notermans SL, Debruyne FM. Erectile dysfunction in diabetic men: the neurological factor revisited. J Urol 151:884-889, 1994.

54. Melman A, Henry DP, Felten DL, O'Connor BL. Effect of diabetes upon penile sympathetic nerves in impotent patients. South Med J 73: 307-309, 317, 1980.

55. Christ GJ. The penis as a vascular organ. The importance of corporal smooth muscle tone in the control of erection. Urol Clin N Ame 22: 727-745, 1995.

56. Lee SW, Wang HZ, Christ GJ. Characterization of ATP-sensitive potassium channels in human corporal smooth muscle cells. Int J Impot Res 11: 189-199, 1999.

57. Lee SW, Wang HZ, Zhao W, Ney P, Brink PR, Christ GJ. Prostaglandin E1 activates the large conductance KCa channel in human corporal smooth muscle. Int J Impotence Res 11:179-188, 1999.

58. Christ GJ, Moreno AP, Melman A, Spray DC. Gap junction-mediated intercellular diffusion of Ca in cultured human corporeal smooth muscle cells. Am J Physiol 263: C373, 1992.

59. Campos de Carvalho AC, Roy C, Moreno AP, Melman A, Hertzberg EL, Christ GJ, Spray DC. Gap junctions formed of connexin43 are found between smooth muscle cells of human corpus cavernosum. J Urol 149: 1568-1575, 1993.

60. Christ GJ, Moreno AP, Parker ME, Gondre CM, Valcic M, Melman A, Spray DC. Intercellular communication through gap junctions: potential role in pharmacomechanical coupling and syncytial tissue contraction in vascular smooth muscle isolated from the human corpus cavernosum. Life Sci 49:PL195, 1991.

61. Rehman J, Chenven E, Brink PR, Grine B, Walcott B, Melman A, Christ GJ. Diminished neurogenic-, but not pharmacologic-induced intracavernous pressure responses in the 3 month Streptozotocin (STZ)-diabetic rat. Am J Physiol 272: H1960-H1971, 1997.

62. Giraldi A, Wen Y, Geliebter J, Christ GJ. Differential gap junction mRNA expression in human corpus cavernosum: a significant regulatory event in cell-to-cell communication? Urol 153:508A, 1995.

63. Andersen J, Grine E, Eng CL, et al. Expression of connexin-43 in human myometrium and leiomyoma. Amer J Obst Gyn 169: 1266-1277, 1993.

64.	Risek B, Guthrie S, Kumar N, Gilula NB. Modulation of gap junction transcript and protein expression during pregnancy in the rat. J Cell Biol 110: 269-282, 1990.

65.	Persson C, Diederichs W, Lue TF, et al. Correlation of altered penile ultrastructure with clinical arterial evaluation. J Urol 142:1462-1468, 1989.

66.	Vernet D, Cai L, Garban H, et al. Reduction of penile nitric oxide synthase in diabetic BB/WORdp (type I) and BBZ/WORdp (type II) rats with erectile dysfunction. Endocrinol 136:5709-5717, 1995.

67.	Kaiser FE, Udhoji V, Viosca SP, et al. Cardiovascular stress tests in patients with vascular impotence. Clin Res 37: 89A, 1989.

68.	Virag R, Bouilly P, Frydman. Is impotence an arterial disorder? Lancet 1: 181-184, 1984.

69.	Jevtich MJ, Edson M, Jarman WD, Herrera HH. Vascular factor in erectile failure among diabetics. Urol 19:163-168, 1982.

70.	Herman A, Adar R, Rubinstein Z. Vascular lesions associated with impotence in diabetic and nondiabetic arterial occlusive disease. Diabetes 27:975-981, 1978.

71.	Akoi I, Shimoyama K, Aoki N, et al. Platelet dependent thrombin generation in patients with diabetes mellitus: effects of glycemic control on coagulopathy in diabetes. J Am Coll Cardiol 27:560-566, 1996.

72.	Jensen T, Bjerre-Knudsen J, Feldt-Rasmussen B, Deckert T. Features of endothelial dysfunction in early diabetic nephropathy. Lancet 1: 461-463, 1989.

73.	Carrier S, Brock G, Kour NW, T.F. L. Pathophysiology of erectile dysfunction. Urology 42: 468-481, 1993.

74.	Rosen MP, Greenfield AJ, Walker TG, et al. Cigarette smoking: an independent risk factor for atherosclerosis in the hypogastric-cavernous arterial bed of men with arteriogenic impotence. J Urol 145:759-63, 1991.

75.	Krane RJ, Goldstein I, Saenz de Tejada I. Medical progress: impotence. N Engl J Med 321: 1648, 1989.

76.	Hakim LS, Goldstein I. Diabetic sexual dysfunction. Endocrinol Metab Clin North America 25: 379-400, 1996.

77.	Mottonen M, Nieminen K. Relation of atherosclerotic obstruction of the arterial supply of corpus cavernosum to erectile dysfunction. Proceedings of the Sixth Biennial International Symposium on Corpus Cavernosum Revascularization and Third Biennial World Meeting on Impotence. Boston: 12, 1988.

78.	Davis-Joseph B, Tiefer L, Melman A. Accuracy of the initial history and physical examination to establish the etiology of erectile dysfunction. Urology 45: 498-502, 1995.

79. Merckx LA, DeBruyne RMG, Goes E, Derde MP, Keuppens F. The value of dynamic color duplex scanning in the diagnosis of venogenic impotence. J Urol 148:318-320, 1992.

80. Kropman RF, Schipper J, Oostayen JA, Nijeholt ABL, Meinhardt W. The value of increased end diastolic velocity during penile duplex sonography in relation to pathological venous leakage in erectile dysfunction. J Urol 148: 314-317, 1992.

81. Melman A, Tiefer L, Pedersen R. Evaluation of first 406 patients in urology department based Cneter for Male Sexual Dysfunction. Urology 32: 6-10, 1988.

82. Haberman S, Bradley WE, Bhatia NN, Johnson BK. Pudendal evoked responses. Arch Neurol 39: 280, 1982.

83. Nisen HO, Larsen A, Lindstrom BL, Ruutu ML, Virtanen JM, Alfthan OS. Cardiovascular reflexes in the neurological evaluation of impotence. Br J Urol 71:199-203, 1993.

84. Sharlip ID. Evaluation and nonsurgical management of erectile dysfunction. Urol Clin N Am 25: 647-659, 1998.

85. Rendell MS, Rajfer J, Wicker PA, Smith MD. Sildenafil for treatment of erectile dysfunction in men with diabetes: a randomized controlled trial. Sildenafil Diabetes Study Group. JAMA 281: 421-426, 1999.

86. Price DE, Gingell JC, Gepi-Attee S, Wareham K, Yates P, Boolell M. Sildenafil: study of a novel oral treatment for erectile dysfunction in diabetic men. Diabetes Med 15: 821-825, 1998.

87. Melman A. Neural and vascular control of erection. In: Rosen RC, Leiblum SR, eds. Erectile Disorder: Assessment and Treatment. New York: The Guilford Press, pp. 55-71, 1992.

88. Kim ED, McVary KT. Topical prostaglandin E-1 for the treatment of erectile dysfunction. Urol 153: 1828-1830, 1995.

89. Beaser RS, Van der Hoek C, Jacobson AM, Flood TM, Desautels RE. Experience with penile prosthesis in the treatment of impotence in diabetic men. JAMA 248:943-948, 1982.

90. Scott FB, Fishman IJ, Light JK. An inflatable penile prosthesis for treatment of diabetic impotence. Ann Intern Med 92:340-342, 1980.

91. McCulloch DK, Young RJ, Prescott RJ, Campbell IW, Clarke BF. The natural history of impotence in diabetic men. Diabetologia 26: 437-440, 1984.

92. Klein R, Klein BE, Lee KE, Moss SE, Cruickshanks KJ. Prevalence of self-reported erectile dysfunction in people with long-term IDDM. Diabetes Care 19: 135-141, 1996.

Chapter 10. Gastrointestinal Manifestations of Diabetes

Christine L. Frissora and Ira M. Jacobson

INTRODUCTION

Diabetes commonly affects every part of the gastrointestinal tract from the esophagus to the rectum. It has been estimated that more than 75% of diabetics may have gastrointestinal symptoms directly related to the effects of diabetic neuropathy. Some gastrointestinal symptoms may be under-reported by diabetic patients and physicians because they appear minor compared to retinopathy, nephropathy and other complications of diabetes. Some patients may be asymptomatic but still have an underlying disorder of gastrointestinal function.

We can divide diabetic patients with gastrointestinal disorders into three groups. The first group consists of patients who suffer from structural or metabolic disorders which also occur in non-diabetic individuals, such as colon cancer or diverticulosis. Thus, an important principle in treating diabetic patients with gastrointestinal disorders is the need to exclude other medical disorders before ascribing symptoms to chronic autonomic dysfunction.

The second group consists of diabetic patients who suffer from gastrointestinal symptoms caused by acute metabolic abnormalities. Metabolic disorders in diabetes cause temporary gastrointestinal problems. Hypermagnesemia from renal insufficiency suppresses intestinal motility. Uremia causes nausea. During diabetic ketoacidosis significant dilation of the stomach can occur, which resolves completely with nasogastric decompression and correction of the acidemia. Neuromuscular function in the gastrointestinal tract will improve when these metabolic abnormalities are corrected.

The third group consists of patients who suffer from chronic autonomic dysfunction. As mentioned above, gastrointestinal disease should not be attributed to autonomic dysfunction until other medical causes have been excluded.

After a review of the neuromuscular functions of the enteric nervous system, this chapter will explore the major effects of diabetes on the gastrointestinal tract and focus on diagnosis and a practical approach to treatment. At this time there are no drugs exclusively indicated for treatment of gastrointestinal disorders in diabetic patients. Therefore the treatment approaches described here can also be applied to non-diabetic patients.

The Enteric Nervous System

Diabetic patients can develop autonomic nervous system dysfunction and diabetic autonomic neuropathy (DAN). This syndrome is caused by metabolic abnormalities from prolonged hyperglycemia. Clinical symptoms of enteric DAN are more common in older patients with long-standing insulin-dependent diabetes, poor glucose control, and peripheral neuropathy. The autonomic nervous system is composed of the parasympathetic and sympathetic nervous system. The sympathetic nervous system is responsible for the "flight or fright" reaction. The parasympathetic nervous system controls homeostatic functions, such as defecation. In animals, classical experiments demonstrated axonal neuropathic changes in the sympathetic neurons supplying the gut, the sympathetic ganglia, postganlionic sympathetic nerves and intramural adrenergic plexuses. [1]

Although not well understood, DAN affects both the vagal input (cholinergic) and sympathetic input (adrenergic) to the enteric nervous system. In order to understand the many gastrointestinal problems associated with diabetes, the relationship between the autonomic nervous system and the enteric nervous system must be understood (Figure 1).

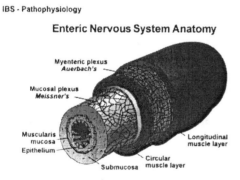

IBS - Pathophysiology

Enteric Nervous System Anatomy

Myenteric plexus Auerbach's

Mucosal plexus Meissner's

Muscularis mucosa

Epithelium

Longitudinal muscle layer

Circular muscle layer

Submucosa

Figure 1. The enteric nervous system (ENS). (From Goyal RK, Hirano I. The enteric nervous system. New Engl J Med 334:1106-15, 1996, with permission.)

The autonomic nervous system actually begins in the amygdala of the brain, which receives stimulatory input from other regions in the brain. The autonomic output goes to the dorsal horn of the spinal cord and then to local neurons which secrete chemicals into local synapses in many parts of the body, including the heart, adrenal glands and the intestine. The enteric nervous system is an intricate system of neurons and muscle that control many functions. The most important are: motility, secretion, the perception of pain (nocioception) and the absorption of water, electrolytes and nutrients.

There are 5 layers of important structures lining the intestine. From the outer layer inward these are:

- The outer longitudinal muscle which is involved in peristalsis.
- The myenteric plexus (Auerbach's plexus): a network of neurons that serve as the "pacemaker of the gut". A loss of inhibitory neurons in the myenteric plexus in the esophagus results in achalasia – a disorder in which the lower esophageal sphnicter fails to relax and patients have difficulty swallowing.
- The inner circular muscle layer.
- The submucosal plexus (Meissner's plexus) of neurons that controls secretion.
- The mucosa of the intestine, lined with enterochromafin cells which release peptides, such as serotonin, from their basolateral membrane in response to food or distention.

Many enterochromaffin cells line the mucosa of the intestine. The villi of the enterochromaffin cell face the lumen. When food stimulates the villi, serotonin is released and causes the intrinsic afferent neuron to secrete acetylcholine and substance P. This results in proximal intestinal contraction. At the same time distal inhibitory neurons release vasoactive inhibitory peptide (VIP) and nitrous oxide (NO), which results in distal relaxation. This is the normal peristaltic reflex, the "bulbring" reflex, which propels food along the tract. When this pattern is interrupted, as in autonomic dysfunction, the motility may be decreased causing constipation, or the motility can increase resulting in diarrhea.

The exquisite regulation of gastrointestinal function of the enteric nervous system is subject to disruption in diabetics for two reasons. First, hyperglycemia can acutely lead to reversible disorders, such as gastroparesis, which resolve upon correction of hyperglycemia. Second, long-standing effects of hyperglycemia can lead to autonomic dysfunction. It has been suggested that glycemic control affects almost every gastrointestinal function, including gastric emptying, myoelectric activity, and the colonic response to feeding. The effects of autonomic nerve damage on release of neurotransmitters, such as vasoactive intestinal peptide (VIP), which normally causes proximal intestinal relaxation and calcitonin G related protein (CGRP), which helps regulate peristalsis, also could contribute to motor dysfunction.

When the enteric nerves do not function properly, peristalsis, the lower esophageal sphincter, gastric emptying, small bowel transit time, and colonic motility can all be affected. The sensory neurons in the enteric nervous system are responsible for the perception of pain. This explains why patients with diabetes may not have symptoms despite gastric distention or severe reflux.

441

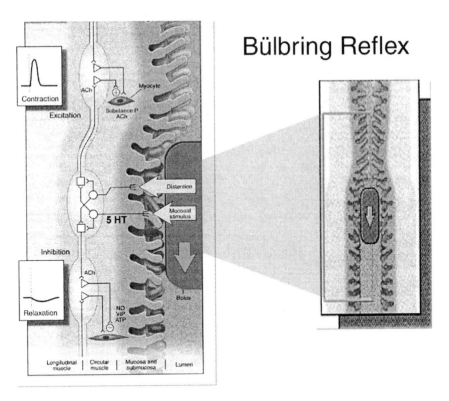

Bülbring Reflex

Figure 2. Normal peristalsis: the bulbring reflex. (Adapted from Goyal RK, Hirano I. *The Enteric Nervous System.* N Engl J Med 334:1106-1115, 1996.)

The approach to treating motility disorders has recently advanced to targeting specific peptide receptors. By modulating a specific receptor, motility can be regulated. Some important pharmacotherapeutic neuroreceptor targets are outlined in Table 1. In order to maximize the safety and efficacy of each drug, the mechanism of action needs to be clearly understood, particularly since certain peptides may have many receptor subtypes. The function of the peptide is determined by the structure of the receptor. Therefore, by binding to several receptor types, one peptide can have many functions.

Serotonin deserves special mention because there are several medications that are being developed to treat motility disorders by moduating serotinin. More than 95% of the serotonin in the body is located in the intestine and only 3% is located in the central nervous system. Serotonin has more than 20 types of receptors located throughout the body. In the intestine, the serotonin type 3 and 4 receptors seem to be the most important. Stimulation of the serotonin type 3 and 4 receptors increases motility and their blockade inhibits motility. For example, tegaserod maleate is a partial serotonin 4 receptor agonist that increases motility.   These functions are important to remember as new motility drugs become available.

Table 1. Targeted Pharmacotherapy for Gastrointestinal Disorders

Drug	Dose	Receptor	Function	Side effect
Alosetron [Lotronex]	0.5 mg – 1mg qd or BID	5-HT3 antagonist	↑ small bowel fluid resorption; ↑ fundic relaxation; ↓ Colon Motility	Constipation Ischemic Colitis ?
Tegaserod [Zelnorm]	2 mg – 6 mg BID	5-HT4 agonist	increases motility	Cholelithiasis ?
Domperidone	10-20 mg before meals and at bedtime	D2 receptor antagonist	improves gastric emptying	↑ prolactin

qd = daily; BID = twice daily
D= Dopamine
5-HT3= 5 hydroxytryptamine or serotonin "3" receptor
5-HT4= 5 hydroxytryptamine or serotonin "4" receptor
Note: Some of these medications have not been approved by the Food and Drug Administration (FDA) in the United States but are available in other countries.

Esophagus

Thirty percent of diabetics have symptoms of esophageal disease. Many others have reflux or other esophageal problems but do not have symptoms because of altered sensory function.   Esophageal symptoms cannot be directly attributed to diabetes until other clinical disorders, including esophageal cancer, have been excluded.

Alarm symptoms in any patient that warrant endoscopy are: hematemesis [vomitus containing blood], dysphagia [difficulty swallowing], odynophagia [pain on swallowing], weight loss, onset of reflux symptoms over the age of 65, chronic reflux for more than five years, and unintentional weight loss. Because coronary atheroslcerosis is common in diabetic patients, chest pain should not readily be attributed to esophageal spasm. Appropriate tests need to be undertaken to exclude coronary artery disease. Specialized tests that assess esophageal motility have a minor role in practice.

Gastroesophageal reflux disease is more common in diabetic patients than in nondiabetic individuals. Several disorders of the esophagus have been described in diabetes. These include decreased lower esophageal sphincter (LES) pressure, slow esophageal transit time, poor peristalsis and weak contractions. All of these can lead to poor esophageal emptying which contributes to reflux. In addition, gastroparesis, which is very common in diabetic patients, contributes to reflux—another factor that makes reflux even more prevalent in diabetic patients.

In some cases reflux is so severe that esophagitis or strictures can occur. Due to sensory abnormalities, a diabetic patient may not feel the acid reflux. If a patient is suspected to have reflux for 5 years, then an endoscopy should be done with special attention paid to the Z-line (the squamocolumnar junction) to exclude Barrett's esophagus.

The term "Barrett's esophagus" implies that the lining of the esophagus has changed from a normal squamocolumnar epithelium to specialized intestinal mucosa with goblet cells. Normally goblet cells are found only in the small intestine. The presence of the goblet cells in the esophagus provides evidence that the acid reflux from the stomach to the esophagus has been severe enough to change the type of cells in the lining- a process called "metaplasia". Barrett's esophagus is thought to be a precurser for esophageal cancer and these patients need surveillance endoscopies more frequently.

The treatment of a diabetic patient with reflux is similar to that of nondiabetics. Anything that empties the esophagus, tightens the lower esophageal sphincter, or empties the stomach will prevent esophageal reflux. The treatment of motility disorders in the United States at this time is challenging because several motility agents have been withdrawn from the market or disapproved by the FDA. Some of the drugs are available in Canada or Mexico. Because effective motility agents are not readily available, lifestyle changes are very important (Table 2).

Table 2. Lifestyle Changes to Improve Reflux

- Sit up properly in a chair whenever eating food and taking pills
- Drink small volumes of liquid throughout the day, between meals, to avoid gastric distention
- Eat small frequent meals
- Avoid "trigger" foods such as onions, pepper, garlic, citrus and tomatoes
- Elevate the head of the bed with 3 inch blocks
- Do not eat anything for 3 hours before lying supine
- Avoid fatty and fried foods
- Drink plenty of water with all pills to avoid pill-induced esophagitis [caused by NSAIDS, iron, digoxin, fosamax]
- Avoid carbonation, alcohol and smoking
- Lose excess weight

Many patients will respond to lifestyle changes alone. However, others will also need suppression of acid secretion for their symptoms to resolve. For patients with mild, intermittent reflux the fastest relief is seen with antacids, such as calcium carbonate (TUMS). If TUMS tablets are sucked, the esophageal contractions promote acid clearance from the esophagus. Products containing magnesium should be avoided in diabetic patients with renal insufficiency. Ranitidine (Zantac) is used 150 mg – 300 mg po qd, but the dose should not exceed 150 mg po qd in patients with renal insufficiency. Ranitidine is appropriate for mild to moderate reflux symptoms and can be taken PRN ("as needed").

For more severe or refractory reflux, there are several proton pump inhibitors available. Proton pump inhibitors work best when taken one hour before the first meal of the day. Proton pump inhibitors must be taken every day to be effective and do not work when taken PRN. No proton pump inhibitor has significant proven clinical benefits over another. Prevacid (lansoprazole) cannot be given to patients with cirrhosis. Prilosec (omeprazole) interacts with coumadin. Protonix (pantoprazole) is available po and IV, can be taken with or without food or antacids, is safe in the elderly, and the least expensive proton pump inhibitor. The only known drug interaction is the decreased absorption of ketoconazole, which is pH dependent.

Table 3. Treatment of Gastroesophageal Reflux Disease

Drug	Mechanism	Dose	Caution
Rantidine [Zantac]	H_2 blocker	150 mg qd, BID or qhs	dose adjustment in renal failure
Famotidine [Pepcid]	H_2 blocker	20-40 mg qd or BID	renal failure
Pantoprazole [Protonix]	PPI	40 mg po or IV qd	Ketoconazole
Omeprazole [Prilosec]	PPI	40 mg po qd	headache, diarrhea (3-5%)
Esomeprazole [Nexium]	PPI	40 mg po qd	headache, diarrhea (3-5%)

H_2 = histamine 2 receptor antagonist
PPI= Proton pump inhibitor
note: H_2 blockers can be taken PRN because they work quickly. Proton pump inhibitors must be taken every morning, 45 minutes before the first meal.

There are minimally invasive procedures, performed endoscopically, which are being developed to treat patients with severe gastroesophageal reflux disease. These techniques have not been proven to be safe and effective in diabetic patients.

Diabetic patients with odynophagia are likely to have candida esophagitis until proven otherwise. Endoscopy with brushings is the most sensitive and specific test. Treatment involves administering fluconazole, 200 mg po for one day, then 100 mg/day for 3 weeks.

Stomach

As many as 50% of patients with type 1 diabetes have delayed gastric emptying or gastroparesis.[2] In gastroparesis, the stomach does not empty quickly enough due to dysrhythmias of the stomach. It is thought that autonomic dysfunction is the most important factor in the pathogenesis of gastric motility. Delayed gastric emptying may be associated with hypoglycemia since there is dysynchrony of insulin administration and emptying of nutrients from the stomach to the small intestine.

Diabetic patients with gastroparesis present with early satiety, nausea and vomiting, abdominal discomfort, postprandial fullness, bloating, reflux, burping and epigastric discomfort. These symptoms are increased by solid meals. Clinical findings include a succussion splash or a large gastric residual after an overnight fast.

Diabetics are prone to form "bezoars" which are balls or conglomerations of undigested food material.[3] Bezoars can cause epigastric discomfort, and even obstruct the pylorus resulting in nausea and vomiting. Gastric bezoars form when antral motor dysfunction is deficient. Pylorospasm and small bowel dysmotility may also contribute to gastric stasis and bezoar formation.[4]

Gastroparesis also contributes to acid reflux. When the stomach does not empty, the retained gastric contents can easily reflux into the esophagus, sometimes causing aspiration. The lifestyle modifications that apply to non-diabetic patients with reflux are even more important in the diabetic patient.

The positive diagnosis of diabetic gastroparesis requires demonstration of a delay in gastric emptying. Measuring the emptying of liquids is of limited use since this is usually normal in diabetics. Assessment of the emptying of solids is more important. Currently gastric scintigraphy, or a "gastric emptying study", a noninvasive measure usually performed by nuclear medicine physicians, is the test of choice.

Diagnostic tests that measure gastric myoelectrical activity and gastric emptying are indicated when the results of standard diagnostic tests are negative and symptoms persist. Electrogastrography (EGG) noninvasively measures fasting and postprandial gastric myoelectricial activity. EGG records activity via electrodes placed on the skin in the epigastrium. EGG accurately reflects the normal 3 cpm electrical rhythm and abnormal gastric dysrythmias termed tachygastria (3.6 – 9.9 cpm) and bradygastria (1.0 – 2.4 cpm). Care must be taken to keep the patient still, since artifacts in the EGG signal may be created by patient movement.[5]

For the few most severe, refractory patients who fail all other treatments, measurement of antroduodenal motility, done only in major referral centers, has a limited role in assessing diabetics with gastroparesis. Patients with selective abnormality of antral motility may tolerate feeding directly into the small bowel; those with a generalized motility disorder may not tolerated enteral feeding.[6]

Helicobacter pylori may be present in patients with diabetes, but is not known to be more common in diabetic patients than in the general population. Whether H. pylori plays a role in diabetic gastroparesis or motility is not established. The indications for treating H. pylori in a diabetic patient are: gastric ulcer, duodenal ulcer or a family history of gastric cancer.

The following conditions need to be excluded when gastroparesis is suspected: gastric outlet obstruction caused by peptic ulcer disease, neoplasm or pyloric stenosis, metabolic derangements, such as ketoacidosis or uremia, and the effects of medications, such as calcium channel blockers and anticholinergic agents.

Table 4. Differential Diagnosis of Gastroparesis

- Mechanical obstruction – bezoar, gastric cancer, pyloric stenosis
- Peptic ulcer disease
- Chronic cholecystitis
- Pancreatitis
- Uremia hypercalcemia – hyperparathyroidism
- Hypokalemia – Addison's disease
- Hypothyroidism
- Medications – anticholinergics, calcium channel blockers, octreotide, levodopa
- Nicotine

Treatment

For mild to moderate disease it is useful to begin the Gastroparesis Diet that was created by Dr. Kenneth Koch (Table 5). The key to enhancing gastric emptying is also to maintain good control of the serum glucose. Even transient hyperglycemia can lead to gastroparesis.

Patients with gastroparesis may not be able tolerate the standard American Diabetic Association diet. High residue foods may lead to bezoar formation in these patients. A low fat diet (< 40 g per day = 360 Kcal) is also recommended since fats delay gastric emptying. Patients should be encouraged to eat six small meals (snacks) a day rather than one or two large meals. This decreases the amount of neuromuscular work the stomach has to do and provides a steady flow of nutrients to the small bowel.

Table 5. The Nausea or Vomiting (Gastroparesis) Diet

Step 1. Gatorade and Bouillon
Diet: Small volume of salty liquids to avoid dehydration
Goal: 1000 to 1500 ml/day in multiple servings e.g. 1-2 oz at a time
Avoid: Citrus and highly sweetened drinks

Step 2. Soup and Crackers
Diet: Soups with noodles or rice and crackers and peanut butter in small amounts in at least six divided meals per day
Goal: 1500 calories per day; avoid dehydration and maintain weight
Avoid: Creamy, milk-based liquids

Step 3. Solid Food: Starches, Chicken and Fish
Diet: Starches such as noodles, pastas, potatoes and rice are easily mixed and emptied by the stomach; chicken breast and fish are usually well tolerated in six divided meals per day; a one-a-day chewable vitamin should be prescribed to be taken with an evening snack; chewable calcium should also be given in the appropriate dose
Goal: To find common foods that evoke minimal nausea or vomiting
Avoid: Fatty Foods which delay gastric emptying and red meats and fresh vegetables which require maximum trituration.

(From Koch KL, Therapy of nausea and vomiting. In *Therapy of Digestive Disorders*. MM Wolfe Ed. WB Saunders, Philaldelphia, pp. 731-746, 2000, with permission.)

For those patients with mild to moderate disease who do not respond to dietary modification alone, targeted pharmacotherapy to empty the stomach can be used (Table 6). To augment gastric emptying, drugs such as metoclopropamide (Reglan), which is a peripheral cholinergic and antidopaminergic agent with central antiemetic activity, can be used. It is helpful to begin with metoclopramide 10 mg po qhs. This can be slowly increased to TID dosing if needed, but the side effects include drowsiness, Parkinson's type movements, and dyskinesia. Sometimes metoclopramide, 5 mg po before lunch and dinner, is enough, especially if the patient is compliant with a low fat, low residue diet.[7]

Domperidone (Motilium) is a peripheral dopamine 2 receptor antagonist that increases gastric emptying. The starting dose of domperidone is 10 mg BID or TID. Central nervous system side effects are observed less frequently with domperidone than with metoclopramide. Other adverse events with metoclopromide and domperidone are hyperprolactinemia and galactorrhea. Domperidone is available in Canada.

Cisapride (propulsid) acts as a partial 5HT$_4$ agonist. Cisapride enhances gastric emptying but is no longer available in the United States due to cardiac arrythmias in certain groups of patients. Erythromycin mimics the effects of motilium and stimulates smooth muscle motilin receptors, which are located in the enteric nervous system. In most patients erthromycin has to be stopped after 5 –7 days due to intolerance or tachyphylaxis.

Table 6. Medications to Stimulate Gastric Emptying

Drug	Dose	Mechanism	Side effects
Metoclopramide	5-10 mg before meals	D2 antagonist 5-HT3 antagonist (peripheral and central)	extrapyramidal, anxiety, drowsiness dystonia, hyperprolactinemia
Erythromycin (suspension)	125-250 mg before meals	Motilin agonist	nausea, diarrhea, cramps, rash
Domperidone*	10-20 mg	D2 antagonist (peripheral)	hyperprolactinemia
Cisapride*	5-20 mg before meals and before bed	5-HT4 agonist (peripheral)	diarrhea, abdominal discomfort

*not available in US
D= Dopamine
5-HT3= 5 hydroxytryptamine or serotonin "3" receptor
5-HT4= 5 hydroxytryptamine or serotonin "4" receptor

The medical treatment of severe gastroparesis (Table 7) involves nasogastric decompression, intravenous fluids, and correction of metabolic derangements (potassium, magnesium, electrolytes and glucose). Bezoars can be mechanically disrupted at the time of endoscopy. Erythromycin (3 mg/kg body weight IV every 8 hours) clears residue, causing a "dumping" from the stomach. One week treatment with oral erythromycin, 250 mg TID, is worth trying once patients tolerate food. Frequent monitoring of blood sugar is essential during this phase. Surgical intervention should be avoided in gastroparesis. Certain patients may be selected for laparoscopic placement of a jejunal feeding tube, but otherwise should not undergo surgery.[6]

Table 7. Management of Diabetic Gastroparesis

Gastric decompression if needed
Upper Endoscopy to exclude bezoar, outlet obstruction
Diet Modification/Glucose Control
    Liquid supplements if solids not tolerated
    Koch's 3 Step Gastroparesis Diet
    Feeding j-tube (only in carefully selected patients)
    Total parenteral Nutrition
Promotility therapy: stimulation of gastric emptying with medication
    Domperidone 10 mg po BID, TID, or QID
    Metoclopramide 5-10 mg po qhs or 30 minutes before meals, if tolerated
Antiemetic therapy
    For moderate symptoms:
    Prochlorperazine (Compazine) 5-10 mg po or IV BID PRN or 25 mg rectal suppository q 12 h PRN
    Antihistamines
    For hospitalized patients with severe gastroparesis:
    Ondansetron (Zofran) 8 – 16 mg IV qd
    Halogenated phenothiazines – Haloperidol, 1-2 mg IM or IV bid
Gastric Pacing (experimental)

Small Intestine

The normal major migratory complex of the small intestine in the fasting state is divided into 3 phases:
I) quiescent; II) discrete clustered contractions [DCC] - small bursts of electrical activity that are uncoordinated and do not propagate; III) prolonged propagated contractions [PCC] - intense contractions of the distal ileum

Phase III activity is called the "intestinal housekeeper" because it expels bacteria from the terminal ileum. Normally, bacteria live in the colon. The ileocecal valve keeps most bacteria from entering the terminal ileum. The Phase III "housekeeper" activity pushes luminal contents, including stray bacteria, from the terminal ileum back into the cecum.

In diabetes, Phase III motility can be impaired and therefore bacteria remain in the distal ileum, leading to small bowel bacterial overgrowth.

Small bowel bacterial overgrowth

Bacterial overgrowth may present with symptoms of periumbilical abdominal discomfort, bloating, gas, distention or diarrhea. Bacterial overgrowth may also be associated with features of malabsorption such as anemia, osteoporosis and coagulopathy. For example, bacteria inhabiting the terminal ileum consume Vitamin B_{12}, leading to B_{12} deficiency. B_{12} deficiency presents as megaloblastic anemia. Bacterial overgrowth also results in bile salt deconjugation and fat malabsoprtion, contributing to diarrhea. Vitamin K is also not absorbed leading to a prolonged prothrombin time. In severe cases, Vitamin D is not absorbed causing osteomalacia.

The gold standard for the diagnosis of bacterial overgrowth is a quantitative culture of jejunal aspirates; a count of more than 10^5 aerobes or $> 10^3$ anaerobes/mL is diagnostic. Alternatively, breath tests can be used measuring the amount of H_2 or $^{14}CO2$ released after oral ingestion of a simple substrate, such as glucose [^{14} C-D-xylose], which is metabolized by enteric bacteria. If the breath test is not available, a therapeutic trial of antibiotics is appropriate if the clinical suspicion is high.

The treatment of bacterial overgrowth includes antibiotics for 10 days to 2 weeks (Table 8).

Table 8. The Treatment of Bacterial Overgrowth

Metronidazole [Flagyl] 250 mg my po TID with meals for 10 – 14 days (Metronidazole cannot be taken during pregnancy or lactation). Amoxicillin and clavulanate potassium (Augmentin), 875 mg orally twice a day for 14 days Doxycycline 100 mg po BID for 10 – 14 days

Celiac Sprue

Celiac disease or "sprue", an allergy to gliadin which is contained in rye, barley and wheat, is more common in diabetics. Patients with sprue can present with a variety of symptoms including rancid gas, oily or floating stools, bloating and constipation or diarrhea. The diarrhea of sprue in diabetics typically improves on a gluten free diet. The gold standard or diagnosis is a small bowel biopsy showing flattening of villi. Antibodies to gliadin, tissue transglutaminase and endomysium can be present. Patients with sprue are often IgA deficient, so one needs to check IgG antibodies as well as IgA levels.

Colon

Constipation is a major gastrointestinal complaint among patients with diabetes. Like gastroparesis, constipation is thought to be caused by decreased colonic motility due to diabetic neuropathy, but the precise pathophysiology is not well understood.[8]

Evaluation begins with a careful rectal examination during relaxation and straining to exclude mucosal lesions, rectocele, prolapse and pelvic floor dysfunction. Medical disorders such as hypercalcemia, hyperthyroidism, diverticular disease, colonic strictures and colon neoplasms need to be excluded as clinically indicated.

If constipation persists, a colonoscopy is needed to exclude structural lesions or malignancy. A flexible sigmoidoscopy with a barium enema is also acceptable as long as the preparation is thorough.

Management is based on an empiric approach (Tables 9 and 10). The first step to treat constipation is to increase water intake to six 8 ounce glasses of water a day, as tolerated. Exercise is very important to stimulate the bowel as well as for the health of the patient. Next, increase fruit intake if allowed. Prunes are often used by patients to treat constipation but should only be used occasionally, as these contain phenolphthalein which can cause dependence over time.

Table 9. Patient Tool: Dietary Guidelines for Functional Disorders

To Improve Constipation:
1. Increase water to six 8 ounce glasses a day
2. Exercise at least 20 minutes per day
3. Encourage the "p" fruits: pears, peaches, pineapple, papaya, plums, pear juice
4. Avoid banana and rice
5. One serving of caffeine may help
6. CaMg tabs (suggest: CVS natural CaMgZinc) with lunch, snack and dinner
7. Prunes can help constipation but contain phenopthalein which causes bowel dependence and may cause worsening of the problem over time
8. Milk of Magnesia in low doses is safe, if you are otherwise healthy
9. Chewable fiber such as equalactin may be helpful by pulling water into the stool
10. Avoid crude fiber: FiberOne/Raisin Bran and Psyllium can all cause bloating, cramping and gas
11. Encourage soluble fiber: lentil soup, split pea, navy bean, oatmeal

Note: make sure the beans are soaked, well cooked and mashed before consuming

To Improve Diarrhea:
1. Encourage bananas, apple, rice, plantains, tea
2. Avoid vitamin supplements containing magnesium, including CaMg tabs
3. Trial of chewable equalactin 1 –2 X/day [or equivalent fiber] which will help pull water into the stool and tone it

To treat bloating/gas:
1. Avoid gum
2. Avoid carbonation, including beer, seltzer and soda
3. Avoid crude fiber such as fiberone, bran, wheat germ
4. Avoid cheese and dairy
5. Encourage bioavailable vitamins only (such as prenatal vitamins) with dinner or a children's chewable (such as Flinstones)
6. Avoid oyster shell calcium and other calcium supplements that are not well absorbed
7. Encourage soluble calcium: Viactive, TUMS, Oscal or Citracal divided into 500 mg at a time (goal for calcium is 1200 mg per day)
8. Common culprits: broccoli, cabbage, cauliflower, cucumber

NOTE: Always consult with your doctor before you begin any supplement or over the counter products. Remember to talk to your doctor if you have intestinal problems!

Soluble fibers are encouraged as opposed to residue (cabbage, bell peppers) which can predispose to bezoar formation. Soluble fibers include oatmeal, lentil soup, split pea soup, navy bean soup and black bean soup. Remember that one serving of bean soup has 15 grms of fiber. That is equivalent to at least 2 heads of broccoli which diabetics cannot have in large quantities due to the indigestion, burping and gas. Fiber supplements may be helpful, such as chewable equalactin (calcium poylcarbophil) which is generally well tolerated. In order for fiber to be effective, the water intake must be increased to 6 glasses a day. Certain crude fibers (fiber one, raisin bran, psyllium) lead to excessive gas, bloating and cramping because these are fermented by bacteria in the colon.

Next, certain medications can be used such as milk of magnesia, and other gentle osmotic laxatives. Rarely, constipation may be severe leading to megacolon. Treatment includes good blood glucose control, fiber supplementation, and implementation of osmotic and prokinetic agents such as cisapride

Table 10. The Treatment of Constipation

1. Diet and Lifestyle Changes: Increase water intake, exercise, functional dietary guidelines (above)
2. Encourage the "p" fruits – pears, papaya, peaches, plums
3. Milk of Magnesia (which comes in a chewable cherry flavor) is effective but check the kidney function to avoid hypermagnesemia
4. Polyethylene glycol powder (Miralax): 1 capful qhs PRN
5. Promotility agents: Tegaserod Maleate [pending FDA approval], Misoprostil [Cytotec] 200 mcg – 400 mcg po qhs PRN

Diarrhea

Diabetic diarrhea is another common gastrointestinal symptom in diabetics with autonomic neuropathy.[9] Diabetic diarrhea is more common in men and is generally most severe at night. Normally adrenergic nerves stimulate resorption of electrolytes and fluids. If these nerves are damaged in diabetes, intestinal resorption may be impaired, leading to diarrhea. This is usually seen in patients with poorly controlled diabetes who have severe autonomic neuropathy.

Whenever a diabetic patient has diarrhea other causes need to be excluded such as infection, a villous adenoma, malignancy and inflammatory bowel disease.

Diagnosis of a patient with diarrhea begins with a detailed review of diet and medication history. Common triggers of osmotic diarrhea are sorbitol, high fructose corn syrup, and antacids that contain magnesium. Ask about fecal incontinence (sometimes patient with incontinence complain of diarrhea even if the stool is formed). One clinical definition of diarrhea is more than 3 bowel movements a day. Often, a patient who has one loose stool in the morning may state that he or she has diarrhea, but his or her bowel movements may actually be normal.

The presence of anemia, macrocytosis, hypoalbuminemia, or excess stool fat suggests intestinal malabsorption. Specific tests are indicated to diagnose small intestinal bacterial overgrowth, celiac disease, or pancreatic exocrine insufficiency which occurs rarely in advanced chronic cases of type 1 diabetes. Quantitation of stool fat over 72 hours may be helpful in certain cases: fecal fat excretion of >15 g day would be indicative of nutrient malabsorption, whereas lower levels of fecal fat [7 to 14 g/day] may not distinguish between an intestinal motor or secretory disorder.

Anorectal Abnormailites

Fecal incontinence in diabetes may be due to autonomic neuropathy. Incontinent patients with diabetes demonstrate decreased anorectal sensation, and decreased rectal sensation to balloon distention.[10] Incontinent diabetics have been reported to have reduced resting anal sphincter pressure (a function of the internal anal sphincter and sympathetic innervation) but usually normal squeeze pressure (a function of the external sphincter). The external anal sphincter function (voluntary) is not usually affected in diabetes. Treatment includes loperamide, and biofeedback aimed at increasing sphincter tone.[11]

Although rare in diabetics, external sphincter dysfunction indicates a pudendal neuropathy and may be associated with dysfunction of the urinary bladder.

The anorectal examination allows assessment of the resting and squeeze anal sphincter pressure. Lack of sensation in the rectum and perianal skin may indicate the presence of a significant neuropathy. Absence of the cutaneous "wink" reflex indicates sacral root dysfunction. Evaluation of anorectal function should include a rectal ultrasound, especially in women who have had vaginal deliveries, to see if the sphincter is intact. Other patients may need anorectal manometry but electromyography or pudendal nerve conduction tests are used mostly as research tools. Defecating proctography evaluates rectal anatomy and may identify defects in the anal canal, rectoceles or intussuseption and the function of the pelvic floor during the process of defecation. Rectoceles are considered to be significant if they fill preferentially and fail to empty during attempted defecation.[8]

Bile Salt Diarrhea

Bile salt diarrhea is reported more commonly in diabetic patients. Bile is normally reabsorbed in the small intestine. If bile reaches the colon, a secretory diarrhea can occur. This is common after a cholecystectomy. Bile salt malabsorption is treated with cholestyramine powder (beginning at 4 to 16 g/day) or by retarding small intestine motility with loperamide [immodium]. Antidiarrheal agents such as loperamide and diphenoxylate [lomotil], are effective, but will exacerbate small bacterial overgrowth. Hence, determining the cause of the diarrhea is important before instituting therapy.

Treatment of Diarrhea in the Diabetic Patient

Management of diabetic diarrhea is often a challenge. Treatment should begin with rehydration, correction of electrolytes, rigorous control of blood glucose, and restoration of nutrition, if necessary, with total parentereal nutrition (TPN),[12] Treatment should be directed at the identified cause of diarrhea rather than by sequential trials. For small bowel bacterial overgrowth antibiotics are effective. Lactose-free diets are recommended for patients with lactase deficiency. For sprue a completely gluten free diet is necessary (patients must avoid all wheat, rye and barley, including beer!). Pancreatic enzymes are useful only in patients with demonstrated exocrine deficiency. Biofeedback techniques aimed at retraining rectal sensation for fecal incontinence can be useful.[13]

As with other gastrointestinal abnormalities, good glucose control is helpful. In diarrhea thought to be due to autonomic dysfunction, clonidine, an alpha 2-adrenoreceptor agonist which stimulates electrolyte and intestinal fluid reabsorption, can be used. This agents also partially improves autonomic neuropathy. Clonidine (0.1 mg to 0.5 mg twice daily) may cause significant adverse effects, such as orthostatic hypotension, and worsening of gastric emptying. Topical clonidine may control diarrhea without causing hypotension.[14] Verapamil (40 mg twice daily) also may help diarrhea by decreasing colonic transit, but hypotension can occur. Lomotil can be used 1 tablet q 12 hours PRN.

For severe, refractory cases, octreotide (a somatostatin analog) has been effective in doses of 50 – 75 mcg subcutaneously twice a day. Octreotide inhibits water secretion in animal and humans, increases gut absorption and suppresses GI hormones that cause diarrhea.[15] Care must be taken when using octreotide since it suppresses exocrine function of the pancreas and can contribute to malabsorption. In addition, octreotide inhibits gallbladder emptying and can lead to gallstone formation.

Biliary Tree

Cholelithiasis is twice as common in diabetes as in individuals who do not have diabetes. This may be due to decreased gallbladder motility and a lithogenic (stone forming) bile composition. Prophylactic cholecystectomy for patients with asymptomatic cholelithiasis is not routinely recommended. Diabetic patients are prone to cholangitis with rare organisms such as Yersinia enterolitica.

Liver Disease

Nonalcoholic fatty liver disease (NAFLD) is the most common liver abnormality seen in diabetes, affecting up to 80% of patients. Patients may present with tender enlargement of the liver. Transaminases are typically elevated 2-3 fold. Coexisting illnesses, such as autoimmune liver disease, hepatitis C, and hemochromatosis should be excluded. Patients with NAFLD who have steatohepatitis are considered to be at risk of progression to fibrosis or even cirrhosis. Treatment is controversial but includes weight loss, if appropriate, low fat diet, and avoiding other hepatotoxins such as Vitamin A and alcohol. Vitamin E 400 IU per day appears to reduce the liver enzymes. There is preliminary evidence that Actigall, 300 mg po qd, may be beneficial. Investigational interest currently centers on metformin because of the pivotal role that insulin resistance appears to play in the pathogenesis of steatohepatitis.

Pancreatic Disease

True exocrine deficiency of the pancreas in diabetes mellitus is rare. Patients with long standing chronic pancreatitis can develop diabetes late in the course of their disease. This situation is usually seen in chronic pancreatitis due to alcohol abuse. In these cases patients develop weight loss due to malabsorption and require treatment with pancreatic enzymes as well as insulin. If a patient with chronic pancreatitis develops new onset diabetes, carcinoma of the pancreas needs to be carefully excluded. Diabetics who drink alcohol have a two to four increased risk of developing adenocarcinoma of the pancreas.[16]

Abdominal Pain

Diabetics are prone to all of the disorders that can affect non-diabetic individuals. These include mesenteric ischemia, diverticular disease, neoplasms, ovarian cysts and torsion, appendicitis, and cholecystitis. Therefore it is always important to exclude other diseases before attributing abdominal pain to diabetes. (Table 11)

In non-diabetic patients pain or distention of the stomach typically is described in the "epigastrium" – the region between the umbilicus and the xiphoid process. The small bowel is referred to the periumbilical area. Colon discomfort is typically manifested in the perimeter of the abdomen. Gallbladder pain normally is referred to the right shoulder or back. In diabetes, the sensory neurons may not function adequately enough to provide these clues to the patient, but, if the patient has abdominal pain, a physician can use these areas to help focus on what part of the gastrointestinal tract is abnormal.

Table 11. Differential Diagnosis of Abdominal Pain by Location

EPIGASTRIC: stomach ulcer, gastroparesis, gastritis, gastric cancer
PERIUMBILICAL: appendicitis, small bowel bacterial overgrowth, sprue
PERIMETER: colon distention, constipation, diverticular disease, colon
      cancer

Mesenteric ischemia, which is a medical and surgical emergency, may occur in diabetics who are at risk for atherosclerosis. Small bowel ischemia is life- threatening and needs to be diagnosed quickly. In these cases, the pain is out of proportion to the findings on examination.

Colonic ischemia, in contrast, is common in people who have a transient low flow state. Colonic ischemia is usually self limited and patients may have low grade pain, diarrhea, and occult blood in the stool. The symptoms may be so transient that patients do not report them to their physicians. In more severe cases, the patient may need to be hospitalized for hydration and treatment with antibiotics, such as ciprofloxacin and metronidazole. Dehydration, antihypertensives and diuretics can all predispose to low flow states.

Chronic abdominal pain may develop as a result of diabetic radiculopathy affecting the thoracic nerve rots. The pain is typically in a girdle distribution and may respond to amitryptiline, 50 mg po qhs. Phenytoin, 100 mg po TID may also be effective.

SUMMARY

Gastrointestinal disorders are common in diabetic patients. It is necessary to exclude structural , neoplastic, infectious and inflammatory disorders before attributing the abnormality to diabetes. Good glucose control is helpful in controlling most gastrointestinal symptoms. Treatment begins with making an accurate diagnosis, educating the patient, initiating permanent lifestyle changes and effective pharmacotherapeutic agents. Medications used to treat depression and hypertension have marked effects on gut function, and alternative drugs may correct disturbances and relieve symptoms. It is hoped that in the future medications to correct the underlying disorders of nerve function will be available.

REFERENCES

1. Chang EB, Fedorak RN, Field M. Experimental diabetic diarrhea in rats: intestinal mucosal denervation, hyposensitivity and treatment with clonidine. Gastroenterology 90:564-9, 1986
2. Horowitz M, Edelbroek M, Fraser R, Maddox A, Wishart J. Disordered gastric motor function in diabetes mellitus: recent insights into prevalence, pathophysiology, clinical relevance, and treatment. Scand J Gastroenterol 26:673-684, 1991
3. Koch KL. Dyspepsia of unknown origin: pathophysiology, diagnosis and treatment . Dig Dis 15:316-329, 1997
4. Mearin F, Camilleri M, Malagelada J-R. Pyloric dysfunction in diabetics with recurrent nausea and vomiting. Gastroenterology 90:1919-1925, 1986.

5. Stern RM, Koch KL, Stewart WR, Vasey MW. Electrogastrography: current issues on validation and methodology. Psychophysiology 24:55-64, 1987.

6. Koch KL. Diabetic gastropathy: gastric neuromuscular dysfunction in diabetes mellitus–a review of symptoms, pathophysiology, and treatment. Digestive Diseases and Sciences 44(6):1061-75, 1999.

7. Koch KL. Unexplained nausea and vomiting. Curr treatment opt in gastroenterol 3:303-313, 2000.

8. Camilleri M. Gastrointestinal problems in diabetes. Endocrin and Metab Clin 25(2):361-78, 1996

9. Saslow SB, Camilleri M. Diabetic diarrhea. Semin gastrointest dis 6:187, 1995.

10. Schiller LR, Santa Ana CA, Schulen AC, et al. Pathogenesis of fecal incontinence in diabetes mellitus. N Engl J Med 307:1666-1671, 1982

11. Wald A, Tunuguntla K. Anorectal sensorimotor dysfunction, fecal incontinence and diabetes mellitus. N Engl J Med 310:1282-1287, 1984

12. Valdovinos MA, Camilleri M, Zimmerman BR. Chronic diarrhea in diabetes mellitus: mechanisms and an approach to diagnosis and treatment. Mayo Clin Proc 68:691-702, 1993

13. Marzuk PM. Biofeedback for gastrointestinal disorders: a review of the literature. Ann Intern Med 103:240-244, 1985

14. Fedorak R, Field M, Chang E. Treatment of diabetic diarrhea with clonidine. Ann Intern Med 102:197-199, 1985

15. Von der Ohe MR, Camilleri M, Thomforde GM, et al. Differential regional effects of octreotide on human gastrointestinal motor function. Gut 36:743-748, 1995

16. Cuzick J, Babiker AG. Pancreatic cancer, alcohol, diabetes mellitus, and gallbladder disease. Int J Cancer 43:415-421, 1989

Other Recommended Review Articles:

Feldman M., Schiller LR. Disorders of gastrointestinal motility associated with diabetes mellitus. Ann Intern Med 98:378-384, 1983

Verne GN, Sninsky CA. Diabetes and the gastrointestinal tract. Gastroenterology Clin 27(4):861-74, 1998

Web Sites and Internet Sources for Patient Information:

www.amwa-online.com
www.healthology.com
www.IBSvillage.com
www.IBSinformation.com

Chapter 11. Hyperlipidemia: Pathogenesis and Management in Diabetes Mellitus

Ira J. Goldberg

INTRODUCTION

Aside from acute complications, care for people with diabetes mellitus requires measures to prevent the secondary complications of this disease. Although hyperglycemia is directly linked to microvascular disease of the eye and kidneys, several lines of evidence suggest that the relationship between macrovascular disease and hyperglycemia is not direct. These data include animal studies of the effects of hyperglycemia on the development and/or progression of atherosclerotic lesions in animals, epidemiological correlations of risk factors and vascular disease, and experimental interventions in humans.[1,2] In most animals, hyperglycemia alone or in the setting of an atherosclerotic lipoprotein profile created by ingestion of a high fat/high cholesterol diet or by genetic manipulation does not increase atherosclerosis unless the diabetes also worsens the lipid abnormalities. In the rabbit alloxan-induced diabetes will actually prevent atherosclerosis; while the rabbits develop hyperglycemia there is also a shift of the lipoprotein profile towards the presence of large particles that are too big to enter the arterial wall.[3] In human populations, multifactorial analysis correlates lipid abnormalities such as elevated LDL and reduced HDL with coronary heart disease (CHD).[4] These lipid parameters are more strongly related to disease development than is fasting glucose or glycosylated hemoglobin. Most important, several intervention trials have clearly demonstrated that reductions in plasma lipoproteins decrease CHD in patients with diabetes.[5] In contrast, intervention trials that have shown a reduction in microvascular disease with better glycemic control have, in general, shown less effect on CHD.

Is the development of excess macrovascular disease in diabetes a result of greater abnormalities of conventional risk factors, or does diabetes accelerate disease under conditions, such as those found in the western world, that allow the development of CHD? Evidence exists for each of these conclusions. The observation that patients with diabetes have more atherosclerosis and that their risk of developing CHD events in some diabetic populations is equivalent to non-diabetics with established CHD[6] supports the hypothesis that the diabetic milieu provides fertile ground for atherosclerosis plaque growth. Other studies showing that the increased risk of CHD occurs in pre-diabetics,[7] patients with normal fasting glucose and glycosylated hemoglobin, implicates non-glucose factors in disease development. Foremost among these are lipoprotein abnormalities.

Regardless of the pathophysiologic processes, reduction of CHD risk by lipoprotein reduction has become one of the central approaches to CHD risk reduction in diabetic patients.

LIPOPROTEINS AND THE PATHWAYS INVOLVED IN INTRACELLULAR LIPID TRANSPORT

Overview

A fundamental process found in all animals is the transport of molecules within the bloodstream. This is needed for communication, regulation, and movement of metabolic substrates and waste. In the case of water-soluble molecules like glucose and insulin, direct secretion into the bloodstream is sufficient. A number of metabolically important substances are, however, hydrophobic; these molecules do not remain in solution in blood. Hydrophobic steroid hormones are transported while associated with specific carrier proteins such as sex hormone binding globulin and cortisol binding globulin. Similarly fat-soluble vitamins such as A and D circulate attached to binding proteins.

Two of the major lipids that are distributed throughout the body are triglycerides and cholesterol. Triglycerides are the major storage form of calories. They are either ingested or synthesized within the liver. Thus transport from the gut or the liver to peripheral tissues is required to deliver fatty acids used as fuel by heart and exercising skeletal muscle and stored as fat in the adipose tissue. Cholesterol is a component of cell membranes and is the basic molecule used for steroid hormone synthesis. Cholesterol circulates both as an alcohol (cholesterol) and as a more hydrophobic ester (cholesteryl ester).

In the bloodstream, most cholesterol and triglyceride are transported in lipoproteins. These spherical particles differ in size, composition and density but have a common structure. The outer surface of the spheres is composed of apolipoproteins; the word "apo" means "without" and these proteins are termed apos to indicate the protein without the lipid moieties. The apolipoproteins are usually amphipathic, meaning that they have hydrophobic domains that interact with lipid and hydrophilic regions that contain charged amino acids and allow the particles to interact with the water phase that is plasma. In addition, these proteins interact with cell surface receptors and act as co-factors for enzymatic reactions. The major apolipoproteins are listed in Table 1. The second major class of surface molecules is phospholipids. Like the apolipoproteins, phospholipids have both a hydrophobic region due to the fatty acid and a charged region due to phosphates. In addition to these major classes of molecules, some cholesterol and a small amount of the core lipids are found on the surface of lipoproteins.

The core of the lipoprotein contains primarily the hydrophobic lipids triglyceride and cholesteryl ester. The ratio of core lipid to surface determines the size and buoyancy of the particles. Smaller particles have relatively more surface area; therefore they have a greater proportion of denser proteins and a smaller percent of less dense core lipids. Larger particles have a greater amount of core: surface; they are larger and less dense. These properties allow for separation of the different classes of lipoproteins by size and density. Historically, isolation of lipoproteins from the blood was performed by centrifugation using solutions containing increasing concentrations of salt. The particles requiring the least salt were termed very low density lipoproteins (VLDL), more salt was need for low density lipoproteins (LDL) to float, and most of the remaining plasma lipid was isolated with a high concentration of salt and was termed high density lipoprotein (HDL). There are two major classes of triglyceride-rich lipoproteins, chylomicrons and VLDL. Both LDL and HDL contain cholesterol as their major core lipid. In addition, other hydrophobic molecules circulate within the core of lipoproteins: retinyl esters (vitamin A) are found in chylomicrons, carotenoids and tocopheral (vitamin E) are in LDL.

Chylomicron metabolism

Chylomicrons are the particles that enable ingested fat-derived calories to enter the body. Following a meal, triglyceride is hydrolyzed to fatty acids that enter the enterocytes and are re-esterified into triglyceride. Via an incompletely understood process, the triglyceride is associated with a large protein apolipoprotein B (apoB). This process of chylomicron assembly requires the actions of an intracellular protein termed the microsomal triglyceride transfer protein (MTP). Another special feature of chylomicrons is that the apoB contained in these particles is formed by the enzymatic insertion of a nucleotide base change to a stop codon leading the translation of apoB48, a protein that is 48% of full-length apoB100.

Chylomicrons are not secreted into the bloodstream, but are conducted away from the gut via the lymphatics (see figure 1). Once they enter the bloodstream via the thoracic duct they become enriched with several apolipoproteins required for their catabolism. One of these is apoCII, the activator of lipoprotein lipase (LpL), the endothelial cell surface associated enzyme that converts triglyceride into free fatty acids. A second is apoE, a ligand to allow association of the partially degraded remnant particle with proteoglycans, heparin-like molecules, within the liver. ApoE is also a ligand for the LDL receptor and LDL receptor related protein (LRP), two endocytic receptors within the liver. Peripheral lipolysis of chylomicron triglyceride provides energy to peripheral, i.e., non-hepatic, tissues. Liver uptake of remnants delivers cholesterol and its esters and esters of vitamin A.

Chylomicron metabolism

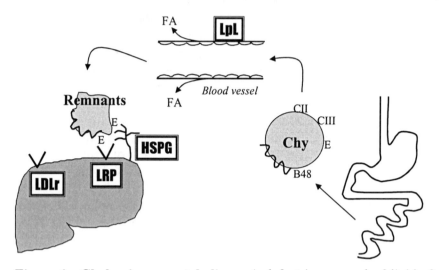

Figure 1. Chylomicron metabolism. A defect in removal of lipids from the bloodstream after a meal is common in patients with diabetes. Chylomicron metabolism requires that these lipoproteins obtain apoCII after they enter the bloodstream from the thoracic duct. Triglyceride within the particles can then be hydrolyzed by lipoprotein lipase (LpL) found on the wall of capillaries. LpL activity is regulated by insulin and its actions are decreased in diabetes. Triglyceride depleted remnant lipoproteins are primarily degraded in the liver. This requires them to be trapped by liver heparan sulfate proteoglycans (HSPG) and then internalized by lipoprotein receptors, LDL receptor and LDL receptor related protein (LRP). Because remnants contain a truncated form of apoB, apoB48, that does not interact with these receptors this uptake is mediated by apoE. (Adapted from Goldberg IJ. J Clin Endocrinol Metab 86:965-9971, 2001.)

VLDL-LDL metabolism

VLDL are produced within the liver and therefore contain triglycerides that are endogenously assembled either from fatty acids that return to the liver on albumin and are de novo synthesized from carbohydrates, or triglyceride that initially enters the liver as a component of other lipoproteins. Regulation of VLDL production is highly dependent on availability of triglycerides. After its secretion from the liver, VLDL like chylomicrons interacts with LpL (figure 2). Some VLDL are partially depleted of triglyceride and then internalized by the liver. Other VLDL undergo a more complete depletion of core lipids due to both LpL and hepatic lipase digestion leading to their conversion to LDL.

LDL are the primary source of circulating cholesterol in primates. Cellular uptake of LDL is accomplished via interaction of apoB with the cell surface LDL receptor. Liver expression of this receptor regulates plasma levels of LDL.

Figure 2. VLDL-LDL metabolism. Poorly controlled type 1 diabetes and type 2 diabetes are associated with increased plasma levels of VLDL. Two factors may increase VLDL production in the liver: the return of more fatty acids

VLDL and its conversion to LDL

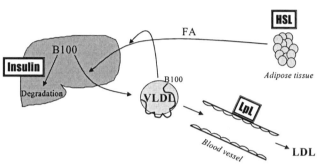

due to increased actions of hormone sensitive lipase (HSL) in adipose tissue and insulin actions directly on apoB synthesis. Both of these processes will prevent the degradation of newly synthesized apoB and lead to increased lipoprotein production. VLDL, like chylomicrons, requires LpL to begin its plasma catabolism leading to production of LDL or return of partially degraded lipoprotein to the liver. (Adapted from Goldberg IJ. J Clin Endocrinol Metab 86:965-9971, 2001.)

Regulation of HDL

Understanding of the metabolic pathways involved in production and catabolism of HDL have evolved significantly. HDL proteins, apoAI and apoAII, are expressed in the gut and liver. Smaller disc-like HDL are initially secreted particles. HDL mature by addition of lipid either by acquisition of surface lipid from triglyceride-rich lipoproteins as they are hydrolyzed by LpL, or by transfer of cellular cholesterol followed by esterification via the actions of the plasma enzyme lecithin cholesterol acyl transferase (LCAT) (see figure 3). Efflux of cholesterol from peripheral tissues is mediated by the ABCA1 transporter.

HDL are catabolized in liver and kidneys. HDL uptake can occur as whole particle endocytosis or HDL lipid can be metabolized without the accompanying protein. Lipid uptake requires the scavenger receptor BI. Hepatic lipase appears to also be involved in this process; this enzyme is a phopholipase for HDL surface lipids. Smaller, lipid depleted HDL and perhaps non-lipid associated apoAI are filtered and then degraded in the kidney.

Lipid transfer

A critical process in regulating the amount of size of HDL and LDL is mediated by cholesteryl ester transfer protein (CETP). This protein transfers cholesteryl ester in the core of LDL and HDL for triglyceride in VLDL (figure 4). Since core triglyceride, unlike cholesteryl ester, can be hydrolyzed by plasma lipases (LpL and hepatic lipase), these particles can be converted to smaller denser lipoproteins. Thus, hypertriglyceridemia i usually associated with reduced HDL cholesterol and small dense LDL

HDL metabolism

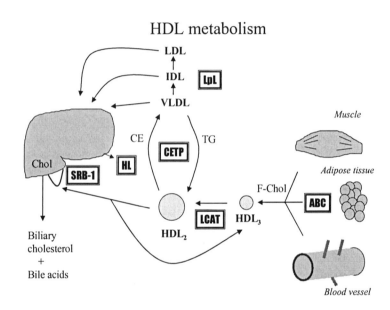

Figure 3. HDL metabolism: *HDL production* requires addition of lipid to small, nascent particles. This lipid arrives via hydrolysis of VLDL and chylomicrons with transfer of surface lipids (phospholipid PL, and free cholesterol, FC) via the actions of phospholipid transfer protein (PLTP). A second pathway is via efflux of cellular free cholesterol (FC), a process that involves the newly described ABC1 transporter, and esterification of this cholesterol by the enzyme lecithin cholesterol acyl transferase (LCAT). *HDL catabolism* may occur through several steps. Hepatic lipase and SRB-1 are found in the liver and steroid-producing cells. HDL lipid can be obtained by these tissues without degradation of entire HDL molecules. In contrast, the kidney degrades HDL protein (apoAI) without lipid, perhaps by filtering non-lipid containing protein. (Adapted from Goldberg IJ. J Clin Endocrinol & Metab 86:965-9971, 2001.)

Figure 4. Plasma lipid exchange: In the presence of increased concentrations of VLDL in the circulation, cholesteryl ester transfer protein (CETP) will exchange VLDL triglyceride for cholesteryl ester in the core of LDL and HDL. This triglyceride can then be converted to free fatty acids by the actions of plasma lipases, primarily hepatic lipase. The net effect is a decrease in size and increase in density of both LDL and HDL. (Adapted from Goldberg IJ. J Clin Endocrinol Metab 86:965-9971, 2001.)

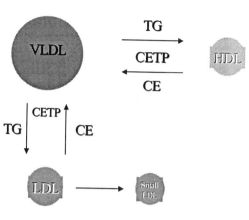

Plasma Lipid Exchange

METABOLIC DERANGEMENTS OF LIPOPROTEIN METABOLISM IN DIABETES

Most patients with either type 1 or type 2 diabetes have lipoprotein levels that are similar to that of age matched controls.[1,8] Although occasional patients with diabetes will have elevated LDL levels that decrease with better glucose control, elevated LDL is associated with more vascular disease but is not the primary reason for the increased CHD in diabetic patients.

The most characteristic lipoprotein abnormality in patients with diabetes, especially type 2, is elevated triglyceride, i.e. VLDL, reduced HDL, and smaller dense LDL. This lipoprotein profile is sometimes referred to as diabetic dyslipidemia. Moreover, in conjunction with obesity, and insulin resistance this lipoprotein profile constitutes part of the "polymetabolic syndrome". The primary lipoprotein abnormality is hypertriglyceridemia. Several processes that are associated with insulin resistance are etiologic in this process. Reduced insulin actions on adipose tissue allows the activation of hormone sensitive lipase; this enzyme hydrolyzes intracellular stores of triglyceride in the adipose tissue and releases free fatty acids into the bloodstream. Liver uptake of the fatty acids leads to increased triglyceride production and greater secretion of VLDL. LpL is also an insulin regulated enzyme and decreased LpL actions reduce plasma clearance of both VLDL and chylomicrons. Thus, a usual but not consistent finding in type 2 diabetes is hypertriglyceridemia, reduced HDL, smaller dense LDL, and a delay in clearance of postprandial lipid.

Although type 1 diabetes out of control is associated with hypertriglyceridemia, well-controlled patients may have elevated HDL.[9]

Occasional patients with diabetes, especially type 2, present with severe hypertriglyceridemia. Triglyceride levels of over 1000 mg/dl usually indicate that in addition to the diabetes the patient has an underlying lipoprotein metabolic disorder. In this context, the best characterized of these disorders is a heterozygous mutation of LpL.[10] In addition to pancreatitis, severe hypertriglyceridemia (usually >10,000) is associated with a syndrome that includes tachypnea and a dementia-like mental status.[11]

Table 1. Apolipoproteins and Lipid Metabolic Enzymes

A. Apolipoproteins		
	MW	Metabolic functions
Apo A-I	28,016	Structural component of HDL; LCAT activator
Apo A-II	17,414	Unknown
Apo A-IV	46,465	Unknown
Apo B-48	264,000	Structural component of chylomicrons
Apo B-100	540,000	Structural component of VLDL and LDL Ligand for the LDL receptor
Apo C-I	6,630	May inhibit hepatic uptake of Chylomicrons and VLDL remnants
Apo C-II	8,900	Activator of lipoprotein lipase
Apo C-III	8,800	Inhibitor of lipoprotein lipase; inhibits Hepatic uptake of chylomicron and VLDL remnants
Apo E	34,145	Ligand for LDL receptor and LRP

B. **Enzymes**

Lipoprotein lipase – hydrolyzes VLDL and chylomicron triglyceride to fatty acids
Hepatic lipase – hydrolyzes triglyceride and phospholipids in VLDL remnants, LDL and HDL
Lecithin cholesterol acyl transferase – converts HDL cholesterol into Esters
Cholesteryl ester transfer protein – shuttles triglyceride and cholesteryl ester between HDL, and LDL and VLDL

C. **Receptors and transporters**

LDL receptor – uptake of LDL and apoE-containing VLDL and chylomicron remnants into liver and other tissues
LDL receptor related protein – uptake of apoE-containing VLDL and chylomicron remnants into the liver
Scavenger receptor—B1—uptake of HDL lipids into the liver
ATP binding cassette A1 – allows efflux of cholesterol from cells

CLINICAL APPROACH TO LIPID DISORDERS

A major philosophic view is that hyperlipidemia is the necessary prerequisite for atherosclerosis development. Moreover, a corollary to this is that levels of plasma lipids that have been considered normal in western diet eating humans are actually elevated. This is why these lipid levels are associated with disease whereas the lower cholesterol levels found in eastern Asian and vegetarian populations are not. Because patients with diabetes have greater risk than average of large vessel disease, they should be viewed as having a lipoprotein abnormality even if their lipid levels are similar to those of normals. Since patients with diabetes have a similar risk for CHD events to patients with established disease, a second basic assumption is that many, perhaps most, people with diabetes either already have or are likely to develop symptomatic atherosclerotic disease. The goals of therapy should then be lipid reduction to levels recommended for other patients with known cardiovascular disease.

One of the first approaches to prevention of macrovascular disease is to reduce plasma LDL in all patients to below 100 mg/dl. This recommendation is made by both the American Diabetes Association (ADA)[8] and the National Cholesterol Education Program, Adult Treatment Panel[12] (http://www.nhlbi.nih.gov/guidelines/cholesterol/index.htm). An additional recommendation is to reduce triglyceride to below 200 mg/dl or non-HDL cholesterol to below 130, the additional 30 points is usually the contribution from a triglyceride level of >150. Although the ADA also sets goals for HDL there is a lack of specific therapeutic measures to achieve this.

Therapeutic lifestyle changes

Because most lipoprotein elevations are seen primarily with western dietary and exercise conditions, the primary approach is often a conversion to a healthier lifestyle. For most patients, if possible this includes more exercise, at least 30 minutes every other day. Maintenance or reduction of weight to ideal is desirable, but is often not achieved. The third objective is to convert the patient from a traditional American diet to one containing a reduced amount of saturated fats and cholesterol. This primarily entails a reduction in meats and whole milk products. In addition, baked goods, snack foods, and restaurant – especially fast food – meals should be reduced. Recently introduced margarines and salad dressing that contain plant sterols that reduce cholesterol absorption, stanol and sterol esters, can reduce cholesterol up to 15%. In addition, fish oil capsules will reduce triglyceride levels. Most clinical trials of fish oil have been relatively short-term and used large numbers of capsules, 10 –12 per day, doses that lead to greater compliance (2-4 per day) appear to be effective if taken for longer periods of time.

There are two basic approaches to lifestyle changes. In one, the patient is confronted with a rather dramatic change. The second is a more gradual behavioral change approach. Each method has its advocates and successful, and unsuccessful, cases.

For exercise, the impediments are usually enjoyment and time. Except for exceptionally disciplined patients, it is often best to find an exercise that the patient finds enjoyable. Unfortunately for some patients this is none! One way to do this is to determine an exercise or sport that the patient played when younger. Sometimes the key to maintaining a program is to do it with a friend or spouse. The timing of the exercise is more important for compliance than for physiological effectiveness. One option is to exercise in the middle of the day, e.g. at lunch hour. There are early morning and evening exercisers, too. For very busy people, a half-hour on a treadmill or exercise bicycle can be an accompaniment to their usually evening television program.

Lipid-lowering medications

Most patients with diabetes mellitus are candidates for lipid-lowering medications. Although a trial of lifestyle changes is appropriate for many patients, especially younger patients, those with established CHD or for whom lifestyle changes are unlikely should be started on medications. These can always be stopped at some later date if the lipid values are markedly reduced and the physician wishes to evaluate the effects of the lifestyle alone.

Medications can often be classified into those that primarily reduce LDL and those that are more effective for triglyceride (VLDL) reduction. In the former category, the easiest and usually most effective therapy is a statin medication. A variety of these drugs are available and they differ by potency; the choice of drug may depend on how much LDL reduction is needed. The drugs are slightly more effective when taken in the evening since most cholesterol biosynthesis occurs overnight. Some are absorbed better with food (lovastatin and simvastatin) and others are best taken before bed. The most common side effects are elevations of liver transaminases (<1-2% of patients), myalgias and myositis. Presumably because these drugs increase liver synthesis of HMG-CoA reductase to try to overcome the effects of the inhibitors, they often lead to slight increases in transaminases. Elevations >3 times the upper limit of normal are an indication to stop the drugs. It should be noted that increases in obstructive liver enzymes, γGTT and alkaline phosphatase, are not characteristic of these drugs and may indicate some other problem, such as excess alcohol or cholelithiasis. Patients will sometime develop aching of the muscles (myalgias) that are either transient during the first few weeks of therapy or are persistent. Occasionally at highest does of medication or when statins are taken with other drugs such as fibric acids, niacin, cylcosporin, and erythromycin, myositis occurs, sometimes with marked elevations of CPK. The patients may wake and complain of flu-like aches. Fluids and discontinuation of the drugs are required. It is best to warn all patients initiating statin therapy of these potential side effects.

As an adjunct to reducing LDL, either bile acid resins or niacin can be added. In general, doubling of the dose of statin will lead to an additional LDL reduction of 6-7%. This is usually the simplest approach. A second medication will reduce LDL by >15%. In non-hypertriglyceridemic patients addition of a resin is a simple way to do this. The drugs can be given up to 3 times a day (with each meal) or only at dinner since for most people that is the time of the largest meal. Occasional patients may feel bloated from the resins and that will reduce their food intake, an added benefit. It is often useful to have patients ingest a high fiber cereal daily before the resins to avoid constipation. New medications that block cholesterol absorption in the gut without the side-effects of resins are in late clinical trials and may soon be on the market.

Niacin is a B vitamin that reduces LDL and triglycerides and is the most effective approach to HDL elevation. Niacin can be purchased over the counter and is a relatively inexpensive therapy. Its major and most consistent side-effect is the development of "flushing", the face and periphery vasodilate. Some patients described a burning or pins and needles-like sensation in their skin. Occasionally, hypotension will occur during the initial flushing. Flushing decreases with aspirin and over time. In an effort to reduce this side effect, a number of slower-acting niacin compounds have been made including niacin inositol and Niaspan®. Niacin therapy has a number of medical problems; it may lead to hyperuricemia and hepatitis. Most important, niacin will worsen glucose tolerance and require the adjustment of diabetic therapy. Therefore although not contraindicated in patients with diabetes, niacin may complicate the management.

Fibric acid medications are a primary therapy for hypertriglyceridemia. The safety and efficacy of these medications to reduce triglycerides and decrease CHD events have been published in the last several years.[13, 14] Fibric acids are relatively easy to take.

A most useful combination, especially in patients with diabetes who have non-optimal LDL and elevated triglyceride levels, is fibric acids and statins. Although this combination must be used with caution since it is associated with a marked increase in myositis, it is used frequently.[15] Use of less than maximal doses of statins is advised in this situation. Some clinicians also reduce the fibric acid dose and give the two medications at different times of the day, the statin at night and the fibric acid in the morning.

SUMMARY

Lipoprotein disorders are common in patients with diabetes mellitus. More importantly, all patients require the clinician to carefully evaluate and in most cases to reduce plasma lipids as perhaps the most effective means to reduce CHD risk. Some patients with hypertriglyceridemia require primarily weight reduction, diet changes, and better glycemic controls. Most others will benefit from LDL reduction. While the initial part of this quote is often true for type 2 diabetes, the second is appropriate for all patients with this disease and, in fact, for most Americans.

"With an excess of fat diabetes begins and from an excess of fat diabetics die"
E. Joslin, 1927

Table 2. Major Lipid-Lowering Drugs

Statins
Lovastatin, simvastatin, pravastatin, fluvastatin atorvastatin, cerivastatin
Mechanisim of action: Inhibits HMG-CoA reductase, the rate limiting enzyme for cholesterol synthesis. Leads to increased LDL receptor expression in the liver
Primary use: Reduction of LDL cholesterol
Side effects: Increased liver function tests, myalgia, myositis
Niacin
Generic niacin, slow release forms including Niaspan®
Mechanism of action: Reduces liver production of apoB-containing lipoproteins. Increases HDL.
Primary use: LDL lowering, triglyceride reduction, HDL increase
Side effects: Flushing, glucose intolerance, hypeuricemia, hepatitis, ulcers
Fibric acid
Gemfibrozil, fenofibrate
Mechanism of action: Decreased VLDL production. Increased triglyceride liposis
Primary use: Hypertriglyceridemia
Side effects: Myositis, especially if used with statins
Bile acid binding resins
Cholestyramine, colestipol, colesevelam
Mechanism of action: Binds bile acids in the gut leading to increase in liver LDL receptor expression
Primary use: LDL reduction
Side effects: Constipation, hypertriglyceridemia

REFERENCES

1. Ginsberg HN. Lipoprotein physiology in nondiabetic and diabetic states. Relationship to atherogenesis. Diabetes Care 14:839-855, 1991.
2. Goldberg IJ. Clinical review 124: Diabetic dyslipidemia: causes and consequences. J Clin Endocrinol Metab 86:965-71, 2001.

3. Nordestgaard BG, Stender S, Kjeldsen K. Reduced atherogenesis in cholesterol-fed diabetic rabbits. Giant lipoproteins do not enter the arterial wall. Arteriosclerosis 8:421-8, 1998.
4. Turner RC, Millns H, Neil HA, Stratton IM, Manley SE, Matthews DR, Holman RR. Risk factors for coronary artery disease in non-insulin dependent diabetes mellitus: United Kingdom Prospective Diabetes Study (UKPDS: 23). Br Med J 316:823-8, 1998.
5. Steiner G. Lipid intervention trials in diabetes. Diabetes Care 23 Suppl 2:B49-53, 2000.
6. Haffner SM, Lehto S, Ronnemaa T, Pyorala K, Laakso M. Mortality from coronary heart disease in subjects with type 2 diabetes and in nondiabetic subjects with and without prior myocardial infarction. N Engl J Med 339:229-34 1998.
7. Haffner SM, Stern MP, Hazuda HP, Mitchell BD, Patterson JK. Cardiovascular risk factors in confirmed prediabetic individuals. Does the clock for coronary heart disease start ticking before the onset of clinical diabetes? JAMA 263:2893-8, 1990.
8. Haffner SM. Management of dyslipidemia in adults with diabetes. Diabetes Care 21:160-78, 1998.
9. Eckel RH, Albers JJ, Cheung MC, Wahl PC, Lindgren FT, Bierman EL. High density lipoprotein composition in insulin-dependent diabetes mellitus. Diabetes 30:132-8 1981.
10. Wilson DE, Hata A, Kwong LK, Lingam A, Shuhua J, Ridinger DN, Yeager C, Kaltenborn KC, Iverius PH, Lalouel JM. Mutations in exon 3 of the lipoprotein lipase gene segregating in a family with hypertriglyceridemia, pancreatitis, and non-insulin- dependent diabetes. J Clin Invest 92:203-11, 1993.
11. Chait A, Brunzell JD. Chylomicronemia syndrome. Adv Intern Med 37: 249-73, 1992.
12. Executive Summary of The Third Report of The National Cholesterol Education Program (NCEP) Expert Panel on Detection, Evaluation, And Treatment of High Blood Cholesterol In Adults (Adult Treatment Panel III). JAMA 285:2486-97, 2001.
13. Effect of fenofibrate on progression of coronary-artery disease in type 2 diabetes: the Diabetes Atherosclerosis Intervention Study, a randomised study. Lancet 357:905-10, 2001.
14. Rubins HB, Robins SJ, Collins D, Fye CL, Anderson JW, Elam MB, Faas FH, Linares E, Schaefer EJ, Schectman G, Wilt TJ, Wittes J. Gemfibrozil for the secondary prevention of coronary heart disease in men with low levels of high-density lipoprotein cholesterol. Veterans Affairs High-Density Lipoprotein Cholesterol Intervention Trial Study Group. N Engl J Med 341:410-8, 1999.
15. Guyton JR. Combination drug therapy for combined hyperlipidemia. Curr Cardiol Rep 1:244-50,1999.

Chapter 12. Dermatological Complications of Diabetes Mellitus; Allergy to Insulin and Oral Agents

Ellen S. Marmur, Fiona R. Pasternack and Matthew C. Varghese

INTRODUCTION

Longstanding diabetes and/or lack of "tight glucose control" over time may result in the development of complications affecting many organ systems, including the skin. In many patients, the first presentation of diabetes may be in the form of dermatitis. Therefore, recognition of skin manifestations of diabetes mellitus is an important aspect of the physical examination. Most cutaneous manifestations of diabetes are attributed either to chronic degenerative changes or to metabolic derangement.

Necrobiotic Disorders

Necrobiosis Lipoidica Diabeticorum. Necrobiosis Lipoidica Diabeticorum (NLD, Figure 1) is a chronic and indolent skin disease that occurs in approximately 0.3 % of diabetic patients and is three times more common in women than in men.[1] Interestingly, compared with the low incidence of NLD in diabetic patients, in two studies of NLD patients, diabetes was subsequently diagnosed in 62%[2] and 42%,[3] respectively. Lesions commonly develop in the third and fourth decades but may develop also in younger patients. NLD, found in both type 1 and type 2 diabetes, may precede the development of diabetes in 15% of patients. In 25% of patients both diseases appear simultaneously.[4] The characteristic lesions of NLD are asymptomatic and are found most commonly on the anterior and lateral surfaces of the lower legs. They may be preceded by trauma. Lesions on other areas of the body are less commonly associated with diabetes.[5] NLD lesions are often painless due to degeneration of cutaneous nerves in the affected region. Lesions may be solitary or multiple. The incidence of NLD is independent of glycemic control. NLD usually resolves in 13 to 19% of patients six to twelve years after onset.[6]

Early lesions of NLD are small red elevated nodules with sharply demarcated borders. As the nodule enlarges, it flattens into a plaque with an irregular outline and eventual depression as the dermis becomes atrophic. The lesion also changes in color to brownish yellow, with the exception of the border, which remains red. The lesions coalesce and sometimes cover the pretibial area completely. Telangiectasias appear as the epidermis becomes scaly and atrophic. Painful shallow ulcers appear in persistent lesions.

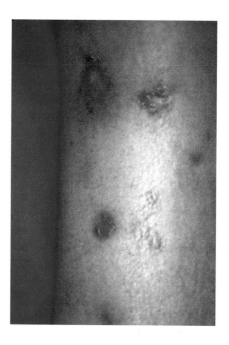

Figure 1. Necrobiosis lipoidica diabeticorum: painful, shallow ulcers and hyperpigmented, yellowish plaques on the pretibial surface.

The differential diagnosis for NLD includes granuloma annulare, sarcoidosis and xanthoma in its early stages.

The exact pathogenesis of NLD has not yet been elucidated. However, since NLD is found in both type 1 and type 2 diabetes, genetic factors are an unlikely cause. Diabetic microangiopathy associated with neuropathy has been implicated in playing a role in the necrobiosis of collagen.[1] Histopathology demonstrates zones of degenerated collagen with loss of normal architecture in dermis, granulomatous changes, palisading of histiocytes around the degenerated collagen, obliteration of dermal blood vessels and sclerosis. The etiology of collagen degeneration is currently under investigation. Immunoreactants, such as IgM, C3, fibrin, IgG and IgA, have been found in vessels of NLD lesions, supporting the theory of an immunologic pathogenesis.[7]

Effective treatments for NLD are still under investigation. Since lesions are independent of glucose levels, glycemic control is an ineffective treatment. Application of topical glucocorticoids under occlusion or by intralesional injections at the periphery of lesions has been beneficial in active lesions. Ulceration may be treated with local wound care or excision of the entire lesion. Some authors suggest increased platelet aggregation as a catalyst for vascular changes.[8] Therefore, studies have attempted to show improvement of lesions with the use of aspirin and dipyridamole, with the dosage being a critical factor. The researchers report therapeutic doses of

However, alteration in collagen metabolism via non-enzymatic glycosylation has been suggested. If this hypothesis is correct, then tight glucose control may be beneficial in limiting the extent of disease.[16]

Scleredema diabeticorum. Scleredema diabeticorum has been found in association with diabetes and is characterized by progressive, painless induration of the skin. Scleredema associated with diabetes has a prevalence of 3% and is more common in obese individuals with vascular complications and non-insulin dependent diabetes.[17] The posterior and lateral neck is usually involved first, with eventual extension to the face, shoulders, anterior neck, arms and torso. Although the exact pathogenesis has yet to be determined, hypotheses suggest decreased insulin levels as the source of derangement of collagen metabolism. Physical examination shows taut indurated, non-pitting areas of skin with poorly demarcated borders. Histopathologic examination reveals marked thickening of collagen bundles that are separated by clear spaces and abundant deposits of mucin in the dermis. There is no effective treatment available for scleredema diabeticorum. Treatment and control of the diabetes have been futile in ameliorating the condition.

Waxy skin, stiff joints and tightness over the skin comprise a *scleroderma*-like syndrome. The condition has been described in 8% to 50% of patients with IDDM and is related to retinopathy, nephropathy and neuropathy. This condition bears no relation to glycemic control, but does increase in incidence with age and duration of diabetes. Skin changes usually begin in the fifth finger and progress toward the first digit, affecting interphalangeal, metacarpal-phalangeal and large joints,[18] leading to limited joint mobility. No treatment other than physical therapy currently exists for this condition.

Infections

Diabetic patients have a greater predisposition for skin infections. Staphylococcal infections, candidiasis, erythrasma and dermatophytosis are the most frequent infections. The reason why diabetics develop more infections compared with healthy controls is still under investigation. Studies of hyperglycemic diabetics have shown decreased chemotaxis, phagocytosis and lysis of organisms in these individuals.[19] Subsequently, a decreased inflammatory and immune response may be the result of thickened capillary walls and compromised vasculature serving as a physical barrier and impeding diffusion of nutrients and movement of leukocytes to the site of injury.[20]

Candida. Candidal infections are more common in diabetic patients than in normal controls. Candidiasis, often seen in poorly controlled diabetics, may also precede the diagnosis of diabetes. Conversely, good glucose control may improve or prevent candidiasis. These infections may present as thrush in the mouth, chronic paronychia in the nailfolds, and intertrigo in the skinfolds. One study reported increased glucose levels in the saliva of diabetic patients with oral candidal infections.[21] *Candida* angular stomatitis is often seen in children with diabetes. Vulvovaginitis is a common complication of poorly controlled diabetes in women and may be accompanied by vulvar pruritus and inflammatory lesions. Genital candidal infections in men, such as balanitis and balanoposthitis, are much less common, but may also be the presenting feature of diabetes. Chronic candidal paronychia usually involves the nailfold and may be associated with inflammation, pain, and loss of the cuticle. Infection between the middle and fourth finger, called erosio interdigitale blastomycetica, is rare.[6] Good glucose control is optimal in the prevention of candidal infections. Topical or systemic antifungal medication may be required in the management.

Bacterial. While most researchers agree that the advent of insulin administration and antibiotics has decreased the incidence of bacterial infections, such as furunculosis, carbunculosis and erysipelas, there is still controversy as to whether infection rates are higher in diabetics than in the general population.[22] However, treatment strategies in the diabetic population can be a challenge.

Staphylococcus aureus and β-hemolytic streptococci are usually the most common bacterial pathogens affecting diabetic skin. They may cause impetigo, folliculitis, furunculosis, carbuncles, ecthyma, cellulitis and erysipelas.[20] Bullous lesions leading to diabetic gangrene and necrotizing fasciitis may complicate bacterial infection of the legs.[23] Diabetic patients may also develop gas gangrene caused by clostridial organisms. Other organisms that cause gas gangrene include *Escherichia coli, Klebsiella and Pseudomonas.*

Diabetic patients may also develop malignant otitis externa due to *Pseudomonas aeruginosa,* which may begin as a cellulitis but progresses to chondritis, osteomyelitis and infectious cerebritis.[6] It is usually seen in elderly patients and often has a fatal outcome.[24]

Corynebacterium minutissimum infection results in erythrasma in diabetic patients. Patients develop erythematous plaques in the upper thigh region, axilla, submammary creases or torso. Plaques may also be confined to the interdigital spaces of the toes.[25] When the lesions progress they become brown, hyperpigmented plaques with scale. Erythrasma may be elucidated by color red fluorescence on Wood's lamp and may be treated with topical or systemic antibiotics.

Phycomycetes infections. Phycomycetes infections may develop in diabetic ulcers or in traumatic wounds as a primary infection or complicating infection. This should be suspected in individuals who do not respond to standard antibacterial or antifungal therapy.[26] Mucormycosis is an example of a deep mycotic infection. This is rare, but has serious consequences. Debilitated patients with diabetic ketoacidosis are predisposed to rhino-

cerebral form and this infection, which may originate in the nasal septum, turbinate or palate, may then extend to involve the cerebrum.[28]
    Therapy for *Phycomycetes* infections must be aggressive due to the high fatality rate. Treatment must be initiated at the earliest opportunity, and includes debridement of all necrotic tissue, intravenous administration of amphotericin B as well as correction of acid-base imbalance and control of hyperglycemia.[6]
    Dermatophytosis. Although dermatophyte infections occur at a similar prevalence when compared with the general population,[27] they are more significant when they occur in diabetics because the lesions may serve as an accessible route for other, mainly bacterial, infections.[28] When these infections are identified, they should be treated.

Miscellaneous

    Diabetic bullae. Diabetic bullae are an uncommon skin condition characterized by the appearance of spontaneous blisters that are usually confined to the hands and feet but also occur on the extensor aspect of forearms and legs. The condition is more common in men than in women as well as in patients with a long history of diabetes.[29] The blisters usually appear suddenly and start as tense, non-erythematous lesions that become flaccid as they enlarge over several days. They vary in size, with some being several centimeters. They may take 6 weeks to heal and can recur.[5] Scarring and atrophy may occur in patients with subepidermal blisters.[30] The exact pathogenesis of blister formation is unclear, although one report documented a reduced threshold for suction-induced blistering.[31] Derangements in carbohydrate metabolism are also implicated.[17]
    Patients with a longstanding history of diabetes may develop bullae as a result of renal failure. Bullae of renal disease, or pseudoporphyria, resemble porphyria cutanea tarda clinically and histologically and are seen in 1-16% of patients undergoing renal dialysis.[32] These patients most commonly develop blisters on the dorsa of their hands, but bullae on other parts of the body are not uncommon. The exact pathogenesis is still unclear, but some proposed etiologic factors include increased serum porphyrin levels,[33] oxidative stress[34] and photosensitivity.
    Acanthosis nigricans. Acanthosis nigricans is a skin manifestation of insulin resistance in several endocrine disorders, including diabetes mellitus. It is non-specific for diabetes. In fact, it occurs in a number of different conditions, including obesity, in response to medications, and as a manifestation of internal disease, such as gastric adenocarcinoma   In diabetics, the high levels of circulating insulin are thought to be responsible for the development of acanthosis nigricans.[35] The condition is characterized

by a black-brown velvety plaques in flexural areas of skin, such as the breast creases, neck-fold, axilla and groin. Some patients also have involvement of the face, hands, elbows, knees and abdominal area.[36]

Lipoatrophy. The group of uncommon disorders that result in a decrease or total absence of subcutaneous fat is referred to as lipodystrophies or lipoatrophies. These conditions are usually seen in conjunction with insulin dependent diabetes mellitus and have a higher prevalence in women compared to men. The lipodystrophies may be congenital or acquired and may result in total or partial loss of subcutaneous fat.

In *total lipoatrophy* of congenital origin, diabetes usually develops in the second decade while the absence of subcutaneous fat is present from birth or develops within the first two years of life. If subcutaneous fat is not absent from birth, it usually disappears over several months. These children usually die from cirrhosis of the liver and their condition has been associated with parental consanguinity. *Acquired total lipoatrophy* starts in childhood or early adulthood. Acquired lipoatrophy may manifest itself after bacterial infections, such as pertussis, or after viral infections. Both forms of total lipoatrophy are often referred to as the Lawrence-Seip syndrome and are considered to be variants of the same disorder, despite differences in presentation. Due to the syndrome's association with consanguineous marriages and the presence of the condition in siblings, it is presumed to have a recessive mode of inheritance.[37]

The syndrome is characterized by total lipoatrophy, insulin resistance, non-ketotic diabetes, increased consumption of oxygen, acceleration of bone and muscle growth, acanthosis nigricans,[38] hepatomegaly due to fatty infiltration from hypertriglyceridemia[39] and finally hepatic failure. Patients with the congenital form may also have the associated features of hirsutism, genital enlargement and central nervous system involvement. Additionally, renal disease or cutaneous xanthomas[40] may be seen. The development of insulin resistant diabetes usually trails the onset of the syndrome by several years.

The cause and pathogenesis of total lipoatrophy have not yet been established. However, hypothalamic dysfunction has been implicated. Upton and Corbin proposed that the defect in this disorder is related to an abnormality in dopamine β-hydroxylase activity and successfully treated a patient with pimozide, a cerebral dopaminergic-blocking agent.[41] Subsequently, Oseid et al reported decreased binding of insulin to its receptor in patients with congenital generalized lipoatrophy.[42]

Partial lipoatrophy develops at any time from childhood to early adulthood and is much more common than the total lipoatrophies. The genetic association is uncertain, although some cases appear to be inherited in an autosomal dominant fashion.[40] The disorder may appear after a febrile childhood illness, such as measles or scarlet fever, or idiopathically. The face is almost always affected, while neck, arm and torso involvement may vary. There is no loss of fat from the hips to the lower extremities and an increase

480

in fat around the hips may also be seen in some individuals. There are several uncommon variants of partial lipoatrophy, which may involve only the buttocks, arms or legs. The adipose loss in lipoatrophy is usually permanent and only reappears in rare instances. As with total lipoatrophy, insulin resistant diabetes may develop several years after partial lipoatrophy has developed. Circulating immune complexes resulting in membranoproliferative glomerulonephritis can be demonstrated in 40 to 50% of patients. Lipoatrophy has also been noted as a local reaction to insulin injections.

Yellow skin or xanthoderma. The nature of yellow skin in diabetes is still under debate. Early studies reported carotenemia in over 50% of diabetic patients[43] and related the change in skin color with this finding. However, a more recent study by Hoerer et al[44] established higher levels of carotene in the blood of non-diabetic controls as compared with diabetics who often had yellow skin, but normal carotene levels. Carotenosis is usually characterized by yellow pigment on the palms, soles and face. Possible causes of yellow skin include elevated serum carotene and nonenzymatic glycosylation of dermal collagen and other proteins that eventually become yellow.[1]

Eruptive xanthoma. This uncommon syndrome in diabetes is characterized by eruptive xanthomas (Figure 4), that are associated with hyperlipidemia, hyperglycemia and glycosuria. The lesions are firm, nontender, yellow papules that erupt in crops on the extensor surfaces. The knees, elbows, buttocks and torso are the most common areas for these lesions. The xanthomas usually resolve once carbohydrate metabolism gets under adequate control.

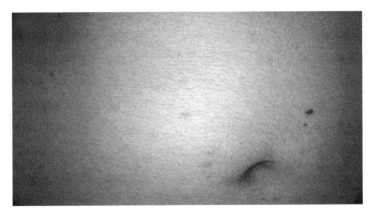

Figure 4. Eruptive xanthoma: firm yellow papules on extensor surfaces.

Acquired perforating dermatosis. Patients with acquired perforating dermatosis (APD, Figure 5) have kidney failure.[45] Lesions usually occur on

481

the extremities, but may also be found on the torso or face. They are usually hyperkeratotic papules less than 1 cm in size. Koebner phenomen can occur and rubbing may cause the papules to coalesce. Patients may be treated with keratolytic agents.

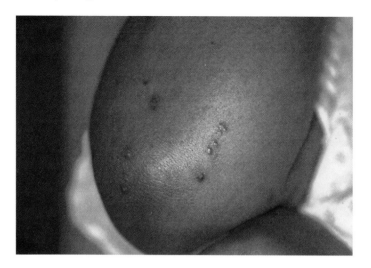

Figure 5. Acquired perforating dermatosis: hyperkeratotic papules on extremities and upper body.

Pigmented purpuric dermatoses. Pigmented purpuric dermatoses (PPD) have been reported in older diabetic patients. Many of these individuals are men and have a history of cardiac decompensation and half have a history of diabetic dermopathy.[46] Whether this condition is a cutaneous marker for microangiopathy is under debate. PPD are caused by erythrocyte extravasation in the superficial vascular plexus. The lesions are usually brown-orange to tan macules or "cayenne pepper" spots in the pretibial area or dorsa of feet.[6]

Lichen planus

Recently, there has been an interest in the association between diabetes mellitus and lichen planus. Reports have shown an increased incidence of abnormal glucose tolerance tests in patients with lichen planus,[47] as well as an increased incidence of lichen planus in diabetics as compared with healthy controls.[48] Higher prevalence was also noted in diabetics who smoke and those with a history of oral candidiasis.[1]

Hemochromatosis

Approximately 80% of patients with hemochromatosis eventually develop diabetes.[49] The main manifestations of hemochromatosis are liver disease, hyperpigmentation, joint disease, hypogonadism and, eventually, diabetes.[6] The classic skin finding is hyperpigmentation which is thought to be due to a general increase in epidermal melanization.[50] Other skin findings in hemochromatosis are spider angiomas in 60-80% of patients, palmar erythema, skin atrophy, ichthyosis and a decrease in body hair.[51]

Vitiligo

Vitiligo is an acquired disorder of pigmentation due to the selective destruction of melanocytes. There is usually a symmetrical depigmentation of the skin that often presents on the dorsa of the hands and on the face. The axillae, genitalia and perianal area may also be involved. Complete depigmentation may occur with progressive involvement. An increased incidence of vitiligo in diabetics has been reported both in type 1 and type 2 diabetes. Treatment of vitiligo can be difficult and prolonged.

Skin tags (Acrochordon)

Recently, an association between skin tags and diabetes mellitus has been reported.[52] Skin tags are small, soft, pedunculated papules that commonly occur on the neck, eyelids and axillae. These lesions have a higher prevalence in women and overweight individuals. Further studies are needed to establish whether skin tags are indeed cutaneous marker for diabetes.

Diabetic Complications

Neuropathy. Diabetic neuropathy is an important condition to diagnose since it may be the presenting manifestation of diabetes in some patients and may also be prevented or slowed with tight glucose control. Older patients with insidious onset of disease are especially at risk. Distal symmetric polyneuropathy is the most common diabetic neuropathy, with motor and sensory involvement.[53] Dorsally subluxed digits, distally displaced plantar fat pads, depressed metatarsal heads, hammer toes and pes cavus (exaggeration of the normal arch) characterize the motor neuropathy. Good foot care plays an important role in the care of these patients and may prevent the formation of debilitating, painless and indolent perforating ulcers (mal perforans)[6]. These lesions are circular, punched out ulcers that occur in a callous or other pressure site. Sensory neuropathies result in numbness, tingling, aching and burning. Restless legs and burning feet may be exacerbated at night. Autonomic nerve damage may initially cause decreased or absent perspiration with compensatory sweating in other parts of the body and may result in erythema, edema and atrophy in advanced cases.[17]
Immunohistochemical analysis has demonstrated a depletion of neuropeptides in the nerve endings of diabetic patients with neurologic dysfunction.[54] Several serotonin-norepinephrine reuptake inhibitors such as

483

desipramine and amitriptyline, have shown some efficacy in treating diabetic neuropathy.[55]

Diabetic foot. The diabetic foot (Figure 6) is the result of a multifactorial pathologic process and requires appropriate care. It is now believed that neuropathy plays as much of a contributory role in foot complications as does vascular pathology. The foot complications of diabetic neuropathy often begin with absence of the ankle jerk reflex, loss of normal foot posture and atrophy of the intrinsic muscles of the foot. As a result, weight is distributed over a much smaller area of plantar skin causing calluses and eventually ulcers.[56] Malalignment of the foot may also lead to ligament tears, minor fractures, loss of bone and a deformed foot. Subsequently, decreased pain perception and dry skin may result in fissuring, cellulitis and deep tissue infection that may go unnoticed by the patient[57].

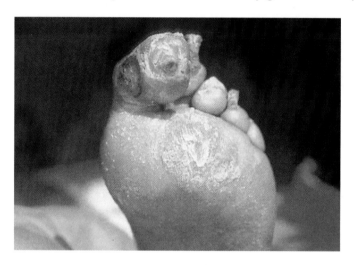

Figure 6. Malalignment of the foot causing calluses, neuropathic ulcers, and dry skin.

In caring for the diabetic patient with peripheral neuropathy of the foot, glucose control is of great importance. Patients should also be educated about the nature of their disease, the recognition of abnormalities and foot care between regularly scheduled visits to the podiatrist. Skin over pressure points should be kept well hydrated with emollients, while ingrown toenails, hallux valgus and claw toes should be managed surgically.[58] Patients should be instructed not to walk around barefoot and should wear special shoes with adequate support and good weight distribution. Recalcitrant ulcers may require debridement, systemic antibiotics or eventual amputation in the case of extensive bone involvement.

Cutaneous Manifestations of Vascular Abnormalities

The most dramatic and debilitating skin complications of diabetes are related to compromise of the vascular system. Derangements affect the small and large blood vessels.

Microangiopathy. Some skin changes can be attributed to small vessel damage. Small vessels usually demonstrate proliferation of endothelial cells, basement membrane thickening and the deposition of PAS-positive material resulting in a decrease of vessel diameter.[59] Pigmented purpuras, periungual telangiectasias,[60] erysipelas-like erythema, NLD, neuropathy and dermopathy may result from microangiopathy.[61] Microvascular impairment can be viewed most easily in the nail fold and retina. Examination of the nail folds may reveal telangiectasias. One study showed nail fold capillary dilatation in 49% of diabetics free of apparent peripheral vascular disease compared with 10% in healthy controls.[62] The relevance of this clinical sign still requires further investigation. According to some data, the eye is more sensitive and reliable in determining microangiopathy.[63] Retinal venous dilatation, microaneurysms, hemorrhages, exudates and neovascularization are considered manifestations of retinal microangiopathy.

Gangrene. The foot is the most common location for tissue necrosis and gangrene due to vascular compromise. Foot gangrene is 50 times more prevalent in diabetics compared with non-diabetics over 40 years of age.[6] While the dry form is caused by the large vessel blockage due to atherosclerosis, wet gangrene is believed to be a late manifestation of microangiopathy. Both may occur in diabetes, but small vessel disease is more common and directly associated with diabetic vascular derangements. Dry gangrene occurs mainly in diabetics with concurrent atherosclerosis. Wet gangrene develops when barely satisfactory perfusion in the extremities becomes insufficient as a result of decreased cardiac output or increased oxygen demand by infected tissue.

Diligent foot care is imperative in these patients, since minor skin abrasions may lead to infection and gangrene. Tinea pedis should also be treated aggressively as the fissures in the skin may be a nidus for infection.

Erysipelas-like erythema. Erysipelas-like erythema is seen most commonly in older individuals with at least a five-year history of diabetes and is also considered to result from small vessel damage. Well-demarcated red areas without fever, leukocytosis or elevated sedimentation rate characterize the disease. Some patients have associated bone destruction due to small vessel insufficiency. Lithner reported the development of erythema in diabetic patients after cardiac decompensation or venous thrombosis.[64]

Diabetic rubeosis. Diabetic rubeosis is a condition seen in patients with a long history of diabetes and is characterized by a reddening of the face and occasionally the hands and feet. The condition is believed to be related to small vessel disease and decreased vascular tone.[18]

Calciphylaxis. Calciphylaxis is observed in the setting of diabetes, end-stage renal disease and hyperparathyroidism and is associated with angiopathy of small and medium vessels. The result of vessel calcification is progressive cutaneous necrosis. Initially plaques appear red to violaceous with a reticulated pattern. There may be bullae formation and eventually a black, bound-down eschar with necrosis of tissues develops. These lesions can become secondarily infected and are slowly progressive despite medical management. Unfortunately, calciphylaxis has a poor prognosis and high fatality rate.[65]

Macroangiopathy. Large vessel disease is usually seen in diabetics in association with microangiopathy. Conversely, microangiopathy is usually seen alone.[17] Atherosclerosis has been shown to have a higher prevalence and incidence in diabetics when compared with the general population.[66] The clinical signs are intermittent claudication, skin atrophy, hair loss, coldness of the toes, nail dystrophy and pallor upon elevation.[67] When the leg is lowered, venous filling is prolonged and dependent mottling rubor and mottling is observed.[6]

Diabetic Drug Reactions

Oral hypoglycemic agents. Sulfonylureas may cause an allergic drug reaction in 1 to 5% of patients with type 2 diabetes. The reaction usually occurs within the first two months of therapy. The reaction is usually in the form of a maculopapular eruption that may be accompanied by generalized erythema or urticarial eruptions. The rash usually disappears on its own while the person continues to maintain the sulfonylurea therapy. Rarely, a generalized pruritus may result in a diffuse exfoliative dermatitis, generalized erythema multiforme, Stevens-Johnson syndrome or toxic epidermal necrolysis that require immediate discontinuation of the drug.

Chlorpropamide, a first generation sulfonylurea, has been shown to cause a disulfiram-like reaction when it is taken in conjunction with alcohol. This reaction occurs in 10 to 30% of patients and results in flushing, headache, tachycardia and dyspnea within 15 minutes of alcohol ingestion.

Insulin. The incidence of allergic reactions caused by insulin may range from 10 to 50% of patients.[68] Some insulin preparations, such as the purified or recombinant types, are much less likely to produce generalized reactions than others. The allergy may be associated with impurities in the insulin, beef or pork protein, the insulin molecule itself[69] or zinc.[70]

Most reactions are localized at the site of injection. Localized, immediate reactions start within 15 minutes to 2 hours of injection with pruritic erythema or urticaria and occasional vesiculation.[71] The reaction, which is mediated by IgG antibodies, may be seen soon after starting insulin therapy or many years thereafter.[67] The best treatment option in this event is to change to a more purified insulin, which has a lower, but not negligible risk for developing an allergic reaction.[72] Local delayed reactions are usually most intense 1 to 2 days after the injection and are characterized by pruritus and burning erythema that is followed by the development of an indurated papule or nodule. Most lesions resolve within a month with continuation of usual insulin administration.[1] Insulin-induced lipoatrophy is most common in children and adolescent girls and may appear at the site of injection within 6 to 24 months of initial administration. While change of injection site alone does not result in resolution of lipoatrophy, incidence of lipoatrophy is decreased when patients are switched to a purer form of insulin or human recombinant insulin. Some children may also develop painless nodules at sites of repeated injections that contain adipose and fibrous tissue.[73]

Systemic allergic reactions to insulin are IgE mediated and may present as generalized urticaria or, rarely, as angioedema or anaphylaxis in less than 1% of insulin-dependent diabetics. Some systemic reactions may be biphasic, developing features of serum sickness-like reaction.

SUMMARY

The skin manifestations of diabetes mellitus are varied and numerous. Often they can present as the initial manifestation of the disease. Occasionally these skin conditions may portend progression of the disease. For these reasons, it is important to be familiar with the cutaneous aspects of diabetes and their diagnosis and therapy.

REFERENCES

1. Perez MI, Kohn SR. Cutaneous manifestations of diabetes mellitus. J Am Acad Dermatol 30:519-31, 1994.
2. Krakowski A, Covo J, Berlin C. Diabetic scleroderma. Dermatologica, 146:193-8, 1973.
3. Rosenbloom AL, Silverstein JM, Lezotte DC, et al. Limited joint mobility in childhood diabetes mellitus indicates increased risk of microvascular disease. N Engl J Med 305:191-4, 1981.
4. Meure M, Szeimies RM. Diabetes mellitus and skin diseases. Curr Probl Dermatol 20:11-23, 1991.
5. Braverman IM, Ed. Skin signs of systemic disease. WB Saunders, Philadelphia, PA, 654-64, 1981.
6. Huntley AC. Cutaneous manifestations of diabetes mellitus. J Am Acad Dermatol 7: 427-55, 1982.
7. Quimby SR, Muller SA, Schroeter AL. The cutaneous immunopathology of necrobiosis lipodica diabeticorum. Arch Dermatol 124:1364-71, 1998.
8. Karkavitsas K, et al. Aspirin in the management of necrobiosis lipodica. Acta Derm 62:183, 1982.

9. Freinkel RK. Diabetes mellitus In Fitzpatrick's Dermatology in General Medicine, 5th Edition. Mc-Graw Hill, New York, p.1969, 1999.
10. Dicken CH, Carrington SG, Winkelmann RK. Generalized granuloma annulare. Arch Dermatol 99:556-63, 1969.
11. Dabski K, Winkelmann RK. Generalized granuloma annulare: clinical and laboratory findings in 100 patients. J Am Acad Dermatol 20:39-47, 1989.
12. Muhlemann MF, Williams DR. Localized granuloma annulare is associated with insulin-dependent diabetes. Br J Dermatol 111: 325-9, 1984.
13. Thyresson HN, Doyle JA, Winkelmann RK. Granuloma annulare: histopathologic and direct immunofluorescence study. Acta Derm Venereol (Stockh) 60:261, 1980.
14. Sherry DD, Rothstein RR, Petty RE, et al. Joint contracture preceding insulin-dependent diabetes mellitus. Arthritis Rheum 25:1362-4, 1982.
15. Starkman HS, Gleason RE, Rand LI, et al. Limited joint mobility of the hands in patients with diabetes mellitus. Ann Rheum Dis 45:130-5, 1986.
16. Lieberman LS, Rosenbloom AC, Riley WJ, et al. Reduced skin thickness with pump administration of insulin. N Engl J Med 303: 940-1, 1980.
17. Weissman K. Skin disorders in diabetes mellitus In Rook/Wilkinson/Ebling's Textbook of Dermatology. Blackwell Science, Inc: Malden, MA, p. 2676, 1998.
18. Brik R, Berant M, Vardi P. The Scleroderma-Like Syndrome of Insulin Dependent Diabetes Mellitus. Diabetes-Metabolism Reviews 7(2): 120-8, 1991.
19. Sabin JA. Bacterial infections in diabetes mellitus. Br J Dermatol 91:481, 1974.
20. Meurer M, Szeimies RM. Diabetes mellitus and skin diseases. Curr Probl Dermatol 20: 11-23, 1991.
21. Knight L, Fletcher J. Growth of candida albicans in saliva: stimulation by glucose associated with antibiotics, corticosteroids and diabetes mellitus. J Infect Dis 123: 371-7, 1971.
22. Oakley WG, Pyke DA, Taylor KW, ed.. Diabetes and its management. Oxford, Blackwell Scientific Publications, Oxford, UK, p.43, 1978.
23. Calhoun JH, Mader JT. Infection in the diabetic foot. Hosp Pract 30:81-104, 1992.
24. Zaky DA, Bentley DW, Lowy K, Betts RF, Douglas RG. Malignant external otitis: a severe form of otitis in diabetic patients. Am J Med 61:298-302, 1976.
25. Montes LF, Dobson H, Dodge BG, Knowles WR. Erythrasma and diabetes mellitus. Arch dermatol 99:674-680, 1969.
26. Tomford JW, Whittlesey D, Ellner JJ, Tomashefski JF. Invasive primary cutaneous phycomycosis in diabetic leg ulcers. Arch Surg 115:770-771, 1980.
27. Alteras I, Saryt E. Prevalence of pathogenic fungi in the toe-webs and toe-nails of diabetic patients. Mycopathologia 67:157-159, 1979.
28. Lugo-Somolinos A, Sanchez JL. Prevalence of dermatophytosis in patients with diabetes. J Am Acad Dermatol 26: 408-10, 1991.
29. Basarab T, Munn SE, McGrath J, Jones RR. Bullous diabeticorum: a case report and literature review. Clin Exp Dermatol 20: 218-20 1995.
30. Bernstein JE, Medenica M, Soltani K, et al. Bullous eruption of diabetes mellitus. Arch Dermatol 115: 324-5, 1975.

31. Bernstein JE, Levine LE, Medenica MM, et al. Reduced threshold to suction-induced blister formation in insulin-epidermolysis bullosa without immunoreactants. J Am Acad Dermatol 8:790-1, 1983.

32. Gilchrest B, Rowe JW, Mihm MC. Bullous dermatosis of hemodialysis. Ann Intern Med 83: 480-3, 1975.

33. Glynne P et al. Bullous dermatoses in end-stage renal failure: porphyria or pseudoporphyria? Amer J Kidney Diseases 34: 155-60, 1999.

34. Vadoud-Sayedi et al. Treatment of hemodialysis-associated pseudoporphyria with N-acetylcysteine: report of two cases. Br J Dermatol 142: 580-1, 2000.

35. Rendon MI, Ponciano PD, Sontheimer RD et al. Acanthosis nigricans: a cutaneous marker of tissue resistance to insulin. J Am Acad Dermatol 21: 461-9, 1989.

36. Sibbald RG, Schachter RK. The skin and diabetes mellitus. Int J Dermatol, 23: 567-584, 1984.

37. Podolsky S. Lipoatrophic diabetes and leprechaunism, in Podolsky S, Viswanthan M, Eds. The Spectrum of the diabetic syndromes. New York, Raven Press, pp. 335-352, 1980.

38. Louis LH, Conn VW, Minick MC. Lipoatrophic diabetes: isolation and characterization of insulin anatagonist from the urine. Metabolism 12:867-886, 1963.

39. Lawrence RD. Lipodystrophy and hepatomegaly with diabetes, lipemia, and other metabolic disturbances. Lancet 250:724-731, 1946.

40. Dunnigan MG. Unusual clinical manifestations of diabetes mellitus. Practitioner 222: 321-330, 1979.

41. Mabry CC, Hollingsworth DR, Upton CV and Corbin A. Pituitary-hypothalamic dysfunction in generalized lipodystrophy. J Pediatrics 82(4): 625-33, 1973.

42. Oseid S, Beck-Nielsen H, Pederson O, Sovik O. Decreased binding of insulin to its receptor in patients with congenital generalized lipodystrophy. N Engl J Med 296: 245-248, 1977.

43. Jelinek, JE. The skin in diabetes mellitus: cutaneous manifestations, complications and associations. In Yearbook of dermatology, 1970. Chicago, Year Book Medical Publishers, Inc., pp. 5-35, 1970.

44. Hoerer E, Dreyfuss F, Herzberg M. Carotenemia, skin color and diabetes mellitus. Acta Diabetol Lat 12: 202-7, 1975.

45. Rapini RP, Herbert AA, Drucker CR. Acquired perforating dermatosis: evidence for combined transepidermal elimination of both collagen and elastic fibers. Arch Dermatol 125: 1074-8, 1989.

46. Lithner F. Purpura, pigmentation and yellow nails of the lower extremities in diabetes. Acta Med Scand 199: 203-8, 1976.

47. Halevy S, Feuerman EJ. Abnormal glucose tolerance associated with lichen planus. Acta Derm Venereol 59: 167-70, 1979.

48. Albrecht M, Banoczy J, Dinya E, et al. Occurrence of oral leukoplakia and lichen planus in diabetes mellitus. J Oral Pathol 21: 364-6, 1992.

49. Muller SA. Dermatologic disorders associated with diabetes mellitus. Mayo Clin Proc 41: 689-703, 1966.

50. Pinkus H, Mehregan AH. A guide to dermatohistopathology. New York, Appleton-Century-Crofts, p. 417, 1976.

51. Chevrant-Breton J, Simon M, Bourel M, Ferrand B. Cutaneous manifestations of idiopathic hemochromatosis. Arch Dermatol 113: 161-5, 1977.
52. Kahana M, Grossman E, Feinstein A, et al. Skin tags: a cutaneous marker for diabetes mellitus. Acta Derm Venereol 67: 175-7, 1986.
53. Bleich HL, Boro ES. Diabetic polyneuropathy: the importance of insulin deficiency, hyperglycemia and alterations in myoinositol metabolism in its pathogenesis. N Engl J Med 295: 1416-20, 1976.
54. Levy DM, Teenghi G, GU XH. Immunohistochemical measurements of nerves and neuropeptides in diabetic skin: relationship to tests of neurological function. Diabetologia 35: 889-97, 1992.
55. Max MB, Lynch SA, Muir J, et al. Effects of desipramine, amitriptyline and fluoxetine on pain in diabetic neuropathy. N Engl J Med 326: 1250-6, 1992.
56. Ellenberg M. Diabetic Foot. NY State J Med, 73: 2778-2781, 1973.
57. Lippman HI, Perotto A, Farrar R. The neuropathic foot of the diabetic. Bull NY Acad Med 52: 1159-1178, 1976.
58. Editorial. Diabetic foot ulcers. Lancet 1:232-233, 1977.
59. Ajam Z, Barton SP, Marks R. Characterization of abnormalities in the cutaneous microvasculature of diabetic subjects. Br J Dermatol 107 (suppl 22): 22-3, 1982.
60. Huntley AC. Cutaneous manifestations of diabetes mellitus. Dermatol Clin 7: 531-46, 1989.
61. Grunfeld C. Diabetic foot ulcers: etiology, treatment and prevention. Adv Intern Med 37: 103-32, 1991.
62. Ditzel J. Functional microangiopathy in diabetes mellitus. Diabetes 17: 388-397, 1968.
63. Landau J, Davis E. The small blood vessels of the conjunctiva and nailbed in diabetes mellitus. Lancet 2: 731-734, 1960.
64. Lithner F, Hietala SO. Skeletal lesions of the feet in diabetics and their relationship to cutaneous erythema with or without necrosis of the feet. Acta Med Scand 200: 155-161, 1976.
65. Fitzpatrick TB et al. Color atlas and synopsis of clinical dermatology. New York, McGraw-Hill, pp. 417-8, 2001.
66. Feingold KR, Siperstein MD. Diabetic vascular disease. Adv Intern Med; 31: 309-40, 1986.
67. Haroon TS. Diabetes and skin: a review. Scott Med J 19: 257-67, 1974.
68. Jegasothy, BV. Allergic reactions to insulin. Int J Dermatol, 19: 139-41, 1980.
69. Galloway JA, Davidson JK. Clinical use of insulin, in Rifkin H, Raskin P, Eds. Diabetes mellitus. Bowie, RJ Brady Co., vol 5, pp 117-27, 1981.
70. Feinglos MN, Jegasothy BV. "Insulin" allergy due to zinc. Lancet 1:122-24, 1979.
71. Galloway, JA, Bressler R. Insulin treatment in diabetes. Med Clin North Am 62: 663-80, 1978.
72. Grammer LC, Metzger BE, Patterson R. Cutaneous allergy to human (recombinant DNA) insulin. JAMA 251: 1459-60, 1984.
73. Edidin DV. Cutaneous manifestations of diabetes mellitus in children. Pediatr Dermatol 2: 161-179, 1985.

Helpful internet source: http://www.dermis.net/index_e.htm.

VII. Therapy of Diabetes Mellitus

Chapter 1. Glycemic Goals

David J. Brillon

INTRODUCTION

Both type 1 and type 2 diabetes are accompanied by microvascular and macrovascular complications. For decades the association between chronic hyperglycemia and the development of long-term eye, kidney, and nerve disease was suspected based on animal models of diabetes[1-3] and the long term observations of clinicians.[4] Nonetheless, the belief that normalization of blood glucose would prevent end organ damage was not universally accepted.[5]

By the 1980's several small prospective multicenter randomized trials were conducted to address this question. These studies were of short duration[6] or had conflicting results regarding the benefits of glycemic control on microvascular disease.[6-8] Indeed the establishment of lower blood glucose levels for 8 months appeared to worsen established retinopathy.[6]

MICROVASCULAR DISEASE

To definitively address the question of glycemic control and the development of diabetic microvascular disease, a large randomized interventional trial, which would eventually involve 29 centers in the US and Canada, was begun. A total of 1441 patients with type 1 diabetes were recruited from 1983 to 1989 to comprise the cohorts of the Diabetes Control and Complications Trial or DCCT.[9] Two cohorts were studied – a primary prevention cohort, to determine if intensive glycemic control would prevent the development of diabetic retinopathy, and a secondary intervention cohort to determine if intensive glycemic control would ameliorate the progression of early diabetic retinal disease. For the primary prevention cohort subjects had to have 1-5 years duration of diabetes, absence of retinopathy by fundus photography and urinary albumin excretion < 40 mg/24 hrs. The secondary intervention cohort criteria were 5-15 year duration of diabetes, mild (one microaneurysm) to moderate nonproliferative retinopathy, and urinary albumin excretion of less than 200 mg/24 hrs. Patients were randomized to either conventional or intensive glycemic control. Intensive therapy included multiple (3 or more) daily insulin injections (MDI) or continuous subcutaneous insulin injection (CSII) via an insulin pump. Insulin doses were adjusted according to fingerstick blood glucose (BG) values (obtained at least 4 times a day), dietary intake, and level of physical activity. The goal of intensive therapy included premeal BG levels 70-120 mg/dl, postprandial levels under 180 mg/dl and hemoglobin A1c (HbA1c) levels within the nondiabetic range (< 6.05%). To help achieve the goals, subjects met monthly with the physician, nurse educator and dietician of the study and were contacted by telephone to review and adjust their regimen as necessary. Subjects randomized to conventional therapy received the usual diabetes treatment of the time, 1-2 insulin injections a day. The goals were to avoid symptomatic hypo- or hyperglycemia but not to achieve specific target glucose levels. Although subjects in the conventional arm also received diet and exercise education, they only performed once daily glucose monitoring and met with the study team on a once every 3 month basis.

Both cohorts of 1441 patients were followed for a mean of 6.5 years. During this time seven field stereoscopic fundus photos, 24 hour urine albumin excretion, clinical neuropathy assessment, peripheral nerve conduction studies and autonomic nerve testing were performed. 99% of the participants completed the study. From an initially statistically identical HbA1c at the beginning of the study, the intensively treated group reached a nadir of 6.9% at 6 months. Throughout the subsequent 6 years a statistically significant separation (approximately 7.2% vs 9.1%) between intensive and conventional therapy was maintained.

The trial was ended prematurely due to significant outcome differences between intensively and conventionally treated subjects. Outcome curves for retinopathy were initially similar but separated after 3 years. Intensive therapy decreased the mean risk of progression of retinopathy by 76% in the primary prevention and by 54% in the secondary intervention cohorts. In addition, the adjusted risk of proliferative or severe nonproliferative retinopathy was reduced by 47% and the need for photocoagulation by 56% in the secondary intervention group. Similarly, with regard to diabetic renal disease, intensive therapy resulted in significant reductions in risk of microalbuminuria of 34% (primary cohort) and 43% (secondary cohort). In the secondary intervention cohort, approximately 10% of whom had microalbuminuria at onset, the risk of albuminuria >300 mg/24 hrs was reduced by 56%. The appearance of clinical neuropathy (defined as the presence of signs or symptoms of peripheral neuropathy accompanied by either abnormal nerve conduction in at least 2 peripheral nerves or abnormal autonomic testing) was reduced with intensive therapy by 69% in the primary cohort and by 57% in the secondary intervention cohort. The reductions were significant for both peripheral and autonomic neuropathy.[10,11]

The positive reductions in cumulative incidence of microvascular complications were also analyzed within subgroups of the DCCT subjects defined on the basis of several baseline covariates to ensure consistency of results. These included age (adolescents versus adults), gender, duration of diabetes, baseline HbA1c, mean blood pressure. The effect of intensive treatment was consistently maintained in all subgroups in both the primary and secondary cohorts. Thus the DCCT conclusively demonstrated that intensive glycemic control therapy delays the onset and slows the progression of diabetic retinopathy, nephropathy and neuropathy in individuals with type 1 diabetes.

The DCCT was the largest and longest duration study of glycemic control in type 1 diabetes. Several months prior to its publication a study involving 102 subjects with type 1 diabetes in Sweden was published. As with the DCCT, subjects participating in the Stockholm Diabetes Intervention Study (SDIS) were randomized to intensive versus standard therapy and followed for 7.5 years[12]. Mean HbA1c levels were reduced from 9.4% to 8.5% in the standard treatment group and from 9.5% to 7.1% in the intensive treatment group. After 7.5 years both progression of nonproliferative retinopathy and the need for laser photocoagulation was less in the group receiving intensive control. There were more patients in the standard group with albumin excretion of at least 300 mg/24 hrs and with nephropathy as defined by subnormal glomerular filtration rates. Peripheral nerve conduction velocities deteriorated more in the standard treatment group. These results were the first to describe the beneficial effects of intensive therapy on retarding the development and progression of microvascular complications in patients with type 1 diabetes.

Based on the DCCT and SDIS studies published in 1993, most diabetes organizations advocated the use of intensive glycemic control therapy for all individuals with type 1 and type 2 diabetes.[13] The latter group was not studied in either trial. However as the microvascular complications were all too similar in both types of diabetes[14-15] the extrapolation was applied. This recommendation was not universally accepted.[16-17] It was felt that the use of intensive insulin therapy in type 2 diabetes may lead to an increase in cardiovascular morbidity and /or mortality due to increased hypoglycemia, higher insulin levels and/or greater weight gain. This concern had some basis in prior epidemiologic studies demonstrating that coronary artery disease (CAD) occurs with greater frequency in type 2 than in type 1 diabetes; a difference attributable to the older age of onset of type 2 diabetes but also to the dysmetabolic state that accompanies the disease.[18-20]

A group of investigators at Kumamoto University in Japan replicated the design of the DCCT but in individuals with type 2 diabetes.[21] 55 subjects with no retinopathy and urine albumin excretion < 30mg/ 24hrs composed the primary prevention group and 55 patients with mild retinopathy and albumin excretion<300 mg/ 24hrs comprised the secondary intervention group. All subjects were then randomized to intensive (>2 insulin injections per day) or conventional (1-2 insulin injections per day) therapy. The goal of the conventional group was the absence of symptomatic hyper- or hypoglycemia. The numeric targets for the intensive group were fasting glucose <140 mg/dl, 2 hour postprandial glucose <200 mg/dl, and HbA1c <

493

7%. Follow-up data were obtained at 3 months and then every 6 months for 6 years. Separation of HbA1c (9.4% in the conventional subjects and 7.1% in those receiving intensive treatment) was maintained through the study. Risk reduction for progression of retinopathy in the combined cohorts was 69%, a result similar to the DCCT (see Table 1). Intensive therapy also reduced the average risk of worsening in retinopathy by 70%. After 6 years nerve conduction velocities were significantly improved in the intensively treated subjects while median nerve conduction velocities deteriorated in the subjects receiving conventional therapy. Intensive glycemic control by MDI delayed the onset and slowed the progression of diabetic retinopathy, nephropathy and neuropathy compared to conventional treatment. This study extended the confirmation of beneficial effects of intensive glycemic therapy seen in the DCCT and in the SDIS to individuals with type 2 diabetes.

Table 1. Risk reductions in microvascular disease

Study	Retinopathy		Microalbuminuria	
	Primary	Secondary	Primary	Secondary
DCCT	76%	54%	34%	43%
Kumamoto	76%	56%	62%	52%

The DCCT was designed as an intervention trial to compare two treatment modalities and not to determine complication risk at various levels of glycemic control. Nonetheless, the data were analyzed and presented in a subsequent paper, which examined the relationship between glycemic levels, as reflected by HbA1c, and the risk of retinopathy progression.[22] There was a continuously increasing risk of retinopathy progression with increasing mean HbA1c levels. Some prior retrospective studies had not found such a relationship for microalbuminuria[23] and retinopathy progression[24] for HbA1c levels below 8%. Analysis of the DCCT data, comprising over 9000 patient-years of observation, found a similar and significant reduction in retinal, renal and neurological complication rates associated with decline in HbA1c. This relationship was consistent over the entire range of HbA1c in the study, even for levels less than 8% (see Figure 1). Thus for a 10% reduction in HbA1c there is a constant 39% decrease in retinopathy progression. As the rate of events per 100 patient year is greater at higher HbA1c values, the absolute reduction in risk is greater with reduction in HbA1c at higher values. Nonetheless there exists no threshold HbA1c value below which a reduction in HbA1c is not accompanied by a reduction in risk for retinopathy and for nephropathy. When the risk of progression of retinopathy is extrapolated over the 9 years of follow-up in the DCCT, then the cumulative incidence of progression is lowered from 20% at a HbA1c of 8% to an incidence of 5.5% at a HbA1c of 6%.[25]

Another question regarding the extrapolation of the DCCT, SDIS, and Kumamoto studies was whether the motivated volunteers screened and selected for enrollment were representative of the general diabetes patient population. In order to address the comparability of the DCCT cohort and the validity of generalizing the DCCT results, a contemporaneous population–based cohort was necessary. The Wisconsin Epidemiologic Study of Diabetic Retinopathy (WESDR) was a large population based incidence study of people with both type 1 and type 2 diabetes conducted concurrently with the DCCT.[26] The measurement of the main endpoint, diabetic retinopathy, was determined using similar methods of classification. Of the patients with type 1 diabetes being followed in the WESDR, 891 subjects underwent baseline and 4 year follow-up assessment. Of these, 39 and 111 met the DCCT inclusion criteria for the primary and secondary cohorts, respectively. The DCCT study cohorts were comparable to the WESDR type 1 population with regard to age, gender, BMI, blood pressure and insulin dose. Because of the DCCT baseline eligibility criteria, retinopathy severity was higher in the WESDR group. Thus the comparison supports the extrapolation of the DCCT results to the general type 1 diabetes population.

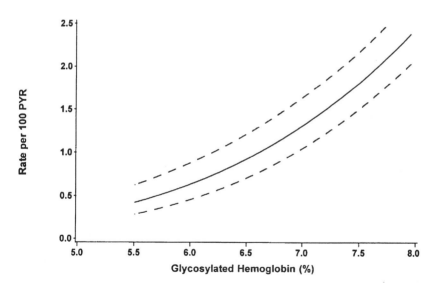

Figure 1. The absolute risk of sustained retinopathy progression (hazard rate per 100 patient-years) in the combined treatment groups as a function of the updated mean HbA1c during follow-up in the DCCT estimated from a Poisson progression model with 95% confidence bands. (From DCCT Research Group. The absence of a glycemic threshold for the development of long- term complications: The perspective of the DCCT. Diabetes 45:1289-98, 1996, with permission.)

495

At the close of the DCCT in 1993 subjects who were in the conventional group were offered intensive treatment and as part of the study closeout were instructed in intensive therapy. Those subjects in both the former intensive and conventional groups were also offered participation in an observational study to continue following the DCCT cohorts. The Epidemiology of Diabetes Intervention and Complications (EDIC) is 10 year follow-up study of the DCCT cohort to continue to monitor the long term micro- and macrovascular complications of type 1 diabetes.[27] One of the study objectives is to compare the effects of the prior intensive or conventional treatments administered during the DCCT on the subsequent development and progression of more advanced retinopathy and nephropathy. 1375 of the 1421 surviving DCCT subjects participated in the EDIC study. During the study all subjects received their diabetes care from their own physicians but were seen yearly for evaluation by the research team. Annual retinal fundus photography was obtained based on year of enrollment in the DCCT, with 1208 (605 in the intensive DCCT group) subjects undergoing evaluation at year 4 of EDIC.

By the end of the first year of EDIC the HbA1c levels in the 1208 subjects had begun to merge (8.1% in the conventional and 7.7% in the intensive). During the first four years of EDIC the median HbA1c values were 8.2% for the conventional and 7.9% for the former intensive groups; a smaller but still statistically significant difference. The year four fundus photography results revealed that 49 % of the subjects from the conventional group had progression of retinopathy from the DCCT baseline, while only 18% of the intensive group had progression. To assess the change in retinopathy during the EDIC years, the level of retinopathy was evaluated for fundus photographs obtained at years 1, 2, 3, and 4 of EDIC and retinopathy progression was compared to the level of retinopathy at the end of the DCCT (see Figure 2). By EDIC year 4 the cumulative incidence of further progression of retinopathy was 70% lower in the intensive than in the conventional treatment group.[28] The significant reduction in retinopathy from end of the DCCT to year four of EDIC was similar regardless of the level of retinopathy at the end of the DCCT. Severe nonproliferative retinopathy, or worse, occurred in 10% of the conventional group but only 2% of the intensive group. This 76% reduction was significant even when adjusting for the level of retinopathy at the end of the DCCT. In addition the risk of progression of retinopathy was highly associated with the mean HbA1c level during both the DCCT and EDIC studies.

Similar results were detected for progression of nephropathy during EDIC. At years 3 and 4, the onset of microalbuminuria was reduced 53%, from 11% in the conventional treatment group to 5% in the intensive group. The risk of new albuminuria was decreased by 86% in the intensive group.

During the four years of EDIC with an increase in the HbA1c of the intensive group and a reduction in the separation in HbA1c between the intensive and conventional DCCT groups, it would be expected, based on the relationship of glycemic control to microvascular disease,[22] that the effects of intensive therapy during the DCCT would be reduced. In contrast the benefits of intensive control on retinopathy and on nephropathy persist for at least 4 years after termination of separation of intensive and conventional treatment and despite rising HbA1c levels. The positive effects of glycemic control appear to have a long lasting duration. These results could be attributed to the effects of chronic hyperglycemia on advanced glycation end products accumulation in end organs, leading to microvascular disease.[29]

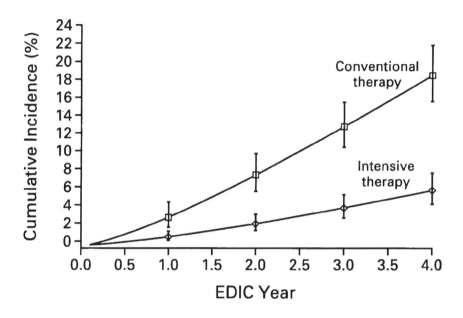

Figure 2. Cumulative incidence of further progression of retinopathy (an increase of at least three steps from the level at the end of the DCCT) in the former conventional therapy and intensive therapy groups. The data are based on regression analysis adjusted for the level of retinopathy at the end of the DCCT, whether patients received therapy as primary prevention or secondary intervention, and both the duration of diabetes and the glycosylated hemoglobin value on enrollment in the DCCT. Patients who underwent scatter photocoagulation during the DCCT were excluded from the analysis (22 in the conventional group and 9 in the intensive therapy group). Bars denote 95 per cent confidence intervals. (From DCCT/EDIC Research Group. Retinopathy and nephropathy in patients with type 1 diabetes four years after a trial of intensive therapy. N Engl J Med 2000; 342:381-89, with permission.)

Intensive glycemic control will delay the onset and slow the progression of diabetic microvascular disease in individuals with both type 1 and in type 2 diabetes. From the DCCT and EDIC study results, the positive benefits of intensive over conventional therapy will be greater the earlier they are implemented and can persist for up to four years after cessation of differential treatment.

MACROVASCULAR DISEASE

Although microvascular disease can lead to substantial morbidity, the major cause of mortality in both type 1 and type 2 diabetes is cardiovascular disease[30-31]. As was the case with microvascular disease, clinicians had long recognized an association of poor glycemic control with the development of macrovascular outcomes in patients with diabetes. Several prospective studies have confirmed that hyperglycemia is a predictor for cardiovascular disease.[32-33] None the less the belief that hyperglycemia causes cardiovascular disease is not universally accepted.[34]

In the DCCT the number of combined major macrovascular events (cardiac, cerebrovascular and peripheral vascular) was twice as high in the conventional treatment (40 events) group as the intensive treatment group (23 events) but this difference was not statistically significant.[35] Lipid risk factors associated with cardiovascular disease such as increased total and LDL cholesterol and elevated triglyceride levels were all significantly reduced in the intensive treatment group. As mentioned above, the DCCT cohorts were of young age at entry (13-39 years). In addition the inclusion criteria eliminated patients with hypertension, hypercholesterolemia and known cardiovascular disease. Such demographics would make it likely that few cardiovascular events would occur by study end. The Kumamoto study evaluated an older age cohort. The total number of combined cardiovascular events in the conventional treatment group was twice that of the intensive treatment group but was not statistically significant due to the small number of patients in the trial.

A much larger group of diabetic patients were studied in the United Kingdom Prospective Diabetes Study. The UKPDS was a multi-center intervention trial of over 5000 patients with new onset type 2 diabetes. The objective of the UKPDS was to determine if intensive glycemic control reduces the risk of micro- and macrovascular complications in individuals with type 2 diabetes and, as a secondary aim, to compare various treatment modalities.[36] The study was conducted by general practitioners in 23 centers throughout the UK between 1977 and 1991. Patients with type 2 diabetes, 25-65 years of age, with FBG >6 mmol/L on 2 occasions were enrolled. All subjects were initially treated with diet modification alone for a 3 month period. At the end of 3 months, those patients who failed to achieve glycemic control (FBG >6.0mmol/L) were randomized to various pharmacologic treatment modalities. Patients with BMI over 120% (N=2187) were randomized to diet alone, sulfonylureas (SU), insulin or metformin. Non-overweight patients (N=2022) were randomly assigned to diet alone, SU or insulin.

The conventional or diet alone subjects received dietary education every 3 months with goals to attain normal body weight, eliminate hyperglycemic symptoms and maintain HbA1c levels < 15 mmol/L. If either symptoms of hyperglycemia or FBG > 15 mmol/L occurred then the subject was again randomized to one of the pharmacologic agents with the aim once more to avoid hyperglycemic symptoms and keep FBG < 15 mmol/L. The goal of intensive therapy was to attain near normal FBG values (< 6 mmol/L). As with the conventional cohort, a second drug was added if the FBG exceeded 15 mmol/L. Median follow-up was 10.7 years.

Unlike the DCCT, SDIS and Kumamoto studies, glycemic separation between the diet and pharmacologic groups was not maintained throughout the trial. HbA1c levels increased in all groups over the duration of the study so that at the end of 10 years, the intensive treatment group median HbA1c level was 7.0% as compared to a 7.9% value for the conventional treatment group. Despite this modest difference, intensive glycemic control with either sulfonylurea or insulin resulted in a significant 21% risk reduction in the progression of retinopathy and a 33% risk reduction in albuminuria[36].The risk reduction for myocardial infarction of 16% was just above statistical significance (p=0.052). Epidemiologic analysis revealed a continuous association between the risk of cardiovascular complications and the level of glycemia. When overweight subjects treated with metformin were compared to the conventional treated overweight group, there were significant risk reductions for diabetes related endpoint and diabetes related death, including myocardial infarction.[37] These results occurred with only a 0.6% HbA1c separation between intensive (7.4%) and conventional (8%) groups, suggesting that the beneficial effects of metformin could have also been due to the drugs ability to improve lipid levels and decrease levels of plasminogen-activator inhibitor type 1. In contrast to the findings with metformin alone, there appeared to be an increase in myocardial infarction when metformin was added to SU to improve glycemic control.

A smaller earlier intervention trial of 153 male subjects with type 2 diabetes also evaluated intensive versus conventional glycemic control. The Veterans Affairs Cooperative Study in Glycemia Control was a feasibility study for a larger trial.[38] Subjects were randomized to intensive therapy, using a stepped multiple insulin injection algorithm plus glipizide, or conventional treatment, using 1 or 2 insulin injections a day. The two groups achieved a HbA1c difference of 2.1% (9.2% vs. 7.1%) for 27 (range 18-35) months. The per cent subjects experiencing a cardiovascular (CV) event was higher, though not statistically so, in the intensive (21.3%) than in the conventional group (11.5%).

The large clinical trials showing beneficial effects of intensive therapy on microvascular disease fail to show a statistical significant benefit on macrovascular disease. In the case of the UKPDS the continually rising glucose levels during the study, resulting in a modest HbA1c separation at study end, probably contributed to the lack of significant reduction in CV

499

disease. It has long been recognized that an increase in CV risk occurs prior to the development of overt type 2 diabetes, at a time when HbA1c may be within the normal range and impaired glucose intolerance is present.[39-40] Much of this increased risk may be related to the lipid, blood pressure and other metabolic abnormalities that occur in individuals with impaired glucose tolerance. On the other hand, the ability of intensive glycemic control to decrease CV disease may require achieving lower glucose levels than those resulting in improvement in microvascular complications. In the case of the DCCT, the age and risk factors of the cohorts resulted in the low CV events. The EDIC study, however, continues monitoring the cohorts and has added CV assessments to further define the clinical course and the potential effects of glycemic control on CV outcomes in type 1 diabetes. B-mode ultrasonography was used to measure carotid intima media wall thickness (IMT), an established index of atherosclerosis[41], at years 1 and 6 of EDIC.[42] Increased IMT was significantly associated with HbA1c both at the time of measurement and during the 6.5 years of the DCCT. Subjects receiving conventional treatment during the DCCT developed greater age related increases in IMT than the intensively treated subjects. In addition to the positive effects on improving cardiovascular risk profile, intensive glycemic control in individuals with type 1 diabetes will result in decreased progression of atherosclerosis, as measured by carotid artery wall thickness.

ADVERSE EFFECTS OF INTENSIVE GLYCEMIC CONTROL

Intensive glycemic control is not without possible side effects. These include weight gain, specific drug side effects, costs in both time and money, and hypoglycemia. The occurrence of low blood sugar carries the greatest risk, including significant morbidity and death. Several fold increases in mild to moderate hypoglycemia occur in all trials utilizing intensive glycemic control. In the DCCT, the incidence of severe hypoglycemia (documented BG<50 mg/dl requiring the assistance of another person for correction) was increased threefold in the intensive treatment group (61.2 episodes/100 patient-years) compared to the conventional group (18.7 episodes/100pt.-yrs).[43] The intensive group did not have an increase in deaths, myocardial infarctions or strokes attributable to hypoglycemia. There was also no difference in the occurrence of neuropsychological changes, as assessed by formal testing, in the intensive treatment group.[44] Similar results regarding the incidence of hypoglycemia were found in the Stockholm Diabetes Intervention Study. The incidence of hypoglycemia, including recurrent episodes, was found to have greater association with the most recent HbA1c than with past values or the average HbA1c during the DCCT trial.[25] There was a 26% (95% C.I. 22-29) increase in the risk in of severe hypoglycemia for each 10% reduction in current HbA1c in the intensive group. The increased risk per 10% lower HbA1c was 58% (95% C.I. 49-60) in the conventionally treated subjects. For both treatment groups, the risk gradient

500

for HbA1c <8% was lower than for values >8%.[25] Over the 6.5 years of the DCCT, 65% of the patients in the intensive group had at least one episode of severe hypoglycemia vs. 35% of the conventionally treated subjects. The number of prior episodes of hypoglycemia was the strongest predictor of future episodes.[43]

In type 2 diabetes, the risk of hypoglycemia and severe hypoglycemia is an order of magnitude less than that in type 1 diabetes. In the UKPDS, the rate of hypoglycemic episodes increases over time in the insulin treated patients but decreases over time in patients treated with oral agents. The percentage of patients with any hypoglycemia was 15.2% for patients on chlorpropramide, for glibenclamide-20.5%, for insulin-25.5%, for metformin- 8.3% and for diet alone- 7.9%. Severe hypoglycemic episodes occurred in 1.8-2% of patients on insulin, 1.0-1.4% on glibenclamide, 1-1.2% on chlorpropramide, 0.6% on metformin and 0.7% on diet alone.[36-37]

Intensive glycemic control also lowers the threshold for hormonal response to hypoglycemia, leading to impaired glucose counter-regulation.[45-46] Patients with type 2 diabetes release counter-regulatory hormones at a higher plasma glucose level and in higher amounts for a similar degree of overall glycemic control.[47] This may account for the lower incidence of hypoglycemia in type 2 diabetes. Weight gain will also accompany intensive glycemic control, with the exception of patients treated with metformin. This is especially troubling in individuals with type 2 diabetes, given the high incidence of associated obesity. In the UKPDS subjects treated with SUs gained 1.7 and 2.6 kg, while patients on insulin gained an average of 4.0 kg.[37] In addition intensive insulin therapy can result in hyperinsulinemia, particularly in type 2 diabetes. The possible adverse effects of high therapeutic insulin levels on vascular injury and atherosclerosis remain controversial.[20-48]

GLYCEMIC CONTROL TARGET LEVELS

The target levels for intensive glycemic control are based on the American Diabetes Association (ADA) recommendations.[49] Clearly patients with both type 1 and type 2 diabetes must be given appropriate dietary and pharmacologic therapy to eliminate the symptoms of hyperglycemia and prevent the consequences of extreme uncontrolled diabetes, i.e. ketoacidosis and hyperosmotic state. The positive effects of intensive glycemic control on the development and the progression of microvascular disease in both type 1 and type 2 diabetes form the basis for the ADA target glucose and HbA1c levels as outlined in Table 2 below.

A case could be made to attempt to achieve glucose levels as close to normal as possible as there is no threshold of HbA1c level below which further reduction in microvascular disease does not occur. Concurrent chronic illness does not limit the achievement of glycemic control.[50] This must be tempered by the fact that the incidence of hypoglycemia will be increased threefold for near-normal glucose levels. For individuals with other diseases where the consequences of severe hypoglycemia may result in morbidity or death, the attainment of normal glycemia with insulin or SU therapy would not be advisable. If the patient has a disease which significantly shortens life expectancy, then the need to prevent long-term complications is absent. Treatment goals must be individualized to account for concomitant disease, the presence of hypoglycemic awareness, and the ability of the patient to monitor glucose levels and follow an intensive treatment plan. For patients with type 2 diabetes it is also important to focus on the concomitant dysmetabolic state and to address any abnormalities in lipids and blood pressure. The ultimate goal of glycemic control is to attain the lowest HbA1c level that will not adversely affect patient safety. Although the ADA goal is a HbA1c <7%, for most patients without other medical illnesses one should attempt to reach a value of 6.0%, providing no severe

TABLE 2. GLYCEMIC CONTROL FOR PEOPLE WITH DIABETES

	Normal	Goal	Additional action suggested
Whole blood values			
Average preprandial glucose (mg/dl)†	<100	80–120	<80/>140
Average bedtime glucose (mg/dl)†	<110	100–140	<100/>160
Plasma values			
Average preprandial glucose (mg/dl)‡	<110	90–130	<90/>150
Average bedtime glucose (mg/dl)‡	<120	110–150	<110/>180
HbA$_{1c}$ (%)	<6	<7	>8

*The values shown in this table are by necessity generalized to the entire population of individuals with diabetes. Patients with comorbid diseases, the very young and older adults, and others with unusual conditions or circumstances may warrant different treatment goals. These values are for nonpregnant adults. "Additional action suggested" depends on individual patient circumstances. Such actions may include enhanced diabetes self-management education, comanagement with a diabetes team, referral to an endocrinologist, change in pharmacological therapy, initiation of or increase in SMBG, or more frequent contact with the patient. HbA$_{1c}$ is referenced to a nondiabetic range of 4.0–6.0% (mean 5.0%, SD 0.5%). †Measurement of capillary blood glucose. ‡Values calibrated to plasma glucose.

(From American Diabetes Association Position Statement Standards of medical care for patients with diabetes mellitus. Diabetes Care 24(S1):S33-S43, 2001, with permission.)

hypoglycemia or treatment side effects occur. For patients with mild diabetes, on diet alone or on pharmacologic agents that cannot cause hypoglycemia, HbA1c levels within the normal range should be readily achievable.

SUMMARY

Intensive glycemic control effectively prevents the occurrence and delays the progression of microvascular complications in both type 1 and type 2 diabetes. Glycemic control will also improve cardiovascular risk factors although positive effects on reducing cardiovascular outcomes has not been conclusively demonstrated. Hypoglycemia incidence is increased threefold with intensive glycemic control. Current recommendations advocate attaining near normal glucose levels when safely feasible.

Helpful internet source for additional information on glycemic goals:
* ADA clinical practice guidelines (http://journal.diabetes.org/CareSup1Jan01.htm)

REFERENCES

1. Engerman R, Bloodworth JM, et al. Relationship of microvascular disease in diabetes to metabolic control. Diabetes 26:760-9, 1977.
2. Engerman RL, Kern TS Progression of incipient diabetic retinopathy during good glycemic control. Diabetes 36:808-12, 1987.
3. Cohen AJ, McGill PD, Rosetti RG, Guberski DL, Like AA. Glomerulopathy in spontaneously diabetic rat: impact of glycemic control. Diabetes 36:944-51, 1987.
4. Pirart J. Diabetes mellitus and its degenerative complications: a prospective study of 4,400 patients observed between 1947 and 1973. Diabetes Care 38:252-61, 1978.
5. Ingelfinger FJ. Debates in diabetes. N Engl J Med 296:1228-30, 1977.
6. Kroc Collaborative Study Group Blood glucose control and the evolution of diabetic retinopathy and albuminuria. N Engl J Med 311:365-72, 1984.
7. Dahl-Jorgensen K, Hanssen KF, Kierulf P, Bjoro T, Sandvik L , Aagenaes O. Reduction of urinary albumin excretion after 4 years of continuos subcutaneous insulin-infusion in insulin-dependent diabetes mellitus. Acta Endocrinologica 117:19-25, 1988.
8. Lauritzen T, Frost-Larsen K, Larsen H-W, Deckert T. Steno Study Group. Effect of 1 year of near- normal blood glucose levels on retinopathy in insulin- dependent diabetes. Lancet 1:200-4, 1983.
9. DCCT Research Group. The effect of intensive treatment of diabetes on the development and progression of long-term complications in insulin-dependent diabetes mellitus. N Engl J Med 329:977-86, 1993.
10. DCCT Research Group. The effects of intensive treatment of diabetes therapy on the development and progression of neuropathy. Ann Int Med 122: 561-68, 1995.
11. DCCT Research Group. The effect of intensive diabetes therapy on measures of autonomic nervous system function in the DCCT. Diabetologia 41:416-23, 1998.
12. Reichard P, Nilsson BY, Rosenquist U. The effect of long term intensified treatment on the development of microvascular complications of diabetes mellitus. N Engl J Med 329:304-9, 1993.

13. Implications of the Diabetes Control and Complications Trial. American Diabetes Association Position Statement. Diabetes Spectrum 6:225- 27, 1993.

14. Klein R, Klein BEK, Moss SE, Davis MD, DeMets DL. Glycosylated hemoglobin predicts the incidence and progression of diabetic retinopathy. JAMA 260:2864-71, 1988.

15. Klein R, Klein BEK, Moss SE, Davis MD, DeMets DL. The Wisconsin Epidemiologic Study of Diabetic Retinopathy: X. Four year incidence and progression of diabetic retinopathy when age at diagnosis is 30 years or more. Arch Opthalmol 107:244-49, 1989.

16. Lasker RD. DCCT: Implications for policy and practice. N Engl J Med 329:1035-36, 1993.

17. Nathan DM. Inferences and implications. Do results from the DCCT apply in NIDDM ? Diabetes Care 18:251-57, 1995.

18. Reaven GM. Pathophysiology of insulin resistance in human disease. Physiol Rev 75:473-86, 1995.

19. Balkau B, Eschwege E, Papoz L, Richard J-L, Claude J-R, Warnet J-M, Ducimetiere P. Risk factors for early death in non-insulin-dependent diabetes and men with known glucose tolerance status. Br Med J 307:295-98, 1993.

20. Hsueh WA, Law RE. Cardiovascular risk continuum: Implications of insulin resistance and diabetes. Am J Med 105(1A)4S-14S, 1998.

21. Ohkubo Y, Kishikawa H, Araki E, Miyata T, Isami S, Motoyoshi S, Kojima Y, Furuyoshi N, Shichiri M. Intensive insulin therapy prevents the progression of diabetic microvascular complications in Japanese patients with non-insulin-dependent diabetes mellitus Diab Res Clin Prac 28:103-17, 1995.

22. DCCT Research Group. The relationship of glycemic exposure (HbA1c) to the risk of development and progression of retinopathy in the DCCT. Diabetes 44:968-83, 1995.

23. Krolewski AS, Laffel LMB, Krolewski M, Quinn M, Warram JH. Glycosylated hemoglobin and the risk of microalbuminuria inpatients with insulin-dependent diabetes mellitus. N Engl J Med 332: 1251-55, 1995.

24. Warram JH, Manson JE, Krolewski AS. Glycosylated hemoglobin and the risk of retinopathy in insulin-dependent diabetes. N Engl J Med 332: 1305-06, 1995.

25. DCCT Research Group. The absence of a glycemic threshold for the development of long- term complications : The perspective of the DCCT. Diabetes 45:1289-98, 1996.

26. DCCT Research Group, Klein R, Moss S. A comparison of the study populations in the DCCT and the WESDR. Arch Int Med 155:745-54, 1995.

27. EDIC Research Group. EDIC: Design, implementation and preliminary results of a long-term follow-up of the DCCT cohort. Diabetes Care 22:99-111, 1999.
28. DCCT/EDIC Research Group. Retinopathy and nephropathy in patients with type 1 diabetes four years after a trial of intensive therapy. N Engl J Med 342:381-89, 2000.
29. Monneir VM, Bautista O, Kenny D et al . Skin collagen, glycoxidation, and cross-linking are lower in subjects with long-term intensive versus conventional therapy of type 1 diabetes: relevance of glycated products versus HbA1c as markers of diabetic complications. Diabetes 45:289-98, 1996.
30. Geiss S, Herman WH, Smith PJ. Mortality in non-insulin-dependent diabetes. In Diabetes in America 2nd edition. Harris M, Editor. Bethesda Md. National Institutes of Health p133-55 (NIH publ.No 95-1468), 1995.
31. Krolewski AS, Kosinski EJ, Warram JH et al. Magnitude and determinants of coronary artery disease in juvenile-onset, insulin-dependent diabetes mellitus. Am J Cardiol 59:750, 1987.
32. Niskanen L,Turpeinen A, Pentilla I, Uusitupa MI. Hyperglycemia and compositional lipoprotein abnormalities as predictors of cardiovascular mortality in type 2 diabetes: a 15 year follow-up from the time of diagnosis. Diabetes Care 21:1861-69, 1998.
33. Wei M, Gaskill SP, Haffner SM, Stern MP. Effects of diabetes and level of glycemia on all cause and cardiovascular mortality. The San Antonio Heart Study. Diabetes Care 21:1167-72, 1998.
34. Barrett-Connor E. Does hyperglycemia really cause coronary heart disease? Diabetes Care 20:1620-22, 1997.
35. DCCT Research Group. Effect of intensive diabetes management on macrovascular events and risk factors in the DCCT. Am J Cardiol 75:894-903, 1995.
36. UKPDS Group. Intensive blood glucose control with sulfonylureas or insulin compared with conventional treatment and risk of complications in patients with type 2 diabetes (UKPDS 33). Lancet 352:837-53, 1998.
37. UKPDS Group. Effect of intensive blood glucose control with metformin complications on in overweight patients with type 2 diabetes (UKPDS 34). Lancet 352:854-65, 1998.
38. Abraira C, Colwell J, Nuttall F, Clark TS, Henderson W, Comstock JP, Emanuele NV, Levin SR, Pacold I, Lee HS. Cardiovascular events and correlates in the Veterans Affairs Diabetes Feasibility Trial. Arch Int Med 157:181-88, 1997.
39. Laasko M, Lehto S. Epidemiology of macrovascular disease in diabetes. Diabetes Review 5: 294-315, 1997.
40. Coutinho M, Gerstein HC, Wang Y, Yusuf S The relationship between glucose and incident cardiovascular events. Diabetes Care 22:233-40, 1999.

41. Burke GL, Evans GW, Riley WA, Sharratt AR, Howard G, Barnes RW et al. Arterial wall thickness is associated with prevalent cardiovascular disease in middle-aged adults: the Artherosclerosis Risk in Communities (ARIC) Study. Stroke 26: 386-91, 1995.

42. Molitch M, Cleary P, Orchard T,Backlund J-Y, O'Leary DH. Change in carotid wall thickness in the DCCT/ EDIC cohort. Diabetes 50 (S2)A74, 2001.

43. DCCT Research Group. Hypoglycemia in the DCCT. Diabetes 46:271-86, 1997.

44. DCCT Research Group. Effects of intensive diabetes therapy in neuropsychological function in adults in the DCCT. Ann Int Med 124:379-88, 1996.

45. Amiel SA, Tamborlane WV, Simonson DC, Sherwin RS. Defective glucose counteregulation after strict glycemic control of insulin-independent diabetes mellitus. N Engl J Med 316:1376-83, 1987.

46. Kinsley BT, Windom B, Simonson DS. Differential regulation of counter-regulatory hormone secretion and symptoms during hypoglycemia in IDDM. Diabetes Care 18:17-26, 1995.

47. Levy CJ, Kinsley BT, Bajaj M, Simonson DS. Effect of glycemic control on glucose counter-regulation during hypoglycemia in NIDDM. Diabetes Care 21:1330-38, 1998.

48. Abraira C, Maki KC. Does insulin treatment increase cardiovascular risk in NIDDM? Clin Diabetes 13:29-31, 1995.

49. American Diabetes Association Position Statement: Standards of medical care for patients with diabetes mellitus. Diabetes Care 24(S1):S33-S43, 2001.

50. El-Kebbi IM, Zeimer DC, Cook C, Miller CD, Gallina DL, Phillips LS. Comorbidity and glycemic control in patients with type 2 diabetes. Arch Int Med 161:1295-1300, 2001.

Chapter 2. Behavioral and Educational Approaches to Diabetes Self-Management

Maria A. Mendoza and Elizabeth A. Walker

INTRODUCTION

Diabetes is a life-long disease managed primarily by the individual.[1] The key to successful self-management of this chronic disease is to provide the individual with knowledge, psychomotor skills, and effective psychological coping to facilitate lifestyle modification.[2] The process of adult learning is not an exact science. It is highly individualized. Oftentimes the clinician would find that strategies successful for one person might not be successful for others.

Adult learning within the process of diabetes self-management education does not occur in a vacuum. Indeed, the medical system, health care providers, and most especially the individual with diabetes must be prepared (educated) and motivated to manage this chronic disease in order to prevent its acute and chronic complications. A recently-developed model for considering a chronic disease like diabetes is presented in Figure 1.[3] This model was developed to highlight a collaborative approach to chronic illness care, so that providers are not thinking that it is only the patient's responsibility for diabetes self-management and patients are not assuming that it is the providers' responsibility to take care of their chronic disease. Productive interactions in the context of a supportive system and surrounding community need both an informed patient and prepared health care providers.[4] We (patients and providers) are all in this together.

Adult learning is a continuous and complex process that involves an interaction between the learner and the material to be learned, usually facilitated by an educator/team.[5] In many instances motivated adults learn through their own efforts. In the traditional sense learning involves an acquisition of knowledge and skills through a variety of media.[6] From the perspective of the diabetes self-management education, learning encompasses a much greater objective. It includes the dimension of behavior change by the individual as a result of the improvement in knowledge.[7]

This chapter addresses practical aspects in diabetes self-management education. It discusses how to evaluate the readiness of the individual to enter the learning process. It describes strategies on how to motivate adults to learn diabetes self-management. The chapter provides practical recommendations on how a physician can facilitate adult learning in a clinical setting. It addresses the issue of adherence to the self-management regimen. It also explores the role of the diabetes team. At the end of the chapter is a sampling of resources for patient teaching.

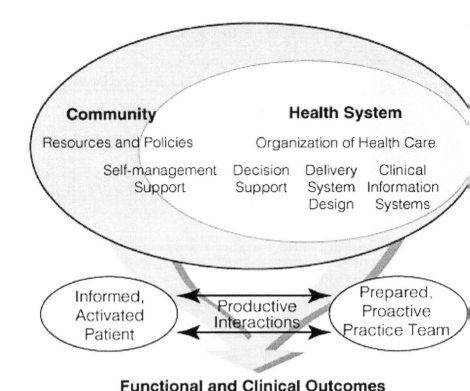

Functional and Clinical Outcomes

Figure 1. Model for the improvement of chronic illness illustrating how the community and health care system must support a productive interaction between patient and provider. Reprinted with permission Wagner, EH. Chronic disease management. Effective Clinical Practice 1:2-4, 1998.

HOW ADULTS LEARN

The learning process in adults is very different from children.[8] Major differences exist in their motivation, self-direction, orientation, participation, and experiences they bring to learning. Table 1 summarizes the characteristics of adult learners.

Adults are very self-directed.[9,10] They want to be active participants in their own learning. Self-learning is very common among adults. They want to choose instructional media that would be comfortable to them. For example, they would rather read materials about diabetes care instead of attending classes if they do not have the time to do so or they feel threatened in a group setting. Some may prefer to watch a video on how to do a fingerstick rather than do it with an educator, because they want the flexibility of watching the film at any time and as many times as they need.

Some want the interaction in a classroom situation rather than self-instruction because they enjoy the group dynamics.

Table 1. Characteristics of Adult Learners

- Self-directed
- Internally motivated
- Problem oriented
- Active participant to learning
- Experienced

Adults are internally motivated to learn.[8] This means that the individual recognizes a *need* and perceives the learning program as a way of meeting this need. This need is derived from something that the individual perceives as important.[11] It is usually problem-oriented. For example, the reason why a person with diabetes would come to a class is to learn a specific skill relevant to meeting a need or goal. It could be as practical as injecting insulin or doing a fingerstick. Or, it could be a desire to solve a problem such as treating or preventing hypoglycemia or how to adjust insulin doses.

Learning among adults is best accomplished through active participation.[12] In general, adults want to be involved in all the stages of learning toward goal accomplishment. It is important for the facilitator and the adult learner to discuss learning needs and goals. These needs and goals should be "learner-centered,"[8-11] i.e., determined by the learner not the educator or team. The ways to acquire the knowledge and skills have to be individualized to the learner's preference. Hands-on learning and group process with active interaction are preferred over passive lecturing. Adults want to ask questions specific to their personal needs; provision for this type of interaction is a good teaching technique.

Adults come into the learning situation with lots of experience.[8,10,12,13] They want to share these experiences with others. The educator must encourage learners to discuss their experiences and provide instructions based on these. Many times sharing experiences would also be a good way to learn. For example, a person who modified the technique of glucose monitoring to deal with decreased sensation in the fingertips should be encouraged to share this with others. Also, having the personal experience provides credibility that is important to adult learners. An instructor who has no diabetes and has not done fingersticks five times a day would not be able to share the pain and apprehension of the person with diabetes going through this experience.

DIABETES SELF-MANAGEMENT EDUCATION PROCESS

Diabetes self-management education (DSME) is an interactive, collaborative, ongoing process involving the learner with diabetes and the educator/team.[6] This process involves (1) assessment of the learner and specific education needs; (2) identification by the patient/learner of self-management goals; (3) provision of education and behavioral interventions to achieve goals; and (4) evaluation of the learning process and outcomes, i.e., attainment of goals.[6] Education does not necessarily translate into behavior change.[7,15] The ultimate goal of DSME is to change behavior. Although knowledge is a necessary component to achieve learning and behavior change, it is not sufficient by itself. Thus, DSME involves not only the provision of knowledge and skills but also psychosocial or psychological counseling, if needed, to facilitate lifestyle modification.[6,15]

Although not expected to be able to teach all the topics recommended by the American Diabetes Association (ADA) as part of the DSME curriculum, the physician should know the scope of the ADA content. The ADA recommends that the competence of each individual with diabetes be assessed in the ten areas outlined in Table 2.

Table 2. ADA Diabetes Self-Management Curriculum

- Describing the diabetes disease process and treatment options
- Incorporating appropriate nutritional management
- Incorporating physical activity into lifestyle
- Utilizing medications (if applicable) for therapeutic effectiveness
- Monitoring blood glucose, urine ketones (when appropriate), and using the results to improve control
- Preventing, detecting, and treating acute complications
- Preventing (through risk reduction behavior), detecting, and treating chronic complications
- Goal setting to promote health, and problem solving for daily living
- Integrating psychosocial adjustment to daily life
- Promoting preconception care, management during pregnancy, and gestational diabetes management (if applicable) [6]

The above list is comprehensive and it is not practical or possible for a busy physician to cover everything. This is where the team approach to teaching becomes important. The physician should at least discuss with the patient and the family, as appropriate, the diabetes disease process and treatment options.

Diabetes self-management education can be provided in a variety of settings depending on availability of resources. Some physicians may be comfortable in providing survival skills instructions to their patients. A survey by the National Institutes of Health revealed that about 41 % of endocrinologists felt that they could adequately handle dietary counseling of their patients.[16] Physicians in a large group practice may hire a certified diabetes educator who may be a nurse, dietitian or psychologist to provide patient teaching onsite. Those in small practice may have to refer patients to other facilities such as hospital-based or free standing privately owned programs. There has to be some mechanism in place for this type of referrals. Knowledge of third-party reimbursement for diabetes education would be helpful to determine where patients could be referred. In some regions diabetes patient education is part of the general medical care and therefore could not be billed separately.[17] Some city or municipal hospitals may offer free educational services to the community for patients with diabetes and their families. This would be a good resource for patients who do not have insurance coverage.

When patients are referred to another institution for patient education, the physician should be aware of the quality of service provided by the agency.[16] The physician should know the general philosophy of the educational program, the curriculum, length and frequency of classes, teaching methodologies used, the credentials of the staff facilitating the program, and the procedure for patient follow-up. Collaborative relationship between the physician and the diabetes education staff is essential for continuity of patient management.[18] Communication, through verbal and written reports, has to be maintained for documentation purposes.[6]

THE DIABETES EDUCATION TEAM

The composition of the diabetes education team varies from one institution to another depending on its size and financial resources. The team may be comprised of nurses, physicians, dietitians, psychologists, social workers, pharmacists, exercise physiologists, and other related disciplines. Coordinating patient education can be a problem in large, complex organizations.[16] The team approach provides the patient with expert perspective on different aspects of diabetes self-care management. For example, the dietitian provides expertise on diet therapy while an exercise physiologist provides an expert perspective on exercise and physical activities. However, like any situation where a variety of people provide patient education, consistency in message conveyed is an important issue to address.[19] Patients get confused if they hear different opinions from a variety of experts. Having a written curriculum and agreeing on the content to be delivered prior to conducting learning sessions can prevent this problem. Regular staff meetings are good channels to resolve conflicting opinions among staff.

In some instances where an institution may not have a significant budget for patient education, one person may be responsible for providing diabetes teaching. Many institutions would prefer to hire a certified diabetes educator. This person is credentialed by the National Certification Board for Diabetes Educators after fulfilling all the criteria for experience in diabetes teaching and mastery of specific body of knowledge in diabetes and adult teaching demonstrated by passing a written examination.[6]

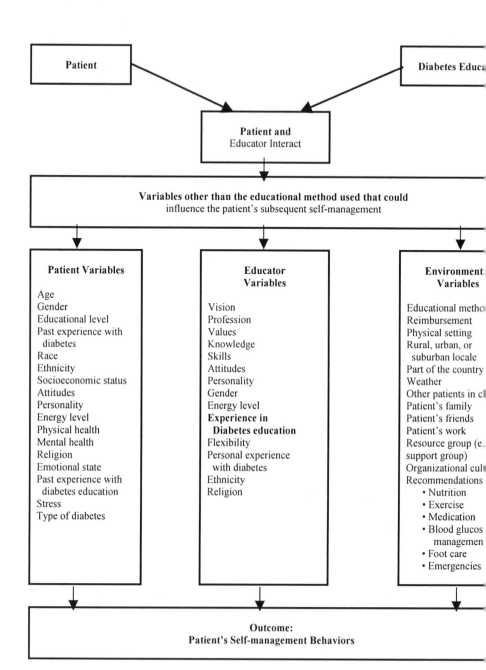

Figure 2. A model depicting the complexity of variables that can influence diabetes management. Reprinted with permission from Anderson B. Funnell M. The Art of Empowerment. Alexandria, VA, American Diabetes Association, p. 27, 2000.

ASSESSMENT OF LEARNING NEEDS

Because adult learners come to the educational experience with a variety of personal, family, and cultural factors there is not one standard for teaching content. Assessment of the individual needs is the first step to facilitate learning. Various factors (physical, psychological, social and cognitive) that may hinder learning should be assessed. (See Table 3 below) Having the diagnosis of diabetes poses an additional stressor to the learning situation.[20] Many may have learned bits and pieces about diabetes self-management over a period of time and experiences and they may be asked to unlearn some things. Furthermore, since learning encompasses more than knowledge acquisition, these patients are also asked to modify their behavior towards a healthier lifestyle.

Table 3. Barriers to Learning

Physical Barriers	Psychological Barriers	Social Barriers	Cognitive Barriers
• Pain • Blindness • Hard of hearing • Poor manual dexterity • Fatigue • Physical symptoms of hyperglycemia and hypoglycemia	• Fear • Denial • Anxiety • Depression • Lack of motivation • Dependency	• Lack of family support • Language barrier • Limited financial resources • Poor access to care • Beliefs and values	• Low literacy skills

The different factors that need to be considered in this assessment process are discussed below. This section only includes the assessment of the adult learner. For information about diabetes teaching in children and adolescents we refer the reader to the end of the chapter for a listing of resources.

Adult literacy

With increasing complexity of the health care system, the subject of health literacy has been the focus of much attention lately. Functional health literacy means the ability to read comprehend and use information to make decisions pertaining to health issues. To be considered health literate the person needs to be able to do tasks such as reading and understanding written health instructions, medicine labels, consent forms, and appointment schedules; understanding written and oral information from health care providers; and act on these information.[21]

The National Adult Literacy Survey estimated that about 44 million (21%) of adult Americans are functionally illiterate, and read at or below a

5th grade level. In addition 50 million or 25% are marginally illiterate.[21] In 1999 the Journal of American Medical Association reported that 46% of American adults are functionally illiterate in dealing with matters pertaining to their health. It is worse among the elderly and patients who perceive their health as being poor, the major consumers of the health care system.[22] The National Academy on an Aging Society reports that low literacy skills is responsible for an additional expenditure of about $73 billion dollars yearly.[23]

Health literacy is an issue in diabetes self management education.[24] The individual with diabetes needs to be able to understand and process the information, and then act on it. In a study of 2,659 low-income patients in an ambulatory center at two public hospitals, it was found that about 42% did not understand the instruction "to take medicine on empty stomach".[25] Diabetes instructions are far more complex than this. For example, when learning insulin dose adjustment according to fingersticks and carbohydrate intake, the individual has to be able to do the mechanical aspect of the task, understand the interaction between blood glucose, carbohydrate intake, physical activity, and insulin, and use this information in making a decision about dose adjustment. This is not a simple task for a patient with low literacy and instructions must be tailored to the individual.

Assessing functional health literacy is not very straightforward. Many adults would not volunteer information regarding their inability to read and write because of shame.[26] Unfortunately, the person's years of schooling do not always predict level of health literacy. Educational and literacy levels are important factors that influence learning. They determine how people learn and the amount of complexity they can tolerate in a learning situation.[27] Some learn best by listening versus reading, while others prefer viewing a video.

There are several methods for measuring literacy, but probably none is practical for use in clinical practice. Physical appearance is an unreliable indicator of literacy skills. Patient's ability to communicate does not measure literacy level. Many patients have average IQ and can be very articulate. Estimating patient's reading-level in a clinical setting is neither practical nor reliable since it does not necessarily translate to comprehension. Patients will attempt to conceal their inability to read and write through avoidance of the situation.[27] There are some red flags that should alert the physician to possible low literacy problem.

- Problem with eyesight: "I forgot my eyeglasses." "My eyes are tired, could you read this for me?"
- Lack of interest in reading instructions: "I'd let my wife read it first." "I don't need these papers. Just show me how."
- Unable to figure out written instructions: "Could you please tell me which one of these papers is for the eye doctor?" "Could you please mark the paper for the eye doctor?"

- Inability to tell you the name of their medicine: "I take one red pill and two white pills."
- Not taking their medications as prescribed. This may not be related to low literacy in many instances. However, inability to read medication labels should be ruled out when patients do not take their medications properly.
- Missing appointments. Again, this may not mean low literacy but a patient who misses many appointments may actually have difficulty reading and following written instructions given by the physician.
- Refuses to fill out forms: "It takes too much time." "I'll take it home and let my daughter do it."
- Underutilization of health care services. Many patients may have other reasons for doing this but those with low literacy almost always underutilize health care services.

Many patients with low literacy have developed coping mechanisms to deal with their learning disability. Many are able to learn diabetes self-management if taught at a level they can comprehend.[28] The physician should be sensitive to the patient's needs by asking questions to verify understanding of the verbal or written instructions. One should never assume that the patient understands. There are a variety of methods to evaluate learning initially and periodically in future visits. Methods used to decrease literacy demands and to evaluate learning are expanded upon below.

Psychosocial Factors

Fear, anxiety, denial, depression and other psychological states can interfere with readiness to learn. The physician and educator should be aware of these problems and refer the patient to the psychiatrist, psychologist, or social worker as appropriate. Social stressors such as lack of insurance, poor access to care, financial problems, housing issues and lack of social support may also interfere with learning and should be part of the routine assessment prior to the learning encounters (see chapter VIII.8).

Cultural Patterns

The prevalence of diabetes is highest among the ethnic minority populations such as African Americans, Hispanic Americans, and Native Americans.[29] Generally these groups also have a lower health status than the majority of the population.[30] The values, beliefs, rules of behavior, and lifestyle practices of the person guide their thinking and actions in particular ways.[31] Culture greatly influences the way the person makes decisions regarding health care. The physician should try to provide culturally-sensitive diabetes instruction to patients. When facilitating learning for a patient who belongs to a particular ethnic group, a cultural assessment needs to be done. This assessment is focused on elements relevant to the medical problem and interventions as well as the evaluation of the effectiveness of treatment.[31,32]

- What language does the patient speak?
- What role does the family play in patient's illness?
- What is the patient's status within the family structure? What are the patient's role/responsibilities/obligations within the family?
- Where does the patient live? With whom? Type of neighborhood (health care resources, environmental stressors)?
- Who does the patient go to for health advice or treatment of his diabetes?
- Does the patient use folk medicines? If so, what are they?
- What does the patient expect from diabetes treatment?
- What is the patient's perception about the health care system?
- Who makes decisions for patients in terms of health care?
- What values does the patient have regarding foods?
- What are the patient's religious or spiritual beliefs and values?
- What are the patient's routine daily activities?

Effective communication, both verbal and non-verbal, is the first step used to engaging the patient from a different culture in a meaningful interaction.[33] Awareness of the ethnic group's rules of conversation such as social introduction, demonstrating respect, and lack of hurried behavior is one of the key communication skills. Knowledge about when to choose a personalized or more detached mode of communication; when to select direct of indirect approaches; and when and how to use silence and touch is needed to interact with different ethnic groups.[32]

Whenever possible, the patient should be referred to an educator with knowledge and skills in dealing with the specific culture. This person has to be able to adapt communication and interaction patterns, make relevant cultural assessment and modify the diabetes education program to suit the patient's needs. Patient's cultural beliefs and values should be considered when facilitating the patient to learn diabetes self-management practices. A common mistake is do nutritional counseling without taking into consideration the patient's values about food, meal preparation, the type of ethnic food he or she eats, dietary patterns, and religious practices involving fasting or feasting.

Special Needs of the Elderly

Diabetes affects the elderly population at a high rate.[29] This group has special needs that have to be considered when providing diabetes self-management education. When assessing the needs of the elderly, one has to keep in mind that there are several factors that may affect their learning. These factors[34-37] are outlined in Table 4.

Table 4. Factors that may affect learning in the elderly include

- Sensory impairment: vision, hearing
- Psychomotor abilities (opening pill bottles, drawing up insulin, testing blood glucose)
- Co-existing medical conditions
- Memory and learning abilities
- Financial issues (fixed income)
- Family and social support
- Access to care (transportation)

In dealing with the elderly with diabetes, it is important not to make assumptions about the patient's mental competence and physical abilities based on age. These have to be assessed individually since the person can learn at any age.[12] Negative attitudes of the health care professionals toward the elderly can affect their behavior and management of diabetes. Stereotypes about the elderly may lead to withholding treatment choices and educational opportunities.

LEARNING STYLES

The individual's preference for teaching-learning experiences in diabetes self-management is a major consideration in planning the diabetes education sessions.[7] Sessions may be conducted in a group, individual settings or may even be self-directed. Learning styles vary from one person to another.[13] A combination of different modalities is frequently used to enhance the learning process. Learning styles may be didactic (lecture) or participatory (group discussion), or a combination of both. To present materials the educator may use a variety of media or techniques such as audio/visual materials, high tech interactive or non-interactive computer programs, Internet, games and simulations, case studies or vignettes, as appropriate.

The Internet is the fastest growing information medium with potentially great impact on health education.[38] The demographics of a typical Internet user are believed to closely resemble an average American.[39] It is estimated that approximately 19 million people use the Internet regularly for health and medical information.[40] As more people take greater initiative in their health care, many use the Internet to explore options and learn about new developments and research about diseases. Although research[38] suggests that there is a slightly greater interest in use of Internet in younger population it was also found that many older patients with diabetes without previous Internet experience are willing to take part in Internet-based self-management programs if barriers to participation are minimized.

There are a number of advantages of the Internet[38] as a medium of support in diabetes self-management education. It is accessible and can potentially reach a great majority of patients with diabetes. It is low cost compared to individual or small group classes. It provides flexibility since it can be done at home at any time as many times as desired. Many Internet sites provide information (some interactive), linkages with other related sites, and forum for people to interact with one another and share experiences. It is not a remote occurrence for a physician to have patients coming in to their office with printed materials about diabetes collected over the Internet. The role of the physicians and diabetes educators in such a situation is to provide the person seeking knowledge through the Worldwide Net the ability to sift through massive amount of information. A list of Internet sites providing diabetes health information is found at the end of this chapter.

Methods to decrease literacy demands

People who have low literacy skills are able to learn diabetes self-management skills. Teaching strategies need to be adjusted to enhance learning. The atmosphere has to be non-threatening for the patient. There are certain things to remember when dealing with patients with low literacy.

- Do not overload patient with information. Provide only the essential information the patient needs to do self-management.
- Make instructions brief and simple. Use simple layman words. Avoid medical terms.
- Introduce one concept at a time. Use common analogies to explain concepts. Provide examples to enhance explanation.
- Avoid distractions and interruptions as much as possible during the learning session.
- Introduce one change at a time. Make sure patient understands and is comfortable with the change before introducing another.
- Use a variety of media to present information. Enhance instructions with use of pictures, charts, models, audiovisual aids, etc.
- Remember to evaluate patient's understanding frequently. Encourage patient to ask questions or seek clarification as needed.

- Reinforce learning through use of drills, practice exercises, and experiential learning. Use patient's real-life problems to facilitate application of concepts learned.

EVALUATION

Paraphrasing is one the easiest methods to evaluate patient understanding.[41] The patient is asked to explain their understanding of the information. This method allows both the patient and the physician to have an interaction about the material taught. The patient is able to clarify the information as needed. The physician is able to assess any gaps in information or areas of misconceptions and provides immediate feedback.

Skills demonstration such as insulin injections, blood glucose monitoring, urine testing, etc. provides knowledge to the physician about the patient's use of the proper techniques. More importantly, the physician is made aware of the patient's psychomotor impairments that may interfere with the proper performance of the skill. For example, a patient with rheumatoid fingers may have difficulty in handling the syringe or the glucometer; a patient with poor eyesight may not be able to accurately draw up the proper dose of insulin. This would provide the opportunity for the physician to recommend some adaptations to ensure safety and accuracy or refer the patient to the educator for further counseling. There are a variety of adaptive devices available to help patient cope with their disabilities.

The physician should ask for frequent *feedback* from the patient to assess the latter's understanding of information. The patient is encouraged to ask questions to enhance their knowledge. The physician also asks questions to verify patient comprehension. Questions answerable by yes or no should be avoided. The examples include questions such as "Do you understand?" or "Do you know how to do this now?" Most patients would answer these questions affirmatively because they may be embarrassed to accept lack of understanding or they do not want "to bother" the busy physician. Examples of questions that yield more information about patient comprehension are: "Explain to me why..." or "Show me how..." Patients who do not know the answer to these questions would feel free to tell the physician to repeat the instruction or procedure if they do not understand.

Because learning diabetes self-management encompasses more than knowledge acquisition *evaluating behavior change* leading to a healthy lifestyle is the ultimate measure of success. There are several methods to measure behavior change. A direct measure is actually observing change in behavior such as self-monitoring of blood glucose, doing physical activities regularly, and consuming healthy diet. In some instances, the physician or the educator may have to rely on self-report, which decreases the reliability and validity of measurement. Indirectly, the effects of behavior change can be measured in terms of metabolic outcomes such as improvement in HbA1c, blood glucose, lipid levels, weight loss, etc.

PATIENT RESOURCES ON THE INTERNET

American Diabetes Association

http://www.diabetes.org

Offers information for medical providers and patients including news, nutrition and exercise guidelines.

Center for Current Research

http://www.lifestages.com/jea;tj/index.html

Offers summaries of recent medical research derived from articles from medical journals. Users may request information on unlisted topics for a fee.

Children with Diabetes

http://www.childrenwithdiabetes.com

Provides support and information for children and families affected by diabetes. Includes an up-to-date headlines related to clinical, nutritional and research reviews about juvenile diabetes. Provides links to news and patient advocacy sites.

Diabetes Action Research and Education Foundation

http://www.daref.org

Offers information about education and program services including a Native American program, an international program, public service, a diabetes camp for children, and a diabetes university program; and information about research projects and upcoming events. Includes a recipe and tip of the week and links to related sites.

Diabetes Digest

http://www.diabetesdigest.com

Provides general information for patients with diabetes such as overview of the disease, types of diabetes, symptoms, treatment, care, and prevalence. Includes information on oral medications, insulin, glucometers, and nutrition. Also includes an online newsletter and links to popular articles from Diabetes Digest.

Diabetes Knowledge

http://people.ne.mediaone.net/dclc/home.html

Offers advocacy information to parents of children with diabetes. Provides access to recent news articles and tips on applying the Individuals with Disability Education Act on behalf of their children. Includes links to product information sites and personal pages.

Diabetes News
http://www.diabetesnes.com
    Home page of the Diabetes News which offers information on new diabetes products and islet cell transplantation as well as reports on current research in related areas. Provides access to current and back issues of Diabetes Forecast, a Health and wellness magazine of the ADA.

Diabetes Research and Wellness Foundation
http://www.diabeteswellness.net
    Provides information on research grants and wellness programs sponsored by the foundation and information on how to develop self-management skills for people with diabetes. Includes articles on weight loss, aspirin, and exercise.

Diabetes Research Institute
http:///www.drinet.org/html/the_diabetes_research_institut.htm
    Provides patient articles on a variety of topics such as islet cell transplantation, encapsulation, genetic engineering, xenotransplantation, immuno genetics, molecular biology, research lipids and cardiovascular research. Also provides information about current clinical trials.

Diabetic Retinopathy Foundation
http://www.retinopathy.org/index.html
    Provides consumer information on how the eye functions, early and advanced stages of retinopathy, treatment, and prevention. Provides links to related sites of interests, including the Juvenile Diabetes Foundation and the American Academy of Ophthalmology.

Family's Guide to Diabetes
http://diabetes.cbyc.com
    This site is part of the Diabetes Web Ring that provides access to other sites in the chain. Includes information about insulin pumps, a chat room, and a bulletin board. Provides articles on symptoms, dietary management, and other Internet resources.

Hypoglycemia Association, Inc.
http://www.silver-bayou.com/hai/index.htm
    Offers information and support to patients about hypoglycemia, causes, diagnosis and treatment. Provides information on how to contact the association to receive a packet of materials with reference lists and useful information. Also provides links to related sites.

Joslin Diabetes Center
http://www.joslin.harvard.edu
    Offers news, information, education and programs for patients with diabetes. It also provides links to articles on diabetes, monitoring, insulin, oral medications, nutrition, exercise, and complications.

National Eye Institute: Diabetic Eye Disease
http://www.buh.gov/publications/diabeye.htm
Offers patients and consumers program materials on diabetic eye disease through brochures, fact sheets, public service announcements, and press releases

NIDDK: National Diabetes Clearinghouse: Diabetes diagnosis
http://www.niddk.nih.gov/health/diabetes/pubs/dignosis/diagnosis.htm
Provides an overview of diagnostic criteria for Type 1 and Type 2 diabetes mainly for consumers and patients. Also provides a link to the Combined Health Information Database (CHID) for additional resources.

NIDDK: Diabetic Neuropathy
http://wwww.niddk.nih.gov/health/diabetes/pubs/neuro/neuro.htm
Offers consumer information on diabetic neuropath including an overview of the condition, incidence, causes, symptoms, types, diagnosis, treatment, foot care, and experimental treatments. Also includes a list of organizations providing support and a suggested list of reading materials.

Exercise:

American Diabetes Association (ADA): Diabetes and Exercise
http://www.diabetes.org/DiabetesCare/Supplement/s30.htm
Discusses the position statement of the ADA in regards to exercise programs in type 1 and type 2 diabetes.

American Diabetes Association (ADA): Exercise: Just the FAQs
http://www.diabetes.org/exercise
Provides general information on the importance of exercise for people with diabetes. Includes a diabetes exercise quiz, fact sheets, and related Diabetes Forecast articles.

International Diabetic Athletes Association (IDAA)
http://www.diabetes-exercise.org
Provides support to patients with diabetes who participate in fitness activities. Offers membership details and information about regional chapters and support groups as well as product catalog and a calendar of upcoming events. Also provides a link to related sites.

Self Monitoring:

American Diabetes Association (ADA): Self-Monitoring of Blood Glucose
http://www.diabetes.org/diabetescare/Supplement/s62.htm

Contains a review of the ADA Consensus Conference on issues dealing with self-monitoring. Includes a review of the current technology and system limitations of various glucose monitors.

Diabetes Monitor: Devices for Glucose Monitoring
http://www.diabetesmonitor.com/other-3a.htm

Presents a wide variety of monitoring system and product Web sites. Provides connections to sites offering new noninvasive and minimally invasive glucometers as well as softwares for patients with diabetes to monitor blood readings and maintain overall control.

Medications:

Insulin Pumpers
http://www.insulin-pumpers.org

Provides support and educational materials on insulin pump therapy to patients with diabetes of all age groups. Provides answers to frequently asked questions about insulin pumps, instructions on how to use pumps, printable log sheets, a directory of physicians who prescribe pumps, and chat forums. Provides links to the home pages of several insulin pump manufacturers, information on carbohydrate content of various foods, and other information on diabetes and insulin pumps.

Medicines for People with Diabetes
http://www.niddk.nih.gov/health/diabetes/pubs/med/omdex.htm

Provides a list of diabetes medications and booklet of information on medicine for people with diabetes. Provides information on types of diabetes, treatments, low blood sugar, and help with recognizing whether or not prescribed medicines are working.

Ray Williams Institute of Paediatric Endocrinology: Devices for Insulin Delivery
http://www.rwi.nch.edu.au/apegbook/diabne33.htm#E9E33

Includes a concise review and illustrations of a variety of insulin delivery devices such as insulin syringes, insulin pen, automatic injectors, jet injectors and pumps.

UTHealth.com: Devices to Take Insulin
http://www.citihealth.com/layout.cfm?hc=O&Body=Articles/00003754

Describes currently available insulin administration devices, including pens, jet injectors, and external pumps. Also includes the delivery system under development such as implantable insulin pumps and the insulin patch. Presents the latest information from the Combined Health Information Database on alternative methods of insulin delivery.

Nutrition:

American Diabetes Association (ADA): Dietary Recommendations for Persons with Diabetes
http://www.hry.info.gifu-u.ac.jp/~diabetes/dietary/mtable2.html
Reviews the dietary recommendations from the ADA using a table format. Includes information on specific nutrients, sugar substitute, sodium, and alcohol.

American Dietetic Association
http://www.eatright.org
Provides patients with diabetes daily nutritional tips, a catalog of publications, a reading list, featured articles, nutrition fact sheets, and information on the food guide pyramid. Also includes a list of dietitian, information of government affairs, and links to related sites.

American Heart Association (AHA): Hyperlipidemia
http://www.americanheart.org/Heart_and_Stroke_A_Z_Guide/hyp.html
Offers a patient guide to hyperlipidemia and a discussion about the various types of this disorder. Includes a list of related AHA publications and access to online guides regarding specific syndromes, treatments and diets.

American Obesity Association (AOA)
http://www.obesity.org
Offers information about the mission of the organization, facts, statistics about obesity, health insurance and treatment of adult obesity, and contact details. Includes a discussion of health problems associated with obesity as well as an interactive Weight Wellness Profile.

Dietary Management of Diabetes Working Group
http://www.clininfo.health.nsw.gov.au/NSWhealth/NSWHEALTH1/nwgroup.htm
Presents a list of six principles of dietary and other lifestyle management strategies. Provides a link to additional useful resources for diabetic patients. Includes a discussion on the physiologic benefits of applying these principles, and practical advice for instituting each suggestion.

NIDDK: I Have diabetes: What Should I Eat?
http://www.niddk.nih.gov/health/diabetes/pubs/nutritn/what/index.htm
Offers nutritional guidelines and details on maintaining good eating habits. Contains a patient education pamphlet for newly diagnosed patients. Presents an overview of use of diet in controlling diabetes. Includes a section on food groups and food pyramids.

Support Group:

NIDDK: Financial Help for Diabetes Care
http://www.niddk.nih.gov/health/diabetes/summary/finanass/finanass.html
Provides information on financial help for diabetes care such as Medicaid programs, the Department of Veterans Affairs, the Hill-Burton Program, the Bureau of Primary Health Care, Health Care Financing Administration Office of Beneficiary Relations, and local public health departments.

Support-Group.com
http://www.support-group.com
Provides ample bulletin boards and online chat opportunities focusing on patient-support-related information on the Internet for over 200 disease categories. Provides access to consumer-oriented background information, organization links, FAQs, and government information sites.

REFERENCES

1. Anderson RM, Funnell MM. Theory is the cart, vision is the horse: reflections on research in diabetes patient education. The Diabetes Educ 25:43-51, 1999.
2. Funnel MM, Anderson RM. The art of empowerment: stories and strategies for diabetes educators. Alexandria, VA. American Diabetes Association, 2000.
3. Wagner EH. Chronic disease management: What will it take to improve care for chronic illness? Effect Clinical Practice 1:2-4, 1998.
4. Wagner EH, Austin B, Von Korff M. Improving outcomes in chronic illness. Manag Care Q 4:12-25, 1996.
5. Redman BK. The process of patient education. 7th ed. St. Louis, Mosby, 1993.
6. Mensing C, Boucher J, Cypress M et al. National Standards for Diabetes Self-Management Education. Diabetes Care 23:682-689, 2000.
7. Walker EA. Characteristics of the adult learner. The Diabetes Educ, 25:16-24, 1999.
8. Knowles M. The adult learner: A neglected species. 4th ed. Houston, TX, Gulf Publishing Co, 1990.
9. Knowles M. Self-Directed Learning. Chicago, Follett; 1975.
10. Tough A. How adults learn and change. The Diabetes Educ 11:21-25, 1985.
11. Brookfield SD. The skillful teacher: on techniques, trust, and responsiveness in the classroom. San Francisco, CA, Jossey-Bass, 1990.

12. Darkenwald GG, Merriam SB. Adult Education Foundation of Practice. NY, Harper Collins Publishing, Inc, 1982.

13. Brookfield SD. Understanding and facilitating adult learning: A comprehensive analysis of principles and effective practices. San Francisco, CA, Jossey-Bass, 1986.

14. Mezirow, J. Transformative Learning: A guide for educators of adults. San Francisco, CA, Jossey-Bass, 1991.

15. Peyrot M. Behavior change in diabetes education. The Diabetes Educ. 25:62-73, 1999.

16. Prospect Associates. Final Report: Survey of physician practice behaviors related to the treatment of people with diabetes mellitus (endocrinologists). Doc#NO1DK82233, NIDDK, NIH, 1991.

17. Walker EA, Wylie-Rosett J, Shamoon H. Health education for diabetes self-management. In Porte D, Sherwin R, Rifkin H. eds. Ellenberg and Rifkin's Diabetes Mellitus, 5th ed. Stanford, Conn, Appleton & Lange 1341-1351, 1997.

18. Anderson RM, Funnell MM. The role of the physician in patient education. Practical Diabetology 9:10-12, 1990.

19. Brown SA. Interventions to promote diabetes self-management: State of the Science, The Diabetes Educ, 26(6) (suppl), 52-61, 1999.

20. Walker EA. Health behavior: from paradox to paradigm. Diabetes Spectrum 14(1):6-8, 2001.

21. Kirsch,I, Jungeblut, A. Jenkins L., Kolstad, A. Adult Literacy in America: A first look at the findings of the National Adult Literacy Survey. Washington, D.C.: National Center for Education Statistics, US Department of Education, 1993.

22. American Medical Association. Health Literacy: Report of the Council on Scientific Affairs. JAMA 281(6):552-557, 1999.

23. National Academy on an Aging Society. Understanding health literacy: New estimates of the costs of inadequate health literacy. 1998.

24. Overland JE, Hoskins PL, McGill MJ, Yue DK: Low literacy: A problem in diabetes education. Diabetic Med 10:847-850, 1993.

25. Williams MV, Parker RM, Baker DW, et al. Inadequate functional health literacy among patients at 2 public hospitals. JAMA 274:1677-682, 1995.

26. Mendoza MA. A study to compare inner city black men and women completers and non-attenders of diabetes self-care classes. Doctoral Dissertation. Teachers College, Columbia University, 1999.

27. Stanley K. Low-literacy materials for diabetes nutrition education. Practical Diabetology 36-44, 1999.

28. Walker EA, Mendoza MA. the strength of many voices: a review of the johns hopkins guide to diabetes. Diabetes Spectrum 11:192-193, 1998.

29. American Diabetes Association. Diabetes 1995 Vital Statistics Alexandria, VA, Author, 1996.

30. United States Department of Health and Human Services. Secretary's Task Force on Black and Minority Health, Vol I-VIII. Washington, D.C., U.S. Government Printing Office, 1985-1986.
31. Leininger M. Leininger's Acculturation health care assessment tool for cultural patterns in traditional and nontraditional pathways. J Transcultural Nurs 2(2):40-42, 1991.
32. Tripp-Reimer T. Cultural assessment. in nursing assessment: a multidimensional approach. Bellack J, Bamford P, Eds. Monterey, CA, Wadsworth Health Services 226-246, 1984.
33. Tripp-Reimer T, Choi E, Kelley S, and Enslein, JC. cultural barriers to care: inverting the problem. Diabetes Spectrum 14(1):13-22, Winter 2001.
34. Glasgow RE, Toobert DJ, Hampson SE, Brown JE, Lewinsohn PM, Donnelly J. Improving self-care among older patients with type II diabetes: the "sixty-something..." study. Patient Educ and Counseling 19:16-24, 1992.
35. Smith DL. Patient education: tuning in to the needs of the elderly. Med Times 114:27-31, 1986.
36. Templeton CL. Nutrition education: the older adult with diabetes. Diabetes Educ 17:355-358, 1991.
37. White JR. The elderly patient with diabetes. Profile, Spring, 3-8, 1992.
38. Feil EG, Glasgow, RE, Boles S, McKay G. Who participates in internet-based self-management programs? A study among novice computer users in a primary care setting. The Diabetes Educ 26(5):806-811, 2000.
39. IntelliQuest, Worldwide Internet/Online Tracking Service (WWITS). 1998. Available at: http://www.intelliquest.com/.
40. Howe L. Patients on the Internet: a new force in healthcare community building. Medicine on the Net. November 1997. Available at: http://www.mednet-i.com.
41. Doak CC, Doak LG, Root J. Teaching patients with low literacy skills. 2nd ed. Philadelphia, Pennsylvania, JB Lippincott Co, 1996.

Chapter 3. Dietary Therapy of Diabetes Mellitus

Gladys Witt Strain

When a new diagnosis of diabetes is established, among the first stressful thoughts experienced by patients are concerns that they will not be able to eat foods they prefer and that their way of living will be compromised. Lifestyle, exercise habits and food preferences must be changed and individual choices will be limited. A patient newly diagnosed with diabetes fears that if certain changes do not occur, he or she will not be able to control blood sugar and he/she will be at risk for the host of complications associated with poorly controlled diabetes. However, the seldom publicized fact is that a person with diabetes should be eating basically similar to all other persons, according to the recommendations of the Dietary Guidelines for all Americans, 2000.[1] These guidelines do not impose a foreboding protocol, but advise how everyone should be eating to consume the nutrients required by the human body and to avoid the weight related illnesses.[2,3] "Healthy eating" and working toward an optimal life style is being encouraged. No longer should a "diabetic diet" or an American Diabetes Association diet (ADA diet) be prescribed by a physician. Rather, it is recommended that a diet prescription be based on careful assessment of food preferences, eating habits and other life style factors. This may require certain expertise that is often beyond the nutrition training of the medical practitioner and can also consume costly medical practice time.   In consultation with the patient, a registered dietitian can develop recommendations that are attainable and consistent with reasonable treatment goals.

A review of the recommended food pyramid emphasizes starches at the base, with vegetables, fruit and milk completing the groups of carbohydrate foods that effect blood sugar. The remainder of the pyramid, the fats and protein foods, meat, poultry, fish and eggs have little direct effect on blood sugar but are important sources of nutrients and calories that can modify weight status and thus the effectiveness of one's endogenouw insulin in helping glucose enter the cell. As mentioned above, the meal plans developed for persons with diabetes, are similar to the dietary guidelines recommended according to sex, age, and activity for the general population.[1]

A more specific Diabetes Food Guide Pyramid has been developed which moves the starchy vegetables out of the vegetable group and the beans and other legumes from the proteins into the starch group for purposes of dietary planning (Fig 1). The Food Pyramid makes it visually possible to see the number of servings of the various food groups recommended and the size of those servings. It should be noted that for purposes of planning the serving sizes have been adjusted so that the servings are relatively similar, between 80 and 100 calories for approximately 15 grams of carbohydrate. (The low calorie vegetables are an exception). This allows for more flexibility in food intake planning.

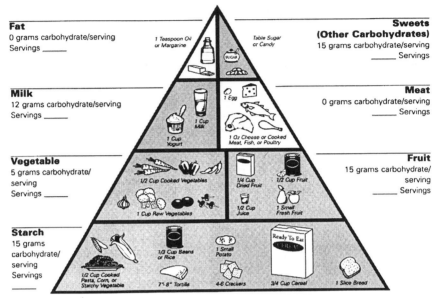

Figure 1. The Food Pyramid. Copyright © Eli Lilly & Company, All Rights Reserved. Reprinted with permission.

The general goal of nutrition intervention (Medical Nutrition Therapy, MNT) is to achieve and maintain near normal blood glucose levels. This is done by balancing carbohydrate intake with insulin administered or present in the body and/or with the use of other medications that modify blood glucose and/or exercise. Adequate calories should be provided to achieve and/or maintain a reasonable weight. This may not be the acceptable weight as defined by a Body Mass Index (Weight/ Height^2) of 18 to 25 (4). Rather, a reasonable weight may be that weight which may be achievable and can be maintained over the long term to provide glycemic control with the incorporation of a modified food and exercise program.

For the patient with type 1 diabetes who is dependent on exogenous insulin, the meal plan should respect the food preferences of the patient as much as possible and encourage a consistent timing of meals. Usually feedings of similar amounts of carbohydrate distributed throughout the day are planned and coordinated with the insulin administration and exercise program. The grams of carbohydrate at a feeding are frequently counted to assure a better distribution of the carbohydrate throughout the day. If blood sugars become unexpectedly high or low, reviewing the actual grams of carbohydrate consumed at the previous feeding may offer an explanation for the blood sugar aberration. When carbohydrate intake and/or the intensity and duration of exercise is modified, the patient must be taught to modify the type and/or dosage of insulin. Some patients prefer extra carbohydrate snacks to balance an increase in exercise rather than modify their medication dosage. As for all persons with diabetes, a reasonable body weight with normalized blood sugars is the treatment goal.

Another group of patients who are managed frequently with the insulin and carefully monitored blood sugar control are the patients who develop gestational diabetes (as discussed in Section V, Chapter 4). The careful regulation of carbohydrate intake and its distribution throughout the day in multiple feedings are the hallmarks of this treatment which seldom presents compliance problems for these well motivated patients. One recent study reports that infants had lower birth weights when their mothers were consuming less than 40% carbohydrate in their diets.[5] Daily caloric needs are generally adjusted in the second half of pregnancy for women of normal weight to 30-32 kcal per kilogram. For overweight women a moderate caloric restriction to 25 kcal per kilogram is advised.[6]

For most persons with type 2 diabetes the importance of caloric deficit in implementing weight change should be emphasized, since at least 80% of such patients are overweight.[7] For most, weight change is best accomplished with a combination of both diet and exercise. And if the control of caloric intake is not stressed in the treatment plan, little weight change generally results.[8,9] (Exercise for the person with diabetes is discussed in Section VIII, Chapter 4 of this volume.) Extreme strategies of starvation and very-low calorie diets seldom achieve longterm weight change.[10] A moderate caloric deficit of 500 calories will produce an average one pound a week decrease in weight; blood sugars generally normalize if the patient achieves a consistent caloric deficit. It is acknowledged that food records are inaccurate and generally under report food intake and over report energy expenditure.[11,12] To estimate energy needs, resting energy requirements (basal needs) can be calculated using a normogram developed by and available in the Mayo Clinic Diet Manual, 1994[13], or various equations including the generally accepted Harris and Benedict equations.[14]

For men: BEE = 66.4 +13.7 (W) + 5 (H) - 6.8 (A)
For women: BEE = 65.5 + 9.6 (W) + 1.8 (H) - 4.7(A)
BEE is basal energy, A is age in years, W is weight in kilograms and H is height in centimeters.

Using height, weight, age, and sex, basal needs can be approximated and modified by a factor for activity and the thermic effect of food [energy needed to process food intake, approximately 7%].[15] Usually total daily energy expenditure is approximately 40% above basal for light activity. After an assessment of the level of daily activity, a range of 30% to 50% above

531

basal is commonly used. From these estimations a potential energy intake can be calculated to achieve the desired rate of weight loss. This should be shared with the patient so the patient can better understand the amount of change necessary to produce the agreed upon energy deficit and diet modifications required to produce a modest weight loss and blood glucose normalization.

Even with all their inaccuracies, the food records do remain an integral part of the treatment protocol. They provide important qualitative information on the individual's *perception* of what they are consuming and their food preferences. In developing a food plan, such records are essential. However, if perfect 1200 calorie food intake records are provided by the weight stable 100 kilogram patient as representative, then basic problems with perception exist and must be explored.[16] It should be understood that such patients are not necessarily withholding or actually distorting what they consume. The interpretation of what constitutes a portion can vary greatly. Perhaps all the "between meal" eating could not be recorded. Others discount the calories from alcohol. For such patients foods of high volume and low energy value (low caloric density) can be particularly helpful.[17] The use of lower fat foods which are less energy dense is achieving more popular support, but the labels of such foods must be reviewed for one can not assume that all such foods are reduced in calories. Increased sugar may be added to help maintain the texture of lower fat products. This increase in carbohydrate certainly may not be helpful to the diabetic patient trying to control his blood glucose. For these reasons many of the foods labeled as reduced in fat or sugars must be carefully evaluated and may not be appropriate.

For most persons with type 2 diabetes a modest weight loss of 5-10% substantially improves glycemic control, but many patients are unwilling to accept such goals.[18] The 200 pound woman is not satisfied weighing 180 pounds and may persist in food restriction efforts until relapse and regain occur. Setting reasonable, maintainable goals in collaboration with the patient is an obligation of the health care provider. For some, blood glucose levels may normalize with moderate, consistent caloric deficit even before much weight loss occurs.[19]

However, for many overweight and obese persons weight loss has remained an elusive goal. Most overweight individuals will not be able to achieve and maintain the standard that has been set for normal body weight. Although a 10% weight change can substantially improve blood glucose control, for those unable to sustain energy restriction, polypharmacy including medications that help produce a caloric deficit may be tried. Currently the choices are limited to the two medications approved for long term usage. Sibutramine is a centrally acting norepinephine, dopamine, and serotonin reuptake inhibitor, and Orlistat acts in the gut to decrease fat absorption by inhibiting pancreatic lipase. These medications are generally used only as part of a comprehensive program including behavior modification, diet instruction and increased physical activity.[20] For those with diabetes and refractory obesity with a BMI over 35, surgery for weight loss is now a viable option.[21,22] Five year follow-up has impressively demonstrated the long term normalization of blood glucose achieved with an acceptable risk benefit ratio.[23,24]

It is of importance to note that type 2 diabetes may also occur and be diagnosed with a normal body mass index of 25 or below. When this occurs factors of body fat distribution, genetics, medications, physical activity, and diet composition (high carbohydrate and low fiber) may play an important role and should be evaluated.

Thus weight status, its modification and maintenance have an important role in diabetes management. It should be noted that treatment protocols to effectively sustain a reasonable body weight are acknowledged as time consuming, costly, and not frequently followed over the long term. However, the costs of the complications of poorly controlled diabetes far out-weigh the cost of the MNT intervention.[25-27] It is also of note that only a limited number of sufficiently trained persons are available to help with the implementation of needed weight change. Another obstacle that contributes to the problem is the frequent lack of third party reimbursement for nutrition services. The necessary changes in perception and behavior will most often not occur with only the handout of a diet sheet in the doctor's office.

The nutrition recommendations for all persons with diabetes have recently been reviewed by the American Diabetes Association and are discussed below.[28] In the past percentages of the macronutrients have been advised, but at the current time the actual amount is determined on the basis of the nutritional assessment and treatment goals. No specific percentage is provided for the amount of carbohydrate or fat. For the fat, no more than 10 % as saturated fat is advised. For proteins, 10-20 % provides a wide range. Again, this focuses the individual prescription on the nutrition assessment.

MACRONUTRIENTS

CARBOHYDRATE: Carbohydrate intake is the dietary focus of blood sugar control. Based on the individual's glucose needs, weight status, lipid profile, and eating habits, carbohydrate intake should be individualized. For years free sugars were banned in the diets of those with diabetes, probably because it was assumed that their quick absorption might contribute to elevated blood sugars. Starches were encouraged as substitutes. Scientific evidence is limited to support this common practice. A systematic approach to the amount a specific food increases blood sugar in comparison with a reference food was developed and called the glycemic index. Since many factors influence the effect of a food on blood sugar, eg. the amount of and types of fiber, rate of ingestion, processing, and cooking, the actual resultant response can be variable. Fruits and milk have been shown to have lower glycemic responses than most starches.[29] Sucrose produces a response similar to common starches like rice, potato, and bread.[30] Although various starches per gram of carbohydrate do have different effects on blood sugar, for purposes of dietary planning it is the total amount of carbohydrate consumed rather than the source that merits primary consideration. Because of the complex nature of the gylcemic response, the glycemic index is seldom used in meal planning. However, it may provide incite into an aberrant effect of a feeding on blood sugar. It should be mentioned that the effects of pizza and Chinese food on elevating blood sugars seem to far surpass the effects of their measured carbohydrate concentration.[31] The variation in responses to different carbohydrates stresses the importance of the patient performing self glucose monitoring to determine the quantities of specific foods that can be tolerated and maintain glycemic control. In dietary planning, the frequency and choice of using sucrose containing foods and/or concentrated sweets must be carefully weighed in the light of their low nutrient density and carbohydrate concentration. Making gram for gram carbohydrate substitutions will work, but frequently such substitutions become additions and then have a negative effect. Fruit is among the most maligned of the carbohydrates and sometimes patients are forbidden fruit even by diabetologists. With fruits, portion sizes and total grams of carbohydrate merit strict attention. For many fruits the defined portion sizes for 15 grams of carbohydrate are much smaller than generally consumed by most people. Again, it merits emphasis that the total amount of carbohydrate at a feeding is a central focus of the dietary plan.

Another dietary sugar, fructose, produces a smaller blood glucose increase than sucrose and has been proposed as a "natural" sweetener. The moderate consumption of fructose containing foods has presented no problem, but when fructose is consumed in large amounts, up to 20% of the calories, it is known to adversely effect blood lipids.[32] The sweeteners that have calories from carbohydrate like fruit juice concentrate, molasses, honey, and corn syrup have direct effects on blood sugar similar to sucrose and offer no advantage to persons with diabetes. Foods are also frequently flavored with the sugar alcohols: sorbitol, mannitol, and xylitol. The sugar alcohols have about one half the calories of table sugar and a reduced glycemic response. Individuals do have different sensitivities to the sugar alcohols, and they are known to have a laxative effect in many persons. Nonnutritive sweeteners are encouraged for people with diabetes to add increased variety to their food choices. One can not help but question if indeed, they have any effect on weight status. However, no adverse effects from using saccharin, aspartame, acesulfame K and sucralose have been demonstrated in humans for many years over a wide range of dosages.

FIBER: For years fiber has received much attention for its disease prevention effects in the general population. Recently the literature is replete with articles demonstrating improved blood glucose management in both type 1 and type 2 diabetes with high fiber diets.[33,34] Both soluble and insoluble fibers are encouraged in amounts similar to the recommendations for the general population (20-35 grams). However, it is the soluble vegetable fibers that are touted for their capacity to slow the absorption of food, inhibit glucose absorption and bind cholesterol.

PROTEIN: At the current time no data is available to indicate that the protein needs of persons with diabetes are different from the dietary reference intake (DRI) for the general population, 0.8 grams /kg of body weight. The American Diabetes Association suggests 10-20% of the total caloric intake from protein sources. Since nephropathy is one of the complications of diabetes (as discussed in Sectioin VII, Chapter 5), special attention may be given to the protein concentration of the diet. Data is available to indicate that with protein restriction the rate of fall inglomerular filtration rate (GFR) can be retarded.[35] However, other studies have contradictory results, possibly due to factors of patient selection and/or compliance with the protocol.[36] As kidney disease progresses further restriction to 0.6 grams/kg is sometimes advised in an attempt to further slow the decline in GFR. Recent research has focused on the type of protein and its effect on the kidney. Diets using soy protein have been shown to reduce hyperfiltration of the kidneys in diabetic individuals.[37] On this basis the substitution of vegetable proteins for animal protein has been suggested as a measure to help prevent the development and/or treatment of kidney disease.

FATS: As for all Americans, less than 10% of the total calories consumed should come from saturated fat. Recommendations on total fat must be left to a matter of individualization depending on weight, lipid status, and treatment goals. People who are at a healthy weight and have normal lipid levels are recommended by the American Diabetes Association to follow the National Cholesterol Education Program (NCEP) and slowly, over an extended time frame of two years, reduce their fat intake to <30%: saturated fat < 10%, polyunsaturated < 10% and monounsaturated <10-15%. If the LDL cholesterol is elevated, saturated fats may be reduced further to the 7% level. Less than 200mg of dietary cholesterol daily is recommended. Omega 3 fatty acids from fish and other seafood are encouraged 3 times per week. However, it must be emphasized that most type 2 diabetics are not at a healthy weight. If weight loss is to be implemented, then total fat reduction may be advised. Fats can easily be identified by patients and decreased to lower energy intake. Even in reduced fat diets the use of fatty fish is encouraged for the benefits of their omega 3 content. Monounsaturated fats like olive oil and canola oil, have been shown not to increase the LDL cholesterol and may improve glycemic control, and triglyceride and HDL-cholesterol levels. However, in type 2 diabetics efforts directed toward weight loss to decrease insulin resistance may be thwarted by these energy dense oils.

For many the texture and flavor of fat are important to eating satisfaction, but as a means of implementing weight loss and improving dyslipidemia, a decrease in total fat is suggested and specifically saturated fats are discouraged. This has resulted in the development of many calorie reduced, low fat and/or fat free products. Are such foods helpful in the achievement of weight loss and the improvement of blood glucose control? The use of foods reduced in fat or produced with a nonabsorbable fat substitute may or may not alter the composition and total calories of the diet. Alternative foods may be consumed in such quantities which can compensate for the changes in fat intake so that total energy is not reduced. To make possible the reduction of fat in certain foods, carbohydrate may be added but this could affect glycemic control. Fat free baked products are a common example of foods that may not be reduced in total calories since carbohydrate if often added. Therefore, the "sugar free" products may not be reduced in either fat or calories. Modified foods can be helpful to increase the variety of food choices, but patients with diabetes must be taught to use them wisely as an aid to calorie, fat, and carbohydrate control in order to foster compliance with their meal plans.

ALCOHOL: Alcohol is metabolized differently than the other macronutrients and for people with diabetes a few words of caution are important. The general recommendations from the Dietary Guidelines for Americans[1] advises two drinks per day for men and no more than one drink for women. It is of note that alcohol is not metabolized to glucose and can inhibit gluconeogenesis. If alcohol is not consumed with food and the patient is taking medication to lower blood glucose, hypoglycemia can result. Alcohol, if taken, should be taken with food. To make a caloric adjustment for alcohol intake, each beverage (12 oz beer, 5 oz wine or 1 ½ oz distilled spirits) is best equated to 2 fat exchanges from the diabetic meal plan. Alcohol is not advised for pregnant women, those with a history of alcohol abuse, and the elderly who may have problems with balance and incoordination. For people with diabetes and other medical problems like pancreatitis, elevated triglycerides, or neuropathy, the consumption of alcohol is discouraged. The use of alcohol is also contraindicated with certain medications, particularly metformin which is frequently prescribed for type 2 diabetes, since alcohol can increase the effects of metformin on lactate metabolism which increases the risk of lactic acidosis.

MICRONUTRIENTS: Vitamins and Minerals
As for the general population, persons with diabetes generally have no need for vitamin and mineral supplementation when the dietary intake is adequate. However, the assessment of an adequate dietary intake requires training and consumes professional time. Many physicians prescribe a pill containing the reference dietary intake (RDI) of the established vitamins as an insurance policy. With the increased risk for heart disease and its adverse outcome in

536

persons with diabetes, antioxidants are frequently prescribed. There is little evidence that this practice is beneficial.[38,39]

Of the minerals, calcium supplementation is frequently advised, particularly after menopause, since dietary calcium may not be sufficient, but as for all the other vitamins and minerals the recommendations are similar to those for the general population.

Chromium has been encouraged because of its positive metabolic role particularly in type 2 diabetes. However, its use remains a topic for research and the American Diabetes Association does not support its use as beneficial to glycemic control.[40] Most people with diabetes have not been found to be chromium deficient unless they have been receiving chromium deficient parenteral nutrition. Magnesium is acknowledged for its role in insulin resistance and its deficiency can contribute to carbohydrate intolerance, however only when low serum magnesium levels can be established is repletion with magnesium appropriate.. The use of diuretics may result in potassium loss that requires supplementation. Hyperkalemia may occur in patients taking angiotensin-converting enzyme (ACE) inhibitors, with renal insufficiency or hyporeninemic hypoaldosteronism.

Sodium is the mineral that receives much attention by both the medical profession and the general public. Dietary recommendations regarding sodium use precipitate frequent medical debate.[41] Recommendations for people with diabetes are no different than for the general population. While the average sodium intake in this country exceeds the 3,000 mg/day suggested by some health authorities, with hypertension 2,400 mg/day or with hypertension and nephropathy <2,000 mg/day is recommended.

IMPLEMENTATION

The above guidelines are simple and straightforward, but their implementation remains complex. Adhering to these guidelines is a challenge not only in diabetes management but for the population in general. From the government's continuing survey of food intake it is reported that approximately 1/3 of the population eat at least some food from all the food groups daily, but only 1-3% of the population eat the recommended number of servings from all the food groups on any given day.[42] If as a people we are all doing so poorly, can we expect those with diabetes to do that much better? Strategies to improve compliance with dietary protocols are under continuous development, however, as with the problem of producing a sustained weight change, patients revert to previous patterns over time and require long term monitoring. Third party payers remain reluctant to cover the needed extended duration of nutrition services.

To approach the development of a workable dietary strategy, first data must be gathered on the food intake pattern that produces the current level of control with a defined exercise program (or lack of it), and the medications prescribed for the management of blood glucose. Blood glucose monitoring is advised with the recording of food intake to identify problems even for those who are managing their diabetes with "diet" only. Many patients fail to identify any sources of carbohydrate other than the free sugars and starches as affecting blood sugars. To distribute carbohydrate throughout the day attention must also be paid to the milk products, fruits, and starchy vegetables that are consumed. If improved blood glucose control is the treatment focus, then the possible interchange of food groups with carbohydrate to increase variety and help enhance dietary compliance needs thorough review with the patient. This must be coordinated with the individual's blood sugar responsiveness to certain foods as ascertained from the food records and blood glucose data. This will help individually determine the portion sizes of certain foods possible to maintain more normalized blood glucose control. However, such expansion of personal knowledge alone may not result in long term dietary behavior change. Food choices are the result of a complex interplay of environment, social, familial, and behavioral factors. To modify food choices, the mediating variables that have been important in the development of food preferences must be changed. With an understanding of the usual eating habits and the factors that influence them, efforts to promote more "healthy eating" have a greater potential for being sustained. Designing dietary protocols to improve diabetes management and blood sugar control is, indeed, complicated. The nutritionist has little published literature to approach the problem. What should be eaten can be defined clearly and succinctly, as above, but motivating the patient sufficiently to activate such an eating plan is the challenge. Techniques incorporating cognitive behavioral principals in treatment protocols have shown promise, but remain in the testing phase as to their efficacy in promoting the needed long-term dietary changes.[43] Very little work has been done with changing preferences and effective prevention in the ethnic minorities who are so rapidly increasing not only in numbers but in their body size which in turn impacts upon their incidence of Type 2 diabetes.

SUMMARY

Exogenous insulin was the magic tool developed for the treatment of type 1 diabetes, but even with this tool, the dietary component of treatment for diabetes remains at the forefront of both effective intervention and the prevention of disease progression for all patients. Diabetes remains a dreaded disease for its feared restrictions on the total life of an individual and the modifications of lifestyle required for glycemic control and to prevent disease progression. It must be stressed that the foods recommended for a person with diabetes are those advised for all Americans to be in good health and to avoid the weight related illnesses. Food selections have been clearly defined in the consensus statement of the American Diabetes Association.

The challenge remains to assist patients to comply with these recommendations by modifying their food choices and their pernicious behaviors regarding food consumption and exercise.

Addendum

As this volume goes to press, an important contribution to the diabetes nutrition literature has been published: the position statement of the American Diabetes Association "Evidence-based nutrition principles and recommendations for the treatment and prevention of diabetes and related complications" (Diab Care 25:202-212, 2002). These recommendations are based on evidence reviewed in the same volume on pages 148-198. The needs of special populations (pregnant women, adolescents, children, the elderly, etc.) are discussed. The lack of adequate studies to support the use of vanadium and chromium is noted. A section has been added on the treatment of co-morbid conditions and acute complications. It is stated that structured programs emphasizing lifestyle changes, reduced fat and energy intake and regular physical activity have now been shown to reduce the risk for developing diabetes in randomized controlled trials. For those interested in nutrition therapy for persons with diabetes, this position statement is a must.

REFERENCES

1. U. S. Dept. of Agriculture, Dietary Guidelines for Americans, 5th edition, 2000. Home and Garden Bull. no. 232, Washington, DC. pp.1-39, 2000.
2. National Institutes of Health, National Heart, Lung, and Blood Institute. Clinical guidelines on the identification, evaluation, and treatment of overweight and obesity in adults—the evidence report. Obes Res 6 (suppl 2):71S-80S, 1998.
3. World Health Organization. Obesity: preventing and managing the global epidemic. Report of a WHO Consultation on Obesity, Geneva, pp 41-72, June 1997.
4. Willett WC, Dietz WH, Colditz GA. Primary care: guidelines for a healthy weight. NEJM 341: 427-434, 1999.
5. Major CA, Henry MJ, Veciana M, Morgan MA. The effects of carbohydrate restriction in patients with diet controlled gestational diabetes. Obstet Gynecol 91: 600-604, 1998.
6. Kjos SL, Buchanan TA. Gestational diabetes. N Engl J Med 341:1749-1756, 1999.
7. Kuczmarski RJ, Flegal KM, Campbell SM, Johnson CL. Increasing prevalence of overweight among US adults: National Health and Nutrition Examination Surveys 1960-1991. JAMA 272:205-11, 1994.

8. Katzel LI, Bleeker ER, Coleman EG, Rogus EM, Sorkin JD, Goldberg AP. Effects of weight loss vs aerobic exercise training on risk factors for coronary disease in healthy, obese, middle-aged and older men. A randomized controlled trial. JAMA 274:1915-1921, 1995

9. Gordon NF, Scott CB, Levine BD. Comparison of single versus multiple lifestyle interventions: are the antihypertensive effects of exercise training and diet-induced weight loss additive? Am J Cardiol 79:763-767, 1997.

10. National Task Force on the Prevention and Treatment of Obesity, NIH. Very low calorie diets. JAMA 967-974, 1993.

11. Lavienja AJ, Braam LA, Ocke MC, Bueon-de-Mesquita HB, Seidell JC. Determinants of obesity-related underreporting of energy intake. Am J Epidemiol 147:1081-1086, 1998.

12. Lichtman SW, Pisarska K, Berman ER, Prestone M, Dowling H, Offenbacher E, Weisal H, Heska S, Matthews DE, Heymsfield SB. Discrepancy between self-reported and actual caloric intake and exercise on obese subjects. New Engl J Med 327: 1893-1896, 1992.

13. Nelson JK, Moxness KE, Jensen MD, Gastineau CF. Mayo Clinic Diet Manual, 7th ed Mosby-Year Book Inc., St. Louis, Missouri, 1994; p.656.

14. Schofield WN, Schofield C, James WPT. Basal metabolic rate. Human Nutr:Clin Nutr 39c(Suppl 1): 1-96, 1985.

15. Ravussin E, Lillioja S, Anderson TE, et.al. Determinants of 24-hour energy expenditure in Man. J Clin Invest 78:1568-1586, 1986.

16. Strain GW. An approach to the diet perscription. Kunstner A, Futterweit W editors. Obesity and Weight Control. Columbia Univ. Press, NYC, New York (in press).

17. Bell EA, Rolls BJ. Energy density of foods affects energy intake across multiple levels of fat content in lean and obese women. Am J Clin Nutr 73: 1010-18, 2001.

18. Foster GD, Wadden TA, Vogt RA, Brewer G. What is a reasonable weight loss? Patients' expectations and evaluation of obesity treatment outcome. J Consult Clin Psychol 65:79-85, 1998.

19. National Institutes of Health: Heart, Lung, and Blood Institute. Clinical Guidelines on the Identification, Evaluation, and Treatment of Overweight and Obesity in Adults—The Evidence Based Report. Obes Res 6 (suppl 2): 110S, 1998.

20. National Institutes of Health, Heart, Lung, and Blood Institute. Clinical Guidelines on the Identification, Evaluation, and Treatment of Overweight and Obesity in Adults—The Evidence Based Report. Obes Res 6 (suppl 2): 100S, 1998.

21. MacLean LD, Rhode BM, Nohr CW. Late outcome of isolated gastric bypass. Ann of Surgery 231: 524-528, 2000.

22. Marceau P, Hould FS, Simard S et al. Biliopancreatic diversion with duodenal switch. World J Surgery 22: 947-954, 1998.

23. Brolin RE, Kenler HA, Gorman JH, Cody RP. Long-limb gastric bypass in the superobese, a prospective randomized study. Ann Surgery 215: 387-395, 1992.
24. Hall JC Watts JM, O'Brein PE et al. Gastric surgery for morbid obesity. The Adelaide Study. Ann Surg 211: 419-427, 1990.
25. Flechtner-Mors M, Ditschuneit HH, Johnson TD, Suchard MA, Adler Metabolic and weight loss effects of long-term dietary intervention in obese patients: four year results. Obes Res 8:399-402, 2000.
26. UK Prospective Diabetes Study Group: Intensive blood glucose control with sulphonylureas or insulin compared with conventional treatment and risk complications in patients with type 2 diabetes (UKPDS 33). Lancet 352: 837-853, 1998.
27. The Diabetes Control and Complications Trial Research Group. The effect of intensive treatment of diabetes on the development and progression of long-term complications in insulin-dependent diabetes mellitus. New Engl J Med 329: 977-86, 1993.
28. American Diabetes Assn. Nutrition recommendations and principles for people with diabetes mellitus. Diab Care 23 (Suppl 1): 543-552, 2000.
29. Hollenbeck CB, Coulston A, Donner C et.al. The effects of variation in percent of naturally occurring complex and simple carbohydrates on plasma glucose and insulin response in individuals with non-insulin-dependent diabetes mellitus. Diabetes 34: 151-155, 1985.
30. Jenkins DAJ, Wolever TMS, Jenkins AL et.al. The glycaemic response to carbohydrate foods. Lancet 2:388-391, 1984.
31. Nuttall FQ, Mooradian AD, DeMarais R, Parker S. The glycemic effect of different meals approximately isocaloric and similar in protein, carbohydrate, and fat content as calculated using the ADA exchange lists. Diabetes Care 6: 432-435, 1983.
32. Franz MJ, Horton ES, Bantle JP et. al. Nutrition principles for the management of diabetes and related complications (technical review). Diabetes Care 17: 490-518., 1994.
33. Giacco R, Parillo M, Rivellese AA, Lasorella G, Giaco A, D'Espiscopo L, Riccardi G. Long-term dietary treatment with increased amounts of fiber-rich low-glycemic index natural foods improves blood glucose control and reduces the number of hypoglycemic events in type 1 diabetic patients. Diab Care 23:1461-74, 2000.
34. Chandalia M, Garg A, Lutjohann D et al. Benefical effects of high fiber intake in patients with type 2 diabetes mellitus. N Engl J Med 342: 1392-98, 2000.
35. Ihle BU, Becker G J, Whitworth JA, et. al. The effect of protein restriction on the progression of renal insufficiency. N Engl J Med 321: 1773-7, 1989.

36. Levey AS, Adler A, Caggiula AW, England BK et al. Effects of dietary protein restriction on the progression of advanced renal disease in the Modification of Diet in Renal Disease Study. Am J Kidney Dis 27: 652-663, 1996.

37. American Diabetes Assn. Diabetic nephropathy (Position Statement). Diabetes Care 23 (Suppl):S69-S72, 2000.

38. Yusuf S, Dagenais G, Pogue J et al. Vitamin E supplementation and cardiovascular events in high risk patients. Heart Outcomes Prevention Evaluation Study Investigators. N Engl J Med 342: 154-160, 2000.

39. GISSI-Prevenione Investigators. Dietary supplementation with n-3 polyunsaturated fatty acids and vitamin E after myocardial infarction: results of the GSSI-Prevenzione trial. Lancet 354: 447-455, 1999.

40. Rendell MS, Kirchain WR. Pharmacotherapy of type 2 diabetes mellitus. Ann Pharmacother 34: 878-95, 2000.

41. Loria CM, Obarzanek E, Ernst N. Choose and prepare foods with less salt: dietary advice for all Americans. J Nutr 131: 536S-551S, 2001.

42. Dixon LB, Cronin FJ, Krebs-Smith SM. Let the pyramid guide your food choices: capturing the total diet concept. J Nutr 313: 461S-472S, 2001.

43. Beck JS. Cognitive Therapy: Basics and Beyond. New York, NY, Guilford Press, 1995.

WEB SITES FOR ADDITIONAL INFORMATION

National Diabetes Education Program
hhtp://ndep.nih.gov

National Institute of Diabetes and Digestive Diseases
www.niddk.nih.gov

Food and Nutrition Information
www.fns.usda.gov/fns

American Diabetes Assn.
http://www.diabetes.org

American Dietetic Assn
hhtp://www.eatright.org

Center for Nutriton Policy and Promotion
www.usda.gov/cnpp

Chapter 4. Exercise in the Therapy of Diabetes Mellitus

Stephen H. Schneider and Rajiv Bhambri

INTRODUCTION

Exercise has been advocated for patients with diabetes for many years but it was only little over a decade ago that the American Diabetes Association felt there was enough evidence of benefit to recommend exercise as a routine part of the treatment of type 2 diabetes mellitus. Our understanding of the complex interactions of exercise with diabetes is still incomplete and the most effective ways to use exercise in the treatment of the disease are still under investigation. During exercise major cardiorespiratory and circulatory responses occur to efficiently supply the increased oxygen and energy needs of the working muscles. Whole body oxygen consumption and glucose turnover may increase more than ten fold and even greater increases may occur in the skeletal muscles.[1] In healthy individuals, a complex hierarchy of hormonal responses regulates the needed alterations in fuel metabolism necessary to maintain normal plasma glucose levels during prolonged activity.[2] This metabolic response to exercise may be severely disordered in patients with diabetes mellitus. In order to understand the effects of diabetes on fuel metabolism during exercise, it is important to first review the normal physiology.

As exercise intensity increases there is a linear relationship between heart rate, oxygen consumption, and workload. Eventually, however, oxygen consumption plateaus in the face of increasing exercise intensity. The point at which oxygen uptake plateaus is known as the maximal aerobic exercise capacity or VO2max. Supra maximal exercise, which can be carried on only for a short time above the VO2max, represents non-aerobic metabolism. The VO2max is important for a number of reasons. It is a useful tool to express the degree of aerobic fitness of an individual. In general, a higher VO2max predicts better performance in endurance type activity. It is also of value in comparing individuals of widely varying fitness levels. At the same percentage of any individuals VO2max, a roughly similar metabolic response will occur. In addition, the VO2max has been useful in generating recommendations for exercise in various groups of individuals. Because the VO2max is rarely directly measured in individual patients, indirect techniques for estimating workloads as a percent of the VO2max have been developed and are discussed later in the chapter. Most of these are based on the linear relationship between heart rate and oxygen consumption throughout mild to moderate degrees of activity.

METABOLIC CHANGES DURING EXERCISE IN NORMAL INDIVIDUALS

Moderate Intensity Exercise (50-75% VO2max)

In the initial stages of exercise muscle glycogen is the chief source of energy.[3] With continued exercise and depletion of muscle glycogen, the working muscles must take up glucose and non-esterified fatty acids (NEFA) from the circulation.[4] Recent evidence suggests that utilization of local triglyceride stores in skeletal muscle may also be an important source of free fatty acid for oxidation during physical activity. In the post-prandial state glucose is derived from an increased hepatic production that closely matches peripheral glucose utilization and which can maintain euglycemia during moderate intensity exercise for long periods of time. However, during prolonged exercise glucose utilization may exceed splanchnic glucose output and hypoglycemia may develop.

The role of neuro-hormonal adaptation during exercise is twofold:

(a) to supply the exercising muscles with their increased fuel and oxygen requirements and,

(b) to maintain whole body glucose homeostasis to supply the brain with adequate substrate. It is not clear what triggers the endocrine response to exercise; it may result from the stimulation of afferent nerves from the working muscles or from subtle deviations in the blood glucose and/or from feed forward mechanisms originating within the hypothalamus.[5] At the start of exercise, a fall in the circulating insulin levels occurs due to an increased alpha adrenergic input to the beta cells.[6] This physiologic decrease in insulin levels promotes peripheral lipolysis and removes the inhibiting effects of insulin on hepatic glycogenolysis and gluconeogenesis. As exercise continues an increase in the level of the counterregulatory hormone glucagon facilitates liver glycogenolysis and later gluconeogenesis, further enhancing hepatic glucose output.[4]

With more prolonged exercise insulin secretion continues to fall and there is a further release of counterregulatory hormones. A rise in catecholamines and falling insulin levels lead to an increase in blood NEFA levels[7] due to both increased lipolysis and decreased NEFA re-esterification in the liver. The liver utilizes the glycerol released during triglyceride breakdown as a substrate for gluconeogenesis and the NEFA are delivered to the working muscles as an energy source. The increased availability of NEFA for muscle metabolism helps restrain the rate of muscle glucose utilization and therefore to limit the fall in glucose during prolonged exercise. In fact, the major role of catecholamines during prolonged exercise is to stimulate lipolysis. Their main impact on hepatic gluconeogenesis is probably via the mobilization of gluconeogenic precursors from peripheral sites.[8] Catecholamines also stimulate glycogenolysis in inactive muscles in the later stages of prolonged exercise.[9] In this situation the glycogen is metabolized to lactate in nonexercising muscle

544

which can then be delivered to exercising muscle where it can be oxidized as fuel and to the liver for gluconeogenesis. This complex and redundant series of hormonal responses regulates blood glucose during exercise with remarkable efficiency and the redundancy of the system insures that glucose homeostasis is robust.

High Intensity Exercise (> 85% VO2max)

During very high intensity exercise the relationship between peripheral glucose utilization and hepatic glucose production may be reversed. Because virtually all of the fuel for high intensity activity is provided by local energy stores of glycogen and to a lesser extent fat, hepatic glucose production often significantly exceeds peripheral glucose utilization leading to hyperglycemia that persists into the post exercise state. The added glucose production most likely originates from hepatic glycogenolysis[5] and epinephrine may be involved in this regulation.[10] There may also be a brief period of relative insulin resistance following very intensive exercise. This transient hyperglycemia is self-correcting and can occur in normal as well as diabetic individuals.

MUSCLE GLUCOSE UPTAKE DURING EXERCISE

The increased muscle glucose uptake during exercise is related to the intensity and not the duration of the exercise once a steady state has been achieved.[5] In general, the greater the exercise intensity the greater the relative utilization of carbohydrate as an energy source. For example, at exercise of roughly 50 percent of an individual's VO2max, half of the energy requirement is supplied by carbohydrate while 80 percent of energy requirements may be supplied by carbohydrate at exercise approaching 80 percent of the VO2max. Since plasma insulin levels fall during exercise, the increased muscle glucose uptake must be mediated by insulin-independent mechanisms or via an increased insulin action on muscle. Exercise probably acts in both ways[5] but the insulin-independent mechanism predominates. During exercise there is an insulin-independent increase in the concentration of the main glucose transporter protein GLUT 4 on the muscle membrane.[11] This is thought to be due to the translocation of the GLUT 4 from the cytoplasm to the sarcolemma.[12] This increase in the number of GLUT 4 on the surface of the cell leads to an increase in the glucose uptake from the circulation into the muscle cell. In addition to changes within the muscle an increased delivery of insulin and glucose to working muscle as a result of enhanced muscle perfusion during exercise is an important determinant of glucose uptake.

POST EXERCISE STATE

In the post exercise period the hormone levels return to basal and glycogen stores are repleted. If exercise is of sufficient intensity and duration to deplete muscle glycogen and adequate carbohydrate is made available, levels of glycogen will rebound to well above pre-exercise levels, a phenomenon called supercompensation. Of great therapeutic importance is the observation that muscle insulin sensitivity is enhanced for prolonged periods of time following a single bout of moderately intense activity. Typically insulin sensitivity is enhanced for 12-24 hours but after sufficient exercise alterations lasting up to 72 hours have been noted. This results in a sustained improvement of insulin sensitivity in individuals who exercise every other day or more. The mechanisms by which exercise results in these sustained benefits are unclear. A relationship to muscle glycogen levels is suggested by the observation that exercise of intensity and duration sufficient for glycogen depletion is required for this effect to occur. In addition, athletes who take in large amounts of glucose following exercise and supercompensate glycogen levels above basal have been reported to have impaired insulin sensitivity. On the other hand, the increase in insulin sensitivity that follows exercise clearly persists at a time when glycogen stores have returned to normal. More recently attention has turned to the enzyme AMP-dependent protein kinase. This enzyme is activated during exercise of the intensity required to lead to improved post exercise glucose uptake. In addition to shifting fuel utilization acutely towards the oxidation of FFA it may also stimulate subsequent glucose utilization by mechanisms independent of insulin action, possibly involving the nitrous oxide system.

ADAPTATIONS TO PHYSICAL TRAINING

Exercise performed on a regular basis with an intensity, duration and frequency sufficient to improve cardiorespiratory fitness, strength, and flexibility is called physical training. Alterations in cardiac and respiratory efficiency and in the neurologic coordination of motor activity are an important factor in improved performance. In addition, there are important cellular adaptations of skeletal muscles with physical training (Table 1).

Table 1: Adaptations to aerobic training

- increase in number of muscle capillaries
- increased muscle perfusion
- increase in size, number and metabolic capacity of mitochondria
- increased availability of muscle glucose transporter GLUT 4
- increase in activity of enzymes hexokinase and glycogen synthase
- transformation of the glycolytic type IIb muscle fibers to type IIa fibers
  with a greater oxidative capacity

This response differs when physical training is primarily aerobic, i.e. low to moderate intensity versus resistance training. The changes associated with aerobic training include:

(a) An increase of the oxidative capacity of the type I slow twitch fibers as well as a change in the type II fast twitch fibers towards the so called type IIa fiber type with a greater oxidative capacity.[13]

(b) an increase in the number of capillaries around muscle fibers[14] which allows for more efficient exchange of nutrients and waste products.

(c) an increase in the size, number and metabolic activity of mitochondria[14a] with a greater capacity for ATP production and oxidative phosphorylation.

(d) an increase in the number of GLUT 4 available for translocation to the cell surface.[15]

(e) an increase in the activity of the enzymes hexokinase and glycogen synthase with an improved capacity for increased glucose uptake, glucose phosphorylation and storage respectively.

These changes occur with little or no muscle hypertrophy and are most obvious in the type 1 and type 2a oxidative fibers.

The adaptive response to resistance training results predominantly in the hypertrophy of type 2b fast twitch fibers with minimal changes in oxidative capacity or vascularization. Much of the early improvement in strength during resistance training is related to more efficient neurologic regulation of fiber recruitment within the muscle.

These changes in muscle function along with the cardiorespiratory and circulatory adaptations to physical training lead to a more efficient use of energy and improvements in aerobic endurance. There is no evidence that the adaptations to exercise in patients with diabetes differ substantially from those of normal individuals.

EXERCISE CAPACITY OF PATIENTS WITH DIABETES

Patients with type 1 diabetes appear to have a normal exercise capacity when metabolic derangements are well controlled. In chronically underinsulinized patients, an inability to store glycogen and a tendency to dehydration can result in poor endurance capacity. In patients with autonomic dysfunction the cardiovascular response to exercise can be further impaired. The situation in patients with type 2 diabetes is more complex. A number of studies suggest that these patients may have a mild impairment of aerobic exercise capacity. Many studies show a VO2max roughly 15% lower than controls with apparently similar levels of physical activity. Interestingly, preliminary studies suggest this difference may be present prior to the onset of overt disease and even in first degree relatives. This is associated with a relatively high percentage of fast twitch fibers, which are less insulin sensitive as well as a decrease in mitochondrial and capillary density. Nevertheless, the relative ability of these patients to improve aerobic exercise capacity during physical training appears to be normal. There is no evidence that resistance training elicits a unique response in patients with diabetes.

FUEL METABOLISM DURING EXERCISE IN PATIENTS WITH DIABETES

Type 1 Diabetes

A number of factors influence the metabolic response to exercise in patients with type 1 diabetes mellitus. These include the adequacy of insulinization, metabolic control, presence or absence of complications, exercise intensity, duration and type and recent food intake.[1] The ability of the body to maintain glucose levels in the face of intense exercise is remarkable. In trained athletes moderate activity of many hours duration may be associated with minimal changes in plasma glucose. Nevertheless , inadequate regulation of plasma glucose levels is common in patients with type 1 diabetes. Similar problems often occur in patients with long-standing type 2 diabetes mellitus who have reached a point of absolute insulin deficiency and are dependent upon exogenous insulin.

One of the major reasons for the sometimes disappointing results of exercise as a means of improving glucose control in type 1 diabetes is hypoglycemia. Hypoglycemia is common in patients with type 1 diabetes during exercise and may require increased carbohydrate intake and a decreased insulin dose which limits potential improvements in glucose control. While the various causes of hypoglycemia during exercise in patients with type 1 diabetes are not always clear there are a number of factors which contribute (Table 2):

(a) Overinsulinization: Exercise is normally associated with a fall in circulating insulin. Subcutaneously injected insulin prior to exercise cannot be shut off and this can lead to a state of relative hyperinsulinemia in patients with type 1 diabetes. Therefore a dose of insulin appropriate at rest may be excessive during exercise. Also, if insulin is injected directly over the exercising muscle its absorption can be accelerated.[16,17] This effect is important for short acting insulins and when exercise occurs within 1 - 2 hours after injection. The absorption of insulin is increased even further if the insulin is injected accidentally directly into the exercising muscle. If the insulin depot is rapidly depleted this can actually result in insulin deficiency later in the day and contribute to hyperglycemia and erratic glucose control.

(b) Impaired counterregulatory response: Patients with type 1 diabetes and relatively long-standing diabetes (> 5 years) may have a blunted glucagon and epinephrine response to hypoglycemia.[18] This may occur in the absence of overt autonomic neuropathy. When combined with the lack of physiological insulin suppression this may be an important contributor to hypoglycemia during exercise.

(c) Increased insulin sensitivity: Hypoglycemia can occur not only during exercise but also many hours after the cessation of exercise. This is because of the exercise-induced increase in insulin action that can persist for hours.[19,20] Post exercise hypoglycemia can occur as long as 6-10 hr following a brisk exercise bout. Such clinically important episodes can be severe and if exercise is performed in the evening, hypoglycemia may occur in the early morning hours while the patient is asleep.

(d) Drugs: Beta-adrenergic blockers may aggravate insulin-induced hypoglycemia. However, because of the redundancy of the hormonal system regulating plasma glucose this problem is generally confined to patients who already have an impaired glucagon response. This is especially true for patients with long standing type 1 diabetes where glucagon secretion is often impaired, but is less common in the larger group of patients with type 2 diabetes.[21] Ethanol, by inhibiting gluconeogenesis, decreasing hepatic glycogen stores and decreasing calorie intake may also predispose the patient with type 1 diabetes to exercise induced hypoglycemia.

Table 2. Contributing Factors Towards Exercise Related Hypoglycemia In Insulin Treated Patients

1. Lack of physiologic suppression of plasma insulin levels
2. Enhanced absorption of insulin injected over exercising muscle
3. Impaired counter regulatory responses of glucagon and epinephrine
4. Increased insulin sensitivity

In contrast to the more common hypoglycemia, some patients in poor metabolic control as a result of absolute insulin deficiency may experience a paradoxical rise in blood glucose with exercise. These patients are insulin deficient, hyperglycemic (fasting blood glucose > 300mg/dl), often ketotic and mildly dehydrated. When these type 1 diabetic patients exercise there is an increase in plasma glucose and ketones.[22,23] This is probably because the insulin deficiency and associated excess of counterregulatory hormones cause an increased hepatic glucose and ketone body production that exceeds peripheral glucose utilization. For practical purposes patients with a fasting blood glucose of > 300 mg/dl or who have evidence of ketones are at risk for paradoxical hyperglycemia. In these patients adequate insulinization needs to be achieved before exercise can exert beneficial effects. Another situation where significant hyperglycemia may occur in patients with type 1 diabetes is following very high intensity exercise.[24] This is usually transient and results from brisk hepatic glycogenolysis at a time when peripheral tissues are using primarily stored glycogen as an energy source. Unlike in healthy individuals, the hyperglycemia may be prolonged in patients with type 1 diabetes because increased endogenous insulin fails to compensate (vide supra).

Type 2 Diabetes
The metabolic response to exercise in most patients with type 2 diabetes is similar to healthy individuals and as noted above it will be modified by a number of factors including drug therapy and exercise intensity.

Patients with type 2 diabetes mellitus have a relatively low incidence of exercise-induced hypoglycemia. This is probably related to intact glucagon and epinephrine responses. However hypoglycemia can occur in patients with type 2 diabetes treated with insulin or insulin secretagogues.

BENEFITS OF EXERCISE TRAINING

The potential benefits of regular physical activity in patients with diabetes include improvements in insulin sensitivity and glycemic control, reduction in cardiovascular risk, improvements in blood pressure, lipid profile and coagulation factors and weight loss[25,26] (Table 3).

Table 3. Benefits of regular exercise in diabetes

- improved insulin sensitivity
- improved glycemic control in type 2 diabetes
- decreased triglycerides
- decreased numbers of small, dense LDL cholesterol particles
- increased HDL cholesterol (with intensive exercise regimens)
- decreased in blood pressure
- increased fibrinolytic activity
- weight loss
- reduced cardiovascular risk
- positive behavior modification
- improved self-esteem and sense of well-being

Insulin Sensitivity
A number of studies have shown an improvement in glucose tolerance following a single exercise bout in normal individuals and patients with patients with type 1 and 2 diabetes.[27,28,29,30] A single episode of exercise in patients with type 2 diabetes can typically improve insulin sensitivity at the liver and muscle up to 16 hours.[31] Individuals undergoing long term physical training regimens with an exercise frequency of three or more sessions per week have improved

insulin stimulated muscle glucose uptake and glucose tolerance and decreased insulin levels.[31,32,33,34] In most studies it is not clear to what extent these improvements are due to the summed effects of acute exercise bouts vs. the trained state per se. In one study after 6 months of physical training insulin sensitivity dramatically improved 12 hours after the last exercise bout but had returned to baseline within a week suggesting that acute exercise effects may predominate.[35] Certainly, more prolonged improvements in metabolic control could result indirectly by changes in body composition that occur during physical training such as decreased visceral fat and increased muscle mass. The mechanisms underlying possible beneficial effects of the trained state include:

(a) Increased insulin-stimulated glucose disposal owing to increased skeletal muscle blood flow.[34]

(b) An increase in insulin-responsive GLUT 4 glucose transporter availability in skeletal muscle with physical training.[12]

(c) An increased activity of mitochondrial enzymes involved in oxidation and storage of glucose in skeletal muscle.

(d) An increased conversion of type IIb to type IIa muscle fibers. Type IIa fibers have higher concentration of glucose transporters, greater capillary density and are more insulin responsive.

(e) Reduced intramuscular triglyceride stores: Intramuscular triglyceride stores have been associated with muscle insulin resistance.[36]

(f) a decrease in intra-abdominal fat stores

(g) An increase in muscle mass during programs of resistance training, which may partially counteract insulin insensitivity through the availability of an increased glucose storage space.[37]

Exercise and Glycemic Control
Type 2 Diabetes

There is substantial evidence that exercise training improves insulin sensitivity and decreases the elevated blood sugars in patients with type 2 diabetes mellitus. Exercise programs performed at 50-70 % $VO_{2\,max}$, for 30-40 minutes, 3-4 times per week consistently show about a 10-20% drop in the HgbA1c from baseline. Long-term studies have shown a sustained effect over as long as 5 years of regular exercise.[38,39] The maximum benefit is seen in patients with impaired glucose tolerance, mild type 2 diabetes and those that are the most insulin resistant.[31,40] This is consistent with the effect of exercise training in improving insulin sensitivity. While the summed effects of individual exercise bouts are clearly a major contributor to improve overall blood glucose control other factors, such as changes in body composition, decreased visceral fat, and other behavioral changes promoted by regular physical activity should not be underestimated.

Type 1 Diabetes

The beneficial effect of exercise on glycemic control in type 1 diabetic patients is less clear. Despite improvements in insulin sensitivity with decreased exogenous insulin requirements[41], studies showing improved glucose control with regular exercise in large patient populations are lacking. One study noted a mild initial improvement in glucose control in 25 type 1 diabetics trained for >3 months that was lost by the third month of observation despite continued adherence to the exercise regimen.[42] The relatively high incidence of hypoglycemia during exercise in type 1 diabetic patients with resultant increased carbohydrate intake and decreased insulin dose probably offset the benefit of the enhanced glucose disposal. Nevertheless, some patients with type 1 diabetes can achieve improved glucose control with exercise although intensive self monitoring and a predictable training regimen are usually required. More importantly, potential beneficial effects of physical training on body composition, psychological state, and cardiovascular risk factors can often be achieved along with a decrease in insulin requirements even in the absence of improvements in HgbA1C. On the other hand, there is no evidence that regular exercise in patients with type 1 diabetes in good metabolic control will lead to worsening of their glucose control. Hence exercise should not be discouraged but instead promoted in these patients.

Exercise and Dyslipidemia

Type 2 diabetes is associated with a characteristic dyslipidemia related to an increased risk of premature atherosclerosis. Most often this consists of hypertriglyceridemia, low levels of HDL cholesterol, and normal or only slightly elevated levels of LDL cholesterol. Additional changes in the composition of LDL cholesterol may also contribute to increased atherogenesis. The mechanisms by which exercise affects lipid metabolism are complex but activation of lipoprotein lipase, changes in hepatic lipase activity, altered caloric balance and changes in body composition and fat distribution may contribute.

Studies have shown that the most consistent effect of exercise training is a reduction in the plasma triglyceride levels, which fall up to 30% from baseline.[43,44,45] Some of the decrease in triglycerides seen with exercise may be transient and related to individual exercise bouts mirroring the effects of exercise on carbohydrate metabolism.[42]

Changes in LDL cholesterol with regular exercise have been less consistently demonstrated. There may be a decrease in the concentration of the small dense LDL particles, which are thought to be more atherogenic.[46] These effects are more pronounced in the patients who are more insulin resistant and have higher initial triglyceride levels. Many studies have not shown an increase in the HDL cholesterol with exercise even when the plasma triglyceride levels decrease. This is probably due to the moderate intensity of the exercise regimens in the studies. In nondiabetic individuals, HDL cholesterol increases are seen only with high intensity exercise performed over a long period of time; many patients with type 2 diabetes are unable or unwilling to exercise to this intensity.

Patients with type 1 diabetes often have a lipid profile very different from their counterparts with type 2 disease. When in good metabolic control HDL-Cholesterol levels may actually be elevated and major abnormalities of cholesterol and triglyceride measurements are unimpressive. Nevertheless, a very high incidence of premature CAD is found in these patents. Regular exercise has a favorable effect on the lipid profile in patients with type 1 diabetes similar to non-diabetic individuals.[5]

Exercise and Hypertension

Hypertension has been associated with the insulin resistance syndrome in patients with impaired glucose tolerance and type 2 diabetes. In trained subjects, both the resting pressure and the blood pressure response to exercise are reduced. Regular exercise in patients with type 2 diabetes may help improve hypertension especially in insulin resistant/ hyperinsulinemic patients.[42,44,47,48] Typically decreases of 5-10 mm Hg of both systolic and diastolic pressure are found with exercise training in subgroups of patients with the insulin resistance syndrome.

Exercise and Fibrinolysis

Many patients with type 2 diabetes have an impaired fibrinolytic system with increased levels of plasminogen activator inhibitor-1 (PAI-1), which is the major inhibitor of tissue plasminogen activator. An acute exercise bout activates the fibrinolytic system and there is an association of aerobic fitness with enhanced fibrinolytic activity. Some of this effect may be mediated indirectly through decreased levels of insulin and triglycerides.[38]

Exercise and Obesity

Weight loss has been shown to improve glucose control and insulin sensitivity, reduce blood pressure and decrease cardiovascular risk. Even moderate weight loss (10-20% from baseline) is generally sufficient to improve glucose tolerance and reduce cardiovascular risk in patients with type 2 diabetes mellitus. Evidence suggests that in order to achieve weight loss, a combination of diet, exercise and behavior modification is essential.[49,50] Exercise alone without dietary restriction is often not effective because of a compensatory increase in appetite and decrease in spontaneous activity. The combination of exercise and moderate caloric restriction is more effective than diet alone.[49,50,51,52] Exercise is also one of the strongest predictors of maintenance of weight loss.[49,50,52]

The beneficial effects of exercise in a weight-reducing program are often underestimated. Exercise increases lean body mass, which can obscure the loss of body fat when body weight is the criterion of success. In addition, exercise may cause a disproportionate loss of intra-abdominal fat, which has been most closely associated with the metabolic abnormalities in the insulin resistance syndrome.

For weight reduction an exercise frequency of at least 5-6 times a week, which burns 250-300 cal/session, is required. This is difficult initially in most patients with type 2 diabetes because of their poor metabolic fitness. Recently there has been an increased interest in resistance exercise as a weight loss tool. Increased muscle mass resulting from resistance exercise results in an increased resting metabolic rate which could help with weight maintenance.

Exercise and Cardiovascular Disease

Insulin resistance is thought to be an important risk factor for premature atherosclerosis in most type 2 diabetic patients. Studies have shown that these patients are more sedentary compared with controls and have an unfavorable cardiovascular risk factor profile. The beneficial effects of physical training on those cardiovascular risk factors which are most common in patients with type 2 diabetes suggest that regular exercise might play an important role in decreasing the very high incidence of premature coronary artery disease.

Although there are no randomized controlled trials assessing reduction in cardiovascular events induced by physical activity in type 2 diabetes, available evidence is consistent with the concept that physical activity may play an important role in reducing cardiovascular risk in type 2 diabetes.[44] Large nonrandomized studies of both men and women with type 2 diabetes and impaired glucose tolerance have found that physical activity is associated with a decreased risk for cardiovascular disease. It also appears that the amount of physical activity is inversely associated with coronary events.[53,54]

RISK OF EXERCISE IN PATIENTS WITH DIABETES

The risks associated with exercise can be divided into metabolic, vascular, neurologic and musculoskeletal (Table 4).

Table 4. Risks of Exercise in Diabetic Patients

1. Metabolic
   a) paradoxical hyperglycemia
   b) hypoglycemia
2. Vascular
   a) vitreous hemorrhage & traction retinal detachment
   b) proteinuria
3. Neurologic
   a) foot injury
   b) excessive increases in blood pressure,
   c) post exercise hypotension
   d) musculoskeletal injuries and degenerative joint disease

Metabolic Derangements

Both hypoglycemia and paradoxical hyperglycemia are important complications of physical activity in patients with type 1 diabetes mellitus and in a smaller group of patients with type 2 disease. The mechanisms responsible for the surprisingly high incidence of hypoglycemia in these patients are discussed above. A number of options are available to avoid hypoglycemia in patients with type 1 diabetes (Table 5). These should be individualized for each patient based on their response to exercise. The options include changing the dose, timing or site of insulin injection in anticipation of exercise or ingesting adequate food during and after exercise. Some of the measures recommended are:

(a) Decreasing the dose of insulin taken prior to exercise. In general, reduction of about 30-50% in the insulin dose can be anticipated with moderate intensity exercise of >30 minutes duration. Greater reductions will be needed for more prolonged exercise.

(b) Avoid injecting short acting insulin into an area where the underlying muscles will be used during exercise within the next 1-2 hours. For example, avoid injecting into the thigh if bicycling is planned.

(c) Often, exercise is spontaneous and a dose of insulin already injected cannot be adjusted. In this situation hypoglycemia may be avoided by consuming snacks of rapidly absorbable carbohydrates. 15-30g of carbohydrates ingested every 30 minutes is generally adequate for moderate intensity exercise.

(d) If possible exercise should be avoided in the late evening as this increases the risk of hypoglycemia in the early morning hours due to increased insulin sensitivity. Delayed hypoglycemia may be avoided by ingesting slowly absorbable carbohydrates and proteins at bedtime.[55] Use of the shorter acting insulin analogs, such as lispro, with evening food intake may also be helpful. Exercise done in the morning prior to the breakfast insulin dose appears to have the lowest risk of hypoglycemia.

Table 5. Recommendations to Avoid Exercise Related Hypoglycemia in Patients with Diabetes

1. Decrease dose of insulin prior to exercise (usually about 30-50%)
2. Avoid injecting short acting insulin 1-2 hours prior to exercise
3. Avoid injecting insulin directly over the exercising muscle
4. Ingest rapidly absorbable carbohydrates (about 15-30 grams every 30 minutes) during exercise to avoid hypoglycemia during exercise.
5. Ingest slowly absorbable carbohydrates and proteins to avoid delayed hypoglycemia.

Similar guidelines to avoid hypoglycemia have been recommended for patients with type 2 diabetes taking insulin and some patients on sulfonylureas.

The variability of the individuals response to physical activity in patients with type 1 diabetes cannot be overemphasized. As a result, self-monitoring of blood glucose (SMBG) by the patient done before, during and after exercise is an essential step in developing personalized exercise recommendations.

When the fasting blood glucose is > 250mg/dl with ketones or >300mg/dl with or without ketones, exercise should be delayed and such patients first should be adequately insulinized.

Microvascular Risks

While controlled studies are not available, observational evidence suggests that physical activity commonly precedes retinal hemorrhage in patients with established advanced retinopathy. Most commonly, this is associated with hypoglycemia; rapid head movements which would increase shear forces, direct trauma to the eyes, or large swings in blood pressure. There is no evidence that regular exercise increases the risks of developing retinopathy or causes retinal hemorrhage in individuals with mild diabetic eye disease. In patients with more advanced retinopathy it is particularly important to avoid exercises that result in Valsalva maneuvers or levels of physical activity that cause a rise in the systolic blood pressure to > 200 mm Hg.

High intensity exercise increases the quantity of protein in the urine for hours after the exercise is completed. In as many as 30 percent of patients with diabetes whose baseline urine protein is normal intense exercise can result in transient proteinuria. Assessments of quantitative urine protein excretion should be done at least 24 hr after the last bout of exercise. Exercises that result in large increases in systolic blood pressure should probably also be avoided in patients with established nephropathy, although no long term studies of the effects of exercise on the progression of nephropathy are available.

Neurological Risks

Peripheral neuropathy: It is prudent to limit weight-bearing exercises in patients with significant peripheral neuropathy as repetitive exercise on insensitive feet will increase the risk for ulcerations and fractures. In addition, loss of proprioception can make some exercises, such as those involving free weights, dangerous.

Autonomic neuropathy: Diabetic patients with autonomic neuropathy are at increased risk for excessive increases in blood pressure during exercise, post exercise hypotension and sudden cardiac death.

Other general measures to reduce the risks from exercise include maintaining adequate hydration during and after exercise and avoiding exercise in extremely hot or cold environments.

EXERCISE RECOMMENDATIONS

Compliance with exercise programs is a major problem. In a study of 255 diabetic patients in a diabetes education program that emphasized exercise, compliance with exercise fell from 80% at six weeks to <50% at three months and <20% at one-year.[42] To improve adherence to exercise programs, the activity should be enjoyable, convenient and the patient should be educated about the physiology of physical activity, its potential benefits and risks. Quantitative indices of progress to provide feedback should be utilized, e.g., measurements of heart rate during submaximal exercise and measurements of body composition.[56] Also, the goals should be realistic. The guidelines and recommendations for exercise in diabetic patients are summarized in Table 6.

Table 6. Guidelines and recommendations for exercise in diabetic patients

1. Pre-exercise evaluation
   A. detailed history, physical examination & appropriate studies with focus on complications of diabetes affecting eyes, heart, blood vessels, kidneys and nervous system
   B. Exercise stress test: for those starting a moderate-high intensity exercise program and those with increased risk for ischemic heart disease including-
      a) patients over the age of 35 years
      b) type 2 diabetes of >10 years duration
      c) type 1 diabetes >15 years duration
      d) presence of peripheral vascular disease
      e) autonomic neuropathy
      f) proliferative retinopathy
      g) nephropathy
      h) presence of multiple traditional risk factors
2. Type of exercise: Aerobic exercise involving large muscle groups (carefully monitored high volume resistance training is also acceptable for appropriate patients).
3. Frequency of exercise: minimum 3-5 times a week
4. Intensity of exercise: 50-75% $VO_{2\,max}$
5. Duration of exercise: 20-45 minutes per session

Pre-exercise evaluation

All patients with diabetes prior to starting an exercise program should undergo a detailed history, physical examination and appropriate studies with the focus on complications of diabetes affecting the eyes, heart, blood vessels, kidneys and nervous system.[38] As noted before, the response to exercise will be influenced by the type and intensity of exercise as well as the presence or absence of complications. The most feared adverse effect of exercise in diabetic patients is sudden death due to arrhythmias or ischemia. Fortunately this is an extremely rare event.

An exercise stress test is recommended for diabetics before starting a moderate-high intensity exercise program who are at an increased risk for ischemic heart disease. This includes patients over the age of 35 years, type 2 diabetes of >10 years duration and type 1 diabetes >15 years duration, and the presence of peripheral vascular disease, autonomic neuropathy, proliferative retinopathy, or nephropathy.[38] The test will help identify silent ischemic heart disease and abnormal blood pressure responses to exercise.

Type of Exercise

Recommendations for the type, intensity and duration of exercise depend on the risks for the individual patient and the desired benefit/outcome such as athletic training, improvements in insulin sensitivity, weight loss and changes in body composition or enhancing muscle strength and flexibility.

The American Diabetes Association recommends repetitive aerobic exercise involving large muscle groups that can be maintained for a prolonged period in patients with diabetes mellitus.[38] Examples of such exercise include brisk walking, jogging, swimming, rowing, dancing and cycling and other endurance activities. The benefits of exercise for a given level of energy expenditure are not dependent on the mode of exercise. Hence, the type of aerobic activity should be determined by patient preference and risks based on complications of diabetes. For example, a patient with severe peripheral neuropathy would be wise to avoid jogging and instead consider exercises such as swimming or cycling.

In addition to aerobic exercise recent research has suggested the benefit of resistance training of a sufficient intensity to build and maintain muscle strength, endurance and fat-free mass in healthy individuals.[57] In patients with diabetes, resistance training has been shown to improve insulin sensitivity in the absence of changes in maximal oxygen uptake ($VO_{2 max}$).[37,58,59] Well designed resistance-training programs with careful monitoring are beneficial and safe[37,60] and light weights with high repetitions can be used to enhance upper body muscle strength in almost all diabetic patients. However, resistance exercise may not be advisable for some older patients, patients with long standing diabetes and increased risk for ischemic heart disease, and patients with diabetic nephropathy and proliferative retinopathy.

Frequency

It is recommended for patients with diabetes to engage in aerobic exercises roughly every other day or 3-5 days each week. It is not yet clear if multiple shorter bouts of activity throughout the day will result in similar improvements in glucose control.

Intensity

The intensity of exercise is usually given to the patient in the form of a recommendation for a specific target heart rate during activity. Most of the studies that show benefit, i.e. improved glucose disposal and insulin sensitivity, are seen with an exercise intensity at 50-75% of an individual's $VO_{2\ max}$. Also, the American Heart Association recommends engaging in activities that use between 700-2000 cal/ week.[61] Lower intensity exercise (<50% $VO_{2\ max}$), which may be associated with improved patient adherence, may also have beneficial cardiorespiratory and circulatory effects but beneficial effects on insulin sensitivity may not occur.[62,63] On the other hand, higher intensity exercise (>75% $VO_{2\ max}$) may be associated with increased cardiovascular risk, musculoskeletal injuries and decreased patient adherence. While most programs emphasize exercises that improve fitness as demonstrated by an increased maximal oxygen uptake, recent studies suggest that regular participation in low-moderate intensity physical activity may reduce the risk of certain diseases such as type 2 diabetes, hypertension and coronary artery disease despite suboptimal effects on $VO_{2\ max}$.[51,64,65]

Heart rate during exercise is linearly related to exercise intensity. If one knows the basal and maximal heart rate, it is possible to estimate a percent of VO2max based on an individual's heart rate during a given activity. Most exercise prescriptions are given as a recommended exercise heart rate. Most patients can learn to measure their own heart rate and for those who cannot inexpensive devices are available that determine heart rate during exercise. The HR_{max} should ideally be determined during formal exercise testing. If the true HR_{max} is not known then one can estimate it from the equation: HR_{max} = 220- patient age (years).

Fifty % of a maximum heart rate can be estimated by the equation:

$$0.5(HR_{max} - HR_{rest}) + Hr_{rest}$$

where HR_{rest} is the basal heart rate which is determined before arising in the morning. Another commonly used approach to prescribing exercise makes use of the rating of perceived exertion. This analog scale can be used by patients to estimate their relative workload with acceptable accuracy after some training.

Resistance exercise programs emphasize what is called high volume resistance exercise. In general a level of resistance is determined which the patient can perform comfortably for 15 repetitions. The patient is then instructed to perform 8 to 12 repetitions of this activity two to three times with a brief rest period between each set. Resistance exercise of this intensity results in changes of pulse and blood pressure similar to aerobic exercise recommended above and appears to be safe for most patients with diabetes.

To reduce the risk of musculoskeletal injuries and prepare the cardiorespiratory system and skeletal muscles for the progressive increase in exercise intensity, a warm up of 5-10 minutes is recommended. The warm up period involves low intensity aerobic exercise such as walking (but not with breath holding). Stretching exercises are quite useful in patients with diabetes who often complain of decreased flexibility. Stretching should be done following a brief aerobic warm up to avoid muscle injury. A cool down period similar to the warm up should be done at the end of the exercise session. This usually involves 10 minutes of activity at an intensity of 30 to 40 percent of that done during the exercise session. This will help gradually reduce the heart rate down to the pre exercise level and reduce the risk of post exercise hypotension and arrhythmias.

Duration

Depending on the intensity of the exercise regimen, the duration of each session will vary in order to provide the optimal benefit. Exercise done at 50-75% $VO_{2\,max}$, 3-5/ week should last 20-45 minutes. Alternative approaches using two or more short exercise sessions of, for example, 10 minutes may also be beneficial but the effectiveness of this approach for improving glucose control is still unclear.

EXERCISE AND THE PREVENTION OF TYPE 2 DIABETES MELLITUS

Decreased physical activity independent of obesity is a risk factor for the development of type 2 diabetes in high-risk individuals. Insulin resistance and visceral adiposity play an important role in the development of impaired glucose tolerance and frank type 2 diabetes. Therefore, physical activity, by decreasing insulin resistance and visceral adiposity in these high-risk patients is likely to be useful to prevent or delay the development of type 2 diabetes.

Individuals at high risk for diabetes mellitus type 2 include those with a family history of type 2 diabetes mellitus and hypertriglyceridemia, a history of gestational diabetes,[66,67] patients with the polycystic ovary syndrome, any individual with android type obesity associated with features of the insulin resistance syndrome such as hypertension and hypertriglyceridemia, patients from ethnic groups such as Native Americans and individuals from the Indian subcontinent. The incidence of type 2 diabetes in young patients from these high risk groups is increasing and may be related to obesity and low levels of physical activity.

Various types of studies have supported the hypothesis that regular physical activity may prevent type 2 diabetes. These include cross-cultural, migrant and other observational studies[68,69,70] and prospective studies in subjects at high risk for developing type 2 diabetes.[71,72,73] Recently, large interventional trials have reinforced the benefits of exercise in reducing the risk for type 2 diabetes. These include the Malmo study from Sweden[45], the Da Quing study from China[74] and the recently concluded Finnish Diabetes Prevention Study.[75] These prospective but not randomized studies show a reduction in the risk of type 2 diabetes of between 15-60% with similar benefits for older and younger individuals and for men and women.

The ongoing Diabetes Prevention Program is a large multicenter prospective trial, which is to be completed in 2002; the preliminary results of this randomized study confirm the benefit of physical activity in the prevention of diabetes.

SUMMARY

Exercise has been shown to be a useful tool in the treatment of diabetes mellitus. Improvements of HgbA1C levels of 1 to 2 percent are generally found in patients with type 2 diabetes mellitus undergoing a modest exercise program three to five times/week. In addition, exercise has beneficial effects on body composition and a variety of cardiovascular risk factors and is associated with a decreased risk of premature coronary artery disease. The benefits of exercise on glucose control are more difficult to attain in patients with type 1 diabetes but beneficial effects on cardiovascular risk factors are likely to be valuable. Aerobic exercises of moderate intensity are generally recommended for patients with diabetes but high volume resistance exercises are also of benefit and should be included for appropriate patients. While the mechanisms remain incompletely understood it is clear that exercise on a regular basis acts through improved insulin sensitivity in liver and skeletal muscle as well as changes in body composition. The risks of initiating a moderate intensity exercise program for most patients with diabetes are minimal. Patients with neurologic and vascular complications of diabetes may need to limit certain activities. Patients treated with insulin and some oral agents are at risk of hypoglycemia related to exercise. These patients require special education and a regimen based on frequent home blood glucose monitoring. In addition to improving the clinical status of patients with established diabetes, exercise may play an even more important role in prevention of type 2 diabetes in high-risk populations. A safe and effective exercise program can be devised for the great majority of patients with diabetes mellitus and should be a part of every comprehensive treatment regimen.

REFERENCES

1. Vitug A, Schneider SH, Ruderman NB. Exercise and type 1 diabetes mellitus. In Exercise and Sport Science Reviews, Vol. 16, pp. 285-304, 1988.
2. Wahren J. Glucose turnover during exercise in healthy man and in patients with diabetes mellitus. Diabetes 28 (suppl 1): 82-88, 1979.
3. Wahren J, Felig P, Ahlborg G, Jorfeldt L. Glucose metabolism during leg exercise in man. J Clin Invest 50: 2715-2725, 1971.
4. Ahlborg G, Felig P, Hagenfeldt L, Hendler R, Wahren J. Substrate turnover during prolonged exercise in man. J Clin Invest 53:1080-1090, 1974.

5. Wasserman DH, Zinman B. Exercise in individuals with IDDM (Technical Review). Diabetes Care 17: 924-937, 1994.

6. Galbo H, Christensen NJ, Holst JJ. Catecholamines and pancreatic hormones during autonomic blockade in exercising man. Acta Physiol Scand 101: 428-437, 1977.

7. Wasserman DH, Lacy DB, Goldstein RE, Williams PE, Cherrington AD. Exercise-induced fall in insulin and the increase in fat metabolism during prolonged exercise. Diabetes 38: 484-490, 1989.

8. Moates JM, Lacy DB, Cherrington AD, Goldstein RD, Wasserman DH. The metabolic role of the exercise-induced increment in epinephrine. Am J Physiol 255: E428- E436, 1988.

9. Ahlborg G. Mechanism for glycogenolysis in nonexercising human muscle during and after exercise. Am J Physiol 248: E540- E545, 1985.

10. Marliss EB, Simantirakis E, Purdon C, Gougeon R, Field CJ, Halter JB, Vranic M. Glucoregulatory and hormonal responses to repeated bouts of intense exercise in normal male subjects. J Appl Physiol 71: 924-933,1991.

11. Goodyear LJ, King PA, Hirshman MF, Thompson CM, Horton ED, Horton ES. Contractile activity increases plasma membrane glucose transporters in absence of insulin. Am J Physiol 258: E667- E672, 1990.

12. Kennedy JW, Hirshman MF, Gervino EV, Ocel JV, Forse RA, Hoenig SJ, Aronson D, Goodyear LJ, Horton ES. Acute exercise induces GLUT4 translocation in skeletal muscle of normal human subjects and subjects with type 2 diabetes. Diabetes 48: 1192-1197, 1999.

13. Saltin B, Henriksson J, Nyaard E, Andersen P, Jansson E. Fiber types and metabolic potentials of skeletal muscles in sedentary man and endurance runners. IN: The Marathon: Physiological, Medical,Epidemiological, and Psychological Studies. Annals of the New York Academy of Sciences, Vol 301, Milvy P (Ed.). New York, NY,1977, pp3-29.

14. Saltin B, Rowell LB. Functional adaptations to physical activity and inactivity. Fed Proc 39: 1506-1513, 1980.

14a. Holloszy JO: Biochemical adaptations to exercise. Aerobic metabolism. In: Exercise and Sport Sciences Reviews, Vol 1, Wilmore JH (Ed.). New York Academic Press, 1973, pp 4471.

15. Hayashi T, Wojtaszewski JF, Goodyear LJ. Exercise regulation of glucose transport in skeletal muscle. Am J Physiol 273:E1039-E1051, 1997.

16. Zinman B, Murray FT, Vranic M, Albisser AM, Leibel BS, McClean PA, Marliss EB. Glucoregulation during moderate exercise in insulin treated diabetics. J Clin Endocrinol Metab 45:741-647, 1977.

17. Koivisto VA, Felig P. Effect of leg exercise on insulin absorption in diabetic patients. N Engl J Med 298: 79-83, 1978.

18. Schneider SH, Vitug A, Mertz MAL, Ananthakrishnan R, Apelian A,Khachadurian AK. Abnormal hormonal response to prolonged exercise in type 1 diabetes. Diabetes 36(suppl I):16A (Abstract), 1987.

19. Wojtaszewski JF, Hansen BF, Kiens B, Richter EA. Insulin signaling in human skeletal muscle: time course and effect of exercise. Diabetes 46: 1775-1781, 1997.

20. Richter EA, Mikines KJ, Galbo H, Kiens B. Effect of exercise on insulin action in human skeletal muscle. J Appl Physiol 66:876-885, 1989.

21. Bolli G, DeFeo P, Compagnucci P, Cartechini MG, Angeletti G, Santeusano F, Brunetti P. Important role of adrenergic mechanism in acute glucose counterregulation following insulin-induced hypoglycemia in type 1 diabetes. Diabetes 31:641-647, 1982.

22. Berger M, Berchtold P Cupper HJ, Drost H, Kley HK, Muller WA, Wiegelmann W, Zimmermann-Telschow H, Gries FA, Kruskemper HL, Zimmerman H. Metabolic and hormonal effects of muscular exercise on juvenile type diabetes. Diabetologia 13:355-365, 1977.

23. Hagenfeldt L. Metabolism of free fatty acids and ketone bodies during exercise in normal and diabetic man. Diabetes 28(suppl 1):66-70, 1979.

24. Mitchell TH, Abraham G, Schiffrin A, Leiter LA, Marliss EB. Hyperglycemia after intense exercise in IDDM subjects during continuous subcutaneous insulin infusion. Diabetes Care 11:311-317, 1988.

25. Kriska AM, Blair SN, Pereira MA. The potential role of physical activity in the prevention of non-insulin dependent diabetes mellitus: The epidemiological evidence. In Exercise and Sports Sciences Reviews. Vol 22. Holloszy JO, Ed., Williams and Wilkins, Baltimore, MD. pp 121-143, 1994.

26. Wallberg-Henriksson H. Exercise and diabetes mellitus. In Exercise and Sport Sciences Reviews. Vol 20. Holloszy JO, Ed., Williams and Wilkins, Baltimore, MD. pp 339-368, 1992.

27. Minuk HL, Vranic M, Hanna AK, Abisser AM, Zinman B. Glucoregulatory and metabolic response to exercise in obese noninsulin-dependent diabetes. Am J Physiol 240: E458-E464, 1981.

28. Giacca A, Groenewoud Y, Tsui E, McClean P, Zinman B. Glucose production, utilization, and cycling in response to moderate exercise in obese patients with Type 2 diabetes and mild hyperglycemia. Diabetes 47:1763-1770, 1998.

29. Martin IK, Katz A, Wahren J. Splanchnic and muscle metabolism during exercise in NIDDM patients. Am J Physiol 269: E583-E590, 1995.

30. Wallberg-Henriksson H, Gunnarsson R, Henriksson J, DeFronzo R, Felig P, Ostman J, Wahren J. Increased peripheral insulin sensitivity and Muscle mitochondrial enzymes but unchanged blood glucose control in type 1 diabetics after physical training. Diabetes 31: 1044-1050, 1982.

31. Schneider SH, Amorosa LF, Khachadurian AK, Ruderman NB. Studies on the mechanism of improved glucose control during exercise in type 2 (non- insulin dependent) diabetes. Diabetologist 26: 355-360, 1984.

32. Hollszy JO, Schultz J, Kusnierkiewic J, Hagberg JM, Ehsani AA. Effects of exercise on glucose tolerance and insulin resistance. Acta Med Scand Suppl 711: 55-65, 1986.

33. Reitman JS, Vasquez B, Dimes I, Nauglesparan M. Improvement of glucose homeostasis after exercise-training in non-insulin-dependent diabetes. Diabetes Care 7: 434-441, 1984.

34. Dela F, Larsen JJ, Mikines KJ, Ploug T, Petersen LN, Galbo H. Insulin-stimulated muscle glucose clearance in patients with NIDDM: effects of one-legged physical training. Diabetes 44: 1010-1020, 1995.

35. Burstein R, Polychronakos C, Toews CJ, MacDoughall JD, Guyda HJ, Posner BI. Acute reversal of enhanced insulin action in trained athletes. Diabetes 34: 750-760, 1985.

36. Pan DA, Lillioja S, Milner MR, Kriketos AD, Baur LA, Bogardus C, Storlein LH. Skeletal muscle lipid composition is related to adiposity and insulin action. J Clin Invest 96: 2802-2808, 1995.

37. Miller WJ, Sherman WM, Ivy JL. Effects of strength training on glucose tolerance and post-glucose insulin response. Med Sci Sports Exerc 16:539-543, 1984.

38. Diabetes mellitus and exercise (ADA position statement). Diabetes Care 24(suppl 1): S51-S55, 2001.

39. Schneider SH Long-term exercise programs. In The Health Professional's Guide to Diabetes and Exercise. Ruderman N, Devlin JT, Eds. American Diabetes Association, Alexandria, VA, pp 123-132, 1995.

40. Krottkiewski M, Lonnroth P, Manrwoukas K, Wrobelwski Z, Rebuffe-Scrive M, Holm G, Smith U, Bjorntrop P. Effects on physical training of insulin secretion and effectiveness and glucose metabolism in obesity and type 2 (non-insulin dependent) diabetes mellitus. Diabetologia 28:881-890, 1985.

41. Yki-Jarvinen H, DeFronzo RA, Koivisto VA. Normalization of insulin sensitivity in type I diabetic subjects by physical training during insulin pump therapy. Diabetes Care 7:520-527, 1984.

42. Schneider SH, Khachadurian AK, Amorosa LF. Ten-year experience with exercise-based outpatient life-style modification program in the treatment of diabetes mellitus. Diabetes Care 15:1800-1810, 1992.

43. Ruderman NE, Ganda OP, Johansen K. The effect of physical training on glucose tolerance and plasma lipids in maturity onset diabetes.Diabetes 28:89-91, 1979.

44. Schneider SH, Vitug A, Ruderman NB. Atherosclerosis and physical activity. Diab Metab Rev 1:513-553, 1986.

45. Eriksson KF, Lindgarde F. Prevention of type II (noninsulin dependent) diabetes mellitus by diet and physical exercise: the six year Malmo feasibility study. Diabetologia 34:891-898, 1991.

46. Houmard JA, Bruno NJ, Bruner RK, McCammon MR, Israel RG, Barakal HA. Effects of exercise training on chemical composition of plasma LDL. Atheroscler Thromb 14: 325-330, 1994.

47. Krotkiewski M, Mandrousask K, Sjostrom L, SuDivan L, Wetterquist H, Bjorntor P. Effects of long term physical training on body fat, metabolism and BP in obesity. Metabolism 28:650-658, 1979.

48. Rocchini AP, Katch V, Schork A, Kelch RP. Insulin and blood pressure during weight loss in obese adolescents. Hypertension 10:267-273, 1987.

49. NHLBI Obesity Education Initiative Expert Panel on the identification, evaluation, and treatment of overweight and obesity in adults. Clinical guidelines on the identification, evaluation, and treatment of overweight and obesity in adults- the evidence report. Obes Res 6:51S-310S, 1998.

50. Wing RR. Physical activity in the treatment of the adulthood overweight and obesity: current evidence and research issues. Med Sci Sports Exerc 31:S547-S552, 1999.

51. Helmirch SP, Ragland DR, Leung RW, Paffenbarger RS. Physical activity and reduced occurrence of non-insulin-dependent diabetes mellitus. N Engl J Med 325: 147-152, 1991.

52. Wing RR: Behavioral Strategies for weight reduction in obese type II diabetic patients. Diabetes Care 12:139-144, 1989.

53. Kohn HW, Gordon NF, Villegas JA, Blair SN. Cardiorespiratory fitness, glycemic status, and mortality risk in men. Diabetes Care 15:184-192,1992.

54. Hu FB, Stampfer MJ, Solomon C, Liu S, Colditz GA, Speizer FE, Willet WC, Manson JE. Physical activity and risk for cardiovascular events in diabetic women. Ann Intern Med 134:96-105, 2001.

55. Nathan DM, Madnek SF, Dellahanty L. Programming pre-exercise snacks to prevent postexercise hypoglycemia in intensively treated insulin-dependent diabetics. Ann Intern Med 102: 483-486, 1985.

56. Schneider SH, Ruderman NB. Exercise and NIDDM (Technical Review). Diabetes Care 13: 785-789, 1990.

57. American College of Sports Medicine. The recommended quantity and quality of exercise for developing and maintaining cardiorespiratory and muscular fitness, and flexibility in healthy adults. (Position Stand)Med Sci Sports Exerc 30: 975-991, 1998.

58. Szczypaczewska M, Nazar K, Kaciwba-Uscilko H. Glucose tolerance and insulin response to glucose load in body builders. Int J Sports Med 10: 34-37, 1989.

59. Smutok MA, Reece A, Goldberg AP, Kokkinos PF, Dawson P, Shulman R. Strength training improves glucose tolerance similar to jogging in middle-aged men (letter). Med Sci Sports Exerc 21 (suppl 2): S33, 1989.

60. Durak EP, Jovanovic-Peterson L, Peterson CM. Randomized crossover study of effect of resistance training on glycemic control, muscular strength and cholesterol in type 1 diabetic men. Diabetes Care 13:1039-1043, 1990.

61. Fletcher GF, Balady G, Froelicher VF, Hartley LH, Haskell WL, Pollock ML. A statement for health professionals from the American Heart Association (Exercise Standards). Circulation 91: 580- 612, 1995.

62. King AC, Haskell WL, Taylor CB, Kraemer HC, DeBusk RF. Home based exercise training in healthy older men and women. JAMA 266: 1535-1542, 1991.

63. Paffenberger RS, Wing AL, Hyde RT. Physical activity as an index of heart attack risk in college alumni. An J Epidemiol 108: 161-175, 1978.

64. Fletcher GF, Balady G, Blair SN, Blumenthal J, Caspersen C, Chaitman B, Epstein S, Sivarajan ES, Froelicher VF, Pina IL, Pollock ML. Benefits and recommendations for physical activity programs for all Americans (Statement on Exercise). Circulation 94: 857-862, 1996.

65. American College of Sports Medicine. Physical activity, physical fitness and hypertension (Position Stand). Med Sci Sports Exerc 25: i-x, 1993.

66. Ruderman NB, Schneider SH, Berchtold P. The metabolically-obese, normal weight individual. Am J Clin Nutr 34:1617-1621, 1981.

67. Ruderman NB, Berchtold P, Schneider SH. Obesity associated disorders in normal weight individuals: some speculations. Int J Obesity 6:151- 157, 1982.

68. Taylor R. Physical activity and prevalence of diabetes in Melanesian and Indian men in Fiji. Diabetologia 27:578-582, 1984.

69. Dowse GK, Zimmet PZ, Gareeboo H, George K, Alberti MM, Tuomilehto J, Finch CF, Chitson P, Tulsidas H. Abdominal obesity and physical activity are risk factors for NIDDM and impaired glucose tolerance in Indian, Creole, and Chinese Mauritians. Diabetes Care 14:271-282, 1991.

70. Kawate R, Yamakido M, Nishimoto Y, Bennett PH, Hamman RF, Knowler WC. Diabetes mellitus and its vascular complications in Japanese migrants on the Island of Hawaii. Diabetes Care 2:161-170, 1979.

71. Kriska AM, Blair SN, Pereira MA. The potential role of physical activity in the prevention of non-insulin dependent diabetes mellitus: The epidemiological evidence. Exerc Sports Sci Rev 22:121-143, 1991.

72. Hu FB, Sibal RJ, Rich-Edwards JW, Colditz GA, Solomon CG, Willett WC, Speizer FE, Manson JE. Walking compared with vigorous physical activity and risk of type 2 diabetes in women: a prospective study. JAMA 282: 1433-1439, 1999.

73. Manson JE, Nathan DM, Krolewski AS, Stampfer MJ, Willett WC, Hennekens CH. A prospective study of exercise and incidence of diabetes among U.S. male physicians. JAMA 268:63-67, 1992.

74. Pan X, Li G, Hu YH. Effects of diet and exercise in preventing NIDDM in people with impaired glucose tolerance. The Da Quing IGT and Diabetes Study. Diabetes Care 20:537-544, 1997.

75. Tuomilehto J, Lindstrom J, Eriksson JG, Valle TT, Hamalainen H, Ilanne-Parikka P, Keinanen-Kiukaanniemi S, Laakso M, Louheranta A, Rastas M, Salminen V, Uusitupa M. Prevention of type 2 diabetes mellitus by changes in lifestyle among subjects with impaired glucose tolerance. The Finnish Diabetes Prevention Study Group. N Engl J Med 344: 1343-1350, 2001.

Chapter 5. Therapy of Type 1 Diabetes Mellitus

Andrew J. Drexler and Carolyn Robertson

INTRODUCTION

The treatment of type 1 diabetes mellitus is both completely clear and extremely complex. Individuals with type 1 diabetes must receive insulin therapy. There are no alternatives and no exceptions. How that insulin should best be administered as well as what blood sugar level should be targeted was unknown prior to 1993. At that time, the Diabetes Control and Complications Trial (DCCT) ended a many decades long debate over the relationship between improved glucose control and the microvascular complications of diabetes.[1] During the DCCT, patients were randomly divided into an intensive control group, which was treated with either insulin injections taken at least three times a day or with an insulin pump, or a conventional group which was treated with only two injections a day. Both groups were given diet instruction, but the former group met with members of a diabetes team on a regular basis. They were taught how to adjust their insulin, manipulate a meal plan and alter their lifestyles to achieve blood glucose levels as close as possible to those seen in non-diabetics. With a difference in hemoglobin A1C of only 1.5% between the two groups, there was an approximately 50% reduction in the microvascular complications (retinopathy, nephropathy and neuropathy). As a result of the strongly affirmative answer from the DCCT, programs of intensive management with blood glucose targets of near normoglycemia became the standard of care for individuals with type 1 diabetes.[2, 3]

Achieving glycemic targets that approach the non-diabetic range requires treatment programs that are designed to reproduce as closely as possible the pattern of glucose and endogenous insulin levels that would have existed if the patient were not diabetic. In the non-diabetic, the pancreas secretes small amounts of insulin directly into the portal vein nearly continuously. This delivery pattern of insulin secretion occurs independent of food and is termed basal insulin secretion. Basal insulin secretion's main role in glucose metabolism is to control hepatic glucose output. The basal secretion of insulin is also necessary for normal protein and lipid homeostasis. While the amount of insulin secreted at any given instant as basal insulin is small, the 24 hour aggregate sum accounts for approximately 50% of the daily insulin requirement[4].

Basal insulin level does not provide the insulin required for proper disposal of meal-ingested carbohydrates. However, the pancreas anticipates a rise in blood sugar associated with eating a meal. Insulin secretion into the portal vein increases in response to food intake as much as ten-fold in a biphasic pattern of insulin release: the first phase of release occurring in the initial five minutes and the second phase occurring 30 minutes later and lasting for 2 or 3 hours.[5] This dramatic increase in insulin arriving at the liver is responsible for converting the liver from an organ of glucose production and release to an organ of glycogen synthesis. Mealtime release of insulin also supports peripheral glucose uptake. As important as the rapid secretion of insulin, is its rapid clearance, which accounts for a return of insulin levels back to baseline within three hours of a meal. Figure 1 represents the pattern of insulin secretion in a non-diabetic individual eating three meals.

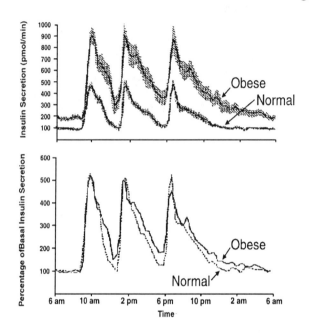

Figure 1. Insulin secretion profiles in normal and obese subjects.
(From Polonsky KS, Sturis J. and Bell GI. Seminars in Medicine of the Beth Israel Hospital, Boston. Non-insulin-dependent diabetes mellitus—a genetically programmed failure of the β-cell to compensate for insulin resistance. New England Journal of Medicine 334:777-83, 1996, with permission).

Current diabetes therapy has not been able to mimic normal physiology. Several problems exist. First, insulin must be injected subcutaneously three or more times per day to achieve the required concentration of insulin both in the pre- and postprandial states. Insulin, once injected, is present in the blood for many hours. Second, since all current therapy is subcutaneous, insulin is delivered initially to the systemic circulation and only secondarily into the portal circulation. Hence, it is not possible to achieve the normal endogenous portal to systemic insulin ratios.

This may have implications for both glucose and lipid metabolism. Finally, much of the insulin injected is not initially soluble, leading to fluctuations in serum insulin levels even after injection of the same dosage.

Recent advances in insulin therapy have been designed to overcome some of these limitations, but we are very far from being able to duplicate the glucose homeostasis found in the non-diabetic. The remainder of this chapter will discuss strategies that provide an approximation of normal physiology.

BLOOD GLUCOSE TESTING AND HEMOGLOBIN A1C MEASUREMENTS

The current era in diabetes treatment can be said to have begun with the introduction of hemoglobin A1C measurements and patient-friendly methods of measuring blood glucose. The understanding of the nature of hemoglobin A1C as an adduct of glucose and hemoglobin defined an objective criterion for measuring overall glucose control. Frequent capillary blood sugar testing was critical to provide the information necessary to validate the use of hemoglobin A1C levels as an integrated average of the mean 24-hour blood sugar value, as well as a technique to improve hemoglobin A1C values in individual patients. Today, both hemoglobin A1C measurements and patient self blood sugar testing are recognized as essential in diabetes care. These parameters provide the patient and the health care provider with immediate feedback that allows for informed change. Despite their advantages, there are some controversies.

How often should blood sugar monitoring be performed?

While a fasting blood sugar may be reflective of the blood sugar values throughout the day in diet controlled type 2 diabetics, data proves that there is a high frequency of wide swings in blood sugar seen in most individuals with type 1 diabetes.[7] When the clinician relies on the testing performed at fixed times of the day, the insulin regimen is designed to optimize blood sugars at only those times and it does not address the unrecognized "highs" and "lows" that can occur at other times of the day. In the absence of continuous glucose monitoring, an individual's glucose profile can be defined by assessing the blood sugar at the times when it would be expected to be either highest or lowest. This would involve testing before each meal, after each meal, at bedtime, as well as overnight (to rule out nocturnal hypoglycemia). Few patients are willing to test that often. Therefore, it becomes necessary to infer the glucose profile. Testing must be scheduled to meet the demands of statistically valid sampling to allow an evaluation of glucose control. This necessitates scattered testing which avoids testing at the same time of the day every day. Most individuals with type 1 diabetes will need to test before each injection of insulin to know how to adjust the dose for fluctuations in blood sugar. Post-prandial blood sugar testing is essential to evaluate the correctness of the dose of short acting insulin used for a specific amount and type of carbohydrate at a meal.[8]

Does the Hgb A1C provide an adequate measure of control?

Hemoglobin A1C measurements remain the benchmark for defining the level of control in people with diabetes. However, in individuals with type 1 diabetes, where wide swings are common throughout the day, the hemoglobin A1C does not define the degree of blood sugar fluctuations.[9]

The DCCT data suggested that patients on more than three injections a day (or a pump) had fewer complications than individuals on two or less injections a day even with the same hemoglobin A1C value. [10] Two individuals with the same hemoglobin A1C levels can have very different mean amplitude of glucose excursions (MAGE). The explanation for this is not clear but one hypothesis is that the people on the three or more injections used more Regular insulin before meals and hence had better post-prandial blood sugar control.[3,8,11] This answer, however, is controversial. If the benefits of the intensive control group with the same hemoglobin A1C as the conventional group described above are due to the decreased MAGE from the use of more Regular insulin, as hypothesized above, then post-prandial testing may be critical for avoidance of complications. While still controversial, some recent data, such as the DECODE study, suggest that post-prandial swings in blood sugar may be important in the development of the microvascular complications of diabetes.[12] If true, this will support the concept that hemoglobin A1C levels alone are not sufficient to define adequate control in individuals with type 1 diabetes. Further, the patients in the intensive control arm of DCCT showed continuing benefits even after their hemoglobin values deteriorated at the conclusion of the study.[13] No accepted explanation of this observation currently exists.

A possible solution to the above problems may come with the wider use of instruments that provide automatic frequent sampling of glucose levels in the interstitial fluid.[14] Two such devices have already been approved for use (Minimed CGM and Cygnus GlucoWatch Biographer) and others are in development. These instruments have limitations and their values may not completely reflect the value obtained with a capillary blood sugar measurement.[15] Specifically, both the time and the magnitude of the peak post-prandial glucose may be different from that obtained by blood sugar testing. More time is needed to fully assess the impact of these devices on diabetes treatment.

INSULIN PREPARATIONS

Insulin preparations can be divided by amino acid sequence into human, analog, or animal insulin and by pharmacokinetics into short-acting, intermediate- acting and long-acting.

Human insulin is created in the laboratory by recombinant DNA technology. It is characterized by having the same amino acid sequence as endogenous human insulin. *Insulin analog* is defined by its amino acid sequence, which is close to, but not the same, as human insulin. Animal insulin is derived from non-human pancreases and, therefore, has an amino acid sequence which is also not identical to human insulin. *Table 1* lists the human and analog insulins currently available in the United States. Animal source insulin is currently used only rarely. Its activity curve differs from human insulin. In general, the onset, peak and duration of animal insulins are longer.

Table 1. Insulin Preparations

Human	Action	Onset	Peak	Duration	Form
Regular	Short to Intermediate	0.5hr	2-4hr	6-12hr	vials,cartridge, pen
NPH	Intermediate	1.5hr	4-6hr	14-16hr	vials, cartridge, pen
Lente	Intermediate	3hr	7-9hr	14- 20hrs	vials
Ultralente	Intermediate to long acting	4hr	8-14hr	24hr	vials
Analogs	**Action**	**Onset**	**Peak**	**Duration**	**Form**
Lispro	Rapid	0.25hr	1.25hr	2.5hr	vials, cartridge, pen
Insulin Aspart	Rapid	0.25hr	1.25hr	2.5hr	Vial
Glargine	Long acting	2hr	None	24+hrs	Vial

Rapid Acting Insulin Preparations

Lispro insulin. This is the first insulin analog to utilize a change in the amino acid sequence of the insulin molecule to alter the insulin kinetics. Its rapid onset and early peak provide the achievement of insulin levels much closer to the levels seen in non-diabetics, making it a true prandial insulin. While it is still unable to completely mimic normal physiology, it does a much better job of covering the carbohydrates ingested with a meal with fewer tendencies to produce 3-hour post-prandial hypoglycemia.[16,17, 18] This is most clear when Lispro is used at dinner in place of Regular insulin: there is a significant decrease in the incidence of 2AM hypoglycemia. Claims have been made that Lispro insulin shows less change in kinetics with increasing dosage than any other insulin. Consequently, taking Lispro and delaying a meal when the pre-prandial sugar is high is not recommended because the meal, when finally eaten, may miss the peak action of the insulin.[19]   In fact, unlike Regular insulin, where a snack is mandatory if the post-prandial sugar is normal, with Lispro insulin snacks will often require an additional insulin injection.   There are potential problems with Lispro insulin. It may not provide sufficient duration of action for a high fat meal.[21] When used at dinner, depending on the insulin regimen, there may be a gap in the basal insulin coverage between bed and the first part of the night.[22] Strategies can be designed to resolve both of these problems when they are recognized.

Insulin Aspart. This insulin is just being introduced into the United States and there is little experience to date with it. In general it is reported to work like Lispro insulin although with a slightly later peak and longer duration of action.[23] This difference is not thought to be clinically significant.

Short-Acting Insulin Preparations

Regular Insulin. The introduction of Lispro insulin has altered our perception of Regular insulin. Originally it was seen as a short-acting insulin designed to cover meals. With the availability of Lispro and now Insulin Aspart, it is recognized that Regular insulin is better seen as a short /intermediate acting insulin. It is better designed to provide some extra duration of prandial coverage for high fat meals or prolonged meals; or as basal insulin to cover gaps between Lispro.   To enhance the effect of preprandial Regular, it is important to also consider the lag time between the injection and the beginning of the meal as well as the composition and volume of the meal.[24] Because of the time necessary for Regular insulin to start to act, it is best taken one half hour before a meal. Some studies have shown that for best post-prandial sugar control, a one-hour wait is even better but this can result in pre-meal hypoglycemia.[25]   When, however, the initial blood sugar is high, delaying the meal after taking Regular insulin can safely take advantage of the late peak of Regular. As discussed below, this strategy is not as efficacious with Lispro insulin and patients need to be advised of the difference. Patients need to be given specific guidelines regarding the need to have sufficient carbohydrate to avoid the risk of postmeal hypoglycemia. The requirement for snacks 3-hours after meals in well-controlled diabetics was a reflection of the observation that with a good 2-hour post-prandial blood sugar and the knowledge that the peak action of the insulin had not passed, a snack to prevent hypoglycemia was essential.[26]

Intermediate Acting Insulin Preparations

NPH Insulin. The most commonly used intermediate-acting insulin in the United States, NPH, can be used to provide basal needs alone. In larger doses it can be used to provide coverage at meals. Of important note, the change from animal source to human insulin significantly altered the kinetics of NPH insulin.[27] While animal source NPH insulin peaked in 8 hours and lasted up to 24-hours, human NPH has very different characteristics - an earlier peak and a shorter duration are common. This has created several problems in the use of NPH insulin. When NPH is administered in the morning in a dose designed to both cover lunch and provide the basal insulin needs of the day, lunch must be eaten within four hours of the administration of the NPH or the patients risk pre-lunch hypoglycemia. Additionally, the shorter duration of action may result in insulin waning in people with late suppers. Similar problems exist when NPH insulin is given at supper. The shortened peak is likely to lower the blood glucose level during the night, increasing the risk of nocturnal hypoglycemia and lack of adequate control of the fasting blood sugar. Since at higher dosages the peak of human insulin is delayed, clinicians are frequently tempted to consider increasing the insulin dose as a strategy to extend its duration. In the type 1 diabetic, the increased insulin dosages of NPH may explain the weight gain and hypoglycemia that is seen in intensive insulin regimens. Usually, this is less of a problem with type 2 diabetes patients who are more insulin resistant and therefore require higher dosages. Moving the administration of the NPH insulin to bedtime may alleviate some of these problems. Even with attention to the time the insulin is administered both problems can still occur based on the kinetics of insulin.[28,29] When NPH is used as basal insulin, it requires 2 to 3 injections of a lowered dose. Even at lowered dosing, caution is necessary because of the insulin's peak. Patients may require a snack to prevent hypoglycemia, especially in the presence of increased or unusual physical activity. In its favor, there is a perception among many clinicians that NPH insulin has a more predictable pattern of action than either Lente or Ultralente insulin.

Lente insulin. In Europe, Lente insulin is often used in place of NPH insulin. The kinetics of Lente was less altered with the conversion to human insulin. In fact, it behaves closer to animal source NPH insulin than does human NPH insulin. For this reason, some groups in the United States use it in preference to NPH insulin. Lente insulin does have, however, some of the same disadvantages as described above for NPH insulin, because it also has a peak. Meals still must be timed to the administration of Lente, though the patient is usually able to delay lunch by up to six hours. Insulin waning overnight continues to be a significant risk. In general, these problems may be less with Lente insulin than NPH. Decreased consistency in timing and the binding of Lente to Regular when they are mixed (due to excess zinc in Lente insulin) are significant disadvantages.[30] Additionally, Lente insulin is not available in a pen form.

Long-Acting Insulin Preparations

Ultralente Insulin. Like NPH insulin, human Ultralente insulin is very different in action compared to animal source Ultralente. The difference is a much shorter duration of action (24 hours versus 36 hours) and a more prominent peak. The criticisms of Ultralente are similar to those of Lente insulin, only more so. While often used as basal insulin, at higher dosages, the tendency to peak can be a significant limitation.

Insulin Glargine. This is the first insulin analog to be developed as basal insulin. It has two major advantages. First, because it is a soluble insulin, its time course is more predictable than any insulin suspension ("cloudy insulin").[31] It also appears to lack a distinct peak in the majority of users. It has the further advantage of having a 24-hour duration of action. These are desirable characteristics for a basal insulin. Since Glargine has just been introduced into the United States, only experience will determine how well it functions as basal insulin. There are disadvantages to this insulin[32]. Because of its acidic base, it cannot be mixed with any other insulin: mixing will cause the insulin to form precipitates and will inactivate the insulin. Additionally, the acid pH may produce a small amount of discomfort at the site of injection.

Insulin Mixtures

In addition to the insulin preparations described above, fixed mixtures of insulin are available. In the United States, NPH and Regular insulin are available as mixtures of 70% NPH and 30% Regular insulin (Humulin 70/30; Novolin 70/30) and 50% NPH and 50% Regular insulin (Humulin 50/50). Mixtures containing Lispro as the short acting insulin required the production of a new intermediate acting insulin. This insulin, called NPL (not available individually), is reported to behave, in terms of its pharmacokinetics, similar to NPH. At present, this is sold as Humalog Mix 75/25 with 75% NPL insulin and 25% Lispro.

Future Insulin Preparations

There are several insulins that are in development. These include additional long acting analogues, Di-arginyl human insulin analogue (Gly, Arg) and a C16 fatty-acid-acylated analogue. Manufacturers are also working on aerosolized formulations of insulin that would replace subcutaneously delivered rapid acting insulin. Early results suggest that inhaled administration of insulin is safe and effective. The concept is an attractive alternative for insulin delivery. However, complete understanding of its safety and efficacy is dependent on analysis of the Phase III studies that are still in progress.

INSULIN ALGORITHMS

Therapy in type 1 diabetes consists of using the above insulins to achieve near-normoglycemia. The attempt to achieve physiologic insulin levels in the diabetic individual needs to be undertaken in a way that is acceptable to the patients and consistent with the limitations of exogenous insulin therapy and glucose monitoring. To meet this requirement, the insulin algorithms must provide a continuous supply of insulin to match the body's basal requirements; they also must provide larger quantities of insulin to assure adequate glucose uptake at meals. In other words, a mixture of insulins that will provide "basal-bolus" insulin therapy needs to be defined [2,3,24,33] Since the DCCT documented the lack of efficacy of a two-injection insulin regimen, the default becomes either three or more insulin injections, or an insulin pump. Basal insulin may be provided as bedtime (HS) Insulin *Glargine*; HS and morning *NPH* or *Lente* insulin; *Ultralente* given in one or two injections; or an insulin pump. Administering either *Regular* or *Lispro* before meals usually provides bolus insulin. A three-injection insulin regimen utilizing AM *NPH* or Lente to provide both the basal dose and to cover lunch, while used in the DCCT, is not a true "basal-bolus" regimen since the intermediate acting insulin is dosed at a level to promote glucose uptake by the muscles. The introduction of short acting analogs, like *Lispro* and *Insulin Aspart,* along with the long acting analog, *Glargine*, has the potential to simplify basal bolus therapy. At present, however, the older strategies need to be considered as well.

In type 1 diabetes mellitus, where insulin resistance is usually not a factor, many studies, including the DCCT, have shown that most patients require approximately 0.5 to 1.0 u/kg though most will require 0.6u/kg of insulin per twenty-four hours.[24,34] Body type (lean patients often require less insulin units /kg); activity; stress; and residual endogenous insulin will determine the actual insulin requirement. 40 to 50% of the total insulin dose provide for the basal insulin requirements and the remainder provides for the boluses of insulin that are needed to cover the meal and to provide adequate postprandial blood sugar control. A 70 kg patient would require a total daily dosage of about 42 u/day. The basal dosage would equal between 16 to 21u. If this insulin was provided by an insulin pump, it translates to an average basal rate of 0.6 to 0.9 u/hr. The remaining insulin of twenty-one to twenty-six units would be distributed for the pre-meal boluses. The skill in treating type 1 diabetes comes from selecting insulins that provide a continuous twenty-four hour basal insulin coverage along with sufficient boluses of insulin at meals to achieve adequate post-prandial control in a way that conforms to the patient's lifestyle. The insulin prescription needs to be individualized for each patient. The same patient may need several different prescriptions, for example, one for weekdays and another for weekends. Women may need one prescription for the first half of their menstrual cycle and a different prescription for the second half. A variety of factors may influence the ambient glucose levels. These factors include the injection site, the depth of penetration, the lag time between injection and the meal, the food consumed, activity and stress levels. In order for blood sugar levels of the individual with diabetes to achieve near-normoglycemia, the insulin dose at any given time will need to be modified by the patient.[3] Therefore, it is necessary to describe more than an exact set of insulin instructions. Patients must be given guidelines for adjusting the insulin dose proactively as opposed to rigid insulin doses. Patient self-blood glucose monitoring accompanied by a program of patient education gives the patient the knowledge and the skills to make these adjustments. In fact, the DCCT showed that without the patient assuming a self-management role, optimal control could not be achieved.[26] A number of starting algorithms are shown in Table 2. These conform to the requirements described above but should only be used in any individual patient as a starting point.

To modify these algorithms, the patients must be aware of the various factors that influence blood sugar and be given strategies for how to adjust the insulin dosage as these other factors change. The most important of these factors are diet, exercise, stress and infections. The patient who alters the content or size of his meals needs a regime that provides for flexibility. Many patients can be taught how to adjust the insulin based on the amount of carbohydrate in the meal (CHO counting); others can be taught how to adjust their insulin dose based on the difference in the meal size from their usual. Patients will benefit from a referral to an experienced and flexible nutritionist to help them master the impact of food on their blood glucose levels.[35,36] Fluctuations in blood sugar without feasible explanation will also often appear in individuals with type 1 diabetes and guidelines for returning the blood sugar to the desired range have to be developed for each individual.[24,37] Ultimately, the use of any insulin prescription/algorithm becomes only one component in the management by the diabetes team. An important component of treating type 1 diabetes is knowing how to anticipate situations when either hypoglycemia or hyperglycemia may occur. More importantly, the patient needs to know how to treat these when they do occur.

Operationally, once a particular regimen has been chosen, the challenge is to adjust it to achieve the desired level of blood sugar control. To determine if the basal insulin or the bolus insulin should be changed, review the blood sugar patterns. If the blood glucose at the next meal is high, note the blood glucose value and compare it to the preceding post meal value. If that glucose value is high, then the bolus of that meal needs to be increased. However, if the post meal value is acceptable then the basal insulin needs to be adjusted. As an example, consider the patient who has an elevated blood sugar at lunch. You determine that it is related to neither the diet nor the activity of the patient; and there is no evidence for a rebound effect after hypoglycemia. To adjust the insulin, you will need to determine if the elevation of blood glucose was related to the inadequate amount of short acting insulin (Humalog) given at breakfast or to the morning basal insulin (NPH). If the 1 to 2-hr post breakfast value is on target, then the

Table 2. Insulin Algorithms

		Breakfast	Lunch	Supper	Bed
Three injection regimen					
Basal	NPH/Lente	40%	None *	None *	20%
Bolus	Lispro/Insulin Aspart	20%	None*	20%	Supplement if bs elevated
Four injection regimen					
Basal	Lente/Ultralente/NPH	20%	None *	None	20%
Bolus	Lispro/Insulin Aspart	20%	20%	20%	Supplement if bs elevated
CSII or Glargine					
Basal	Basal rate or Glargine				40%
Bolus	Bolus	20%	20%	20%	◄————————►
NPO					
Basal	Basal	15% Lente every eight hours or Glargine at 45% once a day in evening or Insulin infusion 40 –60% over 24hr period			
	Coverage	Regular insulin every four hours as needed			
		* Some basal insulin may be needed to cover the gap after the Lispro and before the intermediate insulin begins to work			

higher blood sugar level at lunch is due to the morning NPH. If the post breakfast value is over the target, then the increase of blood glucose at lunch is related to the breakfast Regular.

INSULIN PUMP THERAPY (CONTINUOS SUBCUTEANEUOS INSULIN INFUSION-CSII)

In addition to the described combinations of insulin that can be used to provide basal bolus therapy, the major alternative for insulin delivery is the use of an insulin pump. Insulin pumps are electromechanical devices that release a small amount of insulin on a continuous basis through a catheter to a needle or plastic cannula that is placed under the skin. Usually insulin regimen is prescribed as an amount of insulin that is delivered as units/hour. This amount is programmed into the pump by the patient and corresponds to the estimated basal needs of the individual.[38,39] Pumps can be programmed to provide varying basal rates during the day. This allows the pump to meet the needs of a patient that has varying levels of activity or has hormonal needs that affect the glucose levels throughout the month. No other insulin strategy has this degree of flexibility.[40] The pump can also provide a bolus of insulin to cover meals. Boluses delivered by a pump do not differ from injections of insulin prior to a meal delivered by syringe.

579

CSII has three major advantages. The ability to vary basal rates multiple times throughout the day or night is particularly important in individuals with a pronounced Dawn phenomenon (a significant increase in insulin requirement prior to awakening).[41] The reason for this increased requirement is not clear but may be related to growth hormone secretion overnight. In some individuals, this may require a several fold increase in their hourly basal rate for a 2 to 5 hour period overnight. An insulin pump using Humalog or Insulin Aspart may be the only way to achieve the rapid increase in insulin that is needed without the patient waking up to administer insulin bolus in the middle of the night. A good fasting blood sugar without an unacceptable level of nocturnal hypoglycemia may not be possible in these patients without an insulin pump.[42] Another advantage of the insulin pump includes the certainty of an adequate basal rate even when meals are delayed or activity is altered, as well as the greater predictability of absorption of soluble insulins, either regular or an insulin analog, compared to intermediate acting insulin. While these latter two advantages may be less important with the introduction of Glargine, with its 24-hour duration of action without a peak, the absence of a peak does not meet the need for a spike in insulin overnight for people with a pronounced Dawn phenomenon nor does it allow for a reduction when the individual is more active. Whether this is a significant limitation of Glargine is still to be established.

Ideally, the goal of insulin pump therapy would be to produce a "closed loop system". A closed loop system would involve a glucose sensor capable of automatically monitoring blood sugar and an insulin delivery system that would use the information from the sensor to deliver the correct amount of insulin. Both would need to occur without intervention on the part of the patient. Ideally, the insulin delivery system would transport the insulin to the portal circulation and recreate the normal portal to systemic insulin ratio described previously. Peritoneal insulin delivery systems, which do meet this goal, have been developed but are not yet approved for general use.[43] In addition to the practical barriers to developing a closed loop system, appropriate algorithms that anticipate the rise in blood sugar which occurs as a response to a meal, rather than those that react after the fact to correct the rise in bloods sugar, need to be developed. At present, there is little published data on such insulin algorithms.

TEAM DIABETES MANAGEMENT

The diabetes treatment regimens described above involve the patient as an active participant in decision-making. For this to occur, the patient needs to have information that identifies the different insulins he or she uses and their pharmacokinetics. Patients must also learn how to adjust their insulin regime for more or less food, a delay in meal time or an early meal time, increased activity or exercise, stress, etc. An understanding of nutrition that includes the skill of determining the number of grams of carbohydrate in the meal is essential in knowing how to adjust the amount of bolus insulin for the meal. This approach to diet, called carbohydrate counting, is basic to basal bolus therapy. In general, bolus-dosing focuses only on the carbohydrate eaten at a particular meal while the other contributions to glucose levels are covered by the basal insulin dosage. The Glycemic Index, which is an attempt to better define the effect of different foods on blood glucose level, provides a first approximation that identifies how to alter the insulin for food. Since glycemic index was never modified specifically for patients with type 1 diabetes, it needs to be individualized for each patient.[44] This level of involvement by the patient is unusual in medicine and may require a patient to adopt a unique psychological approach to diabetes.[45] Knowledge by itself is insufficient and is only an initial step to achieve the goal. The patient needs to understand how to integrate that knowledge into behavior. No single profession is capable of providing all the expertise the patient needs for this system to work. Therefore, modern therapy calls for the diabetes team in the treatment of the patient with type 1 diabetes.[46] At the minimum, such a team consists of a physician, diabetes nurse specialist and nutritionist. Ideally, these individuals should all work together in the same facility. When this is not possible, it is critical that they remain in frequent communication and all changes in the treatment regimen made by one member of the team are discussed with the other members of the team. Additional team members often include psychologists, social workers and exercise physiologists.

INSULIN THERAPY DURING SURGERY

Meticulous control of blood glucose during the perioperative period is desirable to avoid the dual risks of hyperglycemia and hypoglycemia. The former exacerbates the risks of electrolyte imbalance, delayed wound healing and prolonged length of stay. The latter is difficult to identify in an anesthetized patient, increasing the potential for an adverse surgical event. The type 1 patient undergoing surgery will require both insulin and glucose replacement to prevent metabolic decompensation. The patient's usual daily dose of insulin should be reduced since the meal-related component of the dose is not required. Emotional stress and a sympathetic discharge are associated with surgery. Therefore, glucose production by the liver is likely to be enhanced and glucose uptake by the muscles reduced, which leads to an increased basal requirement. Appropriate insulin replacement can be assured by prescribing the basal insulin as Q8h subcutaneous delivery of intermediate insulin. By adding small amounts of Regular, either subcutaneously or by intravenous bolus, the ambient blood sugar can be maintained at a range of 100mg – 200mg/dl. Alternatively, the subcutaneous insulin regime can be suspended and an insulin drip initiated at a rate of 0.5 to 1.0 units per hour. With either regime, the patient should also receive an infusion of D5W at 125ml/hr to prevent starvation ketosis. Frequent blood glucose monitoring (Q1h) and assessment of urinary ketones are necessary to titrate each therapy. The duration of the therapy depends on the patient's clinical status. Once the patient is able to ingest food, the usual regime should be initiated. Caution is needed to assure that the initial dose of subcutaneous insulins is given at least 30 to 60 minutes *before* discontinuing the infusion.

HYPOGLYCEMIA

One problem identified in the DCCT was the increased incidence of hypoglycemia associated with improved glycemic control.[47] In the DCCT, there were approximately 61.2 episodes of severe hypoglycemia per 100 patient years in the intensive group versus 18.7 episodes per 100 patient years in the conventional group. Severe hypoglycemia was defined as an event that required the assistance of another person. While the risks of hypoglycemia are real when glucose targets are set as near normal, there is data suggesting that insulin algorithms that utilize the newer insulins (Lispro insulin versus Regular insulin) result in less hypoglycemia for the same level of glycemic control.[48] Additionally, there is data that Glargine results in less hypoglycemia then NPH insulin.[49]

The equally important observation from the DCCT is that many of the patients who have the greatest incidence of severe hypoglycemia do so because of hypoglycemia unawareness. Hypoglycemia unawareness is a condition characterized by the lack of warning signs of hypoglycemia. The response to hypoglycemia is known to occur in two stages. The first is adrenergic, caused by release of epinephrine and presenting as palpitations, sweats, trembling, hunger and fear. The second is neuroglycopenia which may result in impaired consciousness leading to coma. This stage can often be confused with alcohol intoxication. Patients with hypoglycemic unawareness lack the signs typical of the adrenergic phase and slip into neuroglycopenia. Hypoglycemic unawareness can usually be attributed to either of two different causes.[50] The first is a manifestation of autonomic neuropathy and is relatively uncommon. The second is a phenonomen that occurs in patients with frequent episodes of hypoglycemia who lose epinephrine release without developing autonomic neuropathy. Hypoglycemic unawareness caused by frequent episodes of hypoglycemia can be reversed in most cases simply by decreasing the number of episodes of hypoglycemia.[51,52]

PANCREAS AND ISLET TRANSPLANT THERAPY

Pancreas and islet cell transplantation is a complex issue that is usually not managed by the endocrinologists. However, the endocrinologist needs to be aware of the current state of the art in both of these fields since he or she may often be the physician to first initiate discussion of the subject with the patient.

Pancreas transplantation has become a routine procedure in many centers in conjunction with renal transplantation. In general, pancreas transplants fall into three categories in decreasing frequency of performance: simultaneous kidney-pancreas transplant, pancreas transplant after kidney transplant and isolated pancreas transplant. In the first two cases, the patient will require immunosuppressive therapy for the kidney transplant. Since the amount and type of immuno-suppressant is not different for a single or multiple organ transplant, the addition of the transplanted pancreas does not significantly alter the patient risk.[53] In the last case, the risk of immuno-suppression is solely related to the pancreas. In general, while the first two categories are now often standard, the last category is preformed infrequently. When it is performed, it is usually intended to alleviate intractable hypoglycemia that is not responsive to other modes of therapy. Success rates at one year for simultaneous kidney-pancreas transplant are at 90%. The success of pancreas after kidney transplant is somewhat lower.[54]

A key decision in developing pancreas transplantation techniques has involved handling the exocrine pancreatic secretions. Three options have been used, including occlusion of the pancreatic duct, drainage into the bladder and drainage into the intestine. Drainage into the bladder was a popular strategy since it allowed the use of the urinary amylase level to monitor for rejection. The disadvantage of this method, however, was the large volume of fluid lost, including large amounts of bicarbonate, and the irritating nature of the pancreatic secretions to the bladder and external genitalia. As questions have been raised regarding the usefulness of the urinary amylase as indication of rejection, more patients undergo procedures with the enteric drainage of pancreatic secretion.

Islet transplantation has been seen as the eventual goal of therapy for type 1 diabetes. It has the advantage of requiring only minor surgery and allowing the achievement of normal blood sugar values with little risk. The difficulty has been to purify the islets from the pancreatic ascinar cells in a way that leaves them viable and still able to secrete insulin appropriately in response to a rising blood sugar. Until recently, however, there have been only a few isolated incidents of success with islet cell transplant, and then only for a short period of time. Recent work has shown consistent success with islet transplantation using steroid free immuno-suppression regiment.[55] Even if confirmed, there are two issues that will limit the therapy. The first is the availability of human islets. At present, there are only 10,000 pancreases available for transplant per year. Since it takes two to three pancreases per transplant, only between 3,000 and 5,000 patients could be treated per year. Secondarily, the process still requires the use of three separate immuno-suppressive agents. The risk of these drugs limits the use of this procedure to individuals who already have significant morbidity from their diabetes. Methods of developing means of immuno-tolerance not requiring drug therapy are underway along with research to find alternative sources of islets. The new field of stem cell research has in fact focused on provision of islet cell as one of its early goals.

OTHER DRUG THERAPY FOR TYPE 1 DIABETES

Cardiac Disease. The current guidelines, as recommended in the most recent Adult Treatment Panel–III (ATP-III) protocol, suggest that people with diabetes should be treated analogously to individuals who have already had a myocardial infarction.[56] This sets a goal of 100mg/dl for the LDL cholesterol.

Unfortunately, the data associating diabetes with cardiac disease mostly relates to type 2 diabetes. Presumably, individuals with type 1 diabetes do not have the insulin resistance syndrome commonly seen with type 2 diabetes. Nevertheless, it is clear that poorly controlled type 1 diabetes is a risk for cardiac disease. Whether well-controlled type 1 diabetes is a risk for cardiac disease and what defines "well controlled", in this group has not been determined. Until the data is available, caution suggests that the goals for individuals with type 1 diabetes should be the same as those for type 2 diabetes. The same caution suggests that the guidelines for triglyceride and HDL cholesterol levels should also be the same for type 1 and type 2 diabetes. The VA-HIT trial showed benefits from the treatment of hypertriglyceridemia and HDL cholesterol that were comparable to the benefits seen with LDL cholesterol lowering in individuals with diabetes.[57] Since the study included only type 2 diabetics, here again, there is a question whether individuals with well controlled type 1 diabetes who do not have the same dyslipidemia (elevated serum triglycerides and low HDL cholesterol) as individuals with type type 2 diabetes will have the same benefits as shown in the VA-HIT trial.

The same logic concerning cardiac disease suggests that the recommendations for aspirin therapy that apply to individuals with type 2 diabetes should also apply to individuals with type 1 diabetes.[58] The American Diabetes Association (ADA) recommendations do not identify the appropriate dose. Therefore, patients should be advised to take 81 to 325mg day. To minimize the impact on the gastrointestinal system, enteric-coated aspirin should be encouraged.

Renal Disease. The use of ACE inhibitors to slow the progression of renal disease in individuals with diabetes has been standard since 1993, when the benefits of ACE inhibitors were confirmed in a large multi-center study.[59] Many patients are unable to tolerate ACE inhibitors because of the side effect of a cough. The recent RENAL study, confirming similar benefits of angiotensin receptor blockers (ARB's), has justified switching these patients to ARB's.[60] Nevertheless, there are many more studies showing benefits of ACE inhibitors than of ARBs, justifying the continued use of

ACE-inhibitors as the first line of therapy for hypertension and proteinuria in the individual with diabetes.

The more significant current question is the role of ACE inhibitors in the prevention of heart disease in individuals with diabetes and their consequent use in all individuals with diabetes. The HOPE study showed a 22% reduction (p<0.05) in cardiac deaths with the use of ACE inhibitors.[61] This study was carried out in individuals with type 2 diabetes but is thought to apply to individuals with type 1 diabetes as well. The HOPE study has now been essentially confirmed by the ASCAPS/TexCAPS study and suggests that using ACE-inhibitors is a plausible strategy, even in patients without hypertension or microalbuminuria.[62] While such use of ACE inhibitors (or ARB's) is still controversial, it may become standard therapy in the near future.

MONITORING FOR COMPLICATIONS OF DIABETES

While it now appears that for most individuals with type 1 diabetes, complications can be avoided by maintenance of good glycemic control, achievement of tight control is not a certainty over time, nor are all diabetic patients optimally controlled from the onset of their disease. The complications of diabetes can be treated more effectively if identified early. For that reason, the American Medical Association, The Joint Commission on Accreditation of Healthcare Organization and the National Committee for Quality Assurance have joined together and published a consensus statement "Coordinated Performance Measurement for the Management of Adult Diabetes". The sponsors have relied heavily on the recommendations of the American Association of Clinical Endocrinologists (AACE) and the American Diabetes Association (ADA). They have recommended the following schedule of testing for complications.

Ophthalmologic. The ADA recommends a dilated comprehensive eye exam by an ophthalmologist or optometrist who is knowledgeable and experienced in the management of diabetic retinopathy at initial visit and annually for all patients aged 10 years and older who had had diabetes for three to five years; all patients diagnosed after the age of 30 years and any patient with visual symptoms or abnormalities. In addition, poorly controlled patients or those undergoing the initiation and stabilization of treatment may need to be seen by a physician on a quarterly basis. In such cases, the quarterly visit should include a funduscopy and appropriate referral if retinopathy is detected. The AACE guidelines suggest that an ophthalmologist, rather than optometrist, treat the patient.

Renal. The ADA recommends that a routine urinalysis should be performed in all individuals with type 1 diabetes with onset of puberty and after 5 years duration. If the urinalysis is negative for protein, the urine should be screened for microalbumin and then repeated annually. The AACE recommends that the initial assessment include a urinalysis, test for microalbuminuria and creatinine clearance.

Foot Exam. Both the ADA and AACE recommend that a foot examination (visual inspection, sensory exam and pulse exam) be performed during initial assessment. The AACE recommends that the foot examination be part of every follow up visit that should occur quarterly. The ADA recommends an annual foot examination that should include protective sensation, foot structure and biomechanics, vascular status and skin integrity. The ADA does recommend that people with high risk foot conditions be evaluated more frequently and, if neuropathy is present, they should have visual inspection of their feet at every contact with a health professional.

SUMMARY

Insulin therapy for the patient with type 1 diabetes requires a prescription that mimics normal insulin physiology. Since no two individuals are alike, it is not surprising that there are so many different insulin prescriptions. Before designing an insulin regime for these patients, one needs to query the patients about the details of their lifestyle. Are they regimented and willing to maintain a consistent schedule of eating, activity and insulin or do they want or need to vary their schedules daily? If they are more consistent, it is possible to utilize a basic insulin plan. However, if they are variable in their activities of daily living, then they require a more complex insulin prescription.

Creative and flexible insulin plans can accommodate variability in daily activities. However, they increase the likelihood that the patients' blood glucose levels will be unpredictable. Therefore, when flexibility is increased, patients must become more actively involved in the daily management of the disease. In other words, more blood glucose monitoring, record keeping and data analysis are necessary. If patients want to keep their involvement to a minimum, it might be necessary to utilize the more rigid insulin plans that have obvious disadvantages.

REFERENCES

1. DCCT Trial Research Group. the effect of intensive treatment of diabetes mellitus on development and progression of long term complications in insulin dependent diabetes. N Engl J Med 329:977-86, 1993.
2. Skyler JS. Tactics for type 1 diabetes. Endocrinol Metab Clin North Am 26:647-57, 1997.

3. Hirsch IB. Intensive insulin treatment of type 1 diabetes. Med Clin North Am 82:689-719, 1998.
4. Rosenzweig JL. Principles of insulin therapy. In Kahn CR, Weir GC, Joslin EP, Eds. Joslin's Diabetes mellitus. 13th ed., Philadelphia: Lea & Febiger, Philadelphia 460-88, 1994.
5. Binder C, Lauritzen T, Faber O, Pramming S. Insulin pharmacokinetics. Diabetes Care 7:188-99, 1984.
6. Davis SN, Granner DK. In *Goodman & Gilman's The Pharmacological Basis of Therapeutics*. 9th ed., 1487-1517, 1996.
7. McCance DR, Hanson RL, Charles M, Jacobsson LT, Petitt DJ, Bennett PH, Knowler WC. Comparison of tests for glycated haemoglobin and fasting and two hour plasma glucose concentrations in diagnostic methods for diabetes. Brit Med J 308:1323-1328, 1994.
8. Bastyr EJ, Stuart CA, Brodows RG, Schwartz S, Graf CJ, Zagar A, Robertson KE. Therapy focused on lowering postprandial glucose, not fasting glucose, may be superior for lowering HbA1c. Diabetes Care 23:1236-1241, 2000.
9. Ciofetta M, Lalli C, Del Sindaco P, et al. Contribution of postprandial versus interprandial blood glucose to HbA1c in type 1 diabetes on physiologic intensive therapy with lispro insulin at mealtime. Diabetes Care 22:795-800, 1999.
10. The absence of glycemic threshold for the development of long term complications: the perspective of the Diabetes Control and Complications Trial. Diabetes 44:1289-98, 1996.
11. Jovanovic L. Rational for prevention and treatment of postprandial glucose-mediated toxicity. Endocrinologist 9:87-92, 1999.
12. European Diabetes Epidemiology Group. Is fasting glucose sufficient to define diabetes? Epidemiological data from 20 European studies. The DECODE-study group. Diabetes Epidemiology: Collaborative analysis of Diagnostic Criteria in Europe. Diabetologia 42:647-654, 1999.
13. The Diabetes Control and Complications Trial/Epidemiology of Diabetes Interventions and Complications Research Group. Retinopathy and nephropathy in patients with type 1 diabetes four years after a trial of intensive therapy. N Engl J Med 342(6): 381-389, 2000.
14. Updike SJ, Shults MC, Gilligan BJ, Rhodes RK. A subcutaneous glucose sensor with improved longevity, dynamic range, and stability of calibration. Diabetes Care 23:208-214, 2000.
15. Maran A, Crepaldi C, Tiengo A, et al. Continuous subcutaneous glucose monitoring in diabetic patients: a multicentric evaluation. Program and abstracts of the 36th Annual Meeting of the European Association for the Study of Diabetes; September 17-21, 2000; Jerusalem, Israel. Abstract 791.

16. Ilic S, Jovanovic L, Jeng L. What is the optimal postprandial glucose monitoring system in gestational diabetes? Program and abstracts of the 36th Annual Meeting of the European Association for the Study of Diabetes; September 17-21, 2000; Jerusalem, Israel. Abstract 820.

17. Baron AB, Bolli,GB. Use of rapid-acting insulin to restore physiologic insulin levels: avoidance of postprandial hyperglycemia and hypoglycemia http://diabetes.medscape.com/Medscape/ Endocrinology/treatmentUpdate/2000/tu02/public/toc-tu02.html

18. Holleman F, Schmitt H, Rottiers R, Rees A, Symanowski S, Anderson JH. Reduced frequency of severe hypoglycemia and coma in well-controlled IDDM patients treated with insulin lispro. The Benelux-UK Insulin Lispro Study Group. Diabetes Care 20:1827-1832, 1997.

19. Gale EA. A randomized, controlled trial comparing insulin lispro with human soluble insulin in patients with type 1 diabetes on intensified insulin therapy. The UK Trial Group. Diabet Med 17:209-214, 2000.

20. Bolli GB, Di Marchi RD, Park GD, Pramming S, Koivisto VA. Insulin analogues and their potential in the management of diabetes mellitus. Diabetologia 42:1151-1167, 1999.

21. Del Sidaco P, Cioffetta M, Lalli C, Periello G, Pampanelli S, Torlone E, et al. Use of short-acting insulin analogue lispro in intensive treatment of type 1 diabetes: importance of appropriate replacement of basal insulin and time–interval injection–meal. Diabet Med 15: 592-600, 1998.

22. Ahmed AB, Mallias J, Home PD. Optimization of evening insulin dose in patients using the short-acting insulin analog lispro. Diabetes Care 21:1162-1166, 1998.

23. Raskin P, Guthrie RA, Leiter L, Riis A, Jovanovic L. Use of insulin aspart, a fast-acting insulin analog, as the mealtime insulin in the management of patients with type 1 diabetes. Diabetes Care 23:583-588, 2000.

24. Hirsch IB. Diabetes mellitus and the use of flexible insulin regimens. Am J Fam Physician 60:23343-56, 1999.

25. Dimitriadis GD, Gerich JE. Importance of timing of premeal subcutaneous insulin administration in the management of diabetes mellitus. Diabetes Care 6:374-7, 1983.

26. Implementation of treatment protocols in the Diabetes Control and Complications Trial. Diabetes Care 18:361-76, 1995.

27. Scholtz HE, Van Niekerk N, Meyer BH, et al. An assessment of the variability in the pharmacodynamics (glucose lowering effect) of HOE901 compared to NPH and Ultralente human insulins using the euglycaemic clamp technique. Diabetologia 42(suppl 1). Abstract 882, 1999.

28. Bolli GB,Perriello G, Fannelli CG. DeFeo P. Nocturnal blood glucose control in type 1 diabetes mellitus. Diabetes Care 16 (Suppl 3) 71-89, 1993.

29. Francis AJ, Home PD, Hanning I, Alberti KG, Tunbridge WM. Intermediate-acting insulin given at bedtime: effect on blood glucose concentrations before and after breakfast. Brit Med J (Clin Res) 286:1173-6, 1983.

30. Forlani G, Santacroce G, Ciavarella A, et al. Effects of mixing short- and intermediate-acting insulins on absorption course and biological effect of short-acting preparation. Diabetes Care 9:587-590, 1986.

31. Davis SN, Granner DK. In *Goodman & Gilman's The Pharmacological Basis of Therapeutics*. 9th ed., 1487-1517, 1996.

32. Buse J. Insulin glargine (HOE901)—first responsibilities:understanding the data and ensuring safety (editorial comment). Diabetes Care 23:576-8, 2000.

33. Implementation of treatment protocols in the Diabetes Control and Complications Trial. Diabetes Care 18:361-76, 1995.

34. Farkas-Hirsch R, ed. Intensive diabetes management. 2d ed. Alexandria, Va: American Diabetes Association, 1998.

35. Brackenridge BP. Carbohydrate gram counting: a key to accurate mealtime bonuses in intensive diabetes therapy. Pract Diabetol 1:2228, 1992.

36. Dillinger J, Yass C. Carbohydrate counting in the management of diabetes. Diabetes Educ 21:547-552, 1995.

37. Genuth SM. The automatic (regular insulin) sliding scale. Clin Diabetes 12:40-2, 1994.

38. Walsh J, Roberts R. Setting and testing basal rates. *In Pumping Insulin*. San Diego, Torrey Pines Press, p54, 1994.

39. Boland EA, Grey M, Oesterle A, Fredrickson L, Tamborlane WV. Continuous subcutaneous insulin infusion. A new way to lower risk of severe hypoglycemia, improve metabolic control, and enhance coping in adolescents with type 1 diabetes. Diabetes Care 22:1779-1784, 1999.

40. Farkas-Hirsch R, Hirsch IB. Continuous subcutaneous insulin infusion: a review of the past and its implementation for the future. Diabetes Spectrum 7:80-84, 136-138, 1994.

41. Campbell PJ, Bolli GB, Cryer PE, Gerich JE. Pathogenesis of dawn phenomenon in patients with insulin depenedent diabetes mellitus, accelerated glucose production and impaired glucose utilization due to nocturanal surges in growth hormone secretion. N Engl J Med 312:1473-9, 1985.

42. Koivisto VA, Yki-Jarvin H, Helve E, et al. Pathogenesis and prevention of the dawn phenomenon in diabetic patients treated with CSII. Diabetes 35:78-82, 1986.

43. Frei T, Liebl A, Renner R, Hepp KD.Continuous intraperitoneal insulin infusion (CIPII) via the umbilical vein (CIUII) in type 1 diabetic patients: first results. Program and abstracts of the 36th Annual Meeting of the European Association for the Study of Diabetes; September 17-21, Jerusalem, Israel. Abstract 190, 2000.

44. Wolever TM, Day-to-day consistency in amount and source of carbohydrate associated with improved blood glucose control in type 1 diabetes. J Am Coll Nutr 18(3): 242-7, 1999.

45. Anderson RM, Funnell MM, Butler PM, Arnold MS. Fitzgerald JT, Feste CC. Patient empowerment. Results of a randomized control trial. Diab Care 18:943-9, 1995.

46. Skyler JS. Insulin treatment. In Lebovitz HE, ed. Therapy for diabetes mellitus and related disorders. 3d ed. Alexandria, VA, American Diabetes Association 186-203, 1998.

47. The Diabetes Control and Complications Trial Research Group: Hypoglycemia in the Diabetes Control and Complications Trial. Diabetes 46:271-286, 1997.

48. Brunelle RL, Llewelyn J, Anderson JH Jr, Gale EA, Koivisto VA. Meta-analysis of the effect of insulin lispro on severe hypoglycemia in patients with type 1 diabetes. Diabetes Care 21:1726-31, 1998.

49. Baker ABE, Home PD. The effect of insulin analog on nighttime glucose control in type 1 diabetic patients. Diabetes Care 21:32-37, 1998.

50. Cryer PE. Iatrogenic hypoglycemia as a cause of hypoglycemia-associated autonomic failure in IDDM: A vicious cycle. Diabetes 41:255-260, 1992.

51. Dagogo-Jack SE, Rattarasarn C, Cryer PE. Reversal of Hypoglycemia unawareness but not defective glucose counterregulation in IDDM. Diabetes 43:1426-1434, 1994.

52. Fanelli CG, Epifano L, Rambotti AM, et al. Meticulous prevention of hypoglycemia normalizes the glycemic thresholds and magnitude of most neuroendocrine responses to, symptoms of and cognitive function during hypoglycemia in intensively treated patients with short-term IDDM. Diabetes 42:1683-1689, 1993.

53. Humar A, Gruessner R, Sutherland D. Living related donor panreas and pancreas-kidney transplantation. Br Med Bull 53: 879-891, 1997.

54. Farney AC, Cho E, Schweitzer EJ, Dunkin B, Philosophe B, Collonna J, Jacobs S, Jarrell B, Flowers JL, Bartlett ST. Simultaneous cadaver pancreas living-donor kidney transplantation: a new approach for the type 1 diabetic uremic patient. Annals of Surgery 232:696-703, 2000.

55. Ryan EA, Lakey JR, Rajotte RV, Korbutt GS, Kin T, Imes S, Rabinovitch Elliott JF, Bigam D, Kneteman NM, Warnock GL, Larssen I, Shapiro AM. Clinical outcomes and insulin secretion after islet transplantation with the Edmonton protocol. Diabetes 50(4):710-719, 2001.

56. Cholesterol Education Program (NCEP) Expert Panel on Detection, Evaluation, and Treatment of High Blood Cholesterol in Adults (Adult treatment panel iii). JAMA 285:2486-2497, 2001.

57. Rubins HB. Conclusions from the VA-HIT study (editorial). Am J Cardiol 86(5): 543-4, 2000.

58. American Diabetes Association. Clinical practice recommendations 2001aspirin therapy in diabetes. Diabetes Care 24 (Suppl 1): S62-64, 2001.
59. Lewis EJ, Hunsicker LC, Bain RP, Rohde RD. The effect of angiotensin-converting enzyme inhibition on diabetic nephropathy. N Engl J Med 329:1456-62, 1993.
60. Coats AJ. Angiotensin receptor blockers – finally the evidence is coming in. Int J Cardiol 79(2-3:99-103, 2001.
61. Hegele RA. Angiotensin-converting enzyme (ACE) inhibition in the secondary prevention of vascular disease: the Heart Outcomes Prevention Evaluation (HOPE) Trial and its substudies. Curr Atheroscler Rep 2(5):361-2, 2000.
62. Downs JR, Clearfield M, Tyroler HA, Whitney EJ, Kruyer W, Langendor Zagrebelsky V, Weis S, Shapiro DR, Beere PA, Gotto AM. Air Force/Texas Coronary Atherosclerosis Prevention Study (AFCAPS/ TEXCAPS): additional perspectives on tolerability of long-term treatment with lovastatin. Am J Cardiol 87(9):1074-1079, 2001.

Chapter 6. Therapy of Type 2 Diabetes Mellitus

Zachary Bloomgarden

THERAPEUTIC GOALS

Given the relationship between glycemia and the complications of diabetes, a number of recommendations have been put forward regarding the goals of glycemic control for patients with diabetes. The most commonly cited are those of the American Diabetes Association, which has given three ascending sets of levels, those to be considered "normal," those to be used as the "goal" for patients with diabetes, and those above which additional measures are clearly thought to be recommended (Table 1).

Table 1. Glycemic control for people with diabetes*

	Normal	Goal	Additional action suggested
Whole blood values			
Average preprandial glucose (mg/dl)	<100	80-120	<80/> 140
Average bedtime glucose (mg/dl)	<110	100-140	<100/>160
Plasma values			
Average preprandial glucose (mg/dl)	<110	90-130	<90/>150
Average bedtime glucose (mg/dl)	<120	110-150	<110/>180
HbA1c (%)	<6	<6	>8

*The values shown in this table are by necessity generalized to the entire population of individuals with diabetes. Patients with comorbid diseases, the very young and older adults, and others with unusual conditions or circumstances may warrant different treatment goals. These values are for nonpregnant adults. "Additional action suggested" depends on individual patient circumstances. Such actions may include enhanced diabetes self-management education, comanagement with a diabetes team, referral to an endocrinologist, change in pharmacological therapy, initiation of or increase in SMBG, or more frequent contact with the patient HbA1c is referenced to a nondiabetic range of 4.0-6.0% (mean 5.0%, 5D 0.5%). Measurement of capillary blood glucose. Values calibrated to plasma glucose.

Thus, for HbA1c, the normal level is given as below 6%, the desirable goal, based on the level achieved in the intensive treatment group of the DCCT, as below 7%, and the level above which the treating physician must strongly consider additional measures as values above 8%.[1] Recent recommendations have suggested even lower goal for HbA1c levels, that of below 6.5%.[2] Unfortunately, these glycemic goals are not regularly attained in clinical practice. In a cross-sectional analysis of individuals with diabetes in the United States, only 27% and 38% of those treated with insulin and with oral agents had HbA1c <7%, while 51% and 42% of these groups had HbA1c >8%.[3]

Lifestyle changes / Psychosocial factors

Exercise represents an important approach to the treatment of diabetes. The 1994 Behavioral Risk Factor Surveillance System data indicate that in every state surveyed, however, most adults do not engage in regular physical activity.[4] In the United States, 56% of men and 61% of women either never or irregularly engage in physical activity,[5] with 37% of overweight persons reporting no physical activity whatsoever during their leisure time.[6] These factors apply to patients with diabetes. In studies of more than 800 Mexican-American men and women free of diabetes at baseline who participated in the San Antonio Heart Study follow-up, leisure physical activity in men was inversely associated and alcohol consumption, weight control by dieting, and BMI were positively associated with type 2 diabetes. In women, BMI was positively associated with type 2 diabetes and was the strongest lifestyle predictor. Physical activity and weight control by dieting were associated with decreased type 2 diabetes risk in women. Saturated fat and cholesterol avoidance, grams of alcohol consumed per week, and energy intake were also negatively and indirectly associated with type 2 diabetes in women by means of their direct effects on BMI.[7]

Data from the 1989-1990 Australian National Health Survey showed diabetes to be associated with decreased levels of exercise in women, although not in men, along with the expected increased prevalence of obesity, cardiovascular disease, and frequency of hospital admissions, use of outpatient services, and general practitioner consultations.[8] Tessier and colleagues studied obese patients with well-controlled type 2 diabetes enrolled in an exercise program.[9] On the day of the last exercise session, fasting insulin levels and the insulin/glucose ratio were well below baseline as insulin sensitivity improved. These parameters 48 hours later had almost tripled, however, suggesting that the improvement wanes rapidly and that type 2 diabetic patients have to exercise daily for optimal benefit.

A fascinating study compared 35 members of a population of Pima ancestry living in a remote mountainous location in northwestern Mexico with sex-, age- and diabetes status-matched Pimas living in Arizona. Mexican Pimas were more than 25 kg lighter, with average BMI of 24.9 vs 33.4 kg/m^2 in Arizona Pimas. Only two women and one man had type 2 diabetes, contrasting with the expected prevalences of 37% and 54% in age-matched female and male Arizona Pimas. This study suggests a relationship between traditional lifestyle in individuals living in less affluent environments and the lack of diabetes, despite a similar potential genetic predisposition.[10] Another determinant of exercise is social class, with higher social class, as measured by educational level, predicting greater levels of physical activity among individuals with diabetes.[11]

The majority of patients with diabetes, although believing diabetes to be a serious condition, nevertheless fail to follow medical advice about lifestyle modification.[12] Decreased patient satisfaction with health care and with the interpersonal manner of their physicians is common, both in overall patient populations and among patients who are particularly ill. These measures are due to a complex of social and environmental determinants; are also predictive of cigarette smoking, obesity, and overall risk-factor prevalence;[13]

and correlate with decreased compliance with treatment[14,15] and with poorer levels of glycemic control. Anxiety may be another emotional characteristic affecting the control of diabetes. In a study of anxious patients, a 0.8% greater reduction in glycated hemoglobin level was seen with alprazolam, 2 mg daily, than with placebo.[16]

It is noteworthy that a number of recent studies have shown that programs of lifestyle modification are useful in the prevention of diabetes. The Diabetes Prevention Program recruited 3234 individuals whose fasting blood glucose was between 95 and 125 mg/dl, and whose blood glucose 2 hours after ingesting 75 g glucose was between 140 and 199 mg/dl. They were assigned to a program of intensive lifestyle management (exercising 2 ½ hours weekly and attempting to lose 7% of body weight if overweight), to metformin 850 mg twice daily, or to standard care plus a placebo. Over 3 years, 5, 8, and 11% of the three groups developed diabetes.[17] Similar data were reported from studies in Finland[18] and China.[19]

PHARMACOLOGIC THERAPY

This review will address existing treatment approaches. This is a constantly changing field, and new therapeutic modalities, including insulin secretagogues, insulin sensitizers, and novel insulin delivery systems are being developed and will undoubtedly play an important role in the future.

Sulfonylureas (SU)

Glucose uptake by pancreatic islet beta cells leads to adenosine triphosphate (ATP) generation. The increase in cellular ATP levels closes potassium channels (K_{ATP} channels), depolarizing the cells and leading to opening of calcium channels. Increases in cytoplasmic calcium stimulate insulin secretion. SU act by binding to the SU receptor (SUR) adjacent to the K_{ATP} channel, activating this chain of events and causing insulin secretion.[20] Two SUR have been identified, SUR1 and SUR2. SUR1 is found primarily in the beta cells of the pancreas and in the central nervous system. The beta cell K_{ATP} channel is composed of the pore-forming potassium inward rectifier (Kir) 6.2 subunit and the larger SUR1 subunit, which displays high SU affinity and has two sequences showing nucleotide binding. The pore-forming unit has two transmembrane domains linked by a sequence that lines the potassium channel. When expressed, four SUR1 and four Kir 6.2 units link together to form the actual transporter, the Kir subunits around the central channel and the SUR1 subunits arranged at the outer circumference.[21]

SU may also increase plasma insulin levels by decreasing clearance of insulin.[22] There is evidence that SU improve insulin action as well. A crossover study comparing 3 months of glipizide treatment with 3 months of insulin treatment showed higher plasma insulin and C-peptide levels during oral tolerance testing while patients were receiving insulin, as well as higher fasting plasma insulin levels.[23] This leads to the question of whether there are extrapancreatic effects of some or all SU. In vivo, in dogs, after single approximately equipotent blood glucose–decreasing doses, the SU glimepiride increases insulin less than does glipizide, which in turn has a lesser insulin-increasing effect than does glyburide. Studies in hyperglycemic hyperinsulinemic KK-Ay mice under once-daily treatment for 8 weeks showed that glimepiride reduced blood glucose by 40% and HbA1c by 33%, while also decreasing plasma insulin by 50%, whereas glyburide and gliclazide had no effect on these parameters. In vitro, glimepiride and, to a lesser extent, glyburide, also had extrapancreatic effects. In the absence of insulin, both stimulated glucose transport--up to 60% of the maximum insulin response in the rat diaphragm and up to 35% in 3T3 adipocytes. Glycogenesis was stimulated in the rat diaphragm by up to 55% of the maximum insulin effect, and lipogenesis in 3T3 adipocytes by up to 40%. Human studies also have shown that glimepiride potentiates insulin action. These direct insulin-mimetic effects may rely on the induction of GLUT4 translocation from internal stores to the plasma membrane and on the activation of glycogen synthase and glycerol-3-phosphate acyltransferase. The direct effects of SU may ultimately be regulated by a glycosyl-phosphatidylinositol–specific phospholipase C, which is activated by glimepiride in rat adipocytes. Lipolytic cleavage products thereby generated from glycolipidic structures may in turn stimulate specific protein phosphatases, which activate key regulatory proteins/enzymes of glucose and lipid metabolism.[24]

In addition to the beta cells, the heart and vascular tissues have SU receptors and K_{ATP} channels, which may act to protect the myocardium against ischemic damage. Closing of these channels by SU provides a mechanism that could increase coronary disease mortality. A combination of Kir 6.2 with SUR2A is found in cardiac and skeletal muscle, and Kir 6.2, as well as a related protein, Kir 6.1, are found in combination with SUR2B in vascular smooth muscle. The affinity of SU for SUR2A in cardiac tissues is lower than that for SUR1 in the beta-cell. However, animal studies of the effects of glyburide show increased vascular resistance, decreased blood flow, interference with the protective phenomenon of postischemic vasodilatation, and evidence of increased ischemic damage. In humans, there is also evidence of increased systemic vascular resistance, decreased postischemic vasodilatation, and decreased diazide-induced vasodilatation.

Interestingly, different sulfonylureas appear to have different relative binding affinities for SUR1 vs SUR2A, with glyburide having the greatest relative binding affinity for SUR2A. For the rapid-acting secretagogues (vide infra), nateglinide appears to have little affinity for SUR2A, while repaglinide has affinity for SUR2A similar to that of glyburide. Although effects have been demonstrated in experimental ischemia by acutely administering these drugs, it is uncertain whether this applies in individuals with coronary ischemia who are treated with SU in therapeutic doses.[25] Ongoing studies to ascertain whether adverse cardiac effects exist will be of clinical importance.

This important question was addressed in part by the United Kingdom Prospective Diabetes Study (UKPDS) in assessing whether there was a difference between insulin and SU.[26] 896 patients randomized to conventional treatment, 619 treated with chlorpropamide, 615 with glyburide, and 911 with insulin were compared. At 10 years, FBG levels were 175, 160, 155, and 140 mg/dl, with HbA1c 9.0%, 7.9%, 8.1%, and 7.7%. Weight had increased from baseline 2.5, 5, 5, and 7.5 kg. Severe hypoglycemia did not occur with conventional treatment but was seen in around 0.5% of the two SU groups and in around 2% of the insulin treated patients annually. With chlorpropamide, a 4 mm Hg higher systolic and 2 mm Hg higher diastolic blood pressure was seen during the study period. No significant differences were seen between the SU and insulin in total diabetes-related endpoints, diabetes-related mortality, myocardial infarction, microvascular endpoints, retinopathy, or microalbuminuria.

It is interesting to note, in this regard, that SU are highly effective at relatively low doses, and that current maximal recommended dosages probably exceed those required for optimal treatment. A study of glipizide at doses of 10 mg daily, 10 mg twice daily, or 20 mg twice daily for 3 months each, for example, showed mean home glucose levels of 173, 165, and 160 mg/dl on the three dosages. The insulin response to a test meal was greatest after 10 mg/d of glipizide and least after 40 mg/d, suggesting that more than 10 to 20 mg daily produces little or no benefit and may paradoxically reduce beta-cell function.[27] The controlled-release glipizide-GITS (gastrointestinal transit system) preparation may offer particular benefit in allowing somewhat greater degrees of glycemic control with less insulin stimulation than immediate-release glipizide.[28] In an 8-week study, the maximal glycemic response for patients with FBG over 250 mg/dL required a glipizide-GITS dosage of 20 mg daily, while patients with FBG below this level responded optimally to a dosage of 5 mg daily. There was no weight gain with dosages up to 60 mg daily, with symptoms of hypoglycemia seen in 2.9% of patients.[29] Similar arguments have been advanced to suggest that daily dosages of glyburide should not exceed 5 to 10 mg. Peters and Davidson reported in treating patients with markedly symptomatic type 2 diabetes that the majority of patients can be maintained on a daily dose of glyburide of 10 mg or less, although higher doses may play a role in initial treatment.[30]

Replacing insulin with SU rather than discontinuing treatment can be useful in diabetics entering apparent remission. Banerji et al reported such a strategy in patients with initially insulin-requiring diabetes mellitus who had gone into remission, utilizing chronic low-dose SU therapy with glipizide 2.5 mg/d.[57] Thirty African American patients with type 2 diabetes, who had developed near-normoglycemia, were followed with no treatment or were randomly assigned to a 3-year, double-blind glipizide or placebo treatment. Baseline FPG and HbA1c were 107 mg/dL and 4.7%, respectively. Relapse to hyperglycemia, defined as an FPG level >140 mg/dL, occurred in 60% of those not treated but in 20% in the glipizide treatment group.[31] Another important strategy, discussed below (see "combination treatment" section), is the addition of insulin to SU in the treatment of patients with insufficient response to SU alone.

Hypoglycemia is an important consideration when assessing SU therapy. Data from the Tennessee Medicaid Program on a total of 13,963 Medicaid enrollees 65 years of age or older, who were prescribed one of six SU from 1985 to 1989, identified 255 persons with a first episode of serious hypoglycemia during 20,715 person-years of SU use. The rate of serious hypoglycemia was highest in glyburide users at 16.6 per 1,000 person-years and lowest among users of tolbutamide at 3.5 per 1,000 person-years. Users of tolbutamide, tolazamide, and glipizide had lower risks of serious hypoglycemia than did users of chlorpropamide, whereas the risk of serious hypoglycemia among glyburide users did not differ from that of chlorpropamide users. Among second-generation SU, the adjusted relative risk of severe hypoglycemia among glyburide users, compared with glipizide users, was increased 1.9-fold.[32] Population studies have similarly shown lower hypoglycemia frequencies with glimepiride than with glyburide.

Rapidly acting insulin secretagogues

Two additional insulin secretagogues acting at the SUR have been developed. They are nateglinide, an amino acid analogue derived from D-phenylalanine, and repaglinide, a meglitinide showing structural similarity to the non-sulfonylurea moiety of glyburide. Nateglinide has structural similarity to the sulfonylurea and repaglinide to the benzamido portion of glyburide, with nateglinide having different effects in closing the K_{ATP} channel from repaglinide, suggesting that these agents may act differently on SUR1. The affinity of nateglinide for SUR1 is 20-fold lower than that of repaglinide, and there is some evidence that nateglinide may also act through mechanisms other than via SUR and the K_{ATP} channel, such as through changes in intracellular calcium.[33] Both show selectivity of binding to beta cell rather than cardiac SUR.[34] Both show rapid absorption and short plasma half life, contributing to their meal-related potentiation of insulin secretion, and hence have lower incidence of hypoglycemia than seen with sulfonylureas, which have 24-hour action.

Nateglinide is absorbed more rapidly when taken with food, but should be administered just before meals, as the brief plasma half life and rapid turnover at the beta cell SUR allow it to mimic the first phase insulin secretory response to ingested carbohydrate, providing insulin during the period of its maximal efficacy. Its half life is 2.9 hours. The agent has been shown to reduce HbA1c levels to an extent similar to that of metformin, with better response to the two in combination.[35] Other studies with alpha glucosidase inhibitors and thiazolidinediones have shown additive benefit.

Repaglinide shows peak absorption within 1 hour, and a half life in circulation of 1 hour, with a 20% decrease in peak concentration achieved when taken with food.[36] It, too, has been shown to be effective when administered in combination with a variety of other oral antidiabetic agents.

Metformin

Metformin is a biguanide oral hypoglycemic medication that is now widely used in the treatment of type 2 diabetes in the United States.[37] It increases sensitivity to insulin, particularly at the liver, although a definite understanding of its mechanism of action is not yet available. Consistent improvements in triglyceride levels are seen with this agent, and there may be benefits in decreasing LDL and increasing HDL levels.[60] In clinical trials, metformin causes a 50 to 100/mg/dL fall in blood glucose and about a 1% to 2% fall in glycohemoglobin levels. Similar benefit can be seen in patients with an insufficient response to SU alone who are treated with the addition of metformin.[38]

Metformin was one of the drugs used, although as monotherapy only in obese patients, in the UKPDS.[39] Initial results from this study have shown that weight gain is greater with insulin and SU than with diet or with metformin, and fasting insulin levels, which increased with insulin and SU, were stable with diet, and fell with metformin. Hypoglycemia occurred more frequently with insulin than with SU and occurred rarely with diet alone or with metformin. In the metformin substudy of obese patients BMI was 31.6 kg/m2, and other baseline characteristics, including FBG and HbA1c, were similar to those of the overall group. Weight gain with metformin was similar to that with conventional treatment, and less than that with SU or insulin, and there was a lower incidence of severe hypoglycemia than with insulin or SU. The incidence of total diabetes related endpoints with metformin decreased 32% in comparison to that in the conventional treatment group, significantly lower than the 7% reduction in the other intensive treatment groups. There was similarly a 42% lower diabetes related mortality with metformin compared to 20% reduction in the other intensive treatment groups, 36% lower total mortality with metformin compared to 8% reduction in the other intensive treatment groups, and 39% lower myocardial infarction rate with metformin compared to 21% reduction in the other intensive treatment groups. This gives a strong evidence base favoring use of this agent as initial treatment of overweight individuals with diabetes. Indeed, the study authors concluded, "metformin treatment appears to be advantageous as a first-line pharmacological therapy in diet-treated overweight patients with type 2 diabetes. The situation is complex, however, as an additional group of 268 UKPDS patients already treated with SU for whom metformin was added, compared with 269 treated with SU alone, showed an unexpected and significant 60% higher mortality in the combination group. This was suggested by the authors to represent one of the "extremes of the play of chance" rather than true evidence that the combination is disadvantageous.

In randomized controlled studies of 289 patients treated with metformin vs placebo, and of 632 patients treated with metformin and glyburide vs metformin alone vs glyburide alone, metformin monotherapy lowered FBG concentrations to 189 vs 244 mg/dL and glycosylated hemoglobin to 7.1% vs 8.6%. Metformin and glyburide, as compared with either glyburide or metformin alone, similarly lowered FBG concentrations to 187 vs 261 mg/dL and glycosylated hemoglobin to 7.1% vs 8.7%. In both protocols, the patients given metformin had significant decreases in plasma total and low-density lipoprotein cholesterol and plasma triglyceride concentrations.[40] Another study of 48 subjects with type 2 diabetes randomized to receive metformin or glipizide for 1 year showed better glucose control and weight loss rather than weight gain with metformin.[41] It is important to use a sufficient dose of metformin to achieve optimal effect. In a study of 451 diabetic patients treated with 0, 500, 1000, 1500, 2000, or 2500 mg metformin daily, HbA1c decreased 0.8, 1.2, 1.6, 1.9, and 1.5%, suggesting the 2000 mg dose to be optimal.[42] Other studies suggest that some additional benefit may be seen in doses up to 3 g daily, so that further dosage increments may be appropriate for the occasional patient.[43,44]

The major clinical adverse effects of metformin are nausea, seen in about one quarter of patients when treatment is initiated, and diarrhea, seen in about one half. In a study comparing 25 patients treated with 3,000 mg/d of metformin, 25 with 1,500 mg/d, and 23 with placebo, 13 patients were withdrawn from the high-dose treatment group, 8 from the low-dose group, and 2 from the placebo group because of gastrointestinal symptoms.[45] One must therefore use doses over 2 g daily with care, noting that patients who develop adverse symptoms at high doses can often continue to receive some benefit with reductions in the amount administered.

The adverse consequence of metformin of greatest concern is lactic acidosis, which occurs under circumstances of increased plasma metformin concentration when the agent is administered to individuals with decreased renal clearance. It may not be sufficiently appreciated that a number of cationic drugs, including cimetidine, rantidine, digoxin, triamterene, and trimethoprim, eliminated by renal tubular secretion, may have the potential to compete with metformin for renal clearance. Cimetidine has been shown to double metformin levels when the two agents are given to healthy volunteers. Furosemide and nifedipine have both been shown to increase metformin levels by about one quarter after single doses, again in studies of healthy volunteers. These increases are comparable to those seen when metformin is administered to individuals with mild renal insufficiency.[46] The manufacturer currently recommends that the agent not be given to patients requiring pharmacologic treatment for congestive heart failure. In addition, the fall in glomerular filtration rate with age has led to the recommendation that metformin not be used in patients over age eighty unless creatinine clearance has formally been measured.

Both metformin and SU are, then, agents with appreciable potential for adverse effects. Eight hundred forty-three reported cases of SU-induced hypoglycemia had a mortality of 9%, while 42 cases of metformin-associated lactic acidosis had 43% mortality. Forty of the latter cases had documented contraindications, particularly renal impairment, with the remaining two cases due to drug overdosage, one being a suicide. The calculated mortality risks of SU and metformin treatment are 0.0240 and 0.0332 per 1,000 patient-years, respectively. Both groups of drugs should be used with care in type 2 diabetics, particularly in elderly subjects and those with impaired cardiac, renal, or hepatic function.[47]

Alpha glucosidase inhibitors

Acarbose is a pseudotetrasaccharide, binding 1,000 times more avidly than dietary carbohydrates to the intestinal disaccharidases, resulting in a limitation in the postprandial rise of glucose, as well as inhibiting maltase and amylase and decreasing postprandial release of glucagon-like peptide-I (GLP-I) and gastric inhibitory polypeptide (GIP). This effect has persisted at 12 months in clinical studies, with falls in glycohemoglobin by 0.5% to 1.0%, in FBG by 10% to 20%, and in postprandial glucose by 30% to 50%.[48] Acarbose and the related drug miglitol have been reported as having efficacy similar to that of low-dose glyburide in decreasing glucose and HbA1c, without the rise in insulin levels or the possibility of hypoglycemia seen with the latter.[49,50] In Germany, where acarbose has become the most popular prescribed agent in the treatment of type 2 diabetes, post-marketing surveillance of 10,000 patients showed a 1.5% fall in glycohemoglobin, a 40 mg/dL fall in FBG, and a 60 to 80 mg/dL fall in postprandial blood glucose levels. Thus, acarbose appears to be of moderate efficacy for type 2 diabetes.[51] Similar effects have been seen in type 1 diabetes. Adverse effects, usually mild, are frequently seen, with flatulence reported in 20% to 80% of patients in various studies, but with diarrhea occurring less frequently. Abnormal liver chemistries are seen only at doses above the current maximum recommended level of 100 mg three times daily.[52] Greatest effects are seen when the drug is administered immediately prior to the beginning of each meal.[53] The drug does not cause weight loss by inducing malabsorption, but a modest weight decrease, similar to that reported with metformin, is often seen. Combination treatment with metformin,[54] with SU,[55,56] and with insulin[57] leads to additive glucose lowering, with decreases in HbA1c by 0.4% to 0.9% and with reductions in insulin dose requirements. Some studies of patients failing to respond to SU alone suggest that acarbose lowers blood glucose levels less effectively than metformin,[58] while other reports show similar falls in FBG with greater decrements in postprandial glucose levels.[59] It should be recalled that, since other agents may cause hypoglycemia and since sucrose absorption is retarded by acarbose, patients receiving these combinations and developing hypoglycemia must be treated with oral glucose.

A substudy in the UKPDS administered acarbose for a 3-year period. 973 patients were randomized to this treatment and 973 to placebo, with a protocol increasing the dose to 50 mg three times daily over 3 weeks, then to 100 mg three times daily over 4 months. 52% of the patients were treated with SU, insulin, or metformin, 34% with a combination of SU plus metformin, multiple insulin injections, or SU plus insulin, and 14% were on diet alone. The FBG was 160 mg/dl with placebo throughout the 3 year period, 140 mg/dl in the intention-to-treat acarbose group at 1 year, and 150 mg/dl in this group at 3 years. HbA1c was 0.2% lower in the acarbose group. However, compliance was a problem, with 32% of placebo patients but 39% of acarbose patients not taking acarbose during the 3 year period, discontinuation associated with symptoms of flatulence and diarrhea. In patients actually on treatment, HbA1c was 0.5% lower than in the placebo group at 1, 2, and 3 years, similar to the benefit seen with metformin. In this substudy, which was shorter than the overall protocol, there was no change in outcome.[60]

Thiazolidinediones

The thiazolidinediones, a group of insulin sensitizers, enhance insulin action by activating the nuclear peroxisome proliferator activated receptor γ (PPARγ) leading to changes in fatty acid metabolism.[61] The three agents in this class which have been used clinically, rosiglitazone, pioglitazone, and troglitazone, show half-maximal PPARγ binding affinity of 41, 4830, and 7970 nM, proportional to the clinical doses employed of 2-8, 15-45, and 200-600 mg daily.[62] The most notable effect of these agents is in adipocytes, where increased triglyceride synthesis can be demonstrated, along with increased glucose uptake. In vitro studies show increased insulin stimulation of the number and rate of fibroblast conversion into adipocytes.[63] The adipocyte effect leads to a fall in circulating free fatty acids, and it has been theorized that the increase in insulin sensitivity in muscle and, to a lesser extent, in the liver may be caused by an advantageous change in metabolism of these tissues as their degree of "lipotoxicity" decreases.

Alternative suggestions are that thiazolidinediones may change the phenotype of adipocytes in the visceral area of the abdomen to that of subcutaneous fat, thus nullifying one of the principle causes of insulin resistance, or that the agents decrease adipocyte production of cytokines such as tumor necrosis factor-α, which tend to worsen insulin resistance.

A question is whether the potential for adipocyte proliferation may have adverse clinical effect in certain patients. Troglitazone, an agent which has been withdrawn from clinical use because of hepatotoxicity, decreases insulin resistance and hyperinsulinemia, which may be of specific benefit in view of the direct association of insulin resistance with increased coronary artery disease risk.[64] The drug lowers blood glucose, insulin, triglyceride, and blood pressure levels. In 18 patients with type 2 diabetes treated with troglitazone 200 mg twice daily, blood pressure decreased from 164/94 to 146/82 mm Hg, FBG decreased from 159 to 144 mg/dL, and fasting insulin decreased from 9.1 to 6.3 □U/mL. There was a significant correlation between the decrease in blood pressure and that in insulin.[65] In another report of 284 patients with type 2 diabetes, FBG and HbA1c levels fell 24 mg/dL and 0.5% in 136 treated patients but failed to change with placebo. Interestingly, only 46% of the treated patients were classified as responders.[66]

Troglitazone shows additive glycemic benefit when administered in combination with other agents. Ghazzi et al reported a study of 541 patients with type 2 diabetes mellitus with FBG over 140 mg/dl on treatment with micronized glyburide 12 mg daily, randomized to continued glyburide or placebo with addition of troglitazone in dosages of 200, 400, and 600 mg daily. HbA1c increased 1% with 200 mg troglitazone alone, was stable with the 400 and 600 mg dosages, and decreased 1.6%, 1.8%, and 2.7% in patients treated with glyburide plus the three troglitazone dosages. FBG levels were similarly affected, rising 20 mg/dl with troglitazone 200 mg daily alone, and falling 2 and 12 mg/dl with the 400 and 600 mg dosages, but decreasing 54, 61, and 79 mg/dl in patients treated with glyburide plus troglitazone at the three dosages.[67] Inzucchi et al presented a smaller study of 29 patients given combination troglitazone - metformin treatment, with either agent alone showing 20% decreases in FBG levels, and the combination leading to an additional 18% fall.[68] Finally, Schwartz et al reported a study of 350 patients with type 2 diabetes mellitus receiving insulin in dosages of at least 30 units daily, who were randomized to the addition of placebo or troglitazone. HbA1c decreased 0.8% and 1.4%, FBG decreased 35 and 49 mg/dl, and the mean insulin dosage decreased 11 and 29% with 200 mg and 600 mg troglitazone dosages.[69]

There are also data suggesting that the ability of troglitazone to reduce insulin resistance could be useful in preventing type 2 diabetes.[70,71] This may particularly be the case in women with the polycystic ovary syndrome, who also show decreases in the levels of non-sex-hormone-binding globulin-bound testosterone, dehydroepiandrosterone sulfate, estradiol, and estrone with treatment, suggesting a pathogenic role of insulin resistance in the development of this condition.[72] The Troglitazone in Prevention of Diabetes (TRIPOD) study randomized a group of women who had had gestational diabetes, and whose estimated 5-year risk of developing diabetes was 70%, to placebo for 121 and to troglitazone (TGZ) 400 mg daily for 114, with 27 and 29 month follow-up.[73] There was a 60% reduction in diabetes, with a 12.4% annual risk in patients receiving placebo and 5.7% annual risk in those treated with troglitazone. Carotid artery intima-medial thickness in the study showed an increase of .009 vs. .006 mm/year in the placebo vs. troglitazone groups, suggesting another potential benefit. In follow-up, during the first 8 months after stopping treatment, 6 of 40 patients who had received placebo developed diabetes, while only 1 of 41 treated with troglitazone developed disease, suggesting that patients who stop treatment did not "catch-up" but appeared to derive benefit lasting beyond the time of treatment.[74] This observation suggests that an important effect of thiazolidinediones may be found in forthcoming diabetes prevention studies.

Rosiglitazone and pioglitazone have shown efficacy similar to that of troglitazone, with decreases in HbA1c of 0.6-1.2% in monotherapy and in combination with sulphonylureas, metformin, and insulin.[75] A major potential clinical side effect appears to be related to plasma volume expansion. Hemoglobin levels fall on average by 0.5 g, and peripheral edema occurs in 2-4% of persons treated with the thiazolidinediones, a problem particularly in patients receiving insulin, which has led to the recommendation that the agents not be used in those individuals. There remains a recommendation that liver function be monitored during treatment with the drugs, a precaution related to the adverse experience with troglitazone. There is no evidence that either rosiglitazone or pioglitazous is hepatotoxic, however, and when patients with type 2 diabetes do have abnormal liver function it should be recalled that hepatic steatosis is common in this group, and actually improves with thiazolidinedione treatment.

Agents producing weight loss

Clearly, the clinical treatment of overweight patients with diabetes should include a component of weight reduction. Obesity is associated with 1,260 excess deaths per million patient-years per 13-kg weight increase.[76] The 5- to 6-year success rate of diet alone, however, is 2% to 3%.[77] A number of anorexic agents have been shown to improve control of diabetes, but were subsequently withdrawn because of toxicity, including dexfenfluramine[78] and fenfluramine.[79]

The serotonin release inhibitors may be somewhat safer and may offer similar benefit with greater safety. Several randomized studies comparing fluoxetine 60 mg daily with placebo showed improved glycemia in obese patients with diabetes.[80,81] Wise reviewed data from 3,491 obese patients in controlled clinical trials of up to 52 weeks' duration, showing that fluoxetine is effective, well tolerated, and safe in the treatment of obesity and obese diabetics.[82] Sibutramine, another centrally acting agent, inhibits serotonin and norepinephrine reuptake. Potential adverse effects include increases in blood pressure, with diastolic pressures increasing by 10 mm Hg or more in 15-20% of treated patients dry mouth, headache, constipation.[83] Weight loss in patients treated with sibutramine shows a dose response curve, so that with doses of 10 and 15 mg daily, 56 and 65% of patients lose at least 5% and 30 and 38% of patients lose at least 10% of body weight. Modest effects of sibutramine on blood glucose levels in patients with diabetes are, however, discouraging, and long-term studies suggest a falloff in efficacy of these agents over time, with behavioral therapy most useful in the long term, although only for those individuals who persevere.[84]

In addition to the centrally acting drugs, which act by decreasing appetite and increasing satiety, drugs such as methylxanthine, caffeine, ephedrine, and perhaps aspirin increase energy expenditure, and may play a therapeutic role. As with the disaccharidase inhibitors discussed above, inhibitors of intestinal lipase action may be effective in decreasing nutrient absorption, and the agent orlistat is effective in this regard in obese individuals with diabetes.[85] Orlistat inhibits absorption of around 30% of ingested fat, with a recent 2 year study of 743 patients on a hypocaloric diet during year 1 and a weight-maintaining diet during year 2 showing an average weight loss of 10% at 1 year and 8% at 2 years, but a maximum weight loss with placebo of 6% of initial body weight. Weight, waist circumference, lipid profile, and glucose tolerance improved through two years, with 79.8% of patients reporting oily spotting, flatus with discharge, and fecal urgency, generally mild and transient and responding to decreases in fat intake, with mild fall in 25-OH-vitamin D without change in bone density, and without other nutritional deficit. Glucose tolerance testing shows that 25% and 18% of orlistat-treated patients with early diabetes at baseline have normal tests at 52 and 104 weeks, with an additional 44% having IGT at both 52 and 104 weeks.[86] Hollander studied effects of orlistat vs. placebo in 321 obese diabetic patients treated with sulphonylureas. Weight loss at 1 year was 6.2% vs 4.3%, with fall in HbA1c, blood pressure, and total cholesterol levels.[87] We need to learn under which circumstances it is advisable to incorporate agents specifically targeted at weight loss into the treatment of overweight individuals with diabetes.

Treatment of type 2 diabetes during surgery

Because of the many medical conditions associated with diabetes, approximately one quarter of persons with diabetes require a surgical intervention.[88] Retrospective analyses have shown that glucose levels exceeding ~200 mg/dl are associated with adverse postoperative outcome, both in general surgical populations and specifically among individuals undergoing cardiac surgery.[89-92] There are, however, a number of factors which make glycemic control more difficult in the patient undergoing surgery, or, indeed, with any hospitalization. Surgery, particularly with cardiopulmonary bypass, may lead to extreme insulin resistance, with a many-fold range of average insulin requirements depending on the stress of the procedure, as well as patient characteristics such as obesity, liver disease, steroid therapy or sepsis.[93]

Oral hypoglycemic agents, with their potential for causing prolonged glucose-lowering, should not be used in the perioperative period. The continuous administration of insulin, glucose, and potassium is conceptually ideal,[94] either in a single infusion or with separate administration of insulin to allow more precise dose adjustment.[95] Comparison of such approaches with intermittent insulin bolus administration has, however, shown both to give similar levels of glycemic control,[96] given the glucose levels up to 180 mg/dl currently deemed acceptable.[97]

In the postoperative period, patients frequently will miss meals for testing, and meal delivery and medication administration may not be as carefully timed as in the home setting.[98] These considerations favor the use of short-acting insulin secretagogues over that of sulfonylureas, and of rapid-acting insulin analogues over regular insulin for meal administration. For appropriate patients, the somewhat less potent alpha glucosidase inhibitors may also provide flexible preprandial treatment approaches. Metformin should only be given once the patient has been shown to have normal cardiac, renal, and hepatic function, recognizing that there may be a lag of approximately one week between initiation of treatment and full therapeutic effect, and recalling the need to gradually titrate the patient to a full dosage to avoid gastrointestinal side effects. With thiazolidinediones, the lag of several months to full effect presumably means that previously treated patients will continue to show therapeutic effect during a limited stay in hospital even with temporary suspension of treatment. One should not expect these agents to show effect when initiated during a relative brief hospitalization.

Insulin

An important cause of worsening glycemia in type 2 diabetes is the loss of endogenous insulin secretory capacity,[99] implying that insulin treatment should be of value. Insulin therapy in patients with type 2 diabetes has roles both temporarily, when insulin requirements are increased, as during surgery, infection, or pregnancy, and for long-term therapy.[100] Regimens that can be used include evening insulin, use of premixed rapid-plus intermediate-acting insulins, and multiple injections, either alone or in combination with oral agents. Potential concerns are weight gain and hypoglycemia. Among a number of studies of insulin treatment in patients with secondary SU failure, Wolffenbuttel reported a fall in fasting blood glucose of 95 mg/dl and in HbA1c of 3.5%, but an increase in weight of 3.7 kg at 6 months;[101] Birkeland- a fall in HbA1c of 1.6% with an increase in body mass index from 26.4 to 27.8 at one year;[102] and Kudlacek reported a study of 102 patients showing a 1.6% fall in HbA1c but a 10.6 kg weight gain at five year follow-up.[103] Rosengren reported that additional glycemic improvement over conventional insulin treatment can be seen with multiple dose regimens using an insulin pen in type 2 as well as in type 1 diabetic patients, although benefits tended to decrease after one year.[104] In all reports, hypoglycemia occurred much less frequently than in type 1 diabetic patients.

Combination treatment

Several of the previously described studies address the benefits of combinations of hypoglycemic agents. This is a particularly important consideration as it is clear that most individuals with type 2 diabetes fail to respond to single oral agents over time. Assessment of the 5102 patients in the UKPDS showed that at 3 years just over half, at 6 years 35-38%, and at 9 years only 16-21% had HbA1c <8% with monotherapy treatment, suggesting that for the majority of patients multiple agents are required to achieve adequate control.[105] The α-glucosidase inhibitors do not cause hypoglycemia and act locally in the gut, offering the possibility of increased safety. The relatively low cost of SU and the once-daily administration schedule available with glipizide-GITS and glimepiride are important considerations. Metformin may be particularly useful in obese patients, and both thiazolidinediones and metformin have benefit on insulin resistance.

The use of combinations of two or even three oral agents to delay the need for insulin therapy is therefore possible, but we must realize that long-term studies of this approach have not been carried out. The cost of treatment increases from less than $1 per day with SU, to $3 to $6 per day with two agents and to close to $10 per day with three drugs, potentially a major concern.[106] The least-costly combination approach is that of administering SU with insulin. Certainly, this is a logical approach to the treatment of many patients with diabetes. Initially, studies focused on patients receiving high doses of insulin, aiming to see whether these could be decreased. Two reviews of published studies of the addition of SU to insulin both report glycated hemoglobin levels 1.1% lower with combination treatment, suggesting that the approach may be effective.[107,108] Other studies have focused on patients at the stage of failure to achieve adequate control with SU. Decrements in fasting glucose of more than 100 mg/dL and in HbA1c of 2% to 3% can be shown with bedtime intermediate-acting insulin administered in combination with daytime SU.[109-111] Comparing bedtime or morning intermediate insulin with and without SU, however, it appears that the latter lead to only about a 1% fall in HbA1c levels.[112]

Although similar improvements in glycemic control can be seen with multiple insulin dose treatment, the combination treatment may be associated with less weight gain.[113] Furthermore, the combination of SU with a single nighttime insulin dose offers glycemic benefit similar to that seen with the use of multiple insulin dosages. In a study of patients with type 2 diabetes given 10.5 mg of glyburide and randomized to receive treatment with three preprandial doses of regular insulin or a bedtime dose of NPH insulin, HbA1c was lowered similarly, with total daily insulin doses of 29 and 26 units. There was somewhat less weight gain using insulin at bedtime.[114] A similar study using SU treatment with lispro insulin preprandially also showed glycemic improvement over levels with SU alone, although again with weight gain.[115] In a trial of patients with blood glucose of 180 to 300 mg/dL on glimepiride 8 mg twice daily, the combination of glimepiride with an evening dosage of insulin led to more rapid achievement of glycemic control than did administration of insulin alone. Patients with combination treatment had lower insulin dosages and a greater likelihood of achieving target fasting blood glucose levels, with less glycemic variability.[116] Several studies have compared the addition of insulin to that of metformin in patients with secondary SU failure. Improvements in glycemia are similar,[117] but the weight gain seen with insulin does not occur with metformin, a potentially desirable feature.[118]

CLINICAL USE

The clinical dosage pattern and usage of the pharmacologic agents currently used in the United States and discussed above is summarized in Table 2. The manufacturer's prescribing information should be consulted for detailed information prior to prescribing these (or any other) agents.

Table 2. Pharmacological agents currently used in the United States

Agent	Brand name	Dosage and frequency	Adverse effects	Contraindications
Sulphonylureas⁘				
Glyburide	Micronase, Diabeta	0.625*, 1.25, 2.5, 5, 10* mg daily	Hypoglycemia; possible cardiac**	None
Glipizide	Glucotrol	Immediate release form not recommended	"	"
Glipizide GITS	Glucotrol XL	2.5, 5, 10 mg once daily	"	"
Glimepiride	Amaryl	0.5*, 1, 2, 4, 8* mg daily	"	"
Rapidly acting secretagogues				"
Nateglinide	Starlix	60, 120, 180* mg before meals	"	"
Repaglinide	Prandin	0.5, 1, 2, 4* mg before meals	"	"
Biguanide				
Metformin	Glucophage	500, 850, 1000 mg twice or three times daily	Gastrointestinal, lactic acidosis. Should not be administered from ~1 day prior to iodinated contrast media until normal renal function determined	Serum creatinine>1.4 (female), 1.5(male), congestive heart failure, hepatic insufficiency
Metformin extended release	Glucophage XR	500 mg, 1-4 tablets once daily with meal	"	"

Combination agent				
Metformin-glyburide	Glucovance	250 mg plus 1.25 mg, 500 mg plus 2.5 mg, up to two tablets twice daily	See individual agents	
Thiazolidinediones				
Rosiglitazone	Avandia	2, 4 mg once or twice, 8 mg once daily	↑ LDL cholesterol, ↑ fat mass, fluid retention	Concurrent insulin treatment
Pioglitazone	Actos	15, 30, 45 mg once daily	↑ fat mass, fluid retention	None
Alpha glucosidase inhibitors				
Acarbose	Precose	25, 50, 100 mg before meals	Gastrointestinal (flatulence)	Caution with hepatic disease
Miglitol	Glyset	50, 100 mg before meals	"	"
Weight loss agents				
Orlistat	Xenical	120 mg before meals	Gastrointestinal (steatorrhea)	
Sibutramine	Meridia	5, 10, 15 mg daily	↑ blood pressure, dry mouth, headache	Uncontrolled hypertension

(✛The sulfonylureas chlorpropamide, tolazimide, and tolburamide are not as frequently used and are omitted from the table. * Not prepared in this strength; requires portion or combination of existing tablets. ** It is the opinion of this author that adverse cardiac effects may be more likely withglyburide than with the other sulfonylureas listed.)

One can use the information presented in this review to generate the following approach to therapeutic decision-making for patients with type 2 diabetes. First, the goals of treatment should be specified for a given patient. These include glycemic goals, such as HbA1c and pre- and postprandial glucose levels, as well as other metabolic goals, which might be addressed with different therapeutic agents, particularly weight loss, best achieved with metformin, and lipid targets, with metformin lowering LDL cholesterol and the thiazolidinediones increasing HDL cholesterol and lowering triglycerides. Next, one should be careful to assess whether a patient has characteristics that might make it more difficult to use particular agents. Thus, individuals with renal insufficiency might be considered poor candidates for metformin treatment, those with fluid retention might do poorly with thiazolidinediones, a history of gastrointestinal disturbances might cause difficulty with metformin or the alpha-glucosidase inhibitors, glyburide might be avoided for patients with cardiovascular disease, and those with irregular meal schedules might have difficulty with long-acting insulin secretagogues. After eliminating contraindicated agents, one can fairly readily determine with this approach the initial agent and subsequent drugs to be used in glycemic treatment for a given patient.

CONCLUSIONS

New understanding of the pathophysiology of type 2 diabetes and the emergence of novel therapies have led to the potential for enhanced clinical management. This should lead to improved outcomes. It will be important in the future to document such improvement in controlled long-term clinical trials in which the use of appropriate regimens to attain and maintain good glycemic control for periods of many years are studied to assess macrovascular disease, microvascular disease, and other endpoints.

REFERENCES

1. American Diabetes Association Position Statement. Standards of Medical Care for Patients With Diabetes Mellitus. Diabetes Care 24 (Suppl 1), 2001. Downloaded September 15, 2001 from http://www. diabetes.org/clinicalrecommendations/Supplement101/S33.htm.
2. AACE Consensus Conference on Guidelines for Glycemic Control. Endocrine Practice Nov/Dec 2001. Downloaded September 15, 2001 from http://www.aace.com/pub/press/releases/diabetesconsensus whitepaper.php.
3. Harris MI, Eastman RC, Cowie CC, Flegal KM, Eberhardt MS. Racial and ethnic differences in glycemic control of adults with type 2 diabetes. Diabetes Care 22:403-8, 1999.
4. State-specific prevalence of participation in physical activity--Behavioral Risk Factor Surveillance System, 1994. MMWR Morb Mortal Wkly Rep 45:673-675, 1996.
5. Spelsberg A, Manson JE. Physical activity in the treatment and prevention of diabetes. Compr Ther 21:559-562, 1995.
6. Prevalence of physical inactivity during leisure time among overweight persons--Behavioral Risk Factor Surveillance System, 1994. MMWR Morb Mortal Wkly Rep 45:185-188, 1996.
7. Monterrosa AE, Haffner SM, Stern MP, Hazuda HP. Sex difference in lifestyle factors predictive of diabetes in Mexican-Americans. Diabetes Care 18:448-4, 1995.
8. Knuiman MW, Welborn TA, Bartholomew HC. Self-reported health and use of health services: a comparison of diabetic and nondiabetic persons from a national sample. Aust NZ J Public Health 20:241-247, 1996.
9. Tessier D, Menard J, Fulop T, Ardilouze J, Roy M, Dubuc N, Dubois M, Gauthier P. Effects of aerobic physical exercise in the elderly with type 2 diabetes mellitus. Arch Gerontol Geriatr 31:121-132, 2000.
10. Ravussin E, Valencia ME, Esparza J, Bennett PH, Schulz LO. Effects of a traditional lifestyle on obesity in Pima Indians. Diabetes Care 17:1067- 1074, 1994.
11. Chaturvedi N, Stephenson JM, Fuller JH. The relationship between socioeconomic status and diabetes control and complications in the EURODIAB IDDM Complications Study. Diabetes Care 19:423-430, 1996.
12. Murphy E, Kinmonth AL. No symptoms, no problem? Patients' understandings of non-insulin dependent diabetes. Fam Pract 12:184-192, 1995.

13. Connolly VM, Kesson CM. Socioeconomic status and clustering of cardiovascular disease risk factors in diabetic patients. Diabetes Care 19:419-422, 1996.

14. Harris LE, Luft FC, Rudy DW, Tierney WM. Correlates of health care satisfaction in inner-city patients with hypertension and chronic renal insufficiency. Soc Sci Med 41:1639-1645, 1995.

15. Garay-Sevilla ME, Nava LE, Malacara JM, et al. Adherence to treatment and social support in patients with non-insulin dependent diabetes mellitus. J Diab Compl 9:81-86, 1995.

16. Lustman PJ, Griffith LS, Clouse RE, Freedland KE, Eisen SA, Rubin EH, Carney RM, McGill JB. Effects of alprazolam on glucose regulation in diabetes: results of a double-blind, placebo-controlled trial. Diabetes Care 18:1133-1139, 1995.

17. Bailey, CJ. The Diabetes Prevention Program: headline results. Br J Diabetes Vasc Dis 1:62-64, 2001.

18. Tuomilehto J, Lindstorm JH, Erikson JG for the Finnish Diabetes Prevention Study Group. Prevention of type 2 diabetes by changes in lifestyle among subjects with impaired glucose tolerance. N Engl J Med 333:1343-50, 2001.

19. Pan X, Li G, Hu Y, Wang J, Yang With, An Z. Effects of diet and exercise in preventing NIDDM in people with impaired glucose tolerance: the Ga Qing IGT and diabetes study. Diabetes Care 20:537-44, 1997.

20. Aguilar-Bryan L, Nichols CG, Wechsler SW, et al. Cloning of the beta cell high-affinity sulfonylurea receptor: a regulator of insulin secretion. Science 268:423-426, 1995.

21. Bloomgarden, ZT., Perspectives on the News: International Diabetes Federation Meeting, 1997: Issues in the treatment of type 2 diabetes: Sulfonylureas, metformin, and troglitazone. Diabetes Care 21:1024-1026, 1998.

22. Barzilai N, Groop PH, Groop L, DeFronzo RA. A novel mechanism of glipizide sulfonylurea action: decreased metabolic clearance rate of insulin. Acta Diabetol 32:273-278, 1995.

23. Levy J, Vandenberg M, Grunberger G. Insulin versus glipizide treatment in patients with non-insulin-dependent diabetes mellitus: effects on blood pressure and glucose tolerance. Am J Hypertens 8:445-453, 1995.

24. Muller G, Satoh Y, Geisen K. Extrapancreatic effects of sulfonylureas--a comparison between glimepiride and conventional sulfonylureas. Diabetes Res Clin Pract 28(suppl):S115-S137, 1995.

25. Leibowitz G, Cerasi E. Sulfonylurea treatment of NIDDM patients with cardiovascular disease: a mixed blessing? Diabetologia 39:503-514, 1996.

26. UK Prospective Diabetes Study Group. Intensive blood glucose control with sulphonylureas or insulin compared with conventional treatment and risk of complications in patients with type 2 diabetes (UKPDS 33). Lancet 352:837-853, 1998.

27. Stenman S, Melander A, Groop PH, Groop LC. What is the benefit of increasing the sulfonylurea dose? Ann Intern Med 118:169-172, 1993.

28. Berelowitz M, Fischette C, Cefalu W, Schade DS, Sutfin T, Kourides IA. Comparative efficacy of a once-daily controlled-release formulation of glipizide and immediate release glipizide in patients with NIDDM. Diabetes Care 17:1460-1464, 1994.

29. Simonson DC, Kourides IA, Feinglos M, Shamoon H, Fischette C, The Glipizide Gastrointestinal Therapeutic System Study Group. Efficacy, safety, and dose-response characteristics of glipizide gastrointestinal therapeutic system on glycemic control and insulin secretion in NIDDM. Diabetes Care 20:597-606, 1997.

30. Peters AL, Davidson MB. Maximal dose glyburide therapy in markedly symptomatic patients with type 2 diabetes: a new use for an old friend. J Clin Endocrinol Metab 81:2423-2437, 1996.

31. Banerji MA, Chaiken RL, Lebovitz HE. Prolongation of near-normoglycemic remission in black NIDDM subjects with chronic low-dose sulfonylurea treatment. Diabetes 44:466-470, 1995.

32. Shorr RI, Ray WA, Daugherty JR, Griffin MR. Individual sulfonylureas and serious hypoglycemia in older people. J Am Geriatr Soc 44:751-755, 1996.

33. Bokvist K, Hoy M, Buschard K, Holst JJ, Thomsen MK, Gromada J. Selectivity of prandial glucose regulators: nateglinide, but not repaglinide, accelerates exocytosis in rat pancreatic beta cells. Eur J Pharmacol 386:105-11, 1999.

34. Hu S, Wang S, Dunning BE. Tissue selectivity of antidiabetic agent nateglinide: study on cardiovascular and beta cell K(ATP) channels. J Pharmacol Exp Ther 291:1372-9, 1999.

35. Norman P, Rabasseda X. Nateglinide: a structurally novel insulin secretion agent. Drugs of Today 37(Suppl F):1-16, 2001.

36. Package insert, Prandin (repaglinide). NovoNordisk

37. Bloomgarden, ZT. Metformin. Diabetes Care 18:1078-1080, 1995.

38. Hermann LS, Schersten B, Bitzen PO, Kjellstrom T, Lindgarde F, Melander A. Therapeutic comparison of metformin and sulfonylurea, alone and in various combinations: a double-blind controlled study. Diabetes Care 17:1100-1109, 1994.

39. UK Prospective Diabetes Study Group. Effect of intensive blood-glucose control with metformin on complications in overweight patients with type 2 diabetes (UKPDS 43). Lancet 352:854-865, 1998.

40. DeFronzo RA, Goodman AM. Efficacy of metformin in patients with non-insulin-dependent diabetes mellitus: the Multicenter Metformin Study Group. N Engl J Med 333:541-549, 1995.

41. Campbell IW, Menzies DG, Chalmers J, McBain AM, Brown IR One year comparative: trial of metformin and glipizide in type II diabetes mellitus. Diab Metab 20:394-400, 1994.

42. Garber AJ, Duncan TG, Goodman AM, Mills DJ, Rohlf JL. Efficacy of metformin in type 2 diabetes: results of a double-blind, placebo-controlled, dose-response trial. Am J Medication 103:491-7, 1997.

43. Hermann LS, Schersten B, Melander A. Antihyperglycemic efficacy, response prediction and dose-responsee relationships of treatment with metformin and sulphonylureas, alone and in primary combination. Diabet Med 11:953-60, 1994.

44. McIntyre HD, Ma A, Bird DM, Paterson CA, Ravenscroft PJ, Cameron DP. Metformin increases insulin sensitivity and basal glucose clearance in type 2 diabetes. Aust NZ J Medication 21:714-9, 1991.

45. Grant PJ. The effects of high- and medium-dose metformin therapy on cardiovascular risk factors in patients with type II diabetes. Diabetes Care 19:64-66, 1996.

46. Glucophage (metformin) package insert. Bristol-Myers Squibb Company. October 1997.

47. Campbell IW. Metformin and the sulfonylureas: the comparative risk. Horm Metab Res Suppl. 15:105-111, 1985.

48. Acarbose for diabetes mellitus. Med Lett Drugs Ther 38(967):9-10, 1996.

49. Hoffmann J, et al. Efficacy of 24-week monotherapy with acarbose, glibenclamide, or placebo in NIDDM patients: the Essen Study. Diabetes Care 17:561-566, 1994.

50. Pagano G, Marena S, Corgiat-Mansin L, et al. Comparison of miglitol and glibenclamide in diet-treated type 2 diabetic patients. Diab Metab 21:162-167, 1995.

51. Rodger NW, Chiasson JL, Josse RG, et al. Clinical experience with acarbose: results of a Canadian multicentre study. Clin Invest Med 18:318-324, 1995.

52. Coniff RF, Shapiro JA, Robbins D, Kleinfeld R, Seaton TB, Beisswenger P, McGill JB. Reduction of glycosylated hemoglobin and postprandial hyperglycemia by acarbose in patients with NIDDM. Diabetes Care 18:817-824, 1995.

53. Rosak C, Nitzsche G, Konig P, Hofman U. The effect of timing and the administration of acarbose on postprandial hyperglycemia. Diabet Med 12:979-984, 1995.

54. Josse RG. Acarbose for the treatment of type II diabetes: the results of a Canadian multi-centre trial. Diabetes Res Clin Pract 28(suppl):S167-S172, 1995.

55. Johnston PS, Coniff RF, Hoogwerf BJ, et al. Effects of the carbohydrase inhibitor miglitol in sulfonylurea-treated NIDDM patients. Diabetes Care 17:20-29, 1994.

56. Vannasaeng S, Ploybutr S, Nitiyanant W, et al. Effects of alpha-glucosidase inhibitor (acarbose) combined with sulfonylurea or sulfonylurea and metformin in treatment of non-insulin-dependent diabetes mellitus. J Med Assoc Thai 78:578-585, 1995.

57. Coniff RF, Shapiro JA, Seaton TB, Hoogwerf BJ, Hunt JA. A double blind placebo-controlled trial evaluating the safety and efficacy of acarbose for the treatment of patients with insulin-requiring type II diabetes. Diabetes Care 18:928-932, 1995.

58. Calle-Pascual AL, Garcia-Honduvilla J, Martin-Alvarez PJ, Vara E, Calle JR, Munguira ME, Maranes JP. Comparison between acarbose, metformin, and insulin treatment in type 2 diabetic patients with secondary failure to sulfonylurea treatment. Diab Metab 21:256-260, 1995.

59. Bayraktar M, Van Thiel DH, Adalar N. A comparison of acarbose versus metformin as an adjuvant therapy in sulfonylurea-treated NIDDM patients. Diabetes Care 19:252-254, 1996.

60. Bloomgarden, ZT., Perspectives on the News: European Association for the Study of Diabetes Meeting, 1998: Treatment of type 2 diabetes and the pathogenesis of complications. Diabetes Care 22:1209-1215, 1999.

61. Petrie J, Small M, Connell J. Glitazones, a prospect for non-insulin-dependent diabetes. Lancet 349:370-371, 1997.

62. Young PW, Buckle DR, Cantello BC, Chapman H, Clapham JC, Coyle PJ, Haigh D, Hindley RM, Holder JC, Kallender H, Latter AJ, Lawrie KW, Mossakowska D, Murphy GJ, Roxbee Cox L, Smith SA. Identification of high-affinity binding sites for the insulin sensitizer rosiglitazone (BRL-49653) in rodent and human adipocytes using a radioiodinated ligand for peroxisomal proliferator-activated receptor gamma. J Pharmacol Exp Ther 284:751-9, 1998.

63. Whitcomb RW, Saltiel AR. Thiazolidinediones. Exp Opin Invest Drugs 4:1299-1309, 1995.

64. Kuehnle HF. New therapeutic agents for the treatment of NIDDM. Exp Clin Endocrinol Diabetes 104:93-101, 1996.

65. Ogihara T, Rakugi H, Ikegami H, et al. Enhancement of insulin sensitivity by troglitazone lowers blood pressure in diabetic hypertensives. Am J Hypertens 8:316-320, 1995.

66. Iwamoto Y, Kosaka K, Kuzuya T, et al. Effects of troglitazone: a new hypoglycemic agent in patients with NIDDM poorly controlled by diet therapy. Diabetes Care 19:151-156, 1996.

67. Ghazzi M, Radke-Mitchell L, Venable T, The troglitazone study group, Whitcomb R. Troglitazone improves glycemic control in patients with type ii diabetes who are not optimally controlled on sulfonylurea. Diabetes 46 (Suppl 1):44A, 1997.

68. Inzucchi SE, Maggs DG, Spollett GR, Page SL, Rife FS, Walton V, Shulman GI. Efficacy and metabolic effects of metformin and troglitazone in type II diabetes mellitus. N Engl J Med 338:867-72, 1998.

69. Schwartz S, Raskin P, Fonesca V, Graveline JF. Effect of troglitazone in insulin-treated patients with type II diabetes mellitus. N Engl J Med 338:861-6, 1998.

70. Antonucci T, Whitcomb R, McLain R, Lockwood D. Impaired glucose tolerance is normalized by treatment with the thiazolidinedione troglitazone. Diabetes Care 20:188-193, 1997.

71. Nolan JJ, Ludvik B, Beerdsen P, Joyce M, Olefsky J. Improvement in glucose tolerance and insulin resistance in obese subjects treated with troglitazone. N Engl J Med 331:1188-1193, 1994.

72. .Dunaif A, Scott D, Finegood D, Quintana B, Whitcomb R. The insulin-sensitizing agent troglitazone improves metabolic and reproductive abnormalities in the polycystic ovary syndrome. J Clin Endocrinol Metab 81:3299-3306, 1996.

73. Azen SP, Peters RK, Berkowitz K, Kjos S, Xiang A, Buchanan TA. TRIPOD (TRoglitazone In the Prevention Of Diabetes): a randomized, placebo-controlled trial of troglitazone in women with prior gestational diabetes mellitus. Control Clin Trials 19:217-31, 1998.

74. Buchanan TA, Xiang AH, Peters RK, et al. Protection from type 2 diabetes persists in the TRIPOD cohort eight months after stopping troglitazone. Program and abstracts of the 61st Scientific Sessions of the American Diabetes Association; June 22-26, 2001; Philadelphia, Pennsylvania. Diabetes 50(suppl 2):Abstract 327-PP, 2001.

75. Bailey CJ, Day C. Thiazolidinediones today. Br J Vasc Dis 1:7-13, 2001.

76. Manson JE, Faich GA. Pharmacotherapy for obesity--do the benefits outweigh the risks? N Engl J Med 335:659-660, 1996.

77. Albu J, Konnarides C, Pi-Sunyer FX. Weight control: metabolic and cardiovascular effects. Diabetes Reviews 3:335-347, 1995.

78. Chow CC, Ko GT, Tsang LW, Yeung VT, Chan JC, Cockram CS. Dexfenfluramine in obese Chinese NIDDM patients. A placebo-controlled investigation of the effects on body weight, glycemic control, and cardiovascular risk factors. Diabetes Care 20:1122-112, 1997.

79. Connolly HM, Crary JL, McGoon MD, et al. Valvular heart disease associated with fenfluramine-phentermine. N Engl J Med 337:581-588, 1997.

80. Connolly VM, Gallagher A, Kesson CM. A study of fluoxetine in obese elderly patients with type 2 diabetes. Diabet Med 12:416-418, 1995.

81. Gray DS, Fujioka K, Devine W, Bray GA A randomized double-blind clinical trial of fluoxetine in obese diabetics. Int J Obes Relat Metab Disord 16(suppl)4:S67-S72, 1992.

82. Wise SD. Clinical studies with fluoxetine in obesity. Am J Clin Nutr 55(suppl):181S-184S, 1992.

83. Bray GA, Blackburn GL, Ferguson JM, Greenway FL, Jain A, Kaise4r PE, Mendels J, Ryan D, Schwartz SL. Sibutramine dose response and long-term efficacy in weight loss. Int J Obes 18 (suppl 2):60, 1994.

84. Manning RM, Jung RT, Lesse GP, Newton RW. The comparison of four weight reduction strategies aimed at overweight diabetic patients. Diabet Med 12:409-415, 1995.

85. Hollander P. A 57-week study of orlistat in the treatment of obese patients with Type II diabetes. Diabetes 46(Suppl 1):54A, 1997.

86. Heymsfield SB, Segal KR, Hauptman J, Lucas CP, Boldrin MN, Rissanen A, Wilding JP, Sjostrom L. Effects of weight loss with orlistat on glucose tolerance and progression to type 2 diabetes in obese adults. Arch Intern Med 32000;160:1321-6, 1997.

87. Hollander PA, Elbein SC, Hirsch IB, Kelley D, McGill J, Taylor T, Weiss SR, Crockett SE, Kaplan RA, Comstock J, Lucas CP, Lodewick PA, Canovatchel W, Chung J, Hauptman J. Role of orlistat in the treatment of obese patients with type 2 diabetes. A 1-year randomized double-blind study. Diabetes Care 21:1288-94.89, 1998.

88. Jacober SJ, Sowers JR. An update on perioperative management of diabetes. Arch Intern Med 159:2405-11, 1999.

89. Golden SH, Peart-Vigilance C, Kao WH, Brancati FL.Perioperative glycemic control and the risk of infectious complications in a cohort of adults with diabetes. Diabetes Care 22:1408-14, 1999,

90. Pomposelli JJ, Baxter JK 3rd, Babineau TJ, Pomfret EA, Driscoll DF, Forse RA, Bistrian BR.Early postoperative glucose control predicts nosocomial infection rate in diabetic patients. J Parenter Enteral Nutr 22:77-81, 1998.

91. Hugo JM, Ockert DB. Routine peri-operative management of the diabetic patient. S Afr J Surg 30:85-9, 1992.

92. Zerr KJ, Furnary AP, Grunkemeier GL, Bookin S, Kanhere V, Starr A.Glucose control lowers the risk of wound infection in diabetics after open heart operations. Ann Thorac Surg 63:356-61, 1997.

93. Peters A, Kerner W. Perioperative management of the diabetic patient. Exp Clin Endocrinol Diabetes 103:213-8, 1995.

94. Eldridge AJ, Sear JW.Peri-operative management of diabetic patients. Any changes for the better since 1985? Anaesthesia 51:45-51, 1996.

95. Simmons D, Morton K, Laughton SJ, Scott DJ.A comparison of two intravenous insulin regimens among surgical patients with insulin-dependent diabetes mellitus. Diabetes Educ 20:422-7, 1994.

96. Raucoules-Aime M, Lugrin D, Boussofara M, Gastaud P, Dolisi C, Grimaud D. Intraoperative glycaemic control in non-insulin-dependent and insulin-dependent diabetes. Br J Anaesth 73:443-9, 1994.

97. Hemmerling TM, Schmid MC, Schmidt J, Kern S, Jacobi KE.Comparison of a continuous glucose-insulin-potassium infusion versus intermittent bolus application of insulin on perioperative glucose control and hormone status in insulin-treated type 2 diabetics. J Clin Anesth 13:293-300, 2001.

98. Hoogwerf BJ.Postoperative management of the diabetic patient. Med Clin North Am 85:1213-28, 2001.

99. Prando R, Odetti P, Melga P, Giusti R, Ciuchi E, Cheli V. Progressive deterioration of beta-cell function in nonobese type 2 diabetic subjects. Postprandial plasma C-peptide level is an indication of insulin dependency. Diabetes Metab 22:185-191, 1996.

100. Koivisto VA. Insulin therapy in type II diabetes. Diabetes Care 16 (Suppl3):29-39 102, 1993.

101. Wolffenbuttel BH, Weber RF, Weeks L, van Koetsveld PM, Verschoor L Twice daily insulin therapy in patients with type 2 diabetes and secondary failure to sulfonylureas. Diabetes Res 13:79-84, 1990.

102. Birkeland KI, Hanssen KF, Urdal P, Berg K, Vaaler S. A long-term, randomized, comparative study of insulin versus sulfonylurea therapy in type 2 diabetes. J Intern Med 236:305-313, 1994.

103. Kudlacek S, Schernthaner G. The effect of insulin treatment on HbA1c, body weight and lipids in type 2 diabetic patients with secondary-failure to sulfonylureas. A five year follow-up study. Horm Metab Res 24:478-483, 1992.

104. Rosengren A, Adlerberth A, Bresater LE, Ehnberg S, Welin L. Multiple insulin injection therapy using an insulin pen--who benefits? A clinical 3-year follow-up study of 100 type 1 and 51 type 2 diabetic patients. Diabetes Res Clin Pract 20:69-74, 1993.

105. Cull CA, Holman RR, Turner RC for the UK Prospective Diabetes Study (UKPDS) Group. Treatment of NIDDM - progressive requirement for polypharmacy to attain glycaemic goals. Diabetologia 40 (Suppl 1):A1-A722 (abstract 1366), 1997.

106. Mooradian AD. Drug therapy of non-insulin-dependent diabetes mellitus in the elderly. Drugs 51:931-941, 1996.

107. Peters AL, Davidson MB Insulin plus a sulfonylurea agent for treating type 2 diabetes. Ann Intern Med 115:45-53, 1991.

108. Johnson JL, Wolf SL, Kabadi UM. Efficacy of insulin and sulfonylurea combination therapy in type II diabetes: a meta-analysis of the randomized placebo-controlled trials. Arch Intern Med. 156:259-264, 1996.

617

109. Shank ML, Del Prato S, DeFronzo RA. Bedtime insulin/daytime glipizide: effective therapy for sulfonylurea failures in NIDDM. Diabetes 44:165-172, 1995.

108. Miller JL, Salman K, Shulman LH, Rose LI. Bedtime insulin added to daytime sulfonylureas improves glycemic control in uncontrolled type II diabetes. Clin Pharmacol Ther 53:380-384, 1993.

109. Chow CC, Tsang LW, Sorensen JP, Cockram CS. Comparison of insulin with or without continuation of oral hypoglycemic agents in the treatment of secondary failure in NIDDM patients. Diabetes Care 18:307-314, 1995.

110. Niskanen L, Lahti J, Uusitupa M. Morning or bed-time insulin with or without glibenclamide in elderly type 2 diabetic patients unresponsive to oral antidiabetic agents. Diabetes Res Clin Pract 18(3):185-190, 1992.

111. Clauson P, Karlander S, Steen L, Efendic S. Daytime glibenclamide and bedtime NPH insulin compared to intensive insulin treatment in secondary sulfonylurea failure: a 1-year follow-up. Diabet Med 13:471-477, 1996.

112. Landsted-Hallin L, Adamson U, Arner A, Bolinder J, Lins PE. Comparison of bedtime NPH or preprandial regular insulin combined with glibenclamide in secondary sulfonylurea failure. Diabetes Care 18:1183-1186, 1995.

113. Feinglos MN, Thacker CH, English J, Bethel MA, Lane JD. Modification of postprandial hyperglycemia with insulin lispro improves glucose control in patients with type 2 diabetes. Diabetes Care 20:1539-1542, 1997.

114. Riddle MC. Combined therapy with a sulfonylurea plus evening insulin: safe, reliable, and becoming routine. Horm Metab Res 28:430-433, 1996.

115. Klein W. Sulfonylurea-metformin-combination versus sulfonylurea-insulin-combination in secondary failures of sulfonylurea monotherapy. Results of a prospective randomized study in 50 patients. Diab Metab 17:235-240, 1991.

116. Groop L, Widen E. Treatment strategies for secondary sulfonylurea failure. Should we start insulin or add metformin? Is there a place for intermittent insulin therapy? Diab Metab 7:218-223, 1991.

Chapter 7. Prevention of Microvascular Complications of Diabetes

Zachary Bloomgarden and Alina Gouller

INTRODUCTION

There are several approaches to the prevention of complications of diabetes. They include controlling hyperglycemia, controlling blood pressure, utilizing angiotensin converting enzyme (ACE)-inhibitors and angiotensin-receptor blockers (ARBs) and preventing formation of advanced glycosylation end products (AGEs).

The relationship between glycemic control and the complications of Diabetes.

Diabetic retinopathy, nephropathy, and neuropathy occur in all clinical forms of diabetes mellitus, regardless of the cause of the diabetes, with hyperglycemia being the variable shared among these different clinical forms. The results of intervention studies and epidemiological data suggest that hyperglycemia is the major cause of these complications, although the precise mechanisms by which hyperglycemia causes individual complications have not been established.[1] (For a detailed discussion of mechanisms of the development of microvascular complications of diabetes see also chapters VII.3 and VIII.1).

Randomized controlled trials

The findings of the twenty two year long United Kingdom Prospective Diabetes Study (UKPDS) give fascinating insight into the efficacy and safety of treatment of type 2 diabetes and the prevention of macrovascular and microvascular complications. 5102 patients without previous history of type 2 diabetes, severe cardiovascular disease (CVD), renal disease, retinopathy, or other severe illness, who could be randomized to insulin treatment, were entered at the time of diagnosis of diabetes. During a 3 month run-in period the patients were intensively treated with diet, leading to weight loss averaging 4.5 kg and a fall in mean HbA1C to 6.9%. 4209 patients whose fasting blood glucose (FBG) was 110 - 270 mg/dl and who were not symptomatic, allowing randomization to a control group, were enrolled in the study. 1138 patients were placed on "conventional treatment," initially with diet. The FBG fell from 207 mg/dl to 144 mg/dl at the time of randomization at 3 months, increasing at 3 years to 162 mg/dl and at 9 years to 180 mg/dl. In patients treated with diet alone, the FBG remained below 270 mg/dl in 90% at 1 year, 40% at 7 years, and only 20% at 12 years. Body weight increased by 2.5 kg over baseline at 6 years and was stable through 10 years. The "intensive treatment" group included 342 obese patients randomized to metformin with the remaining 2729 either given insulin (with multiple doses, if required for increasing degrees of hyperglycemia), or the sulfonylureas glyburide or chlorpropamide (with metformin and then insulin added, if required). Their FBG was 122 mg/dl at 1 year, 135 mg/dl at 6 years, and 144 mg/dl at 12 years. Body weight increased by 5 kg over baseline at 6 years to reach a level 3.1 kg over the conventional group at 10 years. Hypoglycemia was reported to occur around 25% annually, but severe episodes requiring assistance of another person occurred at a range of around 2%/year. The ten-year average HbA1C was 7.0% for the intensive treatment group and 7.9% for the conventional treatment group.

There were 3277 nonfatal and 927 fatal endpoints during the study period, occurring in 1401 (36%) of the patients. Diabetes-related endpoints including death, myocardial infarction, congestive heart failure, angina, stroke, amputation, renal failure, cataract, blindness, and retinal photocoagulation, occurred 12% less frequently in the intensively treated group. Total microvascular endpoints were decreased 25%, cataracts 24%, retinopathy progression 21%, and microalbuminuria 33%. The risks of requiring photocoagulation and of loss of vibratory sensation were also significantly decreased. The relative risk of myocardial infarction was decreased by 16%, with a borderline statistical significance of $p=.052$. There was no significant difference between the groups in diabetes-related deaths. The investigators concluded that one can "reduce the risk of the diabetic complications that cause both morbidity and premature mortality" with "an intensive glucose-control treatment policy".[2]

It is interesting to compare the UKPDS with the Diabetes Control and Complications Trial (DCCT) of 1,441 patients with type 1 diabetes.[3] 726 had no retinopathy at baseline (the primary prevention cohort) and 715 had mild retinopathy (the secondary intervention cohort). Patients were randomly assigned to receive intensive therapy guided by frequent blood glucose monitoring, with a 6.5 year mean HbA1C value 2% lower than that with conventional insulin therapy. Intensive therapy reduced the adjusted mean risk for the development of retinopathy in the primary prevention cohort by 76%, slowed the progression of retinopathy in the secondary intervention cohort by 54%, and reduced the development of proliferative or severe non-proliferative retinopathy by 47%. In the two cohorts combined, intensive therapy reduced the occurrence of microalbuminuria by 39% and that of macroalbuminuria by 54%. Intensive therapy reduced the development of clinical neuropathy in both cohorts by 64% after 5 years. Nerve conduction velocities increased significantly in patients receiving conventional therapy but remained generally stable for those following the intensive regimen.[4] The initial level of HbA1C observed at eligibility screening and the duration of type 1 diabetes were the dominant baseline predictors of the risk of progression. In each treatment group, the mean HbA1C during the trial was the dominant predictor of retinopathy progression, with every 10% lowering of HbA1C associated with a 43-45% lower risk. Similar results also apply to nephropathy and neuropathy progression.[5] Similarly to the UKPDS, there was a 73% higher risk of becoming overweight in the intensive treatment group, and the frequency of hypoglycemia was threefold greater with intensive than with conventional therapy, both factors which might increase cardiovascular risk in type 2 diabetes.[6]

Several additional studies have shown improved outcomes with treatment of patients with both type 1 and type 2 diabetes. A systematic review of 16 randomized controlled trials of patients with type 1 diabetes over periods of 8 to 60 months with HbA1C 1.4% lower in the intervention groups showed decrease in progression of retinopathy by 49%, and in that of nephropathy by 34%.[7] The prospective Kumamoto study compared 55 Japanese patients with type 2 diabetes treated with an intensive multiple insulin injection regimen similar to that of the DCCT with 55 control patients. Over a 6-year period, rates of appearance or progression of retinopathy, nephropathy, and neuropathy were strikingly similar to those seen in type 1 diabetes in the DCCT. Of those without retinopathy at study onset, 7.7% of the intensively treated group but 32.0% of the control group developed retinopathy, and of those with background retinopathy at baseline, 19.2% and 44.0%, respectively, showed progression of the disorder. The cumulative percentages of development and of progression in nephropathy after 6 years were 7.7% vs 28.0% and 11.5% vs 32.0%, respectively.[8]

A twelve week study compared 192 patients with type 2 diabetes receiving placebo with 377 treated with glipizide GITS (Glucotrol XL, controlled release formulation of glipizide), with HbA1C 9.3% vs. 7.5%. Outcome benefit in terms of quality of life (QOL) was demonstrated in overall symptom scores and in general perceived health. Health economic indicators showed benefit as well, with employed individuals in the placebo group showing a decrease in days worked to 87% of baseline vs. 99% in the glipizide GITS group, with projected absenteeism costs of $115 vs. $24/person/month. The frequency of restricted activity days was 11.6% for the placebo group vs. 7.6% for the glipizide GITS group.[9]

Not all studies show benefit of treatment. The University Group Diabetes Program (UGDP) was initiated in 1959 and reported in the 1970's. In this study, 1027 patients were treated with placebo, a constant insulin dose, a variable insulin dose, phenformin, or tolbutamide. The 9-year follow-up study showed that, despite leading to better glycemic control, insulin failed to improve mortality over that seen with placebo.[10] Plasma glucose levels were maintained at 121 mg/dl in the variable-dose insulin group, 30 to 40 mg/dl lower than in the placebo or fixed insulin treatment groups, a separation similar to that in the UKPDS. No significant differences were found, however, in the final prevalence or the cumulative incidence of total

621

deaths, cardiovascular disease deaths, or myocardial infarctions among the three treatment groups, even when outcomes were adjusted for baseline cardiovascular risk factors. There was a slight suggestion only from post hoc analysis that patients in both insulin treatment groups with good glucose control had fewer cardiovascular events than did those with fair or poor control. In the two additional treatment groups of this study, administration of tolbutamide, a sulfonylurea, and of phenformin, a biguanide, was reported to increase mortality, although the interpretation of these findings remains controversial.[11] Many who have analyzed the UGDP trial believe that it was flawed by inadequate power, insufficient separation of glycemic levels, ignorance of smoking history, and variation in distribution of complications among study centers as possible confounding factor.[12]

As with the UGDP study, the Veterans Affairs Cooperative Study, a feasibility study comparing standard with intensive insulin care of type 2 diabetes, suggests a need for caution in recommending treatment designed to normalize glycemia in patients with insulin-treated type 2 diabetes, particularly those with cardiovascular disease. Of the more than 150 patients enrolled, all on insulin, the "standard care" group administered one morning insulin dose, while the "intensive treatment" group utilized multiple insulin dosages with a goal of normal FBG and HbA1C levels, a much more aggressive approach than that employed in the "intensive" insulin arm of the UKPDS. Over the 2.5-year study period, FBG levels remained at 200 mg/dL in the control group but decreased to about 120 mg/dL with intensive treatment. HbA1C levels were 9.5% with standard treatment, decreasing to 6.8% in the intensive treatment group. Insulin doses increased from about 40 to 50 U/day with standard care, and from about 50 to 90 U/day with intensive treatment. There was no change in weight, lipid levels, or blood pressure. Severe hypoglycemia was seen only twice per 100 patients per year and this, as well as changes in weight, blood pressure, and plasma lipids, did not significantly differ between the groups. There were 61 new cardiovascular events in 40 patients and 10 deaths, 6 due to cardiovascular causes. The overall difference between groups was not statistically significant, with 16 of 77 vs. 24 of 76 having events, but in the subgroup of individuals without prior coronary disease, 6 of 50 with standard treatment, but 14 of 45 with intensive treatment, had a new cardiovascular event, a significant finding which is of some concern. Colwell, discussing the implications of the trial, concluded that it is feasible to achieve excellent glycemic control in men with type 2 diabetes in whom standard pharmacologic therapy has failed, but that the benefit/risk ratio of intensive insulin management in this patient group needs to be established with a long-term prospective clinical trial prior to recommending this approach.[13]

In summary the weight of evidence is that microvascular complications are caused mainly by hyperglycemia and that this is likely to apply in type 2 as well as type 1 diabetes. With macrovascular disease it is /unclear which of the many potentially atherogenic abnormalities, including hypertension, hyperinsulinemia, hyperlipidemia, and the hypercoagulable state, are most important. This is particularly true in view of the clinical observation that macrovascular disease is already well developed in many patients when type 2 diabetes is diagnosed.

Epidemiological studies

In contrast to the somewhat opposing findings of clinical trials of glycemic control in type 2 diabetes, a number of epidemiological studies suggest that improving glycemia may indeed lead to decreased morbidity and mortality.

An important study in an 11-county area in southern Wisconsin followed 674 persons treated with insulin and 696 persons not taking insulin, diagnosed with diabetes at age 30 or older and so presumed to have type 2 diabetes, and 996 persons diagnosed before age 30 and taking insulin, and so presumed to have type 1 diabetes.[14] Patients were studied at a baseline examination from 1980 to 1982, and again between 1984 and 1986 and between 1990 and 1992. The glycosylated hemoglobin level at baseline was strongly related to both the incidence and progression of diabetic retinopathy, to the incidence of gross proteinuria, and to the incidence of loss of tactile sensation or temperature sensitivity in persons with either type 1 or type 2 diabetes. The incidence of macular edema over the 10-year period was 20.1% in the younger onset group, 25.4% in the older onset group taking insulin, and 13.9% in the older onset group not taking insulin and was associated with higher levels of glycosylated hemoglobin in both younger and older onset groups.[15] Within each group, after controlling for other characteristics associated with retinopathy, there was no relationship between higher levels of C-peptide at baseline and lower 6-year incidence or progression of retinopathy. These data suggest that glycemic control, and not hyperinsulinemia, is related to the incidence and progression of diabetic retinopathy.[16] The 10-year cumulative incidence of lower-extremity amputation was 5.4% in younger onset and 7.3% in older onset persons. Multivariate analyses in both groups showed associations of glycosylated hemoglobin levels with amputation, and similar associations were reported with stroke and myocardial infarction.[17]

Two studies of type 2 diabetes from eastern Finland showed that cardiovascular mortality was significantly and linearly associated with glycemic control.[18] The first was of 133 newly diagnosed patients age 45 to 64 years at baseline and followed up to 10 years for cardiovascular mortality, and the second was of 229 newly or previously diagnosed patients age 65 to 74 years at baseline. In another prospective population-based study of the risk of stroke, the levels of cardiovascular risk factors were determined at baseline in 1,059 type 2 diabetic patients and 1,373 nondiabetic control subjects, age from 45 to 64 years, in eastern and western Finland. 34 type 2 diabetics and 5 nondiabetic subjects died from stroke, and 125 type 2 diabetics and 30 nondiabetic subjects had a fatal or nonfatal stroke. The risk of stroke in type 2 diabetic men was about threefold and in women fivefold higher than that in corresponding nondiabetic subjects. Previous history of stroke increased the risk of a new stroke event threefold. Diabetics with FBG > 240 mg/dl and HbA1C >10.7% had about a twofold higher risk of stroke than those with diabetes having better glycemic control. Low levels of high-density lipoprotein cholesterol, high levels of triglycerides, and hypertension were similarly associated with approximately twofold increased risk of stroke mortality or morbidity.[19] In another study of a cohort of newly detected type 2 diabetic individuals diagnosed between 1972 and 1987, clinical data concerning FBG, body mass index (BMI), type of treatment, and concomitant diseases were collected. During a mean follow-up time of 7.4 years, 161 subjects died. In multivariate analysis, higher average FBG was independently related to all-cause, cardiovascular, and ischemic heart disease mortality. Diabetic subjects with average FBG ≥ 140 mg/dl had 50% higher mortality than did those with lower levels.[20]

These studies are complemented by an "epidemiological analysis" of the relationship of events in the UKPDS to the degree of hyperglycemia (Figure 1).[21] Data, adjusted for age, sex, and ethnicity, were analyzed for 4585 patients. Relative to a HbA1C of 6%, a 1% rise increased total diabetes endpoint development by 21%, diabetes-related and total mortality by 25% and 17%, myocardial infarction and stroke by 18% and 15%, microalbuminuria by 35%, and cataract by 18%. All of these outcomes were highly significant, concordant with the results of the intention-to-treat group analysis, without a specific threshold of benefit. Cost effectiveness of glycemic treatment, of follow-up examinations, and of hospitalizations and other treatment of complications suggested that intensive treatment led to higher drug costs but lower hospitalization costs, with a calculated savings of £26/ patient/year in the intensive group. During the study, patients in both groups were seen around 3 times annually, so that a reduction in clinic attendance of the conventional group would be calculated to lead to a £48/patient/year excess cost in the intensive group. If a discount rate of 6% is used to reduce costs of future complications as opposed to past treatment expenditures, the excess cost of intensive treatment per endpoint-free year is between £200 and £550. In comparison, estimates of cardiovascular disease lifestyle advice costs are about £9000, breast cancer screening about £6500, cholesterol treatment in the 4-S study about £3500, and coronary heart disease screening of patients with diabetes about £900, suggesting that glycemic treatment as applied in the UKPDS is highly cost-effective.

Thus, there appears to be a close relationship between glycemic control and microvascular complications of diabetes. However, intensive glycemic control is a challenge and hypoglycemia incidence is increased with intensive glycemic control. Therefore, approaches that focus on non-glycemic factors in the prevention of complications of diabetes have been investigated.

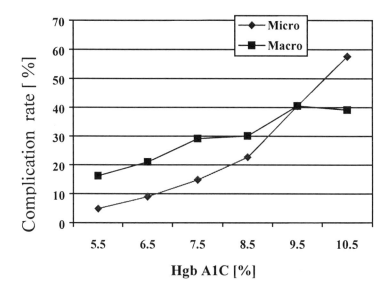

Figure 1. Relationship between mean HbA1C and microvascular and macrovascular complications in UKPDS. (Adapted, with permission, from Stratton IM, Adler AI, Neil HAW et al. Association of glycemia with macrovascular and microvascular complications of type 2 diabetes [UKPDS 35]: prospective observational study. Brit Med J 321: 405-412, 2000).

Can complications of diabetes be prevented by influencing factors independent of glycemia?

Hypertension.

More than 11 million Americans have both diabetes and hypertension. Hypertension substantially contributes to morbidity and mortality in patients with diabetes. The current suggested blood pressure (BP) target is 130/85 mm Hg.[22] Even lower blood pressure levels (less then 125/75 mm Hg) are recommended for patients who have proteinuria greater than 1g/day and renal insufficiency regardless of etiology. More than 65 % of patients with diabetes and hypertension will require two or more antihypertensive medications to achieve this target.

Hypertension Optimal Treatment (HOT) trial was a randomized double-blind, placebo-controlled multinational trial. 1501 diabetic patients , 50-80 years of age, were randomized to diastolic blood pressure (BP) less then 90 mm Hg, less than 85 mm Hg and less than 80 mm Hg. Average follow-up was 3.8 years (3.3-4.9 years). Initial antihypertensive therapy was felodipine (a calcium channel blocker), however 73% of the subjects randomized to lowest blood pressure group required 2.7 different antihypertensive medications, and most participants in this group required an angiotensin converting enzyme (ACE) inhibitor. The group with the lowest BP had 40 % less adverse events (myocardial infarction, strokes and death) (see Fig. 2).[23]

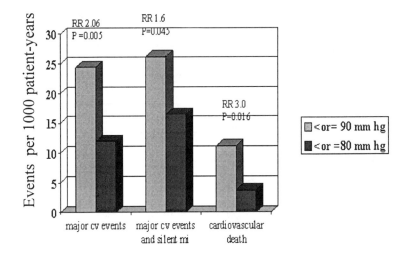

Figure 2. Cardiovascular morbidity and mortality in patients with diabetes mellitus in the HOT trial. RR=relative risk; MI=myocardial infarction; CV=cardiovascular risk. (Adapted, with permission, from Hansson L et al. Effects of intensive blood-pressure lowering and low dose aspirin in patients with hypertension: principal results of the Hypertension Optimal Treatment [HOT] randomized trial. Lancet 351:1755-1762, 1998).

Hypertension in Diabetes study, embedded within the UKPDS, was a multicenter randomized controlled trial including 1148 hypertensive patients with a mean age of 56.4 years and median follow up of 8.4 years. Subjects were randomized to two treatment groups: tight BP control of less than 150/85 mmHg (n=758) vs. less tight control (conventional group), with a BP target of less than 180/105 mmHg (n=390). Atenolol (a beta-blocker), in a maximum dose of 100 mg po qd (n=358) or capoten (an ACE inhibitor), maximum dose 50 mg po bid (n=400), were used as the main two modalities of treatment in tight control group. These agents were avoided in the conventional group. Other agents, such as furosemide, slow release nifedipine, methyldopa and prazosin were added as needed to achieve the target blood pressure.

The study addressed the following questions:

1) Does tight BP control (blood pressure less than 150/85 mm Hg) prevent microvascular complications?

2) Does tight BP control prevent macrovascular complications (myocardial infarction and stroke)?
3) Does the choice of treatment (beta-blockers vs ACE-inhibitors) affect the outcome?
4) Are there particular risks or benefits associated with beta-blockers or ACE inhibitors?

Blood pressure in the tight control group was 144/82 mmHg vs. 154/87 mm Hg in conventional group. Major reduction in all diabetes related endpoints in the tight control group was 24%, in diabetes related death – 32 %, in stroke – 44% and in microvascular complications (mainly due to retinopathy) – 37%. The choice of treatment did not influence the outcome [25] (Fig. 3).

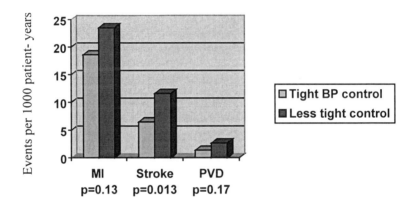

Figure 3. Incidence of clinical endpoints in diabetic patients with tight blood pressure control vs less tight control. MI-myocardial infarction, PVD-peripheral vascular disease. (Adapted, with permission, from UKPDS Group. Tight blood pressure control and risk of macrovascular and microvascular complications in type 2 diabetes: UKPDS 38. Brit Med J 317:703-713, 1998).

In the HOT trial there was a 4 mm Hg difference in the achieved diastolic blood pressure between the intensively treated group and the other target groups (85 vs 81 mm Hg). In the UKPDS trial there was a difference of 5 mm Hg in diastolic and 10 mm Hg in systolic blood pressure between conventional and intensively treated groups. Even these small reductions in blood pressure resulted in significant reduction of macro- and microvascular complications.

Additionally in the UKPDS a comparison of tight blood pressure control vs tight glucose control showed that blood pressure control had greater impact on cardiovascular risk reduction than tight glucose control (Fig. 4).

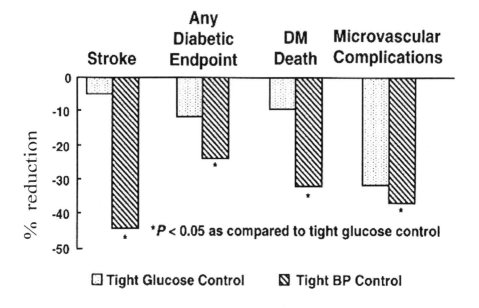

Figure 4. Comparison of the cardiovascular risk reduction between tight glucose control versus tight blood pressure control. While both tight glucose and blood pressure control reduced cardiovascular events, the relative benefit of tight blood pressure control was significantly greater than of tight glucose control. (Adapted, with permission, from UK Prospective Diabetes Study Group. Tight blood pressure control and risk of macrovascular and microvascular complications in type 2 diabetes: UKPDS 38. Brit Med J 317:703-713, 1998).

Advanced glycosylation end products.

It remains unclear how hyperglycemia causes tissue injury. Among proposed mechanisms are the development of advanced glycosylation end products and sorbitol accumulation.

Advanced glycosylation end products (AGEs) comprise a heterogeneous group of molecules that accumulate in plasma and tissues with advancing age, diabetes and renal failure. They are characterized by browning, fluorescence, cross-linking and biological response through specific AGE receptors and were first described in 1912 by French chemist L.C. Maillard (Fig. 5).

AGEs are formed when a carbonyl of a reducing sugar condenses with reactive amino group in a target protein. Studies in animals and humans suggest that AGEs play significant role in pathophisiology of microvascular and macrovascular complications.

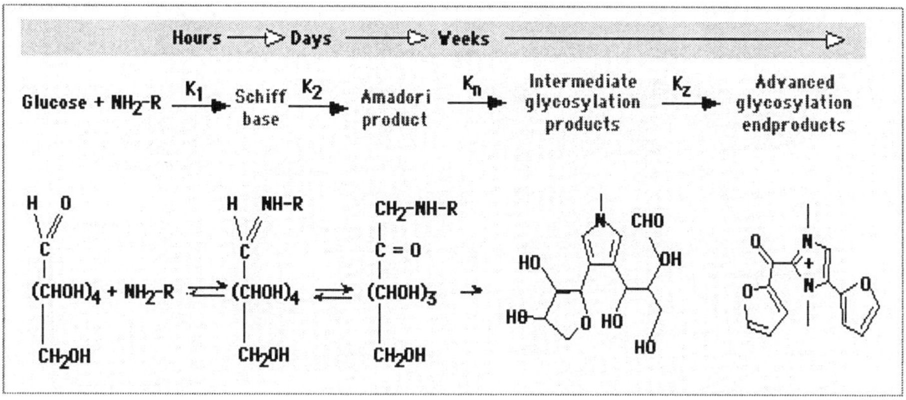

Figure 5. Formation of advanced glycosylation end products in the presence of persistent hyperglycemia. (Adapted, with permission, from Bucala, Vlassara and Cerami. Advanced glycosylation end products – role in diabetic and nondiabetic vascular disease. Drug Development Research 32:77-89, 1994).

Administration of AGEs to nondiabetic rabbits and rats for 2 weeks induced vascular dysfunction similar to that seen in diabetes mellitus (increased vascular permeability, significant mononuclear cell migratory activity, defective vasodilatory responses).[26] AGEs administered to nondiabetic rats for 5 months lead to 50% expansion in glomerular volume, basement membrane widening, increased mesangial matrix indicating significant glomerulosclerosis compared to untreated controls.[27,28]

In human cohort of 125 patients (duration of diabetes 11.6 ± 8.9 years, mean Hb A1C 6.8 ± 1%) with stable blood glucose control and 63 healthy volunteers, serum AGE level was significantly higher in diabetic group and reflected severity of diabetic nephropathy and retinopathy.[29]

AGEs accelerate atherosclerosis through cross-linking of proteins, platelet aggregation, defective vascular relaxation, and abnormal lipoprotein metabolism.[30]

AGEs have a vital role in pathogenesis of diabetic nephropathy and progression of renal failure. Renal failure, in turn, results in decreased excretion and increased generation of AGEs (Figure 6).

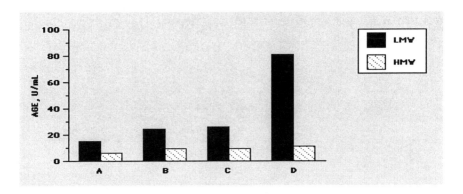

Figure 6. Increased AGE levels in diabetic patients with renal disease.
LMV-low molecular weight advanced glycosylation end products.
HMV-high molecular weight advanced glycosylation end products.
A-normal individuals; B-diabetics with normal renal function;
C-nondiabetics with end stage renal disease (ESRD); D-diabetics with ESRD.
(Adapted, with permission, from Vlassara, H. Serum advanced glycosylation end products: a new class of uremic toxins? Blood Purif 12(1): 54-9, 1994).

Aminoguanidine.

Aminoguanidine is a nucleophilic hydrazine compound, similar in structure to alpha-hydrazinohistidine, which prevents formation of AGEs and glucose-derived collagen cross-links in vitro[31] (Fig. 7). It also blocks the synthesis of nitric oxide, which may be contributing to vascular dysfunction in diabetes, inhibits the oxidant–induced apoptosis and decreases the AGE-induced cross-linking. Aminoguanidine has been shown to have possible therapeutic role in prevention of diabetic complications in animal studies.

In retina of streptozosin induced diabetic rats aminoguanidine reduced the number of acellular capillaries by 80 %. After 75 weeks untreated diabetic animals developed 18.6 fold increase in background diabetic retinopathy comparing to 3.6 fold increase in aminoguanidine treated animals.[32]

Aminoguanidine diminishes proteinuria, mesangial matrix expansion, basement membrane thickness and deposition of AGEs. Benefit is directly related to the duration of treatment in diabetic animals. Thirty two weeks of treatment with aminoguanidine in diabetic rats attenuated increase in gloimeruli fluorescence, decreased the rise of urinary albumin excretion and prevented the mesangial expansion.[33]

Aminoguanidine decreases accumulation of AGEs and increases motor nerve conduction velocity in experimental diabetic rats treated for 12-16 weeks, without any changes in body weight, HbA1C or blood glucose.[34]

In humans high rate of adverse reactions, including hepatotoxicity, prompted early termination of studies.

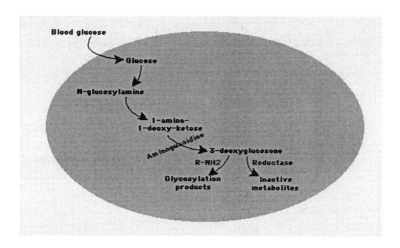

Figure 7. AGE production and possible inhibition by aminoguanidine. (Adapted, with permission, from Clark, CM, Lee, DA et al. Prevention and treatment of the complications of diabetes mellitus. New England Journal of Medicine 332:1210, 1995).[35]

Other agents targeting AGEs are currently under investigation. They are AGE crosslink breakers (clinical role unestablished), such as PTB (N-phenacylthiazolium bromide) and ALT-711 (an ethanol which in one study of diabetic rats resulted in 52% decrease in Hgb-AGE compared with controls) and AGE receptor inhibitors.[36]

Aldose reductase inhibitors.

Glucose that enters cells is metabolized in part to sorbitol via enzyme aldose reductase. Aldose reductase is a broad-specificity aldo-keto reductase with wide species and tissue distribution. The function of the enzyme under euglycemic conditions remains unclear.

Sorbitol production is markedly enhanced by hyperglycemia in experimental diabetes models. The accumulation of sorbitol within the cell results in rise of cell osmolality and a decrease of intracellular myoinositol, leading to decrease in NA-K-ATPase activity.

Drugs that block aldose reductase include spirohydantoins (sorbinil), carboxylic acid derivatives (tolrestat, ponalrestat) and flavonoids.

Animal studies with aldose reductase inhibitors were very promising. In diabetic rats treatment for five month with sorbinil minimized albuminuria and glomerular basement membrane thickening.[37] Aldose reductase inhibitors in this study improved nerve conduction velocity and prevented diabetic cataracts, however, there was no improvement or prevention of retinopathy in diabetic dogs, treated for 5 years.[38]

Aldose reductase facilitates vascular smooth muscle cell growth and proliferation, which is an important feature of atherosclerosis, restenosis and hypertension. Rats fed sorbinil after balloon injury of carotid arteries displayed a 51% and 58% reduction in the ratio of neointima to the media at 10 and 21 days, respectively, after balloon injury.

In humans clinical trials have assessed the efficacy of tolrestat, ponalrestat and sorbinil in the treatment of diabetic retinopathy, neuropathy and nephropathy. The benefits have generally been minimal. It is possible that the drug dose was too small and most studies were too short. Studies with sorbinil have been halted because of severe toxicity. Ponalrestat has not been effective. Tolrestat has been found to be nontoxic and beneficial in the treatment of painful neuropathy. The major side effect was an elevation of liver enzymes, which returned to normal after the discontinuation of the drug.

Sorbinil retinopathy trial was a randomized double blind study of sorbinil in treatment of diabetic retinopathy. 497 patients with type 1 diabetes mellitus, age 18-56 years, 1-15 years of diabetes duration, were treated for average of 41 months with sorbinil or placebo. Worsening of retinopathy occurred in 28% patients on sorbinil and 32 % in placebo group (p=0.34). The number of microaneurisms increased at a slower rate in sorbinil group. However, 7% of subjects developed hypersensitivity in the first 3 months.[39]

Effect of aldose reductase inhibitors on diabetic nephropathy is controversial. Some manifestations may be improved, however these drugs are not effective over the long term. In one study, 20 patients were treated with tolrestat (200 mg po qd) or placebo for 6 months. Tolrestat reversed glomerular hyperfiltration, with glomerular filtration rate (GFR) decreasing from 156 to 124 ml/min. (p<0.001). Urinary albumin excretion decreased from 197 to 158 mg/day (p<0.001).[40] In another study 16 diabetic patients were treated for 12 month with tolrestat (200 mg/day) or ascorbic acid (500 mg bid). Tolrestat had no effect on proteinuria after 9 month.[41]

In diabetic neuropathy aldose reductase inhibitors had inconsistent effect on parestesias, increased nerve conduction in some nerves, but produced no improvement in pain. In one study 372 patients with insulin requiring diabetes mellitus and neuropathy were treated with tolrestat for a mean of 4.2 years. Some were then switched to placebo and showed progression of motor neuropathy and deterioration of vibration threshold, others were continued on tolrestat and remained stable.[42] In another study 200 patients with symptomatic neuropathy were treated with tolrestat (200 mg po qd). 28% had improvement in motor nerve conduction velocity and parestesias vs 5% in placebo group. No benefit in neuropatic pain was established.[43] The sorbinil retinopathy trial demonstrated the lack of consistent benefit on the peripheral nerves: nerve conduction velocity increased in the peroneal nerve, but not in the median motor or sensory nerves, and no improvement in clinical symptoms was observed.[44]

ACE INHIBITORS

The studies available to date provide clear evidence of the beneficial effects of ACE inhibition in patients with microalbuminuria (in both type 1 and type 2 diabetes mellitus) and with overt nephropathy (particularly, in type 1 diabetes mellitus). Overall results clearly show that ACE inhibitors decrease albuminuria or proteinuria independent of blood pressure changes, treatment, duration, and type of diabetes and stage of nephropathy. One study demonstrated decrease in retinopathy progression as well.

The EUCLID (EURODIAB Controlled Trial of Lisinopril in Insulin Dependent Diabetes Mellitus), a randomized, multicenter, controlled clinical trial, enrolled 354 patients with type 1 diabetes, age 20 to 59 years. Patients had normal blood pressure; 85% of patients were normoalbuminuric and 15 % had microalbuminuria. They were randomly assigned to receive placebo or lisinopril (ACE inhibitor). During the 2 year follow-up retinopathy progressed in 13.2% of patients receiving lisinopril and 23.4% of patients receiving placebo (50% risk reduction). Patients with better glycemic control had the most benefit.[45]

HOPE (Heart Outcome Prevention Study) was a randomized double-blind trial to assess the effects of ramipril on cardiovascular death, myocardial infarction and stroke in 9297 patients, mean age 66 years, with a history of coronary artery disease, stroke, peripheral vascular disease or diabetes plus one other major cardiovascular risk factor. The study included 3577 people with diabetes. This study was prematurely terminated because of the clear evidence of beneficial effect of ramipril. Relative risk reductions were the following: for cardiovascular death – 0.75 [confidence interval or CI 0.64-0.87], for MI– 0.8 [CI 0.71-0.91], for stroke – 0.69 [CI 0.56-0.84], for all-cause mortality 0.84 – [CI 0.75-0.95], for revascularization O.84 [CI 0.76-0.93], for complications related to diabetes O.84 [CI 0.72-0.98]. However no adjustments for BP were made.[46]

In the MICRO-HOPE trial 3.577 patients with diabetes and cardiovascular disease (previous event or at least one cardiovascular risk factor) and no proteinuria were assigned to ramipril (10 mg po qd) or placebo. After 4.5 years of follow up there was a 24 % risk reduction of development of overt nephropathy independently of blood pressure control.[46]

ANGIOTENSIN-RECEPTOR ANTAGONISTS.

Until recently it was not known whether angiotensin-receptor blockers (ARBs) slow the rate of progression of nephropathy in patients with diabetes mellitus independently of their capacity to lower the systemic blood pressure. Two randomized trials published in September of 2001 produced convincing evidence that there is a protective effect, which is independent of the reduction in blood pressure.

In one study 1715 patients with hypertension and nephropathy due to type 2 diabetes mellitus were randomized to treatment with irbesartan (300 mg po qd), amlodipine (10 mg po qd) or placebo. Mean duration of follow up was 2.6 years. Target BP was 135/85 mm Hg or less in all groups. The relative risk of end stage renal disease was 23% lower in irbesartan group than in both other groups (14.2 % in irbesartan group vs 18.3 % in amlodipine group and 17.8 % in placebo group). The relative risk of doubling of serum creatinine concentration was 33 % lower in irbesartan group than in placebo group and 37 % lower in irbesartan group than in amlodipine group. The serum creatinine concentration increased 24 % more slowly in the irbesartan group than in the placebo group and 21% more slowly than in the amlodipine group. There were no significant differences in the rates of death from any cause or in the cardiovascular death.[47]

In another study 1513 patients were enrolled and randomized to receive angiotensin-II-receptor blocker losartan or placebo, both taken in addition to conventional antihypertensive treatment for a mean of 3.4 years. Losartan reduced the incidence of end stage renal disease (risk reduction 25%) and the doubling of serum creatinine concentration (risk reduction 28 %). There was no effect on mortality. The level of proteinuria declined by 35 % with losartan.[48]

Both losartan and irbesartan conferred significant renal benefits in patients with type 2 diabetes mellitus and nephropathy independent of the antihypertensive effect of these agents.

SUMMARY

Preventing complications of diabetes mellitus is a challenge for every physician. There is clear evidence that both intensive glycemic control and intensive blood pressure control significantly reduce microvascular and macrovascular complications. Use of ACE-inhibitors and ARBs became a standard of care in patients with diabetes and microalbuminuria, as both classes of drugs were proven to have significant renal benefits independently of their antihypertensive effects. Researches are looking at different mechanisms of tissue injury as the result of hyperglycemia, such as advanced glycosylation end products formation and sorbitol accumulation. However, agents inhibiting formation of these products are still under investigation and early studies in humans have shown a high rate of adverse reactions.

REFERENCES

1. Nathan DM. The pathophysiology of diabetic complications: how much does the glucose hypothesis explain? Ann Intern Med 124: 86-89, 1996.
2. UK Prospective Diabetes Study (UKPDS) Group. Intensive blood-glucose control with sulphonylureas or insulin compared with conventional treatment and risk of complications in patients with type 2 diabetes (UKPDS 33). Lancet 352:837-853, 1998.

3. The Diabetes Control and Complications Trial Research Group. The effect of intensive treatment of diabetes on the development and progression of long term complications in insulin-dependent diabetes mellitus. N Engl J Med 329:977-986, 1993.

4. The Diabetes Control and Complications Trial Research Group. The effect of intensive diabetes therapy on the development and progression of neuropathy. Ann Intern Med 122:561-568, 1995.

5. The Diabetes Control and Complications Research Group. The relationship of glycemic exposure (HbA1c) to the risk of development and progression of retinopathy in the diabetes control and complications trial. Diabetes 44:968-983, 1995.

6. The Diabetes Control and Complications Trial Research Group. Adverse events and their association with treatment regimens in the Diabetes Control and Complications Trial. Diabetes Care 18:1415-1427, 1995.

7. Wang PH, Lau J, Chalmers TC. Meta-analysis of effects of intensive blood glucose control on late complications of type 1 diabetes. Lancet 341:1306-9, 1993.

8. Ohkubo Y, Kishikawa H, Araki E, et al. Intensive insulin therapy prevents the progression of diabetic microvascular complications in Japanese patients with non-insulin-dependent diabetes mellitus: a randomized prospective 6-year study. Diabetes Res Clin Pract 28:103-117, 1995.

9. Testa MA, Simonson DC. Health economic benefits and quality of life during improved glycemic control in patients with type 2 diabetes mellitus. JAMA 280:1490-1496, 1998.

10. Knatterud GL , Klimt CR , Levin ME , Jacobson ME , Goldner MG. Effects of hypoglycemic agents on vascular complications in patients with adult-onset diabetes. VII. Mortality and selected nonfatal events with insulin treatment. JAMA 240:37-42, 1978.

11. The University Group Diabetes Program. A study of the effects of hypoglycemic agents on vascular complications in patients with adult-onset diabetes. V. Evaluation of phenformin therapy. Diabetes 24 (Suppl 1):65-184, 1975.

12. Genuth S. Exogenous insulin administration and cardiovascular risk in non-insulin-dependent and insulin-dependent diabetes mellitus. Ann Intern Med 124: 104-109, 1996.

13. Colwell JA. The feasibility of intensive insulin management in non-insulin-dependent diabetes mellitus: implications of the Veterans Affairs Cooperative Study on Glycemic Control and Complications in NIDDM. Ann Intern Med 124(1, pt 2): 131-135, 1996.

14. Klein R, Klein BE, Moss SE. Relation of glycemic control to diabetic microvascular complications in diabetes mellitus. Ann Intern Med 124(1, pt 2): 90-96, 1996.

15. Klein R, Klein BE, Moss SE, Cruickshanks KJ. The Wisconsin Epidemiologic Study of Diabetic Retinopathy, XV: the long-term incidence of macular edema. Ophthalmology 102:7-16, 1995.
16. Klein R, Klein BE, Moss SE. The Wisconsin Epidemiologic Study of Diabetic Retinopathy, XVI: the relationship of C-peptide to the incidence and progression of diabetic retinopathy. Diabetes 44:796-801, 1995.
17. Moss SE, Klein R, Klein BE. Long-term incidence of lower-extremity amputations in a diabetic population. Arch Fam Med 5:391-398, 1996.
18. Laakso M. Glycemic control and the risk for coronary heart disease in patients with non-insulin-dependent diabetes mellitus: the Finnish studies. Ann Intern Med 124:127-130, 1996.
19. Lehto S, Ronnemaa T, Pyorala K, Laakso M. Predictors of stroke in middle-aged patients with non-insulin-dependent diabetes. Stroke 27:63-68, 1996.
20. Anderson DK, Svardsudd K. Long-term glycemic control relates to mortality in type II diabetes. Diabetes Care 18:1534-1543, 1995.
21. Stratton IM, Adler AI, Neil HAW on behalf of the UKPDS group. Association of glycemia with macrovascular and microvascular complications of type 2 diabetes (UKPDS 35). Br Med J 321:405-412, 2000.
22. The sixth report of the Joint National Committee on prevention, detection, evaluation and treatment of high blood pressure. Arch Internal Medicine 157:2413-46, 1997.
23. Hansson L, Zanchetti A, Carruthers SG, et al, for the HOT Study Group. Effects of intensive blood-pressure lowering and low dose aspirin in patients with hypertension: principal results of the Hypertension Optimal Treatment [HOT] randomized trial. Lancet 351:1755-1762, 1998.
24. UK Prospective Diabetes Study group. Tight blood pressure control and risk of macrovascular and microvascular complications in type 2 diabetes: UKPDS 38. Brit Med Journal 317:703-713, 1998.
25. UK Prospective Diabetes Study group. Efficacy of atenolol and captopril in reducing risk of macrovascular and microvascular complications in type 2 diabetes: UKPDS 39. Brit Med Journal 317:703-713, 1998.
26. Vlassara H, Fuh H, Makita Z, Krungari S, Cerami A, Bucala R. Exogenous advanced glycosylation end products induce complex vascular dysfunction in normal animals: a model for diabetic and aging complications. Proc Nat Acad of Sci 89 (24): 12043-7, 1992.
27. Vlassara H. Serum advanced glycosylation end products. A new class of uremic toxins? Blood Purif 12(1): 54-9, 1994.
28. Yang CW, Vlassara H, Peten EP, et al. Advanced glycation end products up-regulate gene expression found in diabetic glomerular disease. Proc Nat Acad Sci USA 27:9634-9640, 1994.
29. Ono Y, Aoki, et al. Increased serum level of advanced glycation end products and diabetic complications. Diabetes Res. Clinical Practice 41(2), 131-137, 1998.

30. Bucala R. What is the effect of hyperglycemia on atherogenesis and can it be reversed by aminoguanidine? Diabetes Research Clinical Practice Feb; 30 Suppl: 123-130, 1996.

31. Brownlee M, Vlassara H, Koonee T, et al. Aminoguanidine prevents diabetes induced arterial wall protein cross-linking. Science 232:1629-1632, 1986.

32. Hammes HP, Martin S; Federlin K; Geisen K, Brownlee M. Aminoguanidine treatment inhibits the development of experimental diabetic retinopathy. Proc Natl Acad Sci 88(24):11555-11558, 1991.

33. Soulis T, Cooper ME, Vranes D, et al. Effects of aminoguanidine in preventing experimental diabetic nephropathy are related to the duration of treatment. Kidney Intl 50:627-634, 1996.

34. Yagihashi S, Kamijo M, Baba, M, et al. Effect of aminoguanidine on functional and structural abnormalities in peripheral nerve of stz induced diabetic rats. Diabetes 41:47 , 1992.

35. Clark CM, Lee DA, Prevention and treatment of the complications of diabetes mellitus. New England Journal of Medicine 332:1210-1217, 1995.

36. Al-Abed, et al. Inhibition of advanced glycation end product formation by acetaldehyde. Proc Natl Acad Sci 96:2385-2390, 1999.

37. Kassab J, Guillot, R et al. Renal and microvascular effects of an aldose-reductase inhibitor in experimental diabetes. Biochem Pharmacology 48:1003, 1994.

38. Engerman R, Kern, Garment, M, et al. Capillary basement membrane in retina, kidney and muscle of diabetic dogs and galactosemic dogs and its response to 5 years of aldose-reductase inhibition. J Diabetes complications 7: 241-245, 1993.

39. A randomized trial of sorbinil, an aldose reductase inhibitor, in diabetic retinopathy. Sorbinil Retinopathy Trial Research Group Arch Ophthalmol 108:1234-1244, 1990.

40. Passariello N, Sepe J, Marazzo, G, et al. Effect of aldose reductase inhibitor [tolrestat] on urinary albumin excretion rate and glomerular filtration rate in IDDM subjects with nephropathy. Diabetes care 16:789-795, 1993.

41. Mc-Auliffe A, Brooks, B, et al. Administration of ascorbic acid and aldose reductase inhibitor tolrestat in diabetes. Effect on urinary albumin excretion. Nephron 80:277-284, 1998.

42. Santiago J, Sonksen P, Boulton. Withdrawal of the aldose reductase inhibitor tolrestat in diabetic neuropathy. Effect on nerve function. J Diab Compl 7:170-178, 1993.

43. Boulton A, Levin S, et. al. A multicenter trial of aldose reductase inhibitor tolrestat in patients with symptomatic diabetic neuropathy. Diabetologia 33:431-437,1990.

44. Christen WG, Manson JE, Bubes V, Glynn RJ. Risk factors for progression of distal symmetric polyneuropathy in type 1 diabetes mellitus. Sorbinil Retinopathy Trial Research Group. Am J Epidemiol 150(11): 1142-51, 1999.

45. Chaturvedi N, Sjolie AK, Stephenson JM, et al. And the EUCLID Study Group; Effect of lisinopril on progression of retinopathy in normotensive people with type 1 diabetes mellitus. Lancet 351:28-31, 1998.

46. Effects of Ramipril on cardiovascular and microvascular outcomes in patients with diabetes mellitus: results of the HOPE and MICRO-HOPE study. HOPE study investigators. Lancet 355:253-259, 2000.

47. Parving MD, Hendrik L, et al. For the Irbesartan in Patients with type 2 diabetes and microalbuminuria study group. The effect of Irbesartan on the development of diabetic nephropathy in patients with type 2 diabetes. N Engl J Med 345:870-878, 2001.

48. Brenner BM, Cooper ME, et al. for the RENAAL study Investigators. Effects of losartan on renal and cardiovascular outcomes in patients with type 2 diabetes and nephropathy. N Engl J Med 345:861-869, 2001.

Chapter 8. Psychological and Psychiatric Issues in Diabetes Mellitus

Katie Weinger, Garry W. Welch and Alan M. Jacobson

INTRODUCTION

Diabetes mellitus is a chronic endocrine disorder that places significant psychological and physical demands on individuals and their families. Diabetes requires complex treatment involving medication, health-monitoring behaviors, and regulation of lifestyle factors such as dietary intake and exercise. Thus the treatment of diabetes demands active participation of the patient as well as the physician. Consequently, psychological issues surrounding coping with diagnosis, treatment, lifestyle modifications, family stresses, and continued motivation typically arise. Moreover, several psychiatric comorbidities can play a significant role in the course of diabetes and can further complicate treatment.

PREDICTABLE CRISES OF DIABETES

A useful approach to the psychosocial consequences of diabetes is examination of the predictable crises that may occur over the course of this lifelong illness.[1] Four major phases exist, each with its own specific psychological implications for the patient and family.[2]

Onset

Type 1 diabetes. The onset of type 1 diabetes is usually abrupt and immediate care may involve intense medical treatment or hospitalization that requires mobilization of all family resources. The onset of diabetes may be experienced as a loss eliciting grief and mourning for the healthy person. The response to diabetes may be influenced by patients' or family members' prior experience with diabetes, particularly if diabetes resulted in severe complications or death. Often, the emotional crises surrounding the diagnosis of diabetes prevent patients and families from remembering all of the information provided them, further complicating the adaptive process. The physician can provide further support through referrals to other health professionals, nurse educators, nutritionists, exercise physiologists and psychologists. Families with limited emotional and relationship resources are at particular risk in all phases of diabetes treatment. Those families may benefit from referral to a mental health professional. Referral to mental health professionals for support coping with diabetes and normal development issues is helpful for all families of newly diagnosed young children.

Type 2 diabetes. The onset of type 2 diabetes is more insidious with some patients having had the disease for years prior to diagnosis. Patients may present with microvascular or macrovascular complications or may be feeling fine without obvious signs of an illness. Although type 2 diabetes is occurring with increased frequency in children[3], type 2 patients tend to be older, more conditioned to accept chronic illness and medications as a normal part of aging. If diabetes is treated with nutrition and lifestyle or with oral agents, some patients may not realize the seriousness of diabetes or the importance of treatment and may not experience sufficient impetus to alter lifelong eating and activity habits. Others who present with cardiovascular complications at diagnosis may experience a more abrupt crisis at onset.

Prevention of Complications

Once a patient adjusts to the diagnosis of this demanding chronic illness, the next phase entails living with diabetes in the absence of serious consequences. Some patients may not understand the importance or urgency for implementing all of the recommended self-care activities when they are feeling well. In fact, unpleasant symptoms may be more associated with treatment rather than the disease itself, thus dampening motivation.

Helping patients follow treatment recommendations. The goal of therapy at this phase is to maintain healthy living choices and promote adherence to treatment recommendations. During this phase, the person with diabetes learns how to be a patient with a chronic illness. Although health care professionals spend many years learning their roles, patients have not had training in how to be an effective patient. Thus in the therapeutic relationship, one of the provider's roles is to teach the patient how to maximize the value of the time spent at a medical appointment. Suggest that the patient prepares for medical appointments by making lists of all questions before an appointment and not leave until those questions are addressed. When evaluating the success of a treatment plan, consider how well the patient is able to follow self-care recommendations. An important starting point is assessing how well patients know and understand exactly what self-care behaviors their treatment plans recommend. If patients know how many times per day they should check their blood glucose levels, what their meal plans are, how often to take their medications, then the next step is assessing barriers that prevent patients from following recommendations. Finally, consider what support each patient needs to help integrate diabetes treatment into everyday life.[4] Examples of approaches could include simplification of the treatment plan, referral for diabetes education, or referral to a mental health professional for support.

Table 1.   Psychological stages of diabetes

Stage	Consequences	Clinical approaches
I. Onset: adaptive crisis linked to realization "I am ill"	Grief and mourning over loss of health; stress on family. Lack of symptoms or prolonged honeymoon period may lead to denial of illness and its consequences	Establish a therapeutic relationship with patient and family, provide support, answer questions, expect much of information provided to be forgotten, referral for diabetes education, referral of all families with young children for mental health support.
II. Preventive therapy: the challenge of learning and following a complex and demanding therapy when the benefit is distant	Problem integrating treatment recommendations in everyday life; competing concerns resulting in family tension; avoidance of hypoglycemia; driving and safety precautions	Maintain therapeutic relationship. Support patient's self-management efforts. Provide support for healthy patient/ family communication; mental health referral for significant adherence problems. Instruct patients to check glucose levels and treat hypoglycemia before driving or dangerous activities or sports.
III. Development of early medical complications: the frightening facts embed themselves	May lead to anxiety, depression, and return of grief and mourning, may mobilize patient and family to take action	Mental health referral, medical treatment of anxiety and depression.
IV. Complications dominate the illness: 'new' illnesses change the patient's view of self.	Complications may overwhelm diabetes concerns; intensified psychological reactions, change in family roles, medical team assumes a larger role in patient's life, reinvent identity to include heightened isolation, complications, demoralization.	Passing the baton to new medical team members, family therapy and support, mental health referral.

Some diabetes patients approach medical appointments as an evaluation of their behavior and worth. Some may begin the appointment with statements 'I've been bad', others may be reluctant to show their blood glucose logs or have their glucose meters downloaded, and others may simply not come to the appointment. Let patients know that if they are unable to follow their treatment plans, the problem may be that the treatment plan needs adjustment to better suit their lifestyles or that diabetes education and training may be necessary to help them adapt diabetes self-management to their lifestyles. Blame whether real or imagined has no place in the therapeutic relationship. The physician's role includes listening to patients' emotional, physical, and social issues and recognizing patients as collaborative partners in their diabetes care rather than passive recipients.[5]

Fear of hypoglycemia & cognitive effects of hypoglycemia. Many patients fear hypoglycemia and act to avoid hypoglycemic symptoms at the expense of glycemic control. The sweating, tremors, slowed reaction time, cognitive deterioration, and possible seizures[6,7] are unpleasant, frightening, and embarrassing. Patients can become confused and incapacitated so that they require the assistance of others in treating the hypoglycemia. Seizures and coma may require treatment in the emergency department. Hypoglycemia can be dangerous for the patient and others. Therefore, all adolescent and adult patients should be instructed to check blood glucose levels prior to driving, and if below 70 mg/dl, to treat with 15 grams of carbohydrate (6 oz non-diet cola, 3-4 glucose tabs, etc) before driving.[8] This holds true for all adult drivers, including those experienced drivers who have had diabetes for many years. Caution patients to check glucose levels prior to and during performance of any dangerous activity or sport, including using power tools, skiing, running, etc. Patients on insulin and certain oral agents should always have a fast acting glucose source accessible.

Family concerns. The demands of diabetes self-management when no obvious signs of complications are present may frustrate some diabetes patients and prevent them from actively participating in their care. Often problems within the family arise because of family concerns over the lack of diligence in the patient's diabetes self-management or the occurrence of hypoglycemia. Family and friends may be concerned and frightened by symptoms of severe hypoglycemia including impaired cognition, loss of consciousness, and seizures. Fear of complications and hypoglycemia along with frustration with lack of control may trigger family conflict. For example, diabetic adolescents, seeking autonomy and identity with peers, may strive to avoid the unpleasantness and embarrassment of hypoglycemia by keeping blood sugars high while their parents, fearful of future complications, may stress normalizing blood glucose levels.[9] Adult patients may be reluctant to alter long duration lifestyle habits. Patients and families may need help in learning how to channel concern into support by establishing boundaries and improving communication. Patients may need to learn how to discuss what is helpful support and what is detrimental with their family and friends.

Table 2. Guidelines for supporting patient/ family interactions[10]

1. Teach family about diabetes in general.
2. Listen to the family's concerns, worries, and past experiences with diabetes.
3. Educate the family to have realistic and appropriate expectations concerning blood glucose levels and behavior.
4. Model positive helping and prevent destructive family helping that undermines the patient's attempts at healthy diabetes self-care.

Adapted from Anderson B. " Involving Family Members in Diabetes Treatment" (ref. 10).

Diabetes treatment is a team effort with the patient at the center. Meeting all of the patient's health and health education needs in a 15 to 30 minute appointment is not possible. Thus referrals to and communication with other health care professionals are key components of diabetes treatment. Team members including mental health specialists, nutritionists, diabetes nurse educators, and exercise psychologists provide services that are often reimbursed by insurance.

Onset of Medical Complications

The onset of medical complications may stimulate enormous anxiety and fear. Individuals vary in their responses, some may consider early complications as a wake-up call to alter their lifestyles and take charge of their diabetes. They may initiate medical appointments and seek out diabetes education information. Others may become overwhelmed and turn away from the health care system, skipping medical appointments and omitting recommended diabetes self-care behaviors. Family experience with diabetes may influence a patient's response to the onset of complications, whether viewed as inevitable or as a challenge that can be controlled. Although the patient may not overtly show any signs of fear, the assumption that every medical visit contains some anticipatory concern is probably valid. Follow-up calls to reschedule missed appointments can be helpful as clinic attendance is associated with better health outcomes[11] and improved glycemic control not only delays the onset but also delays the progression of diabetes complications.[12] Some patients may want or need help organizing their approaches to diabetes self-care; they may not have the information or planning skills to mount a successful response to complications.

Complications Dominate

This phase typically develops when one or more complications are present to the extent that regular treatment or interventions are necessary. The complications of diabetes can be socially and emotionally devastating: painful neuropathies that interfere with ambulation, digestion, and sexual function, serious cardiovascular disease, blindness, and nephropathy are a few. While adapting to these serious new conditions with additional medical appointments, patients must continue to self-manage their underlying diabetes.

During this phase, some patients may become so focused on the treatment of the complication that diabetes itself is delegated to the background. Successful treatment or remission of the complication, such as with kidney transplantation or retinal laser surgery, still leaves the burden of treating diabetes. The realization of the continuing burden of diabetes may result in a complex response that mixes a sense of relief due to the successful treatment of the complication with sadness and possibly a reinitiation of grieving associated with the diagnosis of diabetes. Patients and their families may require additional support at this time.

PSYCHIATRIC DISORDERS

Individuals with diabetes are at risk of several serious psychiatric disorders that complicate their treatments and their abilities to achieve glycemic targets thus placing them at high risk of the serious microvascular and macrovascular complications of diabetes. Patients with diabetes are at higher than average risk of depression and eating disorders.

Depression and depressive disorders

Depression is a serious psychiatric disorder that interferes with interpersonal relationships, quality of life, and the ability to perform and function. The prevalence of depression among people with diabetes is two to three times that of the general population with estimated rates ranging from 8.5% to 27.3%.[13-15]

Comorbid depression occurs in all age groups and ethnic minorities experience depressive symptoms and depression at approximately rates that equal those of adult Caucasians.[16-19] Depression is associated with poor glycemic control and diabetes complications of retinopathy, nephropathy, hypertension, cardiac disease, and sexual dysfunction.[16, 20-23] In addition, severity of depressive symptoms is associated with poor adherence to dietary recommendations and medication regimen, functional impairment and higher health care costs in primary care diabetes patients.[24] Thus, dysthymia and subclinical depression may influence diabetes treatment. Unfortunately, depression in diabetes is both under-recognized and, when recognized, under-treated.[25, 26]

Table 3. Signs and Symptoms of Depression

Depressive symptoms

Depressed mood	Pessimism
Loss of pleasure or interest in activities	Significant weight or appetite loss
Tearfulness and crying spells	when not dieting; failure to
Irritability *	gain age appropriate weight*
Increased sense of worthlessness or guilt	Indecisiveness
Recurrent thoughts of suicide or death	Social withdrawal
Suicide threats or attempts	Insomnia or hypersomnia *
Decreased concentration *	Psychomotor slowing *
Decreased recent memory*	Psychomotor agitation
Fatigue; loss of energy*	

*Symptoms that may also reflect poorly controlled diabetes and/or hypoglycemia

Depression presents with symptoms that are cognitive, physical, affective, or attitudinal. Rarely will someone present with all the symptoms listed (Table 3). Symptoms of depression are common in everyday life and the physical and cognitive symptoms often overlap with poorly controlled diabetes, making the diagnosis more difficult.[27] However, if a person experiences a depressed mood or loss of interest or pleasure in usual activities and at least four other of the listed symptoms for a duration of at least 2 weeks, then major depression should be considered, particularly if glycemic control also deteriorates and the person is not able to function in the home or occupational roles.[28]

Table 4. Common problems associated with the treatment of depression in diabetes (Ref. 29).

1. Failure to recognize and diagnose
2. Failure to identify target symptoms of the depressed patient.
3. Failure to follow symptom response to treatment over time.
4. Failure to follow patients with sufficient frequency
5. Underdosing of medication
6. Failure to use adjunctive medication when required
7. Premature evaluation of antidepressant therapy

Treatment of Depression in Diabetes
Depressive disorders are usually responsive to treatment, although several barriers to appropriate treatment exist (Table 4). Two types of treatments for depression are readily available: medications and

psychotherapy. Both have been shown to be effective and can be used in combination.[30-31] Choice of treatment depends on an assessment of the patient and the depressive symptoms, the patient's insurance coverage and/or financial situation, patient preference, and experience of the treating physician. Patients with major depressive disorders who are experiencing suicidal ideation are at serious risk and need immediate referral to psychiatric care. Treatment with electroconvulsive therapy is usually reserved for psychotic or intractable depression.[30]

Table 5. Diabetes Implications of Antidepressant Therapy

Classification	Generic	Precautions
Tricyclic	Amitrypiline, clomipramine, desipramine, doxepin, imipramine, nortriptyline, trimipramine	May cause hypoglycemia when used alone or in combination with other drugs such as sulfonylureas.[32] Possible hyperglycemia, increased appetite, weight gain, increased risk of cardiac arrhythmias, blurred vision, urinary hesitancy, sexual dysfunction, constipation, orthostatic hypotension, seizures
Heterocyclics	Amoxapine, maprotiline	Similar to Tricyclics
	Trazodone	Drowsiness, nausea or gastroparesis, impotence, urinary retention or frequency, orthostatic hypotension, seizures
	bupropion	Dizziness, dry mouth, sweating, tremor, decreased appetite, seizures
Selective serotonin reuptake inhibitors (SSRI)	Fluoxetine, paroxetine, sertraline	Possible hypoglycemia, sexual dysfunction, decreased appetite, impaired erectile function, aggravation of gastroparesis, sweating
Serotonin and norepinephrine reuptake inhibitors (SNRI)	Venlafaxine	Sustained hypertension, sexual dysfunction, nausea, sweating, dizziness, anxiety or nervousness, decreased appetite
Monoamine oxidase inhibitors	Isocarboxazid, phenelzine, tranylcypromine	Hypoglycemia (may be severe)[33]; hypertensive crisis; serious/fatal drug interactions such as hyperthermia, rigidity, mycoclonic movements, death

Success of treatment is determined through the evaluation of symptoms, therefore symptoms must be assessed initially and their response to treatment followed over time. As depression improves and symptoms begin to remit, patients are more energetic and therefore at greater risk of suicide. Following patients with sufficient frequency is very important. Adjusting antidepressant medication dosage may be necessary to allow the patient full benefit. The most common reason for treatment failure in a patient who has been started on medication is an insufficient dose; thus, following individualized symptoms for each patient over time is extremely important. Table 5 presents side effects of antidepressant medications that mimic or aggravate diabetes and its complications. Although seizures have been reported with tricylcic and other antidepressants, the most significant risk is with bupropion. Refer to a psychopharmocology text for a more in-depth discussion of antidepressive medications, their actions, and side effects. Tricylic antidepressants have autonomic side effects that can aggravate autonomic neuropathies of diabetes. SSRI's may cause hypoglycemia and worsen impotence. In addition to having serious side effects that may exacerbate diabetes-related conditions, monoamine oxidase inhibitors (MAOI) may interact with many other medications including meperidine, most antidepressants, antiarrythmics, vasoconstrictors, and decongestants with dangerous and potentially fatal consequences.[30] A washout period of approximately 10 days to 5 weeks depending on the antidepressant is necessary prior to switching to or from an MAOI. MAOIs should be used with extreme caution and not as a first line therapy. Some antidepressants have actions that are beneficial to diabetes and these actions may influence the choice of medication. For example, antidepressants that decrease appetite may positively influence an obese type 2 patient's eating habits and weight. Also, tricyclic antidepressants can reduce the pain associated with neuropathy.

Disordered Eating and Diabetes

Weight concerns and dissatisfaction with one's body are common issues for young women in American society. Eating disorders are now recognized as a significant women's health problem and a lethal psychiatric diagnosis.[34] The consequences of these eating disorders are compounded by the severe complications associated with poorly controlled diabetes: retinopathy, neuropathy, and nephropathy.[35] Even subclinical disordered eating in the presence of diabetes may put women at risk by worsening metabolic control and hastening the serious metabolic and microvascular complications of diabetes.[36, 37]

Women with diabetes are at higher risk of developing clinical and subclinical eating disorders including anorexia nervosa, bulimia and binge eating disorder than women in the general population.[38, 39] Several factors associated with type 1 diabetes and its treatment may foster this increased prevalence of disordered eating.[40] In order to prevent serious micro- and macrovascular complications, treatment of diabetes aims to achieve blood glucose ranges as close to normal as possible. This goal requires a complex set of daily patient self-care behaviors such as careful attention to food portions and choices, regular exercise, weight management, multiple insulin injections, and regular blood glucose monitoring. The attention to food portions and weight that is part of routine diabetes management parallels the rigid thinking about food and body image found in women with eating disorders.[40] Also, the institution of insulin therapy and intensive insulin treatment are both associated with weight gain.[12, 41] Recent evidence suggests that women with type 1 diabetes are 2.4 times more at risk of eating disorders and 1.9 times more at risk of subclinical disordered eating than nondiabetic controls.[38] Women with type 1 diabetes and coexisting eating disorders are in poorer glycemic control, with glycosylated hemoglobin levels approximately 2 percentage points (or more) higher than similarly aged women without eating disorders.[35, 42-44]

Growing evidence suggests that as many as 31% of women with type 1 diabetes experiment with insulin omission and approximately 8-10% of women with diabetes reduce or omit necessary insulin injections for the purposes of weight loss at a frequency that warrants diagnosis of an eating disorder.[39, 42, 45, 46] Women reporting intentional insulin misuse had higher HbA$_1$c levels, higher rates of hospital and emergency room visits, higher rates of neuropathy and retinopathy[36,42] and more negative attitudes towards diabetes[47] than women who did not report insulin omission.

Type 2 diabetes and obesity are both recognized as important American public health epidemics (See Section IX Chapter 1). Research evidence indicates that among obese adults there is a distinct subgroup (of 20-46%) who report engaging in recurrent binge eating, defined as consumption of a large amount of food while feeling out of control of the behavior.[48, 49] Striegel-Moore and colleagues[50] found that African American and Caucasian women reported similar rates of single episodes of binge eating (8.4% and 8.8% respectively), however African American women reported significantly more *recurrent* binge eating than Caucasian women (4.5% vs. 2.6%). Additionally, women with recurrent binge eating had a significantly higher body mass index than non-binging controls and reported significantly more psychiatric symptoms.

The literature on binge eating in type 2 diabetes is still in its infancy. Rates of binge eating were substantial among patients with type 2 diabetes, ranging from 14% to 21% in the three small studies that examined this issue [51-53] with women being affected more often than men.[51, 53] When comparing age-, sex-, and weight-matched individuals with and without diabetes, Kenardy and colleagues[52] found that 14% of the patients with newly diagnosed type 2 diabetes experienced problems with binge eating as compared to 4% of the control group.

Therapeutic approaches to eating disorders include prevention, particularly for preadolescent and adolescent girls, but also for diabetes patients of any age and sex. Within the doctor-patient relationship several approaches may be helpful[54]. Avoidance of emphasis on weight loss or, if weight loss is a necessary goal, stressing healthy eating and realistically obtainable short-term goals for both weight and glycemic control supports the development of therapeutic attitudes about diabetes and its treatment. American Diabetes Association guidelines now stress nutritional management and 'healthy eating' instead of 'dieting.' The avoidance of language that may suggest excessive weight loss is key when treating diabetes patients. Allow patients to express their negative feelings about diabetes and their own goals for diabetes treatment without being judgmental. Acknowledging even small improvements in glycemic control when also reaching weight targets (whether that target is to gain or lose weight) is helpful. Family involvement and support is extremely important in the prevention and successful treatment of disordered eating. Women with serious eating disorders require referral to a mental health professional, preferably one who has experience with the treatment of diabetes.

SUMMARY

Diabetes is a chronic illness that places extraordinary demands on the patient and family. Successful treatment of diabetes requires an open and supportive relationship between the patient and provider as well as referral to other health care team members. Patients may experience predictable crises during the treatment of diabetes beginning with the response to diagnosis. The next phase of treatment requires the patient and family to participate in demanding self-care behaviors in the absence of symptoms or complications. The lack of immediacy may interfere with patients' motivation for completing self-care tasks. Continuing poor glycemic control may result in embarrassment over the inability to manage diabetes and in low attendance to medical appointments. Patients and concerned family members may develop relationship problems centered over fears of complications or severe hypoglycemia. At the onset and progression of complications, patients and families may respond with anxiety and grief. Finally, depressive disorders and eating disorders, although more common in diabetes than in the general population, are under-recognized and under-treated. Depression can be treated with medications, however severe depression and eating disorders usually require referral to mental health professionals.

REFERENCES

1. Hamburg BA, Inoff GE. Coping with predictable crises of diabetes. Diabetes Care 6:409-416, 1983.
2. Jacobson AM. The psychological care of patients with insulin-dependent diabetes mellitus. N Engl J Med 334:1249-1253, 1996.

3. Fagot-Campagna A, Pettitt DJ, Engelgau MM, Burrows NR, Geiss LS, Valdez R, Beckles GL, Saaddine J, Gregg EW, Williamson DF, Narayan KM. Type 2 diabetes among North American children and adolescents: an epidemiologic review and a public health perspective. J Pediatr 136:664-72, 2000.

4. Weinger K, Jacobson AM. Psychosocial and quality of life correlates of glycemic control during intensive treatment of type 1 diabetes. Patient Educ Couns 42:123-131, 2001.

5. Glasgow RE, Anderson RM. In diabetes care, moving from compliance to adherence is not enough.: something entirely different is needed. Diabetes Care 22:090-2091, 1999.

6. Draelos MT, Jacobson AM, Weinger K, Widom B, Ryan CM, Finkelstein DM, Simonson, DC. Cognitive function in patients with insulin-dependent diabetes mellitus during hypoglycemia and hyperglycemia. Am J Med 8:35-144, 1995.

7. Weinger K, Jacobson AM. Cognitive impairment in patients with type 1 (insulin dependent) diabetes mellitus: incidence, mechanisms and therapeutic implications. CNS Drugs 9:233-252, 1998.

8. Weinger K, Kinsley BT, Levy CJ, Bajaj M, Simonson DC, Quigely M, Cox DJ, Ryan CM, Jacobson AM. Factors associated with perceptions of safe driving ability during hypoglycemia in type 1 diabetes mellitus. Am J Med 107:246-253, 1999.

9. Weinger K, O'Donnell K, Ritholtz MD. Adolescent views of diabetes-related parent conflict and support: a focus group analysis. Journal Adolescent Health, J Adolesc Health 29:330-336, 2001.

10. Anderson B Involving family members in diabetes treatment. In Practical Psychology for Diabetes Clinicians. Anderson B, Rubin RR (eds). Alexandria, VA: American Diabetes Association, pp 43-50, 1996.

11. Jacobson AM, Adler A, Derby L, Anderson B, Wolfsdorf J. Clinic attendance and glycemic control: a study of contrasting groups of patients with insulin-dependent diabetes mellitus. Diabetes Care 14:599-601, 1991.

12. DCCT Research Group. The effect of intensive treatment of diabetes on the development and progression of long-term complications in insulin-dependent diabetes mellitus. N Eng J Med 329 (14): 977-986, 1993.

13. Anderson RJ, Freedland KE, Clouse RE, Lustman PJ. The prevalence of comorbid depression in adults with diabetes: a meta-analysis. Diabetes Care 24:1069-1078, 2001.

14. Gavard JA, Lustman PJ, Clouse RE. Prevalence of depression in adults with diabetes: An epidemiologic evaluation. Diabetes Care 16:1167-1178, 1993.

15. Goodnick PJ, Henry JH, Buki VM. Treatment of depression in patients with diabetes mellitus. J Clin Psychiatry 56:128-136, 1995.

16. Kovacs M, Mukerji P, Drash A, Iyengar S. Biomedical and psychiatric risk factors for retinaopathy among children with IDDM. Diabetes Care 18:1592-1659, 1995.
17. Roy A, Roy M. Depressive symptoms in African-American type 1 diabetics. Depression and Anxiety 13:28-31, 2001.
18. Gary TL, Crum RM, Cooper-Patrick L, Ford D, Brancati FL. Depressive symptoms and metabolic control in African-Americans with type 2 diabetes. Diabetes Care 23:23-29, 2000.
19. Black SA. Increased health burden associated with comorbid depression in older diabetic Mexican Americans. Results from the Hispanic Established Population for the Epidemiologic Study of the Elderly survey. Diabetes Care 22:56-64, 1999.
20. Lustman PJ, Griffith LS, Gavard JA, Clouse RE. Depression in adults with diabetes. Diabetes Care 15:1631-1639, 1992.
21. Jacobson AM. Psychological care of patients with insulin-dependent diabetes mellitus. N Eng J Med 334: 1249-1253, 1996.
22. Cohen HW, Gibson G, Alderman MH. Excess risk of myocardial infarction in patients treated with antidepressant medications: association of use with tricyclic agents. Am J Med 108:2-8, 2000.
23. de Groot M, Anderson R, Freedland KE, Clouse RE, Lustman PJ. Association of depression and diabetes complications: a meta-analysis. Psychosom Med 63:619-630, 2001.
24. Ciechanowski PS, Katon WJ, Russo JE. Depression and diabetes: impact of depressive symptoms on adherence, function, and costs. Arch Intern Med 160:3278-3285, 2000.
25. Sclar DA, Robison LM, Skaer TL, Galin RS. Depression in diabetes mellitus: a national survey of office-based encounters, 1990-1995. Diabetes Educ 25:331-332, 1999.
26. Jacobson AM, Weinger K. Treating depression in diabetic patients: is there an alternative to medications? Ann Int Med 129:656-657, 1998.
27. Jacobson AM. Psychological perspectives in the care of patients with diabetes mellitus. In Psychiatric Secrets. Jacobson JL, Jacobson AM, Eds., 2nd edition. Philadelphia, Hanley & Belfaus, pp 426-434, 2001.
28. American Psychiatric Association. Diagnostic and Statistical Manual of Mental Disorders, Fourth Edition Test Revision. Washington DC American Psychiatric Association, pp349-397, 2000.
29. Jacobson AM, Weinger K. Psychosocial complications in diabetes. In Medical Management of Diabetes. Leahy J, Clark NG, Cefalu, WT., Eds. New York: Marcel Dekker, Inc., pp 559-572, 2000.
30. U.S. Department of Health and Human Services, Agency for Health Care Policy and Research, Depression Guideline Panel: Depression in Primary Care: Volume 2. Treatment of Major Depression (Clinical Practice guidelines, No. 5) Washington, DC: U.S. Government Printing Office (AHCPR publication #93-0551), 1993.

31. Lustman PJ, Griffith LS, Freedland KE, Kissel SS, Clouse RE. Cognitive behavioral therapy for depression in type 2 diabetes mellitus. A randomized, controlled trial. Ann Intern Med 129:613-621, 1998.

32. Mokshagundam SPL, Peiris AN. Drug induced disorders of glucose metabolism. In Medical Management of Diabetes Mellitus. Leahy JL, Clark NG, Cefalu WT, Eds. New York, Marcel Dekker, Inc., 2000.

33. Pandit MK, Burke J, Gustafson AB, Minocha A, Peiris AN. Drug-induced disorders of glucose tolerance. Ann Intern Med 118:529-539, 1993.

34. Vitiello B, Lederhendler I. Research on eating disorders: current status and future prospects. Biol Psychiatry 47:777-786, 2000.

35. Rydall AC, Rodin GM, Olmsted MP, Devenyi RG, Daneman D. Disordered eating behavior and microvascular complications in young women with insulin-dependent diabetes mellitus. N Engl J Med 336:1849-54, 1997.

36. Affenito SG, Backstrand JR, Welch GW, Lammi-Keefe CJ, Rodriguez NR, Adams CH. Subclinical and clinical eating disorders in IDDM negatively affect metabolic control. Diabetes Care 20:182-184, 1997.

37. Verrotti A, Catino M, De Luca FA, Morgese G, Chiarelli F. Eating disorders in adolescents with type 1 diabetes mellitus. Acta Diabetol 36:21-25, 1999.

38. Jones JM, Lawson ML, Daneman D, Olmsted MP, Rodin G. Eating disorders in adolescent females with and without type 1 diabetes: cross sectional study. BMJ 320:1563-1566, 2000.

39. Fairburn CG, Peveler RC, Davies B, Mann JI, Mayou RA. Eating disorders in young adults with insulin dependent diabetes mellitus: a controlled study. BMJ 303:17-20, 1991.

40. Daneman D, Olmsted M, Rydall A, Maharaj S, Rodin G. Eating disorders in young women with type 1 diabetes. Prevalence, problems and prevention. Horm Res 50 (Suppl 1):79-86, 1998.

41. DCCT Research Group. Weight gain associated with intensive therapy in the Diabetes Control and Complications Trial (DCCT). Diabetes Care 11:567-573, 1988.

42. Polonsky WH, Anderson BJ, Lohrer PA, Aponte JE, Jacobson AM, Cole CF. Insulin omission in women with IDDM. Diabetes Care 17:1178-85, 1994.

43. Wing RR, Nowalk MP, Marcus MD, Koeske R, Finegold D. Subclinical eating disorders and glycemic control in adolescents with type I diabetes. Diabetes Care 9:162-167, 1986.

44. Rodin GM, Daneman D. Eating disorders and IDDM. A problematic association. Diabetes Care 15:1402-1412, 1992.

45. Marcus MD, Wing RR, Guare J, Blair EH, Jawad A. Lifetime prevalence of major depression and its effects on treatment outcome in obese type 2 diabetic patients. Diabetes Care 15:253-255, 1992.

46. Hudson JI, Wentworth SM, Hudson MS, Pope HG Jr. Prevalence of anorexia nervosa and bulimia among young diabetic women. J Clin Psychiatry 46:88-89, 1985.
47. Biggs MM, Basco MR, Patterson G, Raskin P. Insulin withholding for weight control in women with diabetes. Diabetes Care 17:1186-1189, 1994.
48. Wilson, GT, Nonas, CA, Rosenblum, GD. Assessment of binge eating in obese patients. Int J Eat Disord 13:25-33, 1993.
49. de Zwaan M, Mitchell JE, Seim HC, Specker SM, Pyle RL, Raymond NC, Crosby RB. Eating related and general psychopathology in obese females with binge eating disorder. Int J Eat Disord 15:43-52, 1994.
50. Striegel-Moore RH, Wilfley DE, Pike KM, Dohm FA, Fairburn CG. Recurrent binge eating in black American women. Arch Fam Med. 9:83-87, 2000.
51. Wing RR, Marcus MD, Epstein LH, Blair EH, Burton LR. Binge eating in obese patients with type II diabetes. Int J Eat Disord. 8:671-679, 1989.
52. Kenardy J, Mensch M, Bowen K, Pearson SA. A comparison of eating behaviors in newly diagnosed NIDDM patients and case-matched control subjects. Diabetes Care 17:1197-1199, 1994.
53. Crow S, Kendall D, Praus B, Thuras P. Binge eating and other psychopathology in patients with type II diabetes mellitus. Int J Eat Disord 30:222-226, 2001.
54. Rapaport WS, LaGreca A, Levine P. Preventing eating disorders in young women with type 1 diabetes. In Practical Psychology for Diabetes Clinicians. Anderson B, Rubin RR, Eds. Alexandria, VA, American Diabetes Association, pp.133-141, 1996.

Helpful Internet sources for additional information on psychosocial issues in diabetes:

http://www.joslin.org/managing/discussion-board.html/ The Joslin Diabetes Center maintains a psychosocial patient discussion board in its website. A Licensed Social Worker (MSW) answers questions and monitors patients' discussion for accuracy and appropriateness.

http://www.mentalhealth.com/fr13.html -provides links to many mental health sites including those offered by the US government, nonprofit organizations, and some universities.

Additional Helpful Reference

Anderson B, Rubin RR. Practical Psychology for Diabetes Clinicians. Alexandria, VA: The American Diabetes Association, 1996.

VIII. Related Disorders

Chapter 1. Obesity – Genetics, Pathogenesis, Therapy

William C. Hsu and Christos S. Mantzoros

INTRODUCTION

The prevalence of obesity is increasing at alarming rates across all sociodemographic groups in industrialized and developing nations alike. Obesity poses a tremendous clinical challenge, as it contributes to significant morbidity and mortality and carries a staggering economic cost. In this chapter, we examine the current understanding of the epidemiology, etiology, pathophysiology and treatment of obesity.

DEFINITION AND MEASUREMENT OF OBESITY

Obesity is formally defined as an excess of fat mass resulting from the chronic accumulation and storage of excess energy. Although accurate methods of determining the quantity of body fat (including underwater densitometry, dual-energy x-ray absorptiometry, total body water estimate, total body potassium measurement and bioelectrical impedance) have been developed, for practical purposes obesity is classified according to the body mass index (BMI), a ratio of weight in kilograms over height in meters squared. Overweight is defined as a BMI of 25 to 29.9 kg/m² and Class I obesity as a BMI of > 30 – 34.9 kg/m², Class II obesity as a BMI of 35-39.9kg/m²; and Class III obesity as a BMI of >40 kg/m.²

A quarter of the American adults are obese[1] and approximately 60% of U.S. adults are either overweight or obese. Minority populations and those with low incomes or low education are especially susceptible. However, in the past decade, an increase was observed in all age, gender, race and educational levels with the highest magnitude of rise in those who are in their 20's, those with some college education and those of Hispanic ethnicity.[2] More importantly, almost a quarter of the children and adolescents between ages 6 through 17 years are overweight and many have already developed obesity-related complications, such as type 2 diabetes.

CONSEQUENCES OF OBESITY

Obesity now exceeds smoking and poverty as the leading health risk in the United States and is linked to the development of many chronic diseases (Table 1). In general, higher BMIs are associated with higher risk of developing obesity-related comorbidities. For example, a woman with a BMI of 25 has a five-fold relative risk of developing type 2 diabetes than a woman with a BMI of less than 22; a 28-fold higher risk, if the BMI is increased to 30; and a 93 fold higher risk with the BMI of 35 or greater.[3] All cause mortality rises from a BMI nadir of just below 25 kg/m^2 and escalates at a BMI above 30 kg/m^2, accounting for approximately 280,000 to 325,000 deaths annually in the U.S.[4]

Table 1. Medical morbidities associated with obesity

Cardiovascular	**Pulmonary**
Congestive Heart Failure	Hypoventilation syndrome
Coronary heart disease	Sleep apnea
Dyslipidemia	
Hypertension	**Endocrine**
	Diabetes-type 2
Gynecological/Obstetrical	Gestational diabetes
Breast cancer	Hirsutism
Complications of pregnancy	
Endometrial cancer	**Renal**
Menstrual irregularities	Renal cell cancer
Polycystic ovarian syndrome	
	Gastrointestinal
Cerebrovascular	Colon cancer
Stroke	Gallstones
	Gall bladder cancer
Muskuloskeletal	
Osteoarthritis	**Urologic**
Gout	Prostate cancer
	Stress Incontinence
Dermatologic	
Abdominal striae	
Acanthosis nigricans	

Obesity is a highly stigmatized disease. Negative attitudes toward the obese are common and are evident in employment, marriage and educational opportunities.[5] Furthermore, obese patients often experience discrimination from their health care providers, and are less likely to receive preventive care, including screening for cervical and breast cancer.

Given the emphasis on being slim in our society, nearly 40% of Americans attempt to lose weight at any given time, a phenomenon translated into a 30 billion dollar diet industry. Furthermore, the direct medical cost for treating obesity related diseases was estimated to be 51.6 billion in 1995. Combined with the economic value of productivity lost due to obesity related morbidity and mortality, the total economic burden of obesity amounts to a staggering 100 billion dollars per year.[6]

ETIOLOLOGY OF OBESITY

Obesity results from complex interactions between genetic factors and environmental influences. Adoption studies suggest that the BMIs of the adoptees have stronger correlations with the BMIs of the biologic parents, than with that of the adoptive parents. Furthermore, twin studies have shown that identical twins, even when reared apart, have BMIs that are more tightly correlated than fraternal twins. Overall, the genetic contribution to BMI has been estimated to be between 50-90%.[7] Although monogenic defects, as in the classical Prader-Willi, Cohen, and Bardet-Biedl syndromes, or the recently discovered genetic mutations in the locus encoding leptin, leptin receptor, POMC or other enzymes and neuropeptides have been recognized as important causes of obesity, they explain only a distinct minority of common obesity. For example, mutations of the melanocortin-4 (MC4) receptor, considered to be one of the most prevalent mutations responsible for monogenic obesity known to date, are found in approximately 4-5% of obese children and adults with a BMI above 40 kg/m^2.

Table 2. Common drugs that increase weight

Anti-psychotics
Atypical Neuroleptics (clozapine,olanzapine,risperdone)
Conventional Neuroleptics (chlorpromazine, haloperidol, thioridazine)

Anti-Depressants
MAO Inhibitors* (phenelzine)
Lithium
Trazadone
Tricyclics (amitryptyline, immipramine, desipramine)
SSRI* (paroxetine)

Anti-epileptics
Carbamazepine
Valproic Acid

Antidiabetics
Insulin
Sulfonylurea
Thiazolidinediones

Steroids
Corticosteroids
Megesterol Acetate

MAO Inhibitors = Monoamine Oxidase Inhibitors, SSRI = Selective Serotonin Reuptake Inhibitors

The rapidly rising prevalence of obesity in the last decades strongly suggests that environmental factors also play an important role since our genetic makeup has not been altered significantly during this short period. Given the availability of dense caloric food served in ever-larger portions, it is surprising that the correlation between dietary intake and obesity has not been firmly established. In contrast, physical inactivity strongly predicts weight gain in both cross-sectional and longitudinal studies.[8] Other environmental factors, such as smoking cessation and drugs, may also contribute to obesity in susceptible individuals. Smoking cessation is associated with an average weight gain of 3-5 kg due to an increase in appetite and a decline in metabolic rate.[9] Medications, such as tricyclic antidepressants, phenothiazines and certain SSRI such as paroxetine, are commonly associated with weight gain. Among the neuroleptic drugs, "atypical" antipyschotic agents appear to cause greater weight gain than conventional agents[10] (Table 2).

MECHANISMS UNDERLYING WEIGHT REGULATION

Our understanding of the system integrating genetic and environmental factors to regulate energy homeostasis has been greatly advanced by the discovery of leptin, the 167-amino acid product of *ob* gene, discovered in 1994 by positional cloning using the leptin-deficient *ob/ob* mouse model of obesity.[11] Leptin , an anorexigenic hormone produced by the adipocytes, is a member of the cytokine family. Leptin circulates in both free and bound form. Serum leptin levels increase exponentially with an increase in fat mass but decrease in response to hunger or fasting. Comparatively, leptin levels decline with low fat mass and in response to feeding. Leptin acts by crossing the blood-brain barrier to bind to specific receptors in the hypothalamus that in turn modulate the expression of orexigenic and anorexigenic neuropeptides responsible for regulating appetite and energy expenditure. For example, the binding of hypothalamic leptin receptors downregulates the anabolic pathways by inhibiting the expression of orexigenic neuropeptides, including neuropeptides Y (NPY) and agouti-related protein (AgRP), and upregulates the catabolic pathways by stimulating the expression of anorexigenic neuropeptides such as melanocyte stimulating hormone (α-MSH), corticotropin-releasing hormone (CRH) and cocaine-and amphetamine-regulated transcript (CART) in the hypothamalus[12] (Table 3) (Figure 1). In contrast, inhibition of the leptin system, in response to energy deprivation, results in stimulation of appetite, activation of the pituitary-adrenal axis to mobilize energy stores and suppression of both the pituitary-hypothalamic-thyroidal and gonadal axis as well as thermogenesis.[13] The net outcome is a coordinated effort to restore energy balance and return the body to its initial weight.

Activation of the leptin system also affects energy expenditure through the stimulation of the sympathetic autonomic nervous system in mice and has recently been linked with the activation of uncoupling protien

Table 3. Hypothalamic neuropeptides regulating appetite

Anorexigenic	Orexigenic
α-MSH (alpha-melanocyte stimulating hormone)*	AGRP (agouti-related protein)*
CART (cocaine amphetamine-regulated transcript)*	Galanin
CNTF (ciliary neurotrophic factor)	Ghrelin*
CRH (corticotropin releasing hormone)*	MCH(melanin-concentrating hormone)
GLP-1 (glucagon-like peptide-1)*	Noradrenaline
Serotonin	NPY (neuropeptide-Y)*
TRH (thyrotropin releasing hormone)*	Orexin

* Indicates neuropeptides modulated by leptin action

(UCP-1) in the mitochondria of brown adipose tissue in mice and of muscle and fat (UCP-2, UCP-3) in humans.[14] In the animal models, UCP uncouples the cellular oxidation of fuels from the generation of ATP, thereby releasing food energy in the form of heat, a process also known as thermogenesis. The sympathetic nervous system appears to activate thermogenesis by stimulating the beta-adrenergic receptors. Specifically, treatment of multiple animal species with selective agonist of the beta-3 adrenergic receptors caused an increase in energy expenditure. Whether the resulting alterations in thermogenesis are effective for weight loss in human remains the focus of intense investigation.

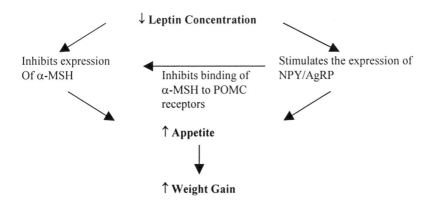

Figure 1. Decreased leptin concentration activates the orexigenic pathway (NPY/AgRP) in the arcuate nucleus and concurrently inhibits the anorexigenic pathway (α-MSH and POMC neurons), together resulting in an increase in food intake.

Although leptin administration has been effective in the limited subjects with absolute leptin deficiency resulting in morbid obesity, common obesity is believed to be associated with high leptin levels and leptin resistance. The apparent resistance may be related to a defect in leptin transport through the brain-blood barrier, binding defect to its receptors, over-expression of hypothalamic inhibitors of leptin action or defective signaling pathways downstream of leptin receptor.

To a certain extent interacting with the leptin system, monoamine neurotransmitters have long been recognized to modulate food intake.[15] The serotonin pathway has traditionally been the target of several anti-obesity drugs that increase serotoninergic signaling and suppresses food intake. The stimulation of serotonin receptors, particularly the $5\text{-}HT_{2c}$ receptors, decreases food intake and the knock out of this receptor, in rodents results in modest obesity. Stimulation of the noradrenergic receptors in the paraventricular nuclei or other hypothalamic areas contributes to hyperphagia and has been the target of current amphetamine-based anorexic agents. Similarly, the stimulation of dopaminergic receptors in the dorsomedial and arcuate nuclei of the hypothalamus decreases food intake whereas mesolimbic dopaminergic pathways may be involved in the pleasurable aspects of feeding. Moreover, pharmacologic depletion and genetic disruption of the dopaminergic pathways results in profound feeding deficits.

Despite clear evidence linking obesity and its complications, such as hypertension and type 2 diabetes, the mechanism by which obesity is related to insulin resistance remains largely elusive. Adipocyte secreted factors, such as leptin and tumor necrosis factor-α, have traditionally been considered to be the mediators of metabolic comorbidities associated with obesity whereas recent data indicate that adiponectin and resistin[16], two recently discovered adipocyte secreted hormones, may also be potential links between obesity and the development of insulin resistance and diabetes.

EVALUATION OF OBESE PATIENTS

Despite the fact that physicians have unique opportunities to play a major role in the prevention and treatment of obesity, concerns about drug safety, the lack of a permanently effective treatment and poor reimbursement have contributed to reluctance of physicians to treat obesity.

BMI is most frequently utilized for the clinical evaluation of obese patients, but it overestimates adiposity in individuals with very short stature or very muscular built and underestimates it in the elderly due to loss of lean body mass. It has also been proposed that abdominal obesity, independent of body weight, maybe a stronger predictor for the development of coronary heart disease. In certain populations, such as Asian Americans, waist

660

circumference may correlate better with morbidity or mortality than the currently established cutoff points for BMI. While a waist circumference of >94 cm in men or >80 cm in women confers increased health risks, when the waist circumference reaches 102 cm in men and 88 cm in women, intervention is definitely justified.[17]

In addition to quantifying the degree of obesity, patient's motivation, expectations and adherence pattern should also be carefully assessed. Obtaining a dietary, smoking and activity history, screening for psychiatric disorders, eating disorders and depression are integral parts of the evaluation. Identifying physical features suggestive of secondary causes of obesity, such as Cushing's syndrome, hypothyroidism or growth hormone deficiency, and detecting and quantifying obesity related co-morbidities are important components of a comprehensive assessment. Finally, since the use of drug therapy for weight loss is contraindicated in pregnancy, a pregnancy test should be considered and contraception recommended for every woman of child-bearing age considering pharmacological therapy.

ESTABLISHING WEIGHT GOALS

Despite initial success, almost all weight loss is regained within 3 to 5 years of completing treatment in more than 90% of treated patients. This common occurrence underlies much of the frustration and fatalism of both patients and clinicians towards obesity treatment, especially when the goal for weight loss has been to achieve ideal body weight. Yet, a weight reduction as little as 5-10% body weight significantly improves blood pressure, lipids, body fat distribution, insulin resistance and glycemic control and may be easier to maintain; therefore, it represents a better goal from the medical point of view. Finally, modest weight loss prevents the development of osteoarthritis and hypertension in normotensive obese subjects and improves the quality of life. Since obesity is a chronic condition, the goal for treatment is not only to reduce weight but also to maintain the reduced weight with the ultimate aim of improving overall health. Given that many obese individuals lose weight for cosmetic reasons, convincing them to set a realistic weight goal and to continue treatment indefinitely is very challenging but also imperative.

CURRENT TREATMENT OPTIONS

Obesity is a chronic disease and requires life-long treatment. Lifestyle modification should be encouraged in all patients who are overweight or obese and specific recommendations have been developed to aid clinicians in the appropriate use of pharmacotherapy or bariatric surgery.

Dietary Therapy

All randomized, controlled studies have documented the efficacy of caloric restriction in weight loss but it remains to be conclusively shown whether food composition has an impact on weight loss as long as calories are fixed. In general, a deficit of 500 kcal/day will result in a weight loss of 1/2 to 1 lb per week. Although for subjects with a BMI greater than 35, a higher caloric deficit of 500-1000 kcal/day may be required, a low calorie diet (LCD), defined as consumption of 1000-1500 kcal/day, generally results in a mean of 8-10% weight reduction during a period of 6 to 12 months. A very low caloric diet (VLCD) i.e. 400-800 kcal/day, produces rapid and significant weight loss during the initial phase but is contraindicated in patients with cardiovascular, hepatic, renal disease and those with eating disorders. It does not achieve a greater weight loss than LCD at 1 year, is associated with high attrition rate and higher cost, and may be associated with nutritional deficiency, electrolyte imbalance, gout, gallstones and cardiac complications including sudden death.[18]

Exercise Therapy

Exercise, when combined with dietary therapy, results in more weight loss than with either therapy alone but most obese patients find it difficult to start a regular exercise program until they have lost first some weight from dieting. In addition to the maintenance of weight loss and the prevention of further weight gain, increasing physical activity results in reduction of abdominal fat, increase in cardiorespiratory fitness and improvement in insulin resistance. Before initiating exercise in obese patients, musculoskeletal and cardiovascular risks must be carefully considered and the intensity and duration should be increased gradually up to the goal of 30 minutes of moderate intensity physical activity (i.e. walking at 3-4 mph) every day, a recommendation endorsed by the Surgeon General, National Institutes of Health and American Heart Association.

Behavior Therapy

Techniques and methodologies designed to improve weight management involve accountability and support through group sessions, keeping food diaries and exercise logs to document caloric intake and energy expenditure, stress management to prevent adverse behaviors that lead to weight gain, and stimulus control, and cognitive restructuring that deals with constructing an appropriate self-image and setting realistic weight goal. Behavior strategies designed to reinforce dietary and exercise treatment generally produce about a 10% reduction in weight within one year. The fear of weight gain may also be an important barrier to smoke cessation, especially among women and teenage smokers, but the emphasis

662

should be placed on the overwhelming health benefits of quitting smoking over the risks associated with the weight gained during cessation.

Drug Therapy

At current development, the role of pharmacotherapy remains supportive to lifestyle modification. If 6-months of lifestyle modification fails to produce adequate weight loss, pharmacotherapy should be considered in patients with a BMI> 30 or a BMI between 27 and 29.9 with co-existing co-morbidities such as hypertension, hyperlipidemia, coronary heart disease, type 2 diabetes and sleep apnea. Currently, the FDA has approved two medications, orlistat and sibutramine, for long-term obesity treatment, but the safety and added efficacy of combination drug therapy, although theoretically plausible, has not yet been tested in large randomized trials.

Orlistat

Orlistat (Xenical) is a pentanoic acid ester that inhibits reversibly pancreatic and gastric lipase. Therefore, about 30% of ingested dietary fat is excreted instead of hydrolyzed to fatty acids and glycerol. The current recommended dose is 120 mg three times a day with meals. In the first large randomized trial[19], the orlistat treated group had an average weight loss of 10.3 kg vs 6.1 kg in the placebo group at one year. By the end of the second year under a eucaloric diet, orlistat treatment results in a smaller weight regain than the placebo group and in a one-year trial greater weight maintenance after dieting. Other studies have shown beneficial effects on low-density lipoprotein cholesterol, insulin levels and abdominal circumference as well as significant improvement in glycemic control in diabetes.

Orlistat is minimally absorbed and generally well tolerated but is contraindicated in chronic malabsorption, cholestasis and hypersensitivity reaction to its components. Flatulence and steatorrhea are the most common adverse effects and absorption of fat-soluble vitamins may be slightly reduced. Thus, vitamin supplementation is recommended at least 2 hours before or after taking orlistat to avoid malabsorption.

Sibutramine

Sibutramine reduces food intake by selectively inhibiting post-synaptic norepinephrine and serotonin reuptake and to a lesser degree dopaminergic reuptake, whereas earlier drugs such as fenfluramine and dexfenfluramine increased serotonin release. In a large randomized multi-center trial lasting 24 weeks, sibutramine was shown to produce weight loss in a dose dependent fashion, ranging from 6.1% up to 9.4% reduction of initial weight.[20] Use of sibutramine for 2 years showed that 43% of the sibutramine-hypocaloric diet group maintained 80% or more of their original weight loss compared in contrast to 16% in the hypocaloric group alone.[21] Sibutramine is also helpful in decreasing and maintaining long-term weight loss achieved by VLCD (220-800 kcal/d).

The use of sibutramine is contraindicated in patients with arrhythmias, coronary artery disease, stroke, congestive heart failure and poorly controlled hypertension, as well as in patients taking monoamine oxidase inhibitors or selective serotonin reuptake inhibitors. Sibutramine has been associated with a small increase of diastolic blood pressure compared with the placebo group and a small increase in the pulse rate. Common side effects of sibutramine are dry mouth, headache, anorexia, constipation and insomnia and are mostly related to sympathomimetic properties of the drug.

Table 4. Drugs that have weight loss effect

Serotoninergics	**Pancreatic Lipase Inhibitor**
Dexfenfluramine	Orlistat*
Fenfluramine	
Fluoxetine	**Hormone**
	Thyroxine
Sympathomimetics	
Benzphetamine*‡	**Antidiabetic**
Bupropion	Metformin
Diethylpropion*‡	
Ephedrine	
Mazindol*‡	
Phendimetrazine*‡	
Phenopropanolamine	
Phentermine*‡	
Sibutramine*	

* Indicates drugs approved by the FDA for weight loss
‡ Indicates Drug Enforcement Agency (DEA) scheduled drugs

Other Agents

Anorexants, currently scheduled as controlled substances, stimulate the adrenergic system by either inhibiting post-synaptic reuptake of norepinephrine or by directly stimulating the pre-synaptic release of noreprinephrine. They are indicated only for short-term use (up to 3 months).

Fenfluramine and dexfenfluramine cause valvular heart disease and pulmonary hypertension resulting in their withdrawal from the market. Phenylpropanolamine, an over-the-counter product for nasal congestion resulting in appetite suppression, was recently linked to the development of hemorrhagic stroke and is being withdrawn from the market. Ephedrine and caffeine induce weight loss by stimulating thermogenesis. Psychotropic medications acting as 5-HT$_{1b}$, 5-HT$_{2c}$ and Dop-2 receptor agonists or as selective serotonin reuptake inhibitors, such as fluoxetine, have weight reducing effects but their action may not be sustainable in the long term. Thyroxine stimulates thermogenesis and reduces body fat but should not be used as an antiobesity agent since it also leads to significant side effects, including the loss of lean body mass, the development of cardiac arrhythmias and osteoporosis. Metformin, an insulin sensitizer, induces anorexia and some weight loss in humans but, due to its rather limited weight reducing effect and potential side effects, its use as anti-obesity agent in the non-diabetic population is not advocated. See Table 4 for a list of drugs with weight loss effect.

Surgical Therapy

Individuals with a BMI exceeding 40 or between 35 and 40 with comorbidities are potential candidates for bariatric surgery after careful evaluation by a multidisciplinary team including internist, surgeon, nutritionist and psychiatrist. Gastric restriction or gastroplasty involves stapling or banding the stomach to decrease the storage capacity of the stomach by constructing a small proximal reservoir with outlet restriction (Figure 1). Gastric bypass involves the partitioning of the stomach by stapling, with an outlet formed by a loop of small intestine proceeding from the proximal stomach, bypassing the distal stomach, duodenum and proximal portion of jejunum (Roux-en-Y) (Figure 1). Long-term weight loss with gastric bypass procedure is considered generally superior. With rapid advances in minimally invasive surgery, laparoscopic gastric bypass may become the procedure of choice in selected patients. Currently, the immediate operative mortality rate has been estimated to be approximately 1%, and early post-operative complications, such as wound infections, deep thrombophlebitis and pulmonary complications can be as high as 10%.[22] After discharge from the hospital, most patients are maintained on liquid diet initially, and are gradually advanced to a full diet. In addition to behavioral modification, exercise and dietary counseling, medical follow-up should be regularly scheduled post-operatively, to monitor for the development of nutrient deficiencies (B12, folate, iron), depression, gastritis, anastomotic ulcer and cholelithiasis.

Bariatric surgery can achieve an average of excess weight reduction of 50% as far as 10 years after surgery. Maximum weight loss is reached approximately 2 years after the operation with significant amount of patients experiencing resolution of the type 2 diabetes, hypertension, hypertriglyceridemia, and obesity hypoventilation syndrome. However, 20-25% of the patients experience weight loss failures mostly due to dietary indiscretion and insufficient follow-up.

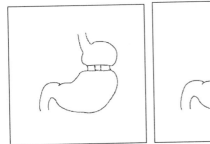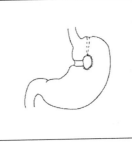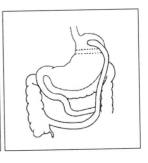

Figure 2. Common procedures of bariatric surgery. Left – gastric banding. Middle – vertical banded gastroplasty. Right – Gastric bypass (Roux-en-Y).

FUTURE DIRECTIONS

New advances in understanding the mechanisms regulating body weight have intensified research efforts and are expected to lead to the development of new treatment options for obesity in the near future.

Leptin and Leptin Analogs

The majority of human obesity is a leptin resistant state. Therefore, efforts to overcome leptin resistance focus on designing leptin agonists that have higher potency, longer serum half-life and ability to cross the blood-brain barrier easier.

Hypothalamic Neuropeptides

The successful weight-loss effects in animal models targeting anorexigenic pathways downstream of the leptin receptor by using melanocortin receptor agonists, such as α-MSH or novel MC3R and MC4R agonists, have generated much interest for their potential use in humans. Alternatively, inhibitors of centrally acting orexigenic molecules, such as AGRP, melanin-concentrating hormone, orexin, opioid receptors and ghrelin are being studied for their potential pharmacological value.

Peripheral Satiety Signals

Molecules such as cholecystokinin, bombesin and glucagon-like peptide-1 that are secreted by the gastrointestinal tract convey satiety signals to the brain. Their analogues may also have suppressive effects on appetite and may be effective against obesity but their development is still in the pre-clinical phase.

Fat Absorption and Metabolism

Blocking molecules in fat digestion or absorption, such as fatty acid transporters in the intestine, or using energy-free substitutes, such as olestra, may reduce contribution of dietary fat to weight gain. Another strategy is to design drugs that inactivate key molecules in fat metabolism.

Thermogenesis

To increase energy expenditure through heat loss, specific beta-3 adrenergic receptor agonists have been tested in multiple animal species and are currently being evaluated for use in humans, whereas the development of drugs that enhance the expression of uncoupling proteins involved in dissipation of energy to heat is still in very early phases.

SUMMARY

Obesity, a chronic disease, has reached epidemic proportions, is associated with overwhelming morbidity, mortality and health care costs. Human and animal studies reveal that energy homeostasis is tightly regulated by highly redundant and complex systems of neuropeptides and neuropathways modulating appetite and energy expenditure. The unmasking of latent genetic predisposition for energy conservation brought on by environmental factors that promote inactivity and high calorie diet is largely responsible for the explosive rise in obesity in recent years. Current treatment options, though limited, are effective in reducing health risks associated with obesity A comprehensive clinical evaluation and setting realistic goals of weight loss are the cornerstones of treatment of obese patients since even a modest weight reduction of 5-10% provides significant health benefits and is reasonably attainable and sustainable. Dietary changes, exercise, behavior modification, pharmacotherapy and surgical therapy are useful tools to achieve this goal, but require life-long efforts to maintain the reduced body weight. As we are entering a new era in understanding the mechanisms of weight regulations, new discoveries hold promise for the development of novel therapeutic agents that will eventually provide tangible benefits to those who are struggling to control excessive body weight.

REFERENCES

1. Flegal KM, Carroll MD, Kuczmarski RJ, Johnson CL. Overweight and obesity in the United States: prevalence and trends. Int J Obes Relat Metab Disord 22:39-47, 1998.
2. Mokdad, AH, Serdula MK, Dietz WH, Bowman BA, Marks JS, Koplan JP. The Spread of the obesity epidemic in the United States. 1991-1998. JAMA 282:1519-22, 1999.
3. Colditz GA, Willett WC, Rotnitzky A, Manson JE. Weigh gain as a risk factor for clinical diabetes mellitus in women. Ann Intern Med 122:481-486, 1995.
4. Allison DB, Fontaine KR, Manson JE, StevensJ, VanItallie TB. Annual deaths attributable to obesity in the United States. JAMA 282:1530-8, 1999.

5. Gortmaker SL, Must A, Perrin JM, Sobol AM, Dietz WH. Social and economic consequences of overweight in adolescence and young adulthood. N Engl J Med 329:1008-12, 1993.

6. Wolf AM, Colditz GA. Current estimates of the economic cost of obesity in the United States. Obes Res 6:97-106, 1998.

7. Maes HH, Neale MC, Eaves LJ. Genetic and environmental factors in relative body weight and human adiposity. Behav Genet 27(4):325-51, 1997.

8. Williamson DF; Madans J; Anda RF; Kleinman JC; Kahn HS; Byers T. Recreational physical activity and ten-year weight change in a US national cohort. Int J Obes Relat Metab Disord 17:279-86, 1993.

9. Williamson DF, Madans J, Anda RF, Kleinman JC, Giovino GA, Byers T. Smoking cessation and severity of weight gain in a national cohort. N Engl J Med 324:739-45, 1991.

10. Allison DB, Mentore JL, Moonseong H, Chandler LP, Cappelleri JC, Infante MC, Weiden PJ. Antipsychotic-induced weight gain: a comprehensive research synthesis. Am J Psychiatry 156:1686-96, 1999.

11. Zhang Y, Proenca R, Maffei M, Barone M, Leopold L, Friedman JM. Positional cloning of the mouse obese gene and its human homologue. Nature 372:425-32, 1994.

12. Ahima RS, Saper CB, Flier JS, Elmquist JK. Leptin regulation of neuroendocrine systems. Front Neuroendocrinol 21:263-307, 2000.

13. Mantzoros CS. The role of leptin in human obesity and disease: a review of current evidence. Ann Intern Med 130:671-80, 1999.

14. Lowell BB, Speigelman BM. Towards a molecular understanding of adaptive thermogenesis. Nature 404:652-60, 2000.

15. Schwartz MW, Woods SC, Porte D Jr, Seeley RJ, Baskin DG. Central nervous system control of food intake. Nature 404:661-70, 2000.

16. Steppan CM, Bailey ST, Bhat S, Brown EJ, Banerjee RR, Wright CM, Patel HR, Ahima RS, Lazar MA. The hormone resistin links obesity to diabetes. Nature 409 (6818):292-3, 2001.

17. National Institutes of Health. Clinical Guidelines on the Identification, Evaluation, and Treatment of Overweight and Obesity in Adults: the Evidence Report. Obes Res 6:51S-209S, 1998.

18. National Task Force on the prevention and treatment of obesity. Very low-calorie diets. JAMA 270:967-74, 1993.

19. Sjostrom L, Rissanen A, Andersen T, Boldrin M, Golay A, Koppeschaar HPF, et al. Randomized placebo-controlled trial of orlistat for weight loss and prevention of weight regain in obese patients. The European Multicentre Orlistat Study Group. Lancet 352:167-72, 1998.

20. Hollander, P, Elbein S, Hirsch I, Kelley D, McGill J, Taylor T, et al. Role of orlistat in the treatment of obese patients with type 2 diabetes: a randomized double-blind study. Diabetes Care 21:1288-94, 1998.

21. James WPT, Astrup A, Finer N, Hilsted J, Kopelman P, Rossner S, Saris WHM, Gaal LFV. Effect of sibutramine on weight maintenance after weight loss: a randomized trial. Lancet 356:2119-25, 2000.
22. NIH Consensus Development Conference. Gastrointestinal surgery for severe obesity. Nutrition 12:397-402, 1996.

Helpful internet source for additional information on obesity:
- NIH clinical guidelines on obesity
  (http://www.nhlbi.nih.gov/guidelines/obesity/ob_home.htm)
- Prevalence of overweight and obesity among adults: United States, 1999. National Center for Health Statistics web site.
  (www.cdc.gov/nchs/products/pubs/pubd/hestats/obese/obse99.htm).

Chapter 2. Hypertension

Samy I. McFarlane, Amal F. Farag and James R. Sowers

INTRODUCTION

Hypertension is a major risk factor for cardiovascular disease (CVD). It substantially increases the risk for coronary heart disease (CHD), stroke and nephropathy. There is a positive association between hypertension and insulin resistance and the evidence of a causal link is growing. When hypertension coexists with diabetes, which it commonly does, the risk of stroke or CVD is doubled and the risk for developing end stage renal disease increases to 5-6 times compared to hypertensive patients without diabetes. In this chapter we discuss the interaction of hypertension, insulin resistance and other CVD risk factors in the context of the metabolic syndrome, emphasizing the unique aspects of hypertension in patients with diabetes. Therapy for hypertension is discussed in the light of the major prospective trials available to-date, such as the HOPE and RENAAL studies.

HYPERTENSION AND CVD IN PATIENTS WITH DIABETES

Cardiovascular diseases are the major cause of mortality in patients with diabetes. Risk factors of CVD that cluster in diabetes are listed in Table 1 and include hypertension, central obesity, dyslipidemia, microalbuminuria and coagulation abnormalities.[1]

Table 1. CVD risk factors associated with diabetes

1. Hypertension
2. Obesity
3. Hyperinsulinemia/insulin resistance
4. Endothelial dysfunction
5. Microalbuminuria
6. Low HDL-cholesterol levels
7. High triglycerides levels
8. Small, dense LDL cholesterol particles
9. Increased Apo-lipoprotein B levels
10. Increased fibrinogen levels
11. Increased plasma activator inhibitor –1 levels
12. Increased C-reactive protein and other inflammatory markers
13. Absent nocturnal dipping of blood pressure and pulse
14. Salt sensitivity
15. Left ventricular hypertrophy
16. Premature coronary artery disease

Among those risk factors, hypertension is approximately twice as frequent in patients with diabetes compared to those without the disease and accounts for up to 75% of CVD risk. Conversely, patients with hypertension are more prone to have diabetes than are normotensive persons.[2] In a large prospective study of 12,550 adults, the development of type 2 diabetes was almost 2.5 times as likely in patients with hypertension as in their normotensive counterparts after adjustment for age, sex, race, education, adiposity, family history with respect to diabetes, physical-activity level and other health-related behavior.[3] The association of hypertension, insulin resistance and the resultant hyperinsulinemia was shown in several studies. In untreated essential hypertensive patients, fasting and postprandial insulin levels were higher than in normotensive controls, regardless of the body mass index (BMI), with a direct correlation between plasma insulin concentrations and blood pressure. In fact authors concluded in this study that essential hypertension is an insulin resistance state.[4] Another study of 24 adults documented that patients with hypertension, whether treated or untreated, are insulin resistant, hyperglycemic, and hyperinsulinemic compared to a well-matched control group.[5] Insulin resistance and hyperinsulinemia also exist in rats with genetic hypertension such as Dahl Hypertensive and spontaneously hypertensive rat (SHR) strains.[6,7] On the other hand, the association of insulin resistance and essential hypertension does not occur in secondary hypertension.[8] This suggests a common genetic predisposition for essential hypertension and insulin resistance – concept that is also supported by the finding of altered glucose metabolism in normotensive offspring of hypertensive patients.[9,10] Therefore hypertension in patients with diabetes must be viewed in the context of the metabolic syndrome. This has important implications in understanding the principles of management of these patients as discussed later. Detailed discussion of the metabolic syndrome (Syndrome X) is presented in chapter IX.5.

UNIQUE ASPECTS OF HYPERTENSION IN PATIENTS WITH DIABETES

Hypertension in patients with diabetes, compared to those without diabetes, has unique features such as increased salt sensitivity, volume expansion, isolated systolic hypertension, loss of nocturnal dipping of blood pressure and pulse, increased propensity to proetinuria and orthostatic hypotension.[2] Most of these features are considered risk factors for CVD (Table 1) and are particularly important for selecting the appropriate antihypertensive medication, for example low dose diuretics for treatment volume expansion, and angiotensin converting enzyme (ACE) inhibitors or angiotensin receptor blockers (ARB) for proteinuria.

Salt sensitivity and volume expansion

Alterations in sodium balance and extracellular fluid volume have heterogeneous effects on blood pressure (BP) in both normotensive and hypertensive subjects. Increased salt intake does not raise BP in all hypertensive subjects and sensitivity to dietary salt intake is greatest in hypertensive patients with diabetes, obesity, renal insufficiency, low renin status, African Americans and elderly. Studies demonstrated that salt sensitivity in normotensive subjects is associated with a greater age-related increase in BP. This is particularly important to consider in management of hypertension in patients with diabetes, especially the elderly persons, since the prevalence of both diabetes and salt sensitivity increases with age.

Isolated systolic hypertension

With the progression of atherosclerosis in patients with diabetes, the larger arteries lose elasticity and become rigid and the systolic BP will thus increase, leading to isolated systolic hypertension which is more common and occurs at a relatively younger age in patients with diabetes.[2]

Loss of nocturnal decline of BP

In normotensive individuals and most patients with hypertension there is a reproducible circadian pattern to BP during 24 hour ambulatory monitoring. Typically, the BP is highest while the patient is awake and lowest during sleep, a pattern called "dipping", in which BP decreases by 10-15%. Patients with loss of nocturnal decline in BP ("non-dippers") have <10% decline of BP during the night compared to daytime BP values.[11] In patients with diabetes, there is a loss of nocturnal dipping as demonstrated by 24 hour ambulatory monitoring of BP. This is particularly important since the loss of nocturnal dipping conveys excessive risk for stroke and myocardial infarction and that ambulatory BP was found to be superior to office BP in predicting target organ involvement, such as left ventricular hypertrophy.[11] About 30 % of myocardial infarctions and 50% of strokes occur between 6:00 AM and noon. This is particularly important in deciding the optimal dosing strategies of antihypertensive medications where drugs that provide consistent and sustained 24 hour BP control will be advantageous.[12]

Microalbuminuria

There is considerable evidence that hypertension in type 1 diabetes is a consequence, rather than a cause, of renal disease and that nephropathy precedes the rise in BP.[2] Persistent hypertension in patients with type 1 diabetes is often a manifestation of diabetic nephropathy as indicated by the concomitant elevation of the urinary albumin. Both hypertension and nephropathy appear to exacerbate each other. In type 2 diabetes, microalbuminuria is correlated with insulin resistance,[13] salt sensitivity, loss of nocturnal dipping and left ventricular hypertrophy.[14] Elevated systolic BP is a significant determining factor in the progression of microalbuminuria. Indeed, there is an increasing evidence that microalbuminuria is an integral component of the metabolic syndrome associated with hypertension.[14] This concept is important to consider in selecting the pharmacologic therapy for hypertension in patients with diabetes where medications that decrease both proteinuria and blood pressure, such as ACE-inhibitors and angiotensin receptor blockers, have evolved as increasingly important tools in reducing the progression of nephropathy in such patients.

Orthostatic hypotension

Pooling of blood in dependent veins during rising from a recumbent position, normally leads to decrease in stroke volume and systolic BP with reflexogenic sympathetic response and resultant increases in systemic vascular resistance and heart rate. In patients with diabetes and autonomic dysfunction, excessive venous pooling can cause immediate or delayed orthostatic hypotension that might cause reduction in cerebral blood flow leading to intermittent lightheadedness, fatigue, unsteady gait and syncope.[15] This is important to recognize in patients with diabetes and concomitant hypertension since it has several diagnostic and therapeutic implications. For example, discontinuation of diuretic therapy and volume repletion might be necessary for the treatment of chronic orthostasis. Also, in a subset of patients with "hyperadrenergic" orthostatic hypertension, as manifested by excessive sweating and palpitation, the use of low dose clonidine might be necessary to blunt excess sympathetic response.[16] Furthermore, increased propensity for orthostatic hypertension in patients with diabetes renders α- adrenergic receptor blockers less desirable and a second line agents for these patients. In addition, doses of all antihypertensive agents must be titrated more carefully in patients with diabetes who have greater propensity for orthostatic hypertension.

MANAGEMENT OF HYPERTENSION IN PATIENTS WITH DIABETES

Joint National Committee VI (JNC VI) guidelines (1997) classify patients with hypertension who also have diabetes (with or without other CVD risk factors) as high risk (group C) or complicated hypertension. All such patients must be started on drug therapy simultaneously with lifestyle modification.[17] The JNC VI recommended a BP goal of <130/85 mmHg for patients with diabetes. However, since its publication in 1997, the results of several major randomized controlled trials, including the Hypertension Optimal Treatment (HOT) trial, the United Kingdom Prospective Diabetes Study (UKPDS), the Appropriate Blood pressure Control in Diabetes (ABCD) trial and the Modification of Diet in Renal Disease (MDRD) trial became available.

After reviewing the data from these trials, the Hypertension and Diabetes Executive Working Group of the National Kidney Foundation recommended lowering the BP goal level to 130/80 mmHg or less in patients with diabetes and/or renal impairment.[18] This treatment goal was also adapted by the Canadian Hypertension Society and by the American Diabetes

674

Association (ADA).[19] The following treatment algorithm (Figure 1) reflects the new treatment goal of BP <130/80mmHg as well as the latest recommendations regarding drug therapy.[20][21] We will also discuss the anticipated changes to JNC VII that is expected in 2002, awaiting the completion of the Antihypertensive and Lipid Lowering Treatment to Prevent Heart Attack (ALLHAT) study.[22]

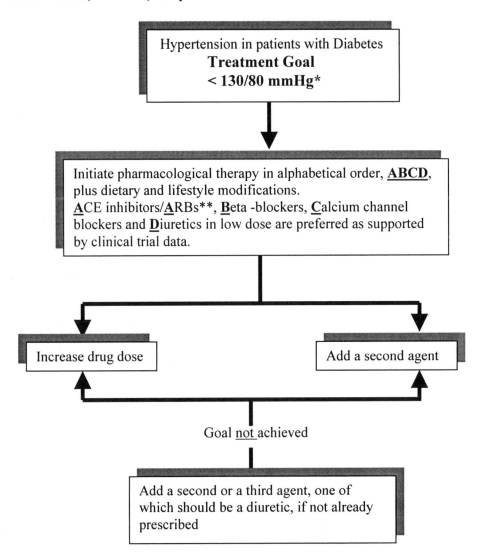

Figure 1. Management of hypertension in patients with diabetes. In patients with >1gram proteinuria and renal insufficiency the treatment goal is BP< 125/75 mmHg. ** ARBs = Angiotensin Receptor Blockers.

Dietary and lifestyle modifications

Both JNC VI and ADA recommend lifestyle and dietary modifications as an integral part of the management of hypertension in patients with diabetes. Addressing other CVD risk factors such as smoking, inactivity and elevated LDL cholesterol, is also emphasized.[17,19] Dietary and lifestyle modifications recommended for patients with hypertension are enlisted in Table 2.

Table 2. Dietary and lifestyle modifications recommended for management of hypertension

1. Weight loss
2. Exercise (aerobic physical activity) 30-45 minutes at least 3 times a week
3. Reduced sodium intake to 100 mmol (2.4 gram) per day
4. Smoking cessation
5. Adequate intake of dietary potassium, calcium and magnesium.
6. Reduced alcohol intake to < 1 oz of ethanol (24 oz of beer) per day.
7. Diet rich in fruits and vegetables but low in fat*

* Based on the results of the Dietary Approaches to Stop Hypertension (DASH) study,[23] the reduction of sodium intake to levels below the current recommendation of 100 mmol per day and the DASH diet both lower BP substantially, with greater effects in combination than singly.[24]

Dietary management and exercise in patients with diabetes are discussed in details in chapters VII.3 and VII.7 respectively. It is important to integrate the above lifestyle and dietary modifications for hypertension in the overall nutritional and lifestyle management of these patients.

Pharmacological therapy for hypertension in patients with diabetes

ACE- inhibitors.

ACE inhibitors were first introduced in the early 1980's as antihypertensive agents. Subsequently, their ability to attenuate albuminuria and renal disease progression led to their use as renoprotective agents in diabetic nephropathy.[25] More recently, randomized controlled trials have shown that ACE inhibitors provide cardiovascular and microvascular benefits and may also improve insulin resistance and prevent the development of diabetes. These cardiovascular benefits were greater than those attributable to the decrease in blood pressure and were particularly demonstrated in people with diabetes.[26] In patients with type 1 diabetes and proteinuria, ACE inhibitor treatment was associated with a 50 percent reduction in the risk of the combined end points of death, dialysis, and transplantation.[25] Furthermore, ACE inhibitors provide considerable benefits in diabetic patients with heart failure. In the Studies of Left Ventricular Dysfunction (SOLVD) trial, ACE inhibitors reduced left ventricular mass and left ventricular dilation and significantly reduced mortality and hospitalization for heart failure.[27]

With these clearly proven benefits, ACE inhibitors are currently recommended as a first line treatment for patients with hypertension and diabetes, particularly those with proteinuria as well as those with heart failure. It its anticipated publication, JNC VII will consider ACE inhibitor as a first line therapy for hypertension.[22]

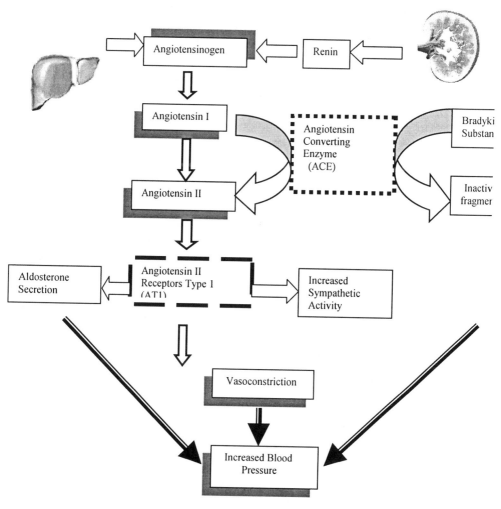

Figure 2. Renin Angiotensin Aldosterone System (RAAS). Site of action for ACE inhibitors ············· and of Angiotensin receptor Blockers (ARBs) ━━ ━

Treatment with ACE inhibitors is associated with cough in a substantial minority of patients (up to 15%). The cough is probably due to the accumulation of bradykinin or substance P (Figure 2). Angioedema is rare and unpredictable but potentially life threatening adverse effect, particularly if the upper airway is involved. It requires immediate discontinuation and supportive care, including airway protection. ACE inhibitors reduce aldosterone secretion (Figure 2) and may cause hyperkalemia, especially at the initiation of therapy. This is of particular concern in patients with diabetes and in those on potassium sparing diuretics. Concomitant use of thiazide or loop diuretics and dietary modification of potassium intake should allow the use of ACE inhibitors without inducing hyperkalemia. It is also important to note that, in patients with normal renal function, ACE inhibitors have little effects on glomerular filtration. However, with reduction in renal function, these agents might precipitate uremia. ACE inhibitors are also relatively contraindicated in patients with bilateral renal artery stenosis and unilateral stenosis and in those with one kidney because of the high risk of renal failure.

Angiotensin II receptor blockers (ARBs)

There are at least four types of angiotensin II receptors, AT1, AT2, AT3 and AT4. Of these, the AT1 receptors mediate most of the effects of angiotensin II, including vasoconstriction, aldosterone release, increased sympathetic outflow and stimulation of sodium resorption. ARBs selectively inhibit the binding of angiotensin II to the AT1 receptors; therefore, they are also called AT1 receptor blockers. Unlike ACE inhibitors, ARBs have no effects on bradykinin system (Figure 2) and therefore they are very well tolerated with lower incidence of side effects such as cough. Angioedema may occur rarely but much less commonly than with ACE inhibitors. Although there are no specific recommendations, ARBs should not be used in patients who developed angioedema on ACE inhibitors, since angioedema is a potentially life threatening condition. In addition, because of inhibition of aldosterone release by ARBs, hyperkalemia is a concern especially in those with renal insufficiency and, as with ACE inhibitors, progressive azotemia and renal failure might occur in those with bilateral renal artery stenosis or those with one kidney and unilateral stenosis of the renal artery.

The JNC VI recommended the use of ARBs as one of several alternative first line therapies for patients with hypertension who cannot tolerate or do not respond to the recommended first line medications. In addition, ARBs were also recommended as an initial therapy for those who could not tolerate ACE inhibitors (usually because of cough) and in whom ACE inhibitors are recommended as first line drugs, such as patients with diabetes and proteinuria, heart failure, systolic dysfunction, post myocardial infarction and those with mild renal insufficiency. However, data from randomized controlled trials in patients with type 2 diabetes suggest that

ARBs may be considered equal to ACE inhibitors for renal protection.[28] Indeed, the Reduction of Endpoints in NIDDM with the Angiotensin Losartan (REENAL) trial[29] demonstrated that angiotensin II receptor blocker combined with conventional antihypertensive treatment as needed confers significant renal protection in patients with type 2 diabetes and nephropathy. The risk of the primary end point (a composite of doubling of serum creatinine, end stage renal disease or death from any cause) was reduced by 16 % with losartan. The risk of doubling of serum creatinine was reduced by 25% and the risk of end stage renal disease was reduced by 28 % over a follow up period of 3.4 years. The study also documented reduction in the initial hospitalization for heart failure. These benefits were above and beyond those attributable to BP reduction alone.

Based on the evidence and because of the better tolerability, it is likely that ARBs will be recommended as a first line therapy for patients with diabetes and hypertension along with ACE-inhibitors.

Beta Blockers

Beta-blockers are very useful antihypertensive agents in the treatment of hypertension in patients with diabetes.[2] In the UKPDS study, atenolol, reduced microvascular complications of diabetes by 37 %, strokes by 44 % and death related to diabetes by 32%. In that study the beta -blocker, atenolol, had equal efficiency compared to the ACE inhibitor, captopril, in reducing the micro- and macrovascular complications of diabetes, most probably secondary to their ability to modulate the RAAS system. In a non-randomized study, hypertensive patients receiving beta- blockers had a 28 % higher risk of diabetes than did those on no medication. In contrast, patients with hypertension who received thiazide diuretics, ACE inhibitors or calcium channel blockers (CCB) were found not to be at increased risk for subsequent development of diabetes compared to patients receiving no medication.[3] However, increased risk for the development of diabetes with beta-blocker therapy was not found in other randomized studies.[30] However, despite the potentially adverse metabolic effects of beta-blockers, they have proved to have significant long –term favorable effects on cardiovascular disease in hypertensive patients with diabetes and therefore, should be used in patients with diabetes, particularly those with coronary disease.

Calcium Channel Blockers (CCBs)

To achieve a target BP of 130/80mmHg, clinical trials suggest that at least 65% of patients require two or more different antihypertensive agents. Additional therapies in people with diabetes (besides ACE inhibitors and diuretics) may include long–acting CCBs. A non-dihydropyridine CCBs, such as verapamil or diltiazem, may have more beneficial effects on proteinuria than a dihydropyridine CCB, such as nifedipine. However , with the use of ACE inhibitors (or ARBs) as a first line treatment, together with a diuretic, the addition of a long acting dihydropyridine, such as amlodipine, nifedipine or felodipine will reduce both proteinuria and CVD events rate. If goal is still not achieved, low dose beta-blocker or alpha/beta blocker can be added. It is important to note that the ABCD trial demonstrated CVD events superiority of ACE inhibitors over calcium channel blockers (Ccbs), however these differences were likely the result of the beneficial effects of ACE inhibitors rather than a negative effect of the Ccbs. The use of Ccbs is particularly helpful in achieving the target BP, especially in patients with isolated systolic BP not responding to the addition of low dose diuretic therapy. Information on whether diuretic/beta-blocker or ACE inhibitor-based treatment is significantly better than a CCB –based regimen awaits results of other studies, such as ALLHAT trial.

Diuretics
Low dose diuretics are effective antihypertensive agents in patients with diabetes as these patients often have expanded plasma volume. Concerns regarding adverse metabolic effects shown with the use of large doses (e.g. 50-200 mg of hydrochlorothiazide) were not substantiated with the use of low dose diuretics. Indeed, a report of 12,500 hypertensive adults did not find any influence of thiazide diuretics on the development of diabetes. Diuretics are also effective and recommended by JNC VI for the treatment of isolated systolic hypertension, which is common and occurs at a younger age in people with diabetes as discussed above. The systolic hypertension in the elderly program (SHEP) trial showed that small doses of chlorothalidone contribute not only safe but also very effective treatment, which is able to reduce the rate of major CVD events, fatal and non-fatal strokes and all cause mortality in patients with diabetes.[31] In addition, diuretics are often a necessary component of combination antihypertensive therapy in people with diabetes who often require 3 or more medications to achieve target BP. Indeed in a report by our group (Diabetes Care, in press,) among 1372 patients with hypertension and diabetes, the average number of medications required to achieve a target BP of 130/85 mmHg was 3.1, consistent with results from other major studies such as UKPDS, MDRD, HOT and ABCD, mentioned above, where more than 2 medications were often required for optimal control of BP.

Fixed dose combination
The use of a fixed dose combination therapy has the potential of enhancing compliance, reducing side effects and cost of medications. Several diuretic- based combinations are available. These include those with beta-blocker, ACE inhibitor and ARB. These agents are being used increasingly. Our above- mentioned report indicates that 23 % of patients with diabetes and hypertension are on a fixed dose combination. Long -term benefits from these fixed-dose combinations remain to be seen. However, a combination of particular interest is that of a dihydropyridine CCB (amlodipine) and an ACE inhibitor (Benazapril). Less pedal edema was reported with this combination than with CCB alone. This observation supports the notion that combination

therapy might reduce side effects. In the above case, CCBs being mainly arteriolar vasodilators, may induce pedal edema, but the addition of an ACE inhibitor with a balanced arterial and venous dilation reduces edema formation. This combination also showed enhanced rate of response compared to either placebo or each component given separately.

SUMMARY

Rigorous treatment of hypertension, a common co-morbid condition in patients with diabetes, is very important to reduce both macrovascular and microvascular complications in this population. Combination therapy is often required to achieve and maintain blood pressure at target level. The currently recommended target BP for patients with diabetes is 130/80 mmHg.

Based on the current evidence from randomized controlled trials, the use of ACE inhibitors/ARBs is recommended as initial therapeutic agents with the addition of other agents as necessary to achieve and maintain target blood pressure.

REFERENCES

1. McFarlane SI, Banerji M, Sowers JR. Insulin resistance and cardiovascular disease. J Clin Endocrinol Metab 86:713-8, 2001.
2. Sowers JR, Epstein M, Frohlich ED. Diabetes, hypertension, and cardiovascular disease: an update. Hypertension 37:1053-9, 2001.
3. Gress TW, Nieto FJ, Shahar E, Wofford MR, Brancati FL. Hypertension and antihypertensive therapy as risk factors for type 2 diabetes mellitus. Atherosclerosis Risk in Communities Study. N Engl J Med 342:905-12, 2000.
4. Ferrannini E, Buzzigoli G, Bonadonna R, et al. Insulin resistance in essential hypertension. N Engl J Med 317:350-7, 1987.
5. Shen DC, Shieh SM, Fuh MM, Wu DA, Chen YD, Reaven GM. Resistance to insulin-stimulated-glucose uptake in patients with hypertension. J Clin Endocrinol Metab 66:580-3, 1988.
6. Kotchen TA, Zhang HY, Covelli M, Blehschmidt N. Insulin resistance and blood pressure in Dahl rats and in one-kidney, one-clip hypertensive rats. Am J Physiol 261:E692-7, 1991.
7. Reaven GM, Chang H. Relationship between blood pressure, plasma insulin and triglyceride concentration, and insulin action in spontaneous hypertensive and Wistar-Kyoto rats. Am J Hypertens 4:34-8, 1991.
8. Sechi LA, Melis A, Tedde R. Insulin hypersecretion: a distinctive feature between essential and secondary hypertension. Metabolism 41:1261-6, 1992.
9. Beatty OL, Harper R, Sheridan B, Atkinson AB, Bell PM. Insulin resistance in offspring of hypertensive parents. Bmj 307:92-6, 1993.

10. Grunfeld B, Balzareti M, Romo M, Gimenez M, Gutman R. Hyperinsulinemia in normotensive offspring of hypertensive parents. Hypertension 23:I12-5, 1994.

11. Verdecchia P, Porcellati C, Schillaci G, et al. Ambulatory blood pressure. An independent predictor of prognosis in essential hypertension. Hypertension 24:793-801, 1994.

12. White WB. A chronotherapeutic approach to the management of hypertension. Am J Hypertens 9:29S-33S, 1996.

13. Bianchi S, Bigazzi R, Quinones Galvan A, et al. Insulin resistance in microalbuminuric hypertension. Sites and mechanisms. Hypertension 26:789-95, 1995.

14. Metcalf TH, Nolan B, Henery M, et al. Microalbuminuria in patients with non-insulin dependent diabetes mellitusrelates to nocturnal systolic blood pressure. Am J Med. 102:531-535, 1997.

15. Streeten DH, Auchincloss JH, Jr., Anderson GH, Jr., Richardson RL, Thomas FD, Miller JW. Orthostatic hypertension. Pathogenetic studies. Hypertension 7:196-203, 1985.

16. Streeten DH. Pathogenesis of hyperadrenergic orthostatic hypotension. Evidence of disordered venous innervation exclusively in the lower limbs. J Clin Invest 86:1582-8, 1990.

17. The sixth report of the Joint National Committee on prevention, detection, evaluation, and treatment of high blood pressure. Arch Intern Med 157:2413-46, 1997.

18. Bakris GL, Williams M, Dworkin L, et al. Preserving renal function in adults with hypertension and diabetes: a consensus approach. National Kidney Foundation Hypertension and Diabetes Executive Committees Working Group. Am J Kidney Dis 36:646-61, 2000.

19. Standards of Medical Care for Patients with Diabetes Mellitus. Diabetes Care, Volume 24, Supplement 1, S33-S43, January 2001.

20. Sowers JR, Williams M, Epstein M, Bakris G. Hypertension in patients with diabetes. Strategies for drug therapy to reduce complications. Postgrad Med 107:47-54, 60, 2000.

21. Bakris G, Sowers J, Epstein M, Williams M. Hypertension in patients with diabetes. Why is aggressive treatment essential? Postgrad Med 107:53-6, 61-4, 2000.

22. Basile JN. Hypertension 2001: how will JNC VII be different from JNC VI? South Med J 94:889-90, 2001.

23. Conlin PR, Chow D, Miller ER, 3rd, et al. The effect of dietary patterns on blood pressure control in hypertensive patients: results from the Dietary Approaches to Stop Hypertension (DASH) trial. Am J Hypertens 13:949-55, 2000.

24. Sacks FM, Svetkey LP, Vollmer WM, et al. Effects on blood pressure of reduced dietary sodium and the Dietary Approaches to Stop Hypertension (DASH) diet. DASH-Sodium Collaborative Research Group. N Engl J Med 344:3-10, 2001.
25. Lewis EJ, Hunsicker LG, Bain RP, Rohde RD. The effect of angiotensin-converting-enzyme inhibition on diabetic nephropathy. The Collaborative Study Group. N Engl J Med 329:1456-62, 1993.
26. Effects of ramipril on cardiovascular and microvascular outcomes in people with diabetes mellitus: results of the HOPE study and MICRO-HOPE substudy. Heart Outcomes Prevention Evaluation Study Investigators. Lancet 355:253-9, 2000.
27. Shindler DM, Kostis JB, Yusuf S, et al. Diabetes mellitus, a predictor of morbidity and mortality in the Studies of Left Ventricular Dysfunction (SOLVD) Trials and Registry. Am J Cardiol 77:1017-20, 1996.
28. Kaplan NM. Management of hypertension in patients with type 2 diabetes mellitus: guidelines based on current evidence. Ann Intern Med 135:1079-1083, 2001.
29. Brenner BM, Cooper ME, de Zeeuw D, et al. Effects of losartan on renal and cardiovascular outcomes in patients with type 2 diabetes and nephropathy. N Engl J Med 345:861-9, 2001.
30. Grimm RH, Jr., Flack JM, Grandits GA, et al. Long-term effects on plasma lipids of diet and drugs to treat hypertension. Treatment of Mild Hypertension Study (TOMHS) Research Group. Jama 275:1549-56, 1996.
31. Hall WD. The Systolic Hypertension in the Elderly Program: Implications for the management of older hypertensive patients. Am J Geriatr Cardiol 1:15-23, 1992.

Helpful Internet sources for additional information on hypertension:

1) The American Society of Hypertension
http://www.ash-us.org

2) Hypertension on line
http://www.hypertensiononline.org

Chapter 3. Coronary Artery Disease and Cardiomyopathy

Jennifer E. Liu and Richard B. Devereux

INTRODUCTION

Cardiovascular disease (CVD) is the leading cause of death in patients with type 2 diabetes. Epidemiological studies have shown that diabetes mellitus is a potent independent risk factor for cardiovascular disease.[1, 2] It has been recognized for several decades that diabetic patients have a 2 to 3 fold higher risk for CVD than their nondiabetic counterparts. CVD accounts for up to 80% of deaths in patients with diabetes, approximately 75% of which are due to ischemic heart disease. More than 25% of diabetic patients have evidence of CVD at diagnosis. Therefore, the American Heart Association has stated that "diabetes is a cardiovascular disease".[3]

Although the cardiovascular disease burden is obvious, the causal pathways are incompletely understood. Two major effects of diabetes on the heart are accelerated coronary artery disease and specific diabetic cardiomyopathy. This chapter reviews the clinical implications of these manifestations of diabetic heart disease and the impact of treatment on cardiovascular mortality and morbidity based on clinical trials.

CORONARY ARTERY DISEASE

The Burden of Coronary Artery Disease in Diabetic Patients. Accelerated coronary artery disease (CAD), accounts for 75 to 80% of deaths and hospitalizations in diabetic individuals and a heavy burden of disability and expense.[4] A large body of epidemiological data documents that diabetes is an independent risk factor for CAD in men and especially in women, who seem to lose most of their inherent protection against CAD.[1,2,5] Diabetic patients with no history of CAD have long-term rates of myocardial infarction and cardiovascular death comparable to those of nondiabetic patients with prior myocardial infarction[6] To make matters worse, when patients with diabetes develop clinical CAD, their survival is worse than that of nondiabetic CAD patients[7] Although cardiovascular mortality is declining in the general US population due to reduction in cardiovascular risk factors and improved treatment of heart disease, the decline is smaller in diabetic men (- 13% vs. -36%), and, worse yet, cardiovascular mortality has actually increased in diabetic women (- 23% vs. + 27%).[8]

Myocardial Infarction: Patients with diabetes are at increased risk of myocardial infarction (MI) compared with the general population. In fact, the incidence of MI among patients with diabetes who did not have CAD was similar to patients without diabetes who had preexisting CAD.[6] Diabetes is associated with a 1.2 to 2.0 fold increase in mortality risk after acute MI after adjusting for known confounding variables (Figure 1).

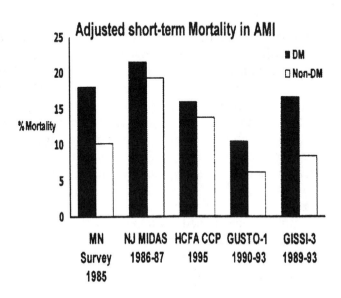

Figure 1. Diabetes and acute myocardial infarction (AMI) outcomes. Diabetes is associated with a 1.2 to 2.0 fold increase in mortality after AMI (Adapted from McGuire DK et al. "Diabetes and ischemic heart disease" Am Heart J 138:S366-S375, 1999, with permission).

The one-year mortality after an MI is also significantly higher in diabetics than non-diabetics (24% vs 14% in men and 33% vs 11% in women). In addition, the prehospitalization mortality rate from acute CHD is higher in diabetics than in non-diabetics. Diabetic patients with MI are less likely to reach the hospital alive (sudden deaths) than nondiabetic patients with MI.[9] The explanation for this high risk is not entirely clear, but may in part be due to a specific coexisting diabetic heart muscle disease which, independent of CAD, impairs myocardial relaxation and contractility. This diabetic cardiomyopathy is discussed later in this chapter.

Silent Ischemia. Myocardial ischemia due to coronary atherosclerosis commonly occurs without symptoms in diabetic patients. As a result, multivessel atherosclerosis often is present before ischemic symptoms occur and treatment is instituted. Diabetic patients have higher prevalences of asymptomatic ischemia on both exercise stress test and 48 h ambulatory ECG monitoring in most,[10,11] but not all[12] studies. The increased rate of silent ischemic episodes is likely due to autonomic neuropathy associated with DM, characterized by loss of sympathetic and parasympathetic innervation to the heart. Therefore, impaired pain perception makes angina a poor discriminating symptom in many diabetic patients with ischemic heart disease.

PATHOPHYSIOLOGY/RISK FACTORS

The increased cardiovascular event rates in diabetes is partially due to independent contributions of the other major cardiovascular risk factors.[1,2,13] Most patients with type 2 DM have the insulin resistance syndrome, also known as Syndrome X or cardiovascular dysmetabolic syndrome, characterized by clustering of metabolic risk factors including hypertension, hyperinsulinemia, glucose intolerance and dyslipidemia.[14] Diabetes is also associated with coagulopathy and endothelial dysfunction, predisposing to thrombosis and vasospasm on top of atherogenesis promoted by the coexisting risk factor of hyperglycemia. However, diabetes has a multiplying effect on cardiovascular risk in the presence of other cardiovascular risk factors.

Dyslipidemia. The Multiple Risk Factor Intervention Trial (MRFIT) showed a curvilinear relationship between total cholesterol and coronary heart disease mortality in diabetic men that was parallel but with about 4-fold greater risk than that in men without diabetes (Figure 2).

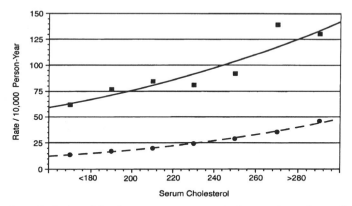

Figure 2. Relationship between serum cholesterol and cardiovascular mortality in diabetic subjects in a 12 year follow-up study from the Multiple Risk Factor Intervention Trial (MRFIT). (Adapted from Goldberg RB. Med Clin North Am 84 (1):81-93, 2000, with permission).

Type 2 diabetic patients have an atherogenic dyslipidemia characterized by three lipoprotein abnormalities: elevated levels of very-low density lipoprotein (VLDL) triglycerides; small, dense low-density lipoprotein (LDL) cholesterol particles; and decreased level of high-density lipoprotein (HDL) cholesterol. Evidence suggests that all elements of diabetic dyslipidemia are atherogenic independent of the commonly elevated serum LDL cholesterol level. Because of frequent changes of glycemic control of diabetic patients and their effects on lipoprotein levels, the American Diabetes Association has recommended that fasting levels of LDL, HDL, total cholesterol, and triglycerides be measured annually in adult patients.[14]

Intervention Trials: No clinical trials have been designed to test specifically whether lipid-lowering treatment reduces CHD events in diabetic patients. Data from subanalyses of clinical trials with lipid-lowering treatment provide some insight into the benefit of treating hyperlipidemia in diabetes. The Helsinki Heart Study found a nonsignificant trend toward lower CHD incidence in diabetic subjects (3.4% vs. 10.5%, p=NS) treated with gemfibrozil as compared to placebo,[15] especially in the subset with high triglycerides and low HDL cholesterol. In addition to the known risks of elevated LDL cholesterol in diabetic as well as non-diabetic patients, diabetes is associated with small, denser LDL cholesterol particles that are especially atherogenic. In subgroup analyses of Scandinavian Simvastatin Survival Study (4S)[16] and the Cholesterol and Recurrent Events (CARE) trial,[17] aggressive LDL lowering therapy reduced recurrent CVD events by 22-25 % in patients with type 2 diabetes.

Based on the most recent National Cholesterol Education Program (Adult Treatment Panel III) guidelines, diabetes is regarded as equivalent to established CHD due to the high risk of new CHD within 10 years. Thus, the primary goal of lipid management in diabetes is to reduce LDL-cholesterol to $\leq$ 100 mg/dl.[18] This goal should be achieved by addition of drug therapy after maximal dietary therapy. Statins are first-line drug therapy for LDL-cholesterol reduction. Triglyceride levels >200 mg/dl should be treated with fibrate therapy. Whether to combine a statin and a fibrate in the treatment of combined hyperlipidemia needs to be carefully considered given the documented, although infrequent, occurrence of rhabdomyolysis with this combination. Although nicotinic acid can effectively reduce triglyceride and raise HDL levels, its potential to worsen hyperglycemia causes it to be relatively contraindicated.

Hypertension. Hypertension is a well-established major risk factor for CVD. The prevalence of hypertension in diabetic patients is at least two-fold increased compared to the non-diabetic population. In addition to the increased risk for coronary events, hypertension also increases the risk of stroke, nephropathy and retinopathy in diabetes. MRFIT demonstrated that the rate of CVD mortality was increased by nearly 3-fold at each level of systolic blood pressure in diabetic as compared to non-diabetic hypertensive men (Figure 3).

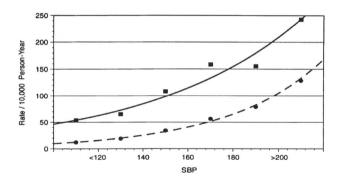

Figure 3. Relationship between systolic blood pressure and cardiovascular mortality in diabetic subjects in a 12 year follow-up study from the Multiple Risk Factor Intervention Trial (MRFIT). (Adapted from Goldberg RB. Med Clin North Am 84 (1): 81-93, 2000, with permission).

Thus, not only is hypertension more prevalent in the diabetic population, it also has a greater impact on the risks of CAD. Clinical trials in hypertensive patients with type 2 diabetes have shown that blood pressure control using several classes of medication is an extremely effective and important preventive therapy.

Intervention Trials. Clinical trial data all support the need to treat hypertension in patients with type 2 diabetes. The Hypertension Optimal Treatment[19] trial evaluated the effect of aggressive lowering of diastolic blood pressure using a calcium channel blocking agent, felodipine. A 51% reduction in cardiovascular events was seen in diabetic patients when diastolic pressure was treated to a mean of 82.6 mm Hg as compared to those treated to a diastolic pressure of 90 mm Hg. In the Systolic Hypertension in the Elderly Trial,[20] antihypertensive treatment with chlorthalidone produced a 34% reduction in CVD events in the diabetic population. A study of tight blood pressure control within the UKPDS[21] showed that a difference of 10/5 mm Hg was associated with a 24% reduction in combined microvascular and macrovascular end points. The Appropriate Blood Pressure Control in Diabetes Trial (ABCD)[22] and the Fosinopril Versus Amlopidipine Cardiovascular Events Randomized Trial (FACET)[23] found that the incidence of CVD events was lower by 8% (p=0.01) and 7% (p=0.03) respectively, in those randomized to an angiotensin-converting enzyme (ACE) inhibitor than in those treated with dihydropyridine calcium channel blockers. In fact, the ABCD trial was terminated one year earlier than scheduled on the basis of recommendations from the independent Data and Safety Monitoring Committee. The committee became concerned with the marked disparity between the two treatment arms in the number of major coronary events that appeared after several years of treatment. The Heart Outcomes Prevention Evaluation (HOPE) and the MICRO-HOPE substudy[24] demonstrated that ACE inhibitors lowered the risk of cardiovascular death by 37% and total mortality by 24% in patients with diabetes. After adjusting for the changes in blood pressure, the risk of cardiovascular and total mortality was still reduced by 25% (p=0.0004). The HOPE study also demonstrated that ACE inhibitors reduced the risk of overt nephropathy (by 24%) as well as microalbuminuria (p=0.02). Albuminuria is not only a marker of nephropathy, but its presence also reflects a higher CVD risk.[25] Another interesting finding, although unexplained, is that there was a 33% reduction in the onset of new diabetes in those not diabetic at baseline over the 4.5 years of the study. Although ACE inhibitors may worsen renal function in patients with bilateral renal artery stenosis and may cause hyperkalemia, they can be used safely with careful titration and measurement of electrolytes and creatinine. Given the powerful protective effect on a range of important cardiovascular outcomes and renal function, ACE inhibitors are emerging as first line antihypertensive treatment in the diabetic population. Recent reports have demonstrated that angiotensin II receptor antagonists also have strong renoprotective effects in patients with type II diabetes.[26] However, future studies are needed to determine whether they have similar cardiovascular protective effects.

Independent of the agent used, aggressive blood pressure control should be a high priority. The Sixth Report of the Joint National Committee (JNC-VI) recommends a target blood pressure of less than 130/85 mm Hg, where possible, in subjects with diabetes.

Hyperglycemia. Chronic hyperglycemia can directly impair vascular endothelial function, which is thought to be one of the underlying mechanism of increased microvascular and macrovascular events in diabetes. Accumulation of advanced glycation end products (AGEs), formed by the glycation of proteins and lipoproteins, in the vessel wall leads to increased vessel stiffness, lipoprotein binding, macrophage recruitment, reduced nitric oxide production and proliferation of vascular smooth muscle cells.[27] All of these contribute to abnormal vasomotion and increased atherogenesis which can lead to arterial thrombosis. Data from clinical trials show that the degree of hyperglycemia in diabetic patients correlates with the risk and severity of microvascular complications, and improving hyperglycemia reduces this risk incrementally. However, the relationship between glycemic control and macrovascular complications is less close. Observational studies that have addressed the relationship of hyperglycemia and the risk of CVD in the diabetic population have yielded conflicting results.[28-32] Available studies are summarized in Table 1.

No adequately powered prospective trials have addressed the impact of glycemic control on cardiovascular outcomes. The Diabetes Control and Complications Trial (DCCT)[33] found a trend towards reduction in cardiovascular events in the intensive treatment group as compared to

Table 1. Hyperglycemia and the risk of CVD

Study	# of DM Subjects	Results
WHO Multinational Study[28]	N=3,583	Neither the degree of hyperglycemia or the duration of DM was related to the onset of CVD
Framingham Study[29]	N=239	No relationship between hyperglycemia and CVD incidence
The Whitehall Study[30]	N=178	Similar risk for CAD in newly diagnosed and previously diagnosed diabetic subjects, suggesting that neither duration nor severity had a major impact on the development of CAD.
Finnish Elderly Study[31]	N=229	The degree of hyperglycemia was independently correlated with CVD occurrence.
The Wisconsin Epidemiological Study of Diabetic Retinopathy[32]	N=10,135	A 1% decrease in hemoglobin A1c predicted 10% fall in CVD events but 50% reduction in retinopathy occurrence or progression, without adjustment for other CVD risk factors.

conventional treatment group (0.5 event per 100 patient years vs. 0.8 event, 95% CI, -10 to 68%). However, the study was conducted among relatively young patients with type 1 diabetes and was not powered to test the hypothesis. The study did find a significant reduction in the microvascular complications in the intensively treated group (76% risk reduction in the development of retinopathy, 39% reduction in microalbuminuria and 60% reduction in clinical neuropathy) . The UKPDS, initiated in the 1970s, reported the effects of intensive treatment of hyperglycemia using sulfonylurea agents, insulin or metformin in newly diagnosed type 2 diabetic patients over a 10 year period.[34] Despite the fact that the hemoglobin A1c was lower in the intensively treated group (7.0% vs. 7.9%, approaching the American Diabetes Association goal of <7%), the reductions in myocardial infarction (14.7 events per 1000 patient-years vs. 17.4 events; p=0.052) and stroke (5.6 events per 1000 patient-years vs. 5.0 events per 1000 patient years; p=0.52) did not attain significance compared with the conventional treatment group. The development of microvascular disease was however, significantly reduced (25%, p<0.01). This study was powered to demonstrate whether improved glycemic control would reduce cardiovascular events, but demonstrated only a modest reduction in myocardial infarction and none for stroke.

Aggressive treatment of hyperglycemia in diabetes has been shown to be extremely beneficial in prevention of microvascular disease. However, reducing HgA1c to <7% is likely to leave a substantial excess risk of cardiovascular disease in diabetic patients. Assessment of all risk factors and aggressive treatment to achieve goal are critical to reduce cardiovascular risk in diabetic patients.

Procoagulant State. Multiple abnormalities in platelet function, coagulation, fibrinolysis and blood viscosity have been described in diabetic patients. Abnormal platelet adhesion and aggregation, increased fibrinogen, factor VII and increased plasminogen activator inhibitor-1 levels are well recognized.[35] These alterations in the coagulation system are particularly seen in those with the metabolic syndrome or Syndrome X. For these reasons, the American Diabetes Association has recommended that aspirin treatment be considered in diabetic patients with two or more risk factors in addition to those with established cardiovascular disease.

Cigarette Smoking and Obesity. Cigarette smoking is a leading risk factor for CVD. In MRFIT,[2] cigarette smoking was a powerful determinant of CVD mortality in men with diabetes and had an additive effect when superimposed on either risk factors. Weight reduction and regular physical activity have beneficial effects on glycemic control, hypertension, dyslipidemia and insulin resistance.

Management of Coronary Artery Disease in Diabetic Patients. Available data, reviewed above, indicates that optimal control of arterial pressure and lipid levels are of substantial benefit, in addition to tight glycemic control for prevention of coronary artery disease events in diabetic patients. Use of aspirin and nephroprotection by ACE inhibitors also appear to reduce CAD risk. After CAD has become manifested by myocardial infarction, optimal glucose control with insulin therapy in diabetic patients was shown to produce a significant 30% reduction in mortality at 12 months as compared to usual glycemic control.[36] Beta blockers are also effective in mortality reduction after myocardial infarction in diabetic patients. Pooled trial results show a 37% reduction in CVD mortality in diabetic patients compared with 13% found in all treated groups.[37] Thus, the management of diabetic patients with acute myocardial infarction should include optimum glycemic control with insulin, immediate coronary reperfusion, aspirin and early beta blockade.

Coronary Revascularization. Coronary artery bypass graft surgery (CABG) and percutaneous coronary angioplasty (PTCA) are both effective revascularization strategies in patients with diabetes. Diabetes is not associated with increased perioperative mortality during bypass graft surgery, although the frequency of wound infection and the length of hospital stay are increased. Although the initial rate of success of PTCA is similar in diabetics and non-diabetics, there is an increased rate of restenosis during the next 6 months. The mechanism of restenosis is thought to be due to exaggerated neointimal hyperplasia rather than increased vessel remodelling.[38] Whether the use of more technologically advanced procedures, such as stenting, will lead to improved outcomes in diabetes remains to be answered by future clinical trials.

Several trials have examined the outcome of PTCA compared to CABG in diabetic patients with multivessel CAD. The Bypass Angioplasty Revascularization Investigation (BARI)[39] demonstrated that 5 year survival was only 65.5% in diabetic patients randomly assigned to PTCA compared to 80.6% survival in the CABG group. For patients without diabetes, the 5-year mortality rates were virtually identical. One limitation of the study, however, was the lack of the use of stents in the angioplasty group, since stenting may improve outcomes in patients with diabetes. One explanation for the higher mortality associated with PTCA is that diabetes is usually associated with more diffuse coronary disease and the vessels are of small caliber. It is likely that angioplasty leaves a higher proportion of myocardium ischemic than does bypass grafting. The issue of whether the findings of the BARI trial are consistent with other revascularization trials has been raised. The Emory Angioplasty Versus Surgery Trial (EAST)[40] found no difference in mortality in diabetic patients treated with PTCA compared with coronary bypass surgery. However, diabetic patients fared no worse than non-diabetic patients in general, which suggest that the diabetic patients in this study represent an unusually low risk group. Also, EAST involved fewer diabetic patients than did BARI and had limited statistical power to detect a treatment difference.

The conclusion which can be drawn from the above two studies is that the form of revascularization for the treatment of multivessel coronary disease in diabetes can be individually tailored to patients, taking into account the clinical and angiographic suitability for each procedure. Those patients with more severe disease should undergo surgery and those with milder form of disease can be treated with angioplasty plus stenting.

CARDIOMYOPATHY

One reason for the poor prognosis in patients with diabetes after myocardial infarction is the increased susceptibility to develop heart failure. Diabetic men have more than twice the frequency of heart failure than non-diabetic cohorts, while diabetic women have a fivefold increased risk of developing heart failure.[41] This excessive risk of heart failure persists despite correcting for age, hypertension, obesity, hypercholesterolemia and coronary artery disease. It has been proposed that a specific diabetic cardiomyopathy exists, independent of coronary artery disease or other coexisting confounding factors, characterized by alteration of left ventricular (LV) structure and function. There are now considerable experimental, pathological and epidemiological data to support the existence of "diabetic cardiomyopathy". The existence of a subclinical or early form of diabetic cardiomyopathy is suggested by a recent study showing abnormal LV structure and function, detected by echocardiography, in newly diagnosed type 2 diabetes.[42] The process of alteration of the myocardium may occur before the degree of abnormality of glucose metabolism reaches the criteria level for the diagnosis of diabetes. Features of this diabetic cardiomyopathy are discussed below.

Left Ventricular Hypertrophy. The association of LV hypertrophy and risk of cardiovascular morbidity and mortality is well established.[43] In one landmark study, LV hypertrophy was associated with a greater relative risk for all-cause mortality than the number of stenotic coronary arteries or the LV ejection fraction.[44] In animal models[45], rats with streptozotocin induced diabetes demonstrate increased LV mass. The combination of hypertension and diabetes mellitus is synergistic in rats, leading to higher mortality, as it does in humans. This finding is confirmed in pathologic studies which showed that human diabetic hearts have higher LV mass, unrelated to the extent of coronary artery disease and hypertension.[46] Other abnormalities noted in human diabetic hearts includes microvascular constriction, interstitial fibrosis and edema. In epidemiological studies, diabetes has been shown to be independently associated with higher prevalences of LV hypertrophy in both the Framingham population and the Strong Heart Study (13 vs 6 %, p<0.05).[47,48] The combination of hypertension and diabetes, which frequently coexist, further increases the prevalence of LV hypertrophy[49] (Figure 4).

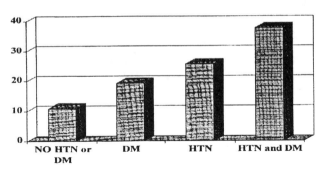

Figure 4. Prevalence of LV hyperthrophy in participants with neither diabetes mellitus (DM) nor hypertension (HTN), DM alone, HTN alone, or both conditions. (Adapted from Bella et al. Am J Cardiol 87:1260-1265, 2001, with permission).

In a population of 1,810 diabetic adults, cardiovascular mortality was significantly higher (OR=2.36, 95% CI 1.18-4.69) in DM participants with as opposed to those without echocardiographic LV hypertrophy, after adjusting for age, gender, body mass index, hypertension, smoking and plasma creatinine.[50] In addition to increasing LV mass, diabetes also impacts cardiac remodeling, with an associated increase in relative wall thickness, a measure of concentricity of the left ventricle.

Left Ventricular Function. Diabetes is associated with systolic and diastolic dysfunction, independent of coronary artery disease or hypertension. Hemodynamic, biochemical and histological studies in alloxan induced diabetic dogs demonstrated a lower stroke volume despite normal LV end diastolic pressure. Chamber stiffness was increased in diabetic dogs compared to control dogs.[51] Isolated papillary muscle studies in diabetic rats indicate prolongation of contraction, prolonged relaxation, and a reduced rate of shortening.[45] A wide range of abnormal biochemical changes have been described in the hearts of diabetic rats including alterations in ATPase, impaired calcium ion transport and alterations in carbohydrate, lipid, and adenine nucleotide metabolism. In clinical studies, Jain et al found increased chamber stiffness in diabetics as compared to non-diabetics.[52] In addition, epidemiolgical studies have found that patients with diabetes have lower fractional shortening (by a mean of 0.7%) and midwall fractional shortening (an index of myocardial contractility) by a mean of 0.9%.[48] Impaired LV systolic function is the strongest predictor of morbid cardiac events in coronary artery disease.[53] Diabetes is also associated with diastolic dysfunction, which appears to predate the onset of systolic dysfunction. The severity of diabetes-associated abnormal LV relaxation is similar to the well known impaired relaxation associated with hypertension.[54] The combination of both diabetes and hypertension induces more severe abnormal LV relaxation than does either condition alone. In addition, abnormal relaxation in subjects with diabetes is associated with worse glycemic control and positively associated with duration of diabetes. Evidence of impaired LV relaxation is associated with higher cardiovascular and all-cause mortality in diabetes.[55] Evidence of diabetic cardiomyopathy is seen early in the course of the disease, often at the onset of diabetes.[42]

Potential Mechanisms. The etiology of diabetic cardiomyopathy characterized by increased LV mass, concentric remodeling, systolic dysfunction and impaired LV relaxation is not entirely clear. It has been proposed that the pathogenic mechanism may be related to metabolic alterations due to hyperglycemia. Interstitial accumulation of advanced-glycated end-products (AGES), collagen deposition and fibrosis in the myocardium have been reported in human diabetic hearts.[46] Animal studies have found p-aminosalicyclic acid-positive material among the muscle fibers and cholesterol and triglyceride deposition in the myocardium.[45] These tissue alterations can increase end-diastolic myocardial stiffness as well as LV mass, and impair systolic function.

The pathogenic mechanism underlying these changes in myocardial tissue composition is unclear. We have recently reported that albuminuria, a strong predictor of cardiovascular mortality and morbidity, is independently associated with increased LV mass and systolic and diastolic dysfunction among diabetic patients.[56] Albuminuria has been proposed to represent a marker of a generalized vascular dysfunction[57] and has been associated with renal alterations, proliferative retinopathy and cardiovascular disease in diabetic and non-diabetic populations. Albuminuria reflects a renal and systemic transvascular albumin leakage that is perhaps due to low vessel wall content of heparin sulfate which has been shown not only in the glomerular basement membrane but also in the atherosclerotic aorta and coronary arteries.[58] This generalized increase of vascular permeability can also cause leakiness of collagen, cholesterol and advanced glycated end-products that have been reported in the myocardium of human hearts[51] Furthermore, this change in permeability causing insudation of lipoproteins into the intima of large vessels can lead to atherosclerosis of the epicardial coronary arteries as well as small arterioles of the heart. Small vessel disease can lead to subendocardial ischemia causing systolic and diastolic myocardial dysfunction. The microvascular changes in the heart are the same as those throughout the rest of the body such as interstitial fibrosis, perivascular thickening and fibrosis and micro-aneurysm formation.

CONCLUSIONS

The high rates of morbidity and mortality associated with diabetes are, most notably due to cardiovascular disease. The risk of developing new coronary heart disease is high in diabetes, in part because of its frequent association with other risk factors for coronary artery disease. In addition, diabetes is associated with higher morbidity and mortality after myocardial infarction. Diabetes is also often associated with a distinct cardiomyopathy which may partially mediate the high mortality associated with coronary heart disease and congestive heart failure. Management goals for the diabetic patient should focus on optimal glucose control and intense modification of coronary disease risk factors, especially optimal control of arterial pressure and lipids. In addition, evaluation to detect subclinical or early clinical evidence of atherosclerosis and diabetic cardiomyopathy may be warranted to target especially intensive intervention most accurately.

REFERENCES

1. Garcia MJ, McNamara M, Gordon T, Kannel WB. 16 year follow-up study. Morbidity and mortality in diabetics in the Framingham population. Diabetes 23: 105, 1976.
2. Kannel WB, McGee DL. Diabetes and Cardiovascular disease; the Framingham Study. JAMA 241: 2035-8, 1979.
3. Grundy SM, Benjamin IJ, Burke GL et al. Diabetes and cardiovascular disease: a statement for healthcare professionals from the American Heart Association. Circulation 100(10):1134-46, 1999.
4. Laakso M, Lehto S. Epidemiology of macrovascular disease in diabetes. Diabetes Rev 5:294-315, 1997.
5. Brezinka V, Padmos I. Coronary heart disease risk factors in women. Eur Heart J 15:1571-1584, 1994.

6. Haffner SM, Lehto S, Ronnemaa T, et al. Mortality from coronary heart disease in subjects with type 2 diabetes and in nondiabetic subjects with and without prior myocardial infarction. N Engl J Med 339(4):229-34, 1998.

7. Stone PH, Muller JE, Hartwell, T, et al. The MILIS Study Group. The effect of diabetes mellitus on prognosis and serial left ventricular function after acute myocardial infarction: contribution of both coronary artery disease and diastolic left ventricular dysfunction to the adverse prognosis. J Am Coll Cardiol 14:49-57, 1989.

8. Gu K, Cowie CC, Harris MI. Diabetes and decline in heart disease mortality in US adults. JAMA 281:1291-1297, 1999.

9. Miettinen H, Lehto S, Salomaa V, et al. Impact of diabetes on mortality after the first myocardial infarction. Diabetes Care 21:69-75, 1998.

10. Naka M, Hiramatsu K, Aizawa T, et al. Silent myocardial ischemia in non-insulin dependent diabetes as judged by treadmill exercise testing and coronary angiography. Am Heart J 123:46-52, 1992.

11. Langer A, Freeman M, Josse R, et al. Detection of silent myocardial ischemia in diabetes mellitus. Am J Cardiol 67: 1073-8, 1991.

12. Caracciolo EA, Chaitman BR, Forman SR et al. Diabetics with coronary disease have a prevalence of asymptomatic ischemia during exercise treadmill testing and ambulatory ischemia monitoring similar to that of non-diabetic patients. Circulation 1996; 93: 2097-2105.

13. Stamler J, Vaccaro O, Neaton JD et al. Diabetes, other risk factors, and 12-year cardiovascular mortality for men screened in the Multiple Risk Factor Intervention Trial (MRFIT). Diabetes Care 16:434-444, 1993.

14. ADA Consensus Panel. Role of cardiovascular risk factors in prevention and treatment of macrovascular disease in diabetes: American Diabetes Association. Diabetes Care 12: 573-579, 1989.

15. Koskinen P, Manttari M, Manninen V, et al. Coronary heart disease incidence in NIDDM patients in the Helskinki Heart Study. Diabetes Care15(7):820-5, 1992.

16. Pyorala K, Pedersen TR, Kjekshus J, et al. Cholesterol lowering with simvastatin improves prognosis of diabetic patients with coronary heart disease. A subgroup analysis of the Scandinavian Simvastatin Survival Study (4S). Diabetes Care 20(4): 614-20, 1997.

17. Goldberg RB, Mellies MJ, Sacks FM et al. For the CARE investigators. Cardiovascular events and their reduction with pravastatin in diabetic and glucose-intolerant myocardial infarction survivors with average cholesterol levels: subgroup analyses in the Cholesterol and Recurrent Events (CARE) trial. Circulation 98: 2513-2519, 1998.

18. Executive Summary of the Third Report of the National Cholesterol Education Program (NCEP) Expert Panel on Detection, Evaluation, and Treatment of High Blood Cholesterol in Adults (Adult Treatment Panel III). JAMA 285: 2486-2497, 2001.

19. Hansson L, Zanchetti A, Carruthers SG, et al. Effects of intensive blood-pressure lowering and low-dose aspirin in patients with hypertension: principal results of the Hypertension Optimal Treatment (HOT) randomized trial. HOT Study Group. Lancet 351(9118):1755-62, 1998.

20. Curb JD, Pressel SL, Cutler JA, et al. for the Systolic Hypertension in the Elderly Program Cooperative Research Group: Effect of diuretic-based antihypertensive treatment on cardiovascular disease risk in older diabetic patients with isolated systolic hypertension. Systolic Hypertension in the Elderly Program Cooperative Research Group. JAMA 276:1886-1892, 1996.

21. UK Prospective Diabetes Study Group. Tight blood pressure control and risk of macrovascular and microvascular complications in type 2 diabetes: UKPDS 38. Br Med J 317 (7160):703-13, 1998.

22. Estacio RO, Jeffers BW, Hiatt WR et al: The effect of nisoldipine as compared with enalapril on cardiovascular outcomes in patients with non-insulin dependent diabetes and hypertension. N Engl J Med 338:645-652, 1998.

23. Tatti P, Pahor M, Byrington RB, et al: Outcome results of the Fosinopril Versus Amlopidine Cardiovascular Events Randomized Trial (FACET) in patients with hypertension and NIDDM. Diabetes Care 21:597-603, 1998.

24. Effects of ramipril on cardiovascular and microvascular outcomes in people with diabetees mellitus: results of the HOPE study and MICRO-HOPE substudy. Heart Outcomes Prevention Evaluation Study Investigators. Lancet 355:253-9, 2000.

25. Mogensen CE. Microalbuminuria predicts clinical proteinuria and early mortality in maturity-onset diabetes. N Engl J Med 310:356-360, 1994.

26. Brenner BM, Cooper ME, de Zeeuw D, et al. Effects of losartan on renal and cardiovascular outcomes with type 2 diabetes and nephropathy. N Engl J Med 345:861-869, 2001.

27. Brownlee M. Glycation and diabetic complications. Diabetes 43:836-41, 1994.

28. West KM, Ahuja MM, Bennet PH, et al. The role of circulating glucose and triglyceride concentrations and their interactions with other "risk factors" as determinants of arterial disease in nine diabetic population samples from the WHO Multinational Study. Diabetes Care 6:361-369, 1983.

29. Wilson WF, Cupples AD, Kannel WB. Is hyperglycemia associated with cardiovascular disease? The Framingham Study. Am Heart J 2:586-590, 1991.

30. Jarrett RJ, Shipley MJ. Type 2 (non-insulin-dependent) diabetes mellitus and cardiovascular disease: Putative association via common antecedents: Further evidence from the Whitehall Study. Diabetologia 31:737-740, 1988.

31. Kuusisto J, Mykkanen L, Pyorala K, et al. NIDDM and its metabolic control predict coronary heart disease in elderly subjects. Diabetes 43:960-967, 1994.

32. Klein R: Kelly West Lecture 1994: Hyperglycemia and microvascular and macrovascular disease in diabetes. Diabetes Care18:258-268, 1995.

33. Diabetes Control and Complications Trial Research Group (DCCT): The effect of intensive treatment of diabetes on the development and progression of long-term complications in insulin-dependent diabetes mellitus. N Engl J Med 329:977-986, 1993.

34. UK Prospective Diabetes Study (UKPDS) Group: Intensive blood-glucose control with sulfonylureas or insulin compared with conventional treatment and risk of complications in patients with type 2 diabetes (UKPDS33). Lancet 352:837-852, 1998.

35. Colwell JA: Aspirin therapy in diabetes. Diabetes Care 20:1767-1771, 1997.

36. Malmberg K, Ryden L, Efendic S, et al. Randomized trial of insulin-glucose infusion followed by subcutaneous insulin treatment in diabetic patients with acute myocardial infarction (DIGAMI Study): effects on mortality at 1 year. J Am Coll Cardiol 26: 57-65, 1995.

37. KendallMJ, Lynch KP, Hjalmarson A, et al. Beta-blockers and sudden cardiac death. Ann Intern Med 123:358-67, 1995.

38. Kornowski R, Mintz GS, Kent KM, et al. Increased restenosis in diabetes mellitus after coronary interventions is due to exaggerated intimal hyperplasia. Circulation 95:1366-69, 1997.

39. The Bypass Angioplasty Revascularization Investigation (BARI) Investigators. Comparison of coronary bypass surgery with angioplasty in patients with multivessel disease. N Engl J Med 335:217-25, 1996.

40. King SB, Lembo NJ, Weintraub WS, et al, for the Emory Angioplasty Versus Surgery Trial (EAST). A randomized trial comparing coronary angioplasty with coronary bypass surgery. N Engl J Med 331:1044-50, 1994.

41. Abbott RD, Donahue RP, Kannel WB, et al. The impact of diabetes on survival following myocardial infarction in men vs. women. The Framingham Study. JAMA 260:3456, 1988.

42. Liu JE, Robbins DC, Sosenko J, et al. Abnormal LV Structure and Function are Associated with Recent Conversion from Normal Glucose Tolerance to Diabetes Mellitus – the Strong Heart Study (SHS). Diabetes Suppl 2:50:147, 2001.

43. Levy D, Garrison RJ, Savage DD, Kannel WB, Castelli WP: Prognostic implications of echocardiographically determined left ventricular mass in the Framingham Heart Study. N Engl J Med 322:1561-1566, 1990.

44. Liao Y, Cooper RS, McGee DL, Mensah GA, Ghali JK: The relative effects of left ventricular hypertrophy, coronary artery disease, and ventricular dysfunction on survival among black adults. JAMA 273:1592-1597, 1995.

45. Fein FS, Sonnenblick EH. Diabetic cardiomyopathy. Cardiovascular Drugs Ther 8:65-73, 1994.
46. Van Hoeven KV, Factor SM. A comparison of the pathological spectrum of hypertensive, diabetic, and hypertensive-diabetic heart disease. Circulation 82:848-855, 1990.
47. Galderisi M, Anderson KM, Wilson PW et al. Echocardiographic evidence for the existence of a distinct diabetic cardiomyopathy (The Framingham Heart Study). Am J Cardiol 68:85-89, 1991.
48. Devereux RB, Roman MJ, Paranicas M, et al. Impact of diabetes on cardiac structure and function. The Strong Heart Study Circulation 101:2271-2276, 2000.
49. Bella JN, Devereux RB, Roman MJ, et al. Separate and joint cardiovascular effects of hypertension and diabetes: The Strong Heart Study. Am J Cardiol 87:1260-5, 2001.
50. Liu JE, Palmieri V, Roman MJ et al. Cardiovascular disease and prognosis in adults with glucose disorders: The Strong Heart Study. J Am Coll Cardiol 35:263A, 2000.
51. Regan TJ, Wu CF, Yeh CK, Oldewurtle HA, Haider B. Myocardial composition and function in diabetes: the effect of chronic insulin use. Circ Res 49:1268-1277, 1981.
52. Jain A, Avendano G, Dharamsey S, et al. Left ventricular diastolic function in hypertension and role of plasma glucose and insulin. Comparison with diabetic heart. Circulation 93:1396-1402, 1996.
53. Mock MB, Ringqvist I, Fischer LD, and Participants in the Coronary Artery Surgery Study (CASS) Registry. Survival of medically treated patients in the coronary artery surgery study (CASS) registry. Circulation 66:562-571, 1982.
54. Liu JE, Palmieri V, Roman MJ, et. al. The impact of glycemia and diabetes on left ventricular filling pattern: The Strong Heart Study. J Am Coll Cardiol 37:1943-9, 2001.
55. Bella JN, Palmieri V, Roman MJ, et al. Prognostic significance of abnormal peak early to late diastolic filling ratio in middle-aged to elderly American Indians: The Strong Heart Study. J Am Coll Cardiol 35:293A, 2000.
56. Liu, J.E., Palmieri V, Roman MJ, et al. Association of albuminuria with systolic and diastolic left ventricular dysfunction in type 2 diabetes: The Strong Heart Study. J Am Coll Cardiol 37:221A, 2001.
57. Deckert T, Feldt-Rasmussen B, Borch-Johnsen K, Jensen T, Kofoed-Enevoldsen. Albuminuria reflects widespread vascular damage – The Steno Hypothesis. Diabetologia 32:219-226, 1989.
58. Yla-Herrtuala S, Sumuvuori H, Karkola K, Mottonen M, Nikkari T.Glycosaminoglycans in normal and atherosclerotic human coronary arteries. Lab Invest 61:231-236, 1986.

Chapter 4. Polycystic Ovary Syndrome

Susan B. Zweig, Marsha C. Tolentino, Leonid Poretsky

DEFINITION, CLINICAL MANIFESTATIONS, AND PREVALENCE

Polycystic ovary syndrome (PCOS) is a common disorder affecting (depending on the population studied and the definition of the syndrome) between 5 to 20% of reproductive age women.[1] If the middle of this range is considered as a realistic prevalence, then PCOS may be the most prevalent endocrine disorder in women. In spite of the widespread presence of PCOS, its precise definition still eludes both investigators and practitioners. Most consensus definitions describe PCOS as a disorder characterized by *chronic anovulation* and the presence of some degree of *hyperandrogenism,* with the exclusion of specific disorders that may lead to similar phenotypes, particularly, 21-hydroxylase deficiency and other forms of congenital adrenal hyperplasia. The definition proposed in 1990 by the National Institutes of Health Conference on PCOS requires a minimum of two criteria: menstrual abnormalities due to oligo- or anovulation, and hyperandrogenism of ovarian origin. Other disorders, such as 21-hydroxylase deficiency, androgen secreting tumors, and hyperprolactinemia, must be excluded.[2]

Presence of polycystic ovaries on pelvic sonogram is not a necessary criterion for establishing the diagnosis of PCOS.[3] If polycystic ovaries are detected sonographically in a patient without anovulation or hyperandrogenism, the term "polycystic ovaries" (PCO) rather than "polycystic ovary *syndrome*" (PCOS) is used.[4]

Clinical manifestations vary widely among women with this disorder. Chronic anovulation may present as infertility or some form of menstrual irregularity, such as amenorrhea, oligomenorrhea or dysfunctional uterine bleeding. Signs of hyperandrogenism include hirsutism, seborrhea, acne and alopecia. Evidence of virilization, including clitoromegaly, may be present in severe cases. Obesity and acanthosis nigricans are clinical features that are commonly seen in PCOS women and are associated with insulin resistance.

Epidemiological data and prospective controlled studies have reported an increased prevalence of insulin resistance, impaired glucose tolerance, and undiagnosed type 2 diabetes mellitus in these women.[5] In this chapter, we will discuss the role of insulin resistance in the pathogenesis of PCOS, the risk of diabetes mellitus in this population and the role of insulin sensitizing agents in treating patients with polycystic ovary syndrome.

STEIN-LEVENTHAL SYNDROME

Although reports of disorders resembling PCOS date prior to the 17th century, the first clear description belongs to Chereau, who in 1844 described "sclerocystic degeneration of the ovaries".[6] The modern era of PCOS began with a report by two gynecologists, Irving F. Stein and Michael L. Leventhal, who in 1935 described a syndrome of amenorrhea, hirsutism, and enlarged polycystic ovaries in anovulatory women. After observing the restoration of menstruation following ovarian biopsies in patients with this syndrome, Stein and Leventhal performed one-half to three-fourths wedge-resection of each ovary in 7 women. During the operation the ovarian cortex containing the cysts was removed. All of the patients who underwent wedge resection in Stein and Leventhal's series experienced the return of their menses and two became pregnant.

Stein and Leventhal established both the term "polycystic ovary syndrome" and the theory attributing the origin of this disorder to endocrine abnormalities.[7] In 1949, Culiner and Shippel coined the term "hyperthecosis ovarii" for polycystic ovaries comprised of nests of theca cells. Wedge resection performed in patients with this condition did not result in amelioration of hyperandrogenism. These women were masculinized, and often had diabetes and hypertension. The hyperthecosis ovarii was characterized by familial clustering. The polycystic ovaries in these patients were found to have not only hyperplasia of the theca cells but also atretic follicles.[8]

Hormonal studies in PCOS women were performed only after the clinical manifestations and anatomical abnormalities of this disorder were well reported. In one of the first studies that measured hormone levels in PCOS patients, McArthur et al., in 1958, reported increased urinary levels of luteinizing hormone (LH).[9] Reports of elevated circulating androgen levels followed.[10]

During the last two decades PCOS has been identified as a metabolic disorder in which underlying insulin resistance and consequent hyperinsulinemia contribute to hyperandrogenism.

MAIN HORMONAL ABNORMALITIES

The two main endocrine theories of PCOS attribute its pathogenesis to the primary role of either central (hypothalamic, pituitary) or ovarian hormonal abnormalities.[11]

The central theory proposes that the initial pathogenic event is an abnormally increased pulsatile secretion of gonadotropin releasing hormone (GnRH) from the hypothalamus that causes a tonically increased secretion of LH instead of the normal pulsatile pattern with a surge during ovulation.[12] It has been proposed that LH levels may rise further because of hyperandrogenism: after androstenedione is converted in the peripheral fat to estrone by aromatase, estrone enhances LH secretion by increasing LH-producing gonadotroph sensitivity to GnRH.[13] In response to increased LH, ovarian thecal cells undergo hypertrophy and their androgen secretion is further increased, thus establishing a vicious cycle. On the contrary, follicle stimulating hormone (FSH) secretion is normal or decreased due to negative feedback from increased estrogen levels produced through aromatization of androgens. Thus, the LH:FSH ratio is often increased.

The ovarian theory attributes primary pathogenic role in the development of PCOS to the ovary, where the production of androgens is increased.[11] According to this theory, dysregulation of the enzyme cytochrome P450c17-alpha, which comprises 17-hydroxylase and 17/20 lyase activities, results in increased amount of androgens. Increased levels of androstenedione and estrone could also be secondary to reduced levels of the enzyme 17-ketosteroid reductase, which converts androstenedione to testosterone and estrone to estradiol.[14]

When ovarian theca cells from women with PCOS were propagated *in-vitro*, it was shown that the activity of 17 α-hydroxylase/C17,20 lyase and 3β-hydroxysteroid dehydrogenase levels were elevated. This results in increased production of testosterone precursors, and, ultimately, causes increased testosterone production. Thus, thecal cells from PCOS patients, when cultured *in-vitro*, possess intrinsic ability to produce increased amounts of testosterone.[15]

In summary, main hormonal abnormalities in PCOS include elevated androgen and estrogen levels and commonly, although not always, an elevated LH:FSH ratio. Hyperinsulinemia, commonly observed in patients with PCOS, contributes to the development of these hormonal abnormalities.[16]

INSULIN RESISTANCE IN PCOS

In 1921, Archard and Thiers described "the diabetes of bearded women", the first reference to an association between abnormal carbohydrate metabolism and hyperandrogenism.[17] Since then, several syndromes of extreme insulin resistance have been described in patients with distinctive phenotypes which include acanthosis nigricans, hyperandrogenism, polycystic ovaries or ovarian hyperthecosis and, sometimes, diabetes mellitus. These syndromes (described in detail in Chapter V.6) are rare and include leprechaunism, type A and B syndromes of insulin resistance, lipoatrophic diabetes and Rabson-Mendenhall syndrome. Severe insulin resistance observed in these rare syndromes can be due to a mutation of the insulin receptor gene or other genetic defects in insulin action. In the type B syndrome of insulin resistance, anti-insulin receptor antibodies have been identified.[18,19,20]

Euglycemic hyperinsulinemic glucose/insulin clamp studies are used to quantify insulin resistance. After a priming dose of insulin, euglycemia is maintained by a constant dose of insulin infusion and simultaneous glucose infusion, the rate of which is adjusted to achieve normal circulating glucose levels. When stable glucose levels are achieved, the rate of peripheral glucose utilization, measured in grams glucose/m^2 of body surface area, is equal to the rate of glucose infusion. Insulin clamp studies in PCOS subjects have demonstrated significant reduction in insulin-mediated glucose disposal similar to that seen in diabetes mellitus, thus proving that many patients with PCOS are insulin resistant.[21]

Insulin sensitivity is affected by several independent parameters, including obesity, muscle mass and the site of body fat deposition (central versus peripheral obesity).[21] When insulin clamp studies are performed in PCOS women who are matched to non-PCOS controls for body mass index and body composition, insulin resistance is demonstrated in PCOS women independent of these parameters. Thus, lean PCOS women are more insulin resistant than lean controls. However, body fat does have a synergistically negative effect on insulin sensitivity in PCOS, so that lean PCOS women are usually less insulin resistant than the obese PCOS subjects. The etiology of insulin resistance in polycystic ovary syndrome is unknown, although abnormalities of insulin receptor signaling have been reported in some patients.[22]

It has been hypothesized that elevated serum insulin levels in patients with PCOS result in excessive ovarian androgen production, as well as ovarian growth and cyst formation. Several in-vitro studies have demonstrated the presence of insulin receptors in the ovary[23,24,25] and the stimulation of androgen production in ovarian cells by insulin.[26] Continuous stimulation of the ovary by hyperinsulinemia in synergism with LH over a prolonged period of time may produce morphological changes in the ovary, such as ovarian growth and cyst formation.[27] The effects of insulin on the ovary can be mediated by the binding of insulin to its own receptor or to the type 1 IGF receptor in what is known as the "specificity spillover" phenomenon. The latter could be an important mechanism in cases of extreme insulin resistance with severe hyperinsulinemia.[28,29]

ROLE OF INSULIN IN OVARIAN FUNCTION

Despite Joslin's early observations of abnormal ovarian function in women with type 1 diabetes mellitus,[30] insulin was not thought to play a significant role in ovarian function until the late 1970s, when patients with extreme forms of insulin resistance were described.[18,19] Manifestations of ovarian hypofunction (primary amenorrhea, late menarche, anovulation, and premature ovarian failure) in untreated type 1 diabetes mellitus can be understood if it is accepted that insulin is necessary for the ovary to reach its full steroidogenic and ovulatory potential. Thus, patients with insulin deficiency commonly exhibit hypothalamic-pituitary and ovulatory defects, but not hyperandrogenism.[16,21] On the other end of the clinical spectrum, women with syndromes of severe insulin resistance exhibit anovulation associated with hyperandrogenism, as discussed above.

If insulin is capable of stimulating ovarian androgen production in insulin resistant patients, one has to postulate that ovarian sensitivity to insulin in these patients is preserved, even in the presence of severe insulin resistance in the classical target organs, such as liver, muscle, and fat.[29] To explain this paradox, we will briefly review cellular mechanisms of insulin action in the ovary and the relationships between insulin, insulin-like growth factors (IGFs) and their receptors.

The term "insulin-related ovarian regulatory system" has been proposed to describe a complex system of ovarian regulation by insulin and IGFs (11). The components of this system include insulin, insulin receptors, insulin-like growth factor I (IGF-I), insulin-like growth factor II (IGF-II), type 1 IGF receptors, type 2 IGF receptors, IGF binding proteins (IGFBPs) 1-6, and IGFBP proteases. The relationships among the various components of this system are illustrated in Figure 1 and are discussed in detail in reference 11.

Insulin receptors are widely distributed in the ovaries. These ovarian insulin receptors are structurally and functionally similar to insulin receptors found in other organs (see Chapter II.3). Regulation of insulin receptor expression, however, may be somewhat different in the ovaries compared to other target tissues. While in classical target tissues insulin receptors are downregulated by hyperinsulinemia, there is evidence that circulating factors other than insulin may regulate insulin receptor expression in the ovaries of premenopausal women.[32,33] These factors may include sex steroids, gonadotropins, IGFs, and IGFBPs. The phenomenon of differential regulation of ovarian insulin receptors, with their preservation in spite of hyperinsulinemia, may provide one explanation for the ovarian responsiveness to insulin in premenopausal women with insulin resistance in peripheral target organs.

The ovarian insulin receptors have heterotetrameric $\alpha_2\beta_2$ structure; possess tyrosine kinase activity and may stimulate the generation of inositolglycans. After insulin binds to the α-subunits of the insulin receptor, the β-subunits are activated via phosphorylation of the tyrosine residues and acquire tyrosine kinase activity, e.g. the ability to promote phosphorylation of other intracellular proteins. The intracellular proteins phosphorylated under the influence of the insulin-receptor tyrosine kinase are the insulin receptor substrates (IRS) (see Chapter II.3).

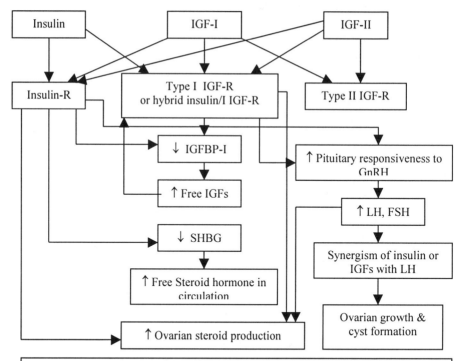

Figure 1. The relationships among the various components of the insulin-related ovarian regulatory system. Insulin, IGF-I, and IGF-II, acting through insulin receptors or type I IGF receptors, increase pituitary responsiveness to GnRH; stimulate gonadotropin secretion directly; stimulate ovarian steroidogenesis; inhibit IGFBP-1 and SHBG production; and act synergistically with gonadotropins to promote ovarian growth and cyst formation. (Adapted, with permission, from L. Poretsky et al. The insulin-related ovarian regulatory system in health and disease. *Endocrine Reviews* 20(4): 535-582, 1999. ©The Endocrine Society)

The insulin receptor activation and IRS phosphorylation result in the activation of phosphatidylinositol-3 kinase (PI-3-kinase). This activation is necessary for transmembrane glucose transport. Mitogen-activated protein kinase (MAPK), responsible for DNA synthesis and gene expression, is also activated by insulin; MAPK activation does not require activation of PI-3-kinase.

Tyrosine kinase activation is the earliest postbinding event and is necessary for many of the effects of insulin. Although it is believed to be the main signaling mechanism of the insulin receptor, an alternative-signaling pathway involving the generation of inositolglycan second messengers has been described[34,35] (see Figure 2). This alternative pathway has been found to mediate several of the effects of insulin, including, possibly, ovarian steroid production. Thus, activation of MAP-kinase and inositolglycan signaling cascades follows pathways that are distinct from those involved in glucose transport. This phenomenon of postreceptor divergence of insulin signaling pathways helps explain how some of the effects of insulin may be normally preserved, or even over-expressed, in the presence of hyperinsulinemia observed in insulin resistant states. In fact, it has been recently demonstrated that some of the ovarian effects of insulin are PI-3 –kinase independent.[36]

Finally, the ovaries may remain sensitive to the actions of insulin in the presence of insulin resistance because, as mentioned above, insulin, when present in high concentration, can activate type 1 IGF-receptors. This pathway of insulin action may be operative in patients with syndromes of extreme insulin resistance whose insulin receptors are rendered inactive by a mutation or by anti-insulin receptor antibodies. There is evidence that type 1 IGF-receptors may be up-regulated in the presence of hyperinsulinemia both in animal models and in women with PCOS.[37,38,39]

In summary, the paradox of preserved ovarian sensitivity to insulin in insulin resistant states can be explained by differential regulation of insulin receptors in the ovaries of premenopausal women; by activation of signaling pathways distinct from those involved in glucose transport (inositolglycan and MAP-kinase pathways, rather than tyrosine kinase and PI-3 kinase pathways); and by the activation of type 1 IGF-receptors which may be up-regulated in the presence of hyperinsulinemia (Table 1).

Table 1. Possible mechanisms of preserved ovarian sensitivity to insulin in insulin resistant states.

1. Differential regulation of ovarian insulin receptors in premenopausal women
2. Activation of alternative insulin signaling pathways (MAP-kinase and inositol-glycan), rather than PI-3 kinase pathway of glucose transport
3. Activation of type 1 IGF-receptors which may be up-regulated by hyperinsulinemia

INSULIN EFFECTS RELATED TO OVARIAN FUNCTION

Potential mechanisms underlying the gonadotropic activity of insulin include direct effects on steroidogenic enzymes, synergism with FSH and LH, enhancement of pituitary responsiveness to GnRH, and effects on SHBG and on the IGF/IGFBP systems (see Table 2). Investigations focused on these mechanisms have provided insights not only into normal ovarian physiology, but also into the pathogenesis of ovarian dysfunction in a wide spectrum of clinical entities, such as obesity, diabetes mellitus, PCOS and syndromes of extreme insulin resistance.

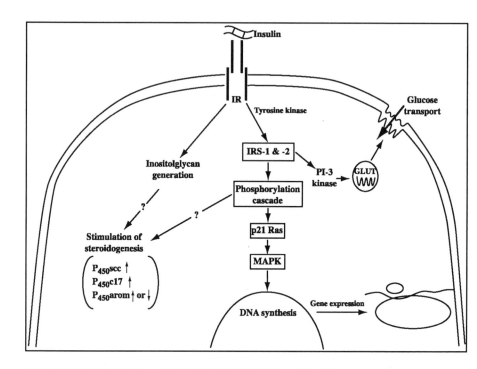

Fig. 2. Insulin receptor, its signaling pathways for glucose transport, and hypothetical mechanisms of stimulation or inhibition of steroidogenesis. The main pathways for the propagation of the insulin signal include the following events: after insulin binds to the insulin receptor α-subunits, the β-subunit tyrosine kinase is activated; IRS-1 and -2 are phosphorylated; PI-3 kinase is activated; GLUT glucose transporters are translocated to the cell membrane, and glucose uptake is stimulated. An alternative signaling system may involve generation of inositolglycans at the cell membrane after insulin binding to its receptor. This inositolglycan signaling system may mediate insulin modulation of steroidogenic enzymes. (Adapted, with permission, from L. Poretsky et al. The insulin-related ovarian regulatory system in health and disease. *Endocrine Reviews* 20(4): 535-582, 1999. ©The Endocrine Society)

Effects on steroidogenesis. In vitro, insulin acts on the granulosa and thecal cells to increase production of androgens, estrogens and progesterone. This action is likely mediated by the interaction of insulin with its receptors. Several in vitro studies, however, have demonstrated that supraphysiologic concentrations of insulin are needed to achieve this steroidogenic effect on the ovary, suggesting that, under some circumstances, insulin action may be mediated via the type 1 IGF receptor.[16,29]

Studies that attempted to determine whether insulin stimulates or inhibits aromatase or 17-α-hydroxylase have resulted in contradictory conclusions. For example, Nestler et al reported that 17-α-hydroxylase activity appears to be stimulated by insulin,[40] but Sahin et al in a later study

Table 2. Insulin effects related to ovarian function:

Effect	Organ
Directly stimulates steroidogenesis	Ovary
Acts synergistically with LH and FSH to stimulate steroidogenesis	Ovary
Stimulates 17 α-hydroxylase	Ovary
Stimulates or inhibits aromatase	Ovary, adipose Tissue
Up-regulates LH receptors	Ovary
Promotes ovarian growth and cyst formation synergistically with LH/hCG	Ovary
Down-regulates insulin receptors	Ovary
Up-regulates type I IGF receptors or hybrid insulin/type I IGF receptors	Ovary
Inhibits IGFBP-I production	Ovary, liver
Potentiates the effect of GnRH on LH and FSH	Pituitary
Inhibits SHBG production	Liver

Adapted, with permission, from L. Poretsky et al. The insulin-related ovarian regulatory system in health and disease. *Endocrine Reviews* 20(4): 535-582, 1999. ©The Endocrine Society

found no relation between insulin levels and 17-hydroxyprogesterone (17-OHP) after treatment with GnRH agonist.[41] One study showed that, after gonadotropin infusion, hyperinsulinemic women with PCOS had an increased estradiol/ androstenedione ratio compared with women with PCOS and normal insulin levels,[36] thus suggesting insulin's stimulatory effect on aromatase. However, in other studies increased circulating levels of androstenedione were found during insulin infusions, suggesting that insulin inhibits aromatase.[43, 44]

Ovarian androgen production in response to insulin has also been extensively studied *in-vivo* both directly, in the course of insulin infusions, and indirectly, after a reduction of insulin levels by insulin sensitizers or other agents, such as diazoxide. While insulin infusion studies did not produce consistent evidence of increased androgen production, reduction of insulin levels has consistently resulted in decreased androgen levels.[11]

Synergism with LH and FSH on the stimulation of steroidogenesis. At the ovarian level, insulin has been demonstrated to potentiate the steroidogenic response to gonadotropins.[16,39] This effect is possibly caused by an increase in the number of LH receptors that occurs under the influence of hyperinsulinemia.[16,45]

Enhancement of pituitary responsiveness to GnRH. Another area of uncertainty is whether insulin enhances the sensitivity of gonadotropes to GnRH in the pituitary. Several investigators have demonstrated increased responsiveness of gonadotropes to GnRH in the presence of insulin in cultured pituitary cells.[46,47] Nestler showed decreased circulating levels of LH in patients treated with insulin sensitizers.[48] But in another study, gonadotropin responsiveness to GnRH did not change after insulin infusion.[49] Similarly, in rats with experimentally produced hyperinsulinemia, response of gonadotropins to GnRH does not appear to be altered.[37]

The effect on SHBG. Insulin has been shown to suppress hepatic production of sex hormone-binding globulin (SHBG).[50,51,52,53] Lower levels of SHBG result in increased serum levels of unbound steroid hormones, such as free testosterone. In PCOS and other hyperinsulinemic insulin-resistant states, insulin may increase circulating levels of free testosterone by inhibiting SHBG production. When insulin sensitizers are used, SHBG levels rise, thereby decreasing free steroid hormone levels.[48]

The effect on IGFBP-1. Insulin has been found to regulate insulin-like growth factor-binding protein-1 (IGFBP-1) levels. In both liver and ovarian granulosa cells, insulin inhibits IGFBP-1 production.[28,54,55] Lower circulating and intraovarian IGFBP-1 concentrations result in higher circulating and intraovarian levels of free IGFs that may contribute to increased ovarian and adrenal steroid secretion.[11, 56]

Type 1 IGF receptor. Insulin increases ovarian IGF-I binding in rats, suggesting an increase in the expression of ovarian type 1 IGF receptors or hybrid insulin/type 1 IGF-receptors.[37] In these studies, ovarian type 1 IGF receptors are up-regulated even though insulin receptors are either down-regulated or preserved. Studies in women with PCOS appear to confirm this phenomenon.[38,57]

Ovarian growth and cyst formation. It has been shown that insulin enhances theca-interstitial cell proliferation in both human and rat ovaries.[58,59,60, 61,62] In a report of a patient with the type B syndrome of insulin resistance, infusion of insulin resulted in a significant increase of ovarian volume with sonogram demonstrating that the ovaries doubled in size.[63] Experimental hyperinsulinemia in synergism with hCG produces significant increase in ovarian size and development of polycystic ovaries in rats (Figure 3).

In summary, in a number of in-vitro animal and human ovarian cell systems and *in-vivo* experiments in animals and in women a variety of insulin effects related to ovarian function have been demonstrated. These effects can account for many features of PCOS in hyperinsulinemic insulin resistant women.[11] Insulin effects related to ovarian function are summarized in Table 2.

1 cm

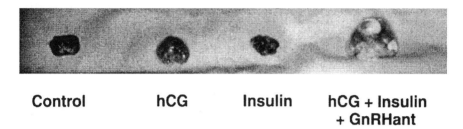

Control	hCG	Insulin	hCG + Insulin
			+ GnRHant

Fig. 3. The effects of 23 days of daily injections of normal saline (control), hCG, insulin, or insulin plus hCG and GnRHant on gross ovarian morphology in rats. Female Sprague-Dawley rats were randomized into the following treatment groups: vehicle; high-fat diet (to control for the effects of weight gain); insulin; hCG; GnRH antagonist (to control for possible central effects of insulin *vs.* direct effects on the ovary); GnRHant and hCG; insulin and GnRHant; insulin and hCG; insulin, hCG, and GnRHant. Ovarian morphology in the group treated with insulin and hCG (not shown) did not differ from that seen in the group treated with insulin, hCG, and GnRHant (shown above). [Reproduced with permission from L. Poretsky et al.: Metabolism 41:903-910, 1992 (20). ©W.B. Saunders Co.]

RISK OF DIABETES MELLITUS; PREVENTION OF DIABETES

A major risk factor for the development of type 2 diabetes mellitus in PCOS is insulin resistance. However, a defect in pancreatic β-cell function resulting in deficient insulin secretion has also been reported in PCOS patients.[64]

The prevalence and predictors of risk for type 2 diabetes mellitus have been studied in PCOS women. In prospective studies of glucose tolerance in women with hyperandrogenism and chronic anovulation, the prevalence of undiagnosed diabetes mellitus was 7.5% and that of impaired glucose tolerance (IGT) was 31.1%. Further analysis of the non-obese subgroup demonstrated that the risk for diabetes decreased to 1.5% and for IGT to 10.3%. However, these rates were still significantly increased compared to a population-based study of women in the U.S. in whom the prevalence rate of undiagnosed diabetes mellitus was 1.0% and that of IGT was 7.8%.[65]

A study of women with previous history of gestational diabetes revealed a greater prevalence of polycystic ovaries (PCO) compared to controls (39.4% versus 16.7%), higher serum levels of adrenal androgens and significantly impaired glucose tolerance. Oral glucose tolerance testing in these women uncovered a decreased early phase insulin response while euglycemic clamp studies demonstrated impaired insulin sensitivity. The investigators theorized that a dual component of insulin resistance plus impaired pancreatic insulin secretion could explain the vulnerability of PCOS patients to diabetes.[66]

PCOS, and not PCO (in which the polycystic ovarian morphology is not associated with anovulation), has been found to be a substantially more significant risk factor for diabetes mellitus than race or ethnicity.[65] Factoring in obesity, age, family history of diabetes and waist/hip ratios, the prevalence of glucose intolerance increases. This suggests that the pathogenesis of diabetes mellitus in PCOS is a result of underlying genetic defects, resulting in insulin resistance and pancreatic β- cell dysfunction, and an interplay of various environmental factors.

Primary prevention of type 2 diabetes mellitus was the focus of the Diabetes Prevention Program (DPP). The DPP, a National Institutes of Health-sponsored clinical study, targeted preventive measures at specific individuals or groups at high risk for the future development of type 2 diabetes (See Section X). The study interventions included intensive lifestyle modification or pharmacological intervention versus placebo. The primary outcome was the development of diabetes mellitus in these high-risk groups. The results of this study showed that both lifestyle modification and treatment with metformin prevented or delayed the onset of type 2 diabetes in individuals with impaired glucose tolerance (IGT).[67,68] Thus, specific interventions may be implemented at an early enough time period to prevent the development of diabetes mellitus and its accompanying complications in high-risk individuals. PCOS, with its dual defect of insulin resistance and β-cell dysfunction, is a significant risk factor for diabetes mellitus. When effective protocols for prevention of diabetes mellitus are established, PCOS patients may become one target group for such measures.

ROLE OF INSULIN SENSITIZERS

There are numerous treatment modalities for signs and symptoms of PCOS. However, traditional approaches, although often successful, do not address insulin resistance.

Hyperandrogenism and its consequences, such as hirsutism and acne, have many treatment modalities. Hirsutism can be treated with depilatories, shaving, waxing, electrolysis, or laser therapy. Oral contraceptives can be used to decrease androgen levels, and anti-androgen medications, such as spironolactone[69] or cyproterone acetate,[70] may be used as well to reduce manifestations of hyperandrogenism.

Oral contraceptive pills may also be used to treat menstrual irregularities. This treatment leads to a reduction in LH and an increase in SHBG. The increased SHBG binds the excess androgens, thereby decreasing the amount of free circulating androgens.[71] Progestins may be used to regulate the menstrual cycle, however they do not affect the hair growth or metabolic abnormalities.

Weight loss, when successful, is a very effective measure which addresses insulin related abnormalities of PCOS by decreasing insulin resistance and circulating insulin levels. One report studied 18 obese women who were hyperandrogenic and insulin-resistant. A weight reduction diet resulted in a decrease in plasma androstenedione and testosterone levels.[72] Pasquali et al found decreased concentrations of LH, fasting insulin and testosterone levels after weight loss in 20 obese women with hyperandrogenism and oligo-ovulation.[73] In another study, 67 obese anovulatory women were treated with weight reduction. 60 of these women ovulated and 18 became pregnant.[74]

When weight loss is not achieved, insulin resistance can be reduced with the help of insulin sensitizers, such as biguanides, thiazolidinediones, and d-chiroinositol. The goal of these approaches is to decrease the amount of circulating insulin, thereby decreasing insulin's stimulatory effect on androgen production and gonadotropin secretion. Circulating levels of SHBG and IGFBP-1 are increased, leading to clinical improvement via mechanisms described above.[75]

Metformin (Glucophage®) decreases hepatic gluconeogenesis and increases fat and muscle sensitivity to insulin. There are many reports showing meformin's efficacy in PCOS, however most of the studies have been short-term only. One long-term study followed women with PCOS treated with metformin (500 mg p.o. tid) for 6-26 months. These women not only had a reduction in insulin and androgen levels, independent of any change in weight, but also a sustained increase in menstrual regularity.[76]

Nestler and co-workers showed that when insulin secretion is decreased by metformin administration either alone or in combination with clomiphene in obese women with PCOS, the ovulatory response is increased.[77] In analysis of 14 studies of metformin treatment of PCOS, 57% of women had ovulatory improvement with metformin.[78] The improvement in ovulation may have been only due to weight loss. However, lean women with PCOS, who had increased P450c17 alpha activity and whose circulating insulin levels were reduced while on metformin, experienced a decline in P450c17-alpha activity and improvement in hyperandrogenism.[40] In another study, women with PCOS who were given metformin demonstrated decreased circulating levels of LH, free testosterone, and a decreased LH/FSH ratio, as well as a reduced body mass index (BMI).[79]

In one study of women with PCOS given metformin, improved endometrial function and intrauterine environment were found. This observation suggests that metformin can be used to improve implantation and pregnancy maintenance in women with PCOS.[80]

A thiazolidinedione (TZD) Troglitazone (Rezulin®) was shown to improve insulin action in patients with PCOS.[81] Studies with troglitazone in patients with PCOS showed improvements in ovulation, insulin resistance, hyperandrogenemia and hirsutism.[82] However, troglitazone was taken off the market because of hepatotoxicity. Additional studies with other TZDs (rosiglitazone and pioglitazone) are needed to determine their efficacy in PCOS.

One of insulin's actions in the metabolism of glucose involves activation of inositol phosphoglycan mediators. It has been hypothesized that insulin resistance and hyperinsulinemia may occur when there is a deficiency of these mediators. In one study, obese women with PCOS were given either D-chiroinositol or placebo. Patients in the treatment group demonstrated improved insulin sensitivity, reduced circulating triglyceride levels and blood pressure, and an improved ovulatory rate compared with patients given placebo. Declines in circulating levels of free and total testosterone and DHEAS were also observed, but these changes were not significantly different from the control group. D-chiroinositol treatment also decreased serum levels of 17α-hydroxyprogesterone (a marker of ovarian androgen production) in response to leuprolide (a GnRH analog).[83]

Patients and physicians should be aware that at this time insulin sensitizers are not approved by the Food and Drug Administration for use in PCOS. Women with PCOS who think that they are infertile and therefore do not use contraception may become pregnant while on these medications. Thus it is important to discuss contraception before prescribing these drugs. Further studies are needed before insulin sensitizers are widely used in patients with PCOS.

CONCLUSIONS

PCOS is a compilation of multiple endocrine and metabolic abnormalities. The main features of PCOS include chronic anovulation, hyperandrogenemia, and polycystic ovaries. Many patients have insulin resistance and hyperinsulinemia of unknown etiology, although often related to obesity. Besides the hirsutism, acne, and infertility, these women are at an increased risk for diabetes.

New therapeutic strategies addressing insulin resistance in PCOS are rapidly developing. As research elucidates specific ovarian effects of insulin and specific pathways of insulin signaling in the ovary, new targets will be identified for emerging therapies.

REFERENCES

1. Knochenhauer ES, Key TJ, Kahsar-Miller M, Waggoner W, Boots LR, Azziz R. Prevalence of the polycystic ovarian syndrome in unselected black and white women of the Southeastern United States: a prospective study. J Clin Endocrinol Metab 83:3078-3082, 1998.
2. Zawadzki JK, Dunaif A. Diagnostic criteria for polycystic ovary syndrome: towards a rational approach. In: Dunaif A ed. Polycystic Ovary Syndrome. Boston: Blackwell Scientific, 337-384, 1995.
3. Speroff L, Glass RH, Kase NG, eds. Anovulation and the polycystic ovary. In: Clinical gynecologic endocrinology and infertility, 6th ed. Baltimore: Lippincott Williams & Wilkins; 487-522, 1999.

4. Kovacs GT, ed. Polycystic ovary syndrome. Cambridge University Press, Cambridge, UK, 2000.

5. Dunaif A. Hyperandrogenic anovulation (PCOS): a unique disorder of insulin action associated with an increased risk of non-insulin-dependent diabetes mellitus. Am J Med [Suppl] 98:33S-39S, 1995.

6. Chereau, A. Mémoires pour servir a l'étude des maladies des ovaries. Paris: Fortin, Masson and Cie, 1844.

7. Stein IF, Leventhal ML. Amenorrhea associated with bilateral polycystic ovaries. Am J Obstet Gynecol 29:181-186, 1935.

8. Culiner A, Shippel S. Virilism and thecal cell hyperplasia of the ovary syndrome. J Obstet Gynaecol Br Comm 56:439-445, 1949.

9. McArthur JW, Ingersoll FW, Worcester J. The urinary excretion of interstitial-cell and follicle-stimulating hormone activity by women with diseases of the reproductive system. J Clin Endocrinol Metab 18:1202-1215, 1958.

10. De Vane GW, Czekala NM, Judd HL, Yen SS. Circulating gonadotropins, estrogens, and androgens in polycystic ovarian disease. Am J Obstet Gynecol 121:496-500, 1975.

11. Poretsky L, Cataldo N, Rosenwaks Z, Giudice L. The insulin-related ovarian regulatory system in health and disease. Endocr Rev 20:535-582, 1999.

12. Zumoff B, Freeman R, Coupey S, Saenger P, Markowitz M, Kream J. A chronobiologic abnormality in luteinizing hormone secretion in teenage girls with the polycystic-ovary syndrome. N Engl J Med 309:1206-1209, 1983.

13. McLachlan RI, Healy DL, Burger HG. The ovary. In: Felig P, Baxter JD, Broadus AE, Frohman LA, eds. Endocrinology and Metabolism. 2nd ed. New York: McGraw-Hill Book Company; 951-983, 1987.

14. Pang S, Softness B, Sweeney WJ, New MI. Hirsutism, polycystic ovarian disease, and ovarian 17-ketosteroid reductase deficiency. N Engl J Med 316:1295-1301, 1987.

15. Nelson VL, Qin K-N, Rosenfeld RL, Wood JR, Penning TM, Legro RS, Srauss JF III, McAllister JM. The biochemical basis for increased testosterone production in theca cells propagated from patients with polycystic ovary syndrome. J Clin Endocrinol Metab 86:5925-5933, 2001.

16. Poretsky L and Kalin M. The gonadotropic function of insulin. Endocr Rev 8:132-141, 1987.

17. Archard C, Thiers J. Le virilisme pilaire et son association a l'insuffisance glycolytique (diabete des femmes a barbe). Bull Acad Nat Med 86:51, 1921.

18. Kahn CR, Flier JS, Bar RS, Archer JA, Gorden R, Martin MM, Roth J. The syndromes of insulin resistance and acanthosis nigricans: insulin-receptor disorders in man. N Engl J Med 294:739-745, 1976.

19. Flier JS, Kahn CR, Roth J, Bar RS. Antibodies that impair insulin receptor binding in an unusual diabetic syndrome with severe insulin resistance. Science 190:63-65, 1975.
20. Taylor SI, Moller DE. Mutations of the insulin receptor gene. In: Moller DE ed. Insulin Resistance. New York: John Wiley & Sons; 83-121, 1993.
21. Dunaif A. Insulin resistance and the polycystic ovary syndrome: mechanism and implications for pathogenesis. Endocr Rev 18:774-800, 1997.
22. Dunaif A, Book CB, Schenker E, Tang Z. Excessive insulin receptor serine phosphorylation in cultured fibroblasts and in skeletal muscle: a potential mechanism for insulin resistance in the polycystic ovary syndrome. J Clin Invest 96:801-810, 1995.
23. Poretsky L, Smith D, Seibel M, Pazianos A, Moses AC, Flier JS. Specific insulin binding sites in the human ovary. J Clin Endocrinol Metab 59:809-811, 1984.
24. Poretsky L, Grigorescu F, Seibel M, Moses AC, Flier JS. Distribution and characterization of the insulin and IGF-I receptors in the normal human ovary. J Clin Endocrinol Metab 61:728-734, 1985.
25. El-Roeiy A, Chen X, Roberts VJ, Shimasaki S, Ling N, LeRoith D, Roberts Jr CT, Yen SS. Expression of the genes encoding the insulin-like growth factors (IGF-I and II), the IGF and insulin receptors, and IGF-binding proteins 1-6 and the localization of their gene products in normal and polycystic ovary syndrome ovaries. J Clin Endocrinol Metab 78:1488-1496, 1994.
26. Barbieri RL, Makris A, Ryan KJ. Effects of insulin on steroidogenesis in cultured porcine ovarian theca. Fertil Steril 40:237-241, 1983.
27. Poretsky L, Clemons J, Bogovich K. Hyperinsulinemia and human chorionic gonadotropin synergistically promote the growth of ovarian follicular cysts in rats. Metabolism 41:903-910, 1992.
28. Poretsky L, Chandrasekher YA, Bai C, Liu HC, Rosenwaks Z, Giudice L. Insulin receptor mediates inhibitory effect of insulin, but not of insulin-like growth factor (IGF)-1, on binding protein 1 (IGFBP-1) production in human granulosa cells. J Clin Endocrinol Metab 81:493-496, 1996.
29. Poretsky L. On the paradox of insulin-induced hyperandrogenism in insulin-resistant states. Endocr Rev 12:3-13, 1991.
30. Joslin EP, Root HF, White P. The growth, development and prognosis of diabetic children. JAMA 85:420-422, 1925.
31. Zumoff B, Miller L, Poretsky L, Levitt C, Miller E, Heinz U, Denman H, Jandorek R, Rosenfeld R. Subnormal follicular-phase serum progesterone levels and elevated follicular-phase serum estradiol levels in young women with insulin-dependent diabetes. Steroids 55:560-564, 1990.

32. Poretsky L, Bhargava G, Kalin MF, Wolf SA. Regulation of insulin receptors in the human ovary: *in vitro* studies. J Clin Endocrinol Metab 67:774-778, 1988.

33. Poretsky L, Bhargava G, Saketos M, Dunaif A. Regulation of human ovarian insulin receptors in vivo. Metabolism 39:161-166, 1990.

34. Saltiel AR. Second messengers of insulin action. Diabetes Care 13:244-256, 1990.

35. Nestler JE, Jakubowicz DJ, De Vargas AF, Brik C, Quintero N, Medina F. Insulin stimulates testosterone biosynthesis by human thecal cells from women with polycystic ovarian syndrome by activating its own receptor and using inositolglycan mediators as the signal transduction system. J Clin Endocrinol Metab 83:2001-2005, 1998.

36. Poretsky L, Seto-Young D, Shrestha A, Dhillon S, Mirjany M, Liu H-C, Yih MC, Rosenwaks Z. Phosphatidyl-inositol-3 kinase-independent insulin action pathway(s) in the human ovary. J Clin Endocrinol Metab 86:3115-3119, 2001.

37. Poretsky L, Glover B, Laumas V, Kalin M, Dunaif A. The effects of experimental hyperinsulinemia on steroid secretion, ovarian [^{125}I] insulin binding, and ovarian [^{125}I] insulin-like growth factor I binding in the rat. Endocrinology 122:581-585, 1988.

38. Samoto T, Maruo T, Matsuo H, Katayama K, Barnea ER Mochizuki M. Altered expression of insulin and insulin-like growth factor-I receptors in follicular and stromal compartments of polycystic ovarian ovaries. Endocr 40:413-424, 1993.

39. Willis D, Mason H, Gilling-Smith C, Franks S. Modulation by insulin of follicle-stimulating hormone and luteinizing hormone actions in human granulosa cells of normal and polycystic ovaries. J Clin Endocrinol Metab 81:302-309, 1996.

40. Nestler JE, Jakubowicz DJ. Decreases in ovarian cytochrome P450c17 alpha activity and serum free testosterone after reduction of insulin secretion in polycystic ovary syndrome. N Engl J Med 335:617-23, 1996

41. Sahin Y, Ayata D, Kelestimur F. Lack of relationship between 17-hydroxyprogesterone response to buserelin testing and hyperinsulinemia in polycystic ovary syndrome. Eur J Endocrinol 136:410-415, 1997.

42. Fulghesu AM, Villa P, Pavone V, Guido M, Apa R, Caruso A, Lanzone A, Rossodivita A, Mancuso S. The impact of insulin secretion on the ovarian response to exogenous gonadotropins in polycystic ovarian syndrome. J Clin Endocrinol Metab 82:644-648, 1997.

43. Stuart CA, Nagamani M. Acute augmentation of plasma androstenedione and dehydroepiandrosterone by euglycemic insulin infusion: evidence for a direct effect of insulin on ovarian steroidogenesis. In: Dunaif A, Givens JR, Haseltine FP, Merriam GR eds. Polycystic Ovary Syndrome. Boston: Blackwell Scientific Publications; 279-288, 1992.

44. Stuart CA, Prince MJ, Peters EJ, Meyer WJ. Hyperinsulinemia and hyperandrogenemia: in vivo androgen response to insulin infusion. Obstet Gynecol 69:921-925, 1987.

45. Poretsky L, Piper B. Insulin resistance, hypersecretion of LH, and a dual-defect hypothesis for the pathogenesis of polycystic ovary syndrome. Obstet Gynecol 84:613-621, 1994.

46. Adashi EY, Hsueh AJW, Yen SSC. Insulin enhancement of luteinizing hormone and follicle-stimulating hormone release by cultured pituitary cells. Endocrinology 108:1441-1449, 1981.

47. Soldani R, Cagnacci A, Yen SS. Insulin, insulin-like growth factor I (IGF I) and IGF-II enhance basal and gonadotropin-releasing hormone-stimulated luteinizing hormone release from rat anterior pituitary cells *in vitro*. Eur J Endocrinol 131:641-645, 1994.

48. Nestler JE, Jakubowicz DJ. Lean women with polycystic ovary syndrome respond to insulin reduction with decreases in ovarian P450c17 alpha activity and serum androgens. J Clin Endocrinol Metab 82:4075-9, 1997.

49. Dunaif A, Graf M. Insulin administration alters gonadal steroid metabolism independent of changes in gonadotropin secretion in insulin-resistant women with polycystic ovary syndrome. J Clin Invest 83:23-29, 1989.

50. Plymate SR, Matej LA, Jones RE, Friedl KE. Inhibition of sex hormone-binding globulin production in the human hepatoma (HepG2) cell line by insulin and prolactin. J Clin Endocrinol Metab 67:460-464, 1988.

51. Peiris AN, Stagner JL, Plymate SR, Vogel RL, Heck M, Samols E. Relationship of insulin secretory pulses to sex hormone-binding globulin production in normal men. J Clin Endocrinol Metab 76:279-282, 1993.

52. Fendri S, Arlot S, Marcelli JM, Dubreuil A, Lalau JD. Relationship between insulin sensitivity and circulating sex hormone-binding globulin levels in hyperandrogenic obese women. Int J Obes Relat Metab Disord 18:755-759, 1994.

53. Nestler JE, Powers LP, Matt DW, Steingold KA, Plymate SR, Rittmaster RS, Clore JN, Blackard WG. A direct effect of hyperinsulinemia on serum sex hormone-binding globulin levels in obese women with the polycystic ovary syndrome. J Clin Endocrinol Metab 72:83-89, 1991.

54. Pao CI, Farmer PK, Begovic S, Villafuerte BC, Wu G, Robertson DG, Phillips LS. Regulation of insulin-like growth factor-I (IGF I) and IGF-binding protein I gene transcription by hormones and provision of amino acids in rat hepatocytes. Mol Endocrinol 7:1561-1568, 1993.

55. Lee PD, Giudice LC, Conover CA, Powell DR. Insulin-like growth factor binding protein-1: recent findings and new directions. Proc Soc Exp Biol Med 216:319-357, 1997.

56. Giudice LC. Insulin-like growth factors and ovarian follicular development. Endocr Rev 13:641-669, 1992.

57. Nagami M, Stuart CA. Specific binding sites for insulin-like growth factor I in the ovarian stroma of women with polycystic ovarian disease and stromal hyperthecosis. Am J Obstet Gynecol 163:1992-1997, 1990.

58. Duleba AJ, Spaczynski RZ, Olive DL, Behrman HR. Effects of insulin and insulin-like growth factors on proliferation of rat ovarian theca-interstitial cells. Biol Reprod 56:891-897, 1997.

59. Duleba AJ, Spaczynski RZ, Olive DL. Insulin and insulin-like growth factor I stimulate the proliferation of human ovarian theca-interstitial cells. Fertil Steril 69:335-340, 1998.

60. Watson H, Willis D, Mason H, Modgil G, Wright C, Franks S. The effects of ovarian steroids, epidermal growth factor (EGF), insulin (I), and insulin-like growth factor-1 (IGF-I), on ovarian stromal cell growth. Program of the 79th Annual Meeting of the Endocrine Society, Minneapolis, MN, (Abstract 389), 1997.

61. Bogovich K, Clemons J, Poretsky L. Insulin has a biphasic effects on the ability of human chorionic gonadotropin to induce ovarian cysts in the rat. Metabolism 48:995-1002, 1999.

62. Damario M, Bogovich K, Liu HC, Rosenwaks Z, Poretsky L. Synergistic effects of IGF-I and human chorionic gonadotropin in the rat ovary. Metabolism 49:314-320, 2000.

63. De ClueTJ, Shah SC, Marchese M, Malone JI. Insulin resistance and hyperinsulinemia induce hyperandrogenism in a young type B insulin-resistant female. J Clin Endocrinol Metab 72:1308-1311, 1991.

64. Dunaif A, Finegood DT. Beta-cell dysfunction independent of obesity and glucose intolerance in the polycystic ovary syndrome. J Clin Endocrinol Metab 81:942-947, 1996.

65. Legro R, Kunselman A, Dodson W, Dunaif A. Prevalence and predictors of risk for type 2 diabetes mellitus and impaired glucose tolerance in polycystic ovary syndrome: a perspective, controlled study in 254 affected women. J Clin Endocrinol Metab 84:165-169, 1999.

66. Koivunen RM et al. Metabolic and steroidogenic alterations related to increased frequency of polycystic ovaries in women with a history of gestational diabetes. J Clin Endocrinol Metab 86: 2591-2599, 2001.

67. The Diabetes Prevention Program Research Group. The Diabetes Prevention Program: baseline characteristics of the randomized cohort. Diabetes Care 23(11):1619-1629, 2000.

68. Fujimoto W. Background and recruitment data for the U.S. Diabetes Prevention Program. Diabetes Care 23:B11-B13, 2000.

69. Board JA, Rosenberg SM, Smeltzer JS. Spironolactone and estrogen-progestin therapy for hirsuitism. South Med J 80:483-486, 1987.

70. Falsetti L. Gamera A, Tisi G. Efficacy of the combination ethinyl oestradiol and cyproterone acetate on endocrine, clinical and ultrasonographic profile in polycystic ovarian syndrome. Human Reproduction 16:36-42, 2001.

71. Dewis P, Petsos P, Newman M, Anderson DC. The treatment of hirsuitism with a combination of desogestrel and ethinyl oestradiol. Clin Endocrinol 22:29-36, 1985.

72. Bates GW, Whitworth NS. Effect of body weight reduction on plasma androgens in obese infertile women. Fertil Steril 38:406-409, 1982.

73. Pasquali R, Antenucci D, Casimirri F, Venturoli S, Paradisi R, Fabbri R, et al. Clinical and hormonal characteristics of obese and amenorrheic women before and after weight loss. J Clin Endocrinol Metab 68:173-9, 1989.

74. Clark AM, Thornley B, Tomlinson L, Galletley C, Norman RJ. Weight loss in obese infertile women results in improvement in reproductive outcome for all forms of fertility treatment. Hum Reprod 13:1502-5, 1998.

75. Crave JC, Fimbel S, Lejeune H, Cugnardey N, DeChaud H, Pugeat M. Effects of diet and metformin administration on sex hormone-binding globuliln, androgens, and insulin in hirsute and obese women. J Clin Endocrinol Metab 80:2057-2062, 1995.

76. Moghetti P. Castello R. Negri C. Tosi F. Perrone F. Caputo M. Zanolin E. Muggeo M. Metformin effects on clinical features, endocrine and metabolic profiles, and insulin sensitivity in polycystic ovary syndrome: a randomized, double-blind, placebo-controlled 6-month trial, followed by open, long-term clinical evaluation. J Clin Endocrinol Metab 85:139-46, 2000.

77. Nestler JE, Jakubowicz DJ, Evans WS, Pasquali R. Effects of metformin on spontaneous and clomiphene-induced ovulation in the polycystic ovary syndrome. N Engl J Med 338:1876-1880, 1998.

78. Bloomgarden ZT, Futterwiet W, Poretsky L. The use of insulin-sensitizing agents in patients with polycystic ovary syndrome. Endocr Pract. 7:279-286, 2001.

79. Velazquez E. Acosta A, Mendoza SG. Menstrual cyclicity after metformin therapy in polycystic ovary syndrome. Obstetrics & Gynecology 90:392-395, 1997.

80. Jakubowicz DJ, Seppala M, Jakubowicz S, Rodriguez-Armas O, Rivas-Santiago A, Koistinen H, Koistinen R, Nestler JE. Insulin reduction with metformin increases luteal phase serum glycodelin and insulin-like growth factor-binding protein 1 concentrations and enhances uterine vascularity and blood flow in the polycystic ovary syndrome. J Clin Endocrinol Metab 86:1126-1133, 2001.

81. Dunaif A, Scott D, Finegood D, Quintana B, Whitcomb R. The insulin-sensitizing agent troglitazone improves metabolic and reproductive abnormalities in the polycystic ovary syndrome. J Clin Endocrinol Metab 81:3299-3306, 1996.

82. Azziz R, Ehrmann D, Legro RS, Whitcomb RW, Hanley R, Fereshetian AG, O'Keefe M, Ghazzi MN. Troglitazone improves ovulation and hirsutism in the polycystic ovary syndrome: A multicenter, double blind, placebo-controlled trial. J Clin Endocrinol Metab 86: 1626-1632, 2001.

83. Nestler JE, Jakubowicz DJ, Reamer P, Gunn RD, Allan G. Ovulatory and metabolic effects of D-chiro-inositol in the polycystic ovary syndrome. N Engl J Med 340:1314-1320, 1999.

Chapter 5. Insulin Resistance and the Metabolic Syndrome

Rochelle L. Chaiken

INTRODUCTION

Insulin resistance is defined as an impaired biological response to the actions of insulin.[1] It was classically described as resistance to insulin mediated glucose uptake in peripheral cells. However, as the metabolic and mitogenic processes of insulin action are better understood, abnormal insulin action in these pathways is being elucidated. Thus, impaired biological response to insulin may be associated with either endogenous or exogenous insulin and can be quantified by changes in several metabolic processes, including carbohydrate, lipid, or protein metabolism or by changes in mitogenic processes.[2]

Historically insulin resistance was first identified by Himsworth and Kerr in the 1930s. They observed that obese subjects with diabetes had insulin insensitivity and did not respond normally to exogenous insulin.[3] But it was not until the 1960s, with the development of the first insulin assay, that there could be greater understanding of the relationship between circulating insulin levels and the stimulation of various metabolic processes, in particular glucose metabolism.[4] It became clear that to maintain normal glucose tolerance in the presence of insulin resistance compensatory hyperinsulinemia had to develop.[5-6]

In the late 1980s Modan described an association between hyperinsulinemia and atherogenic lipid profiles, impaired glucose tolerance, obesity, and hypertension.[7-9] Reaven put forth the concept that insulin resistance may play a central role in the pathogenesis of a variety of disease states, including type 2 diabetes, hypertension and coronary artery disease, and described this constellation of clinical and laboratory findings as Syndrome X.[10] Syndrome X was defined as: 1) resistance to insulin-stimulated glucose uptake; 2) glucose intolerance; 3) hyperinsulinemia; 4) increased very-low-density lipoprotein triglyceride; 5) decreased high-density lipoprotein cholesterol; and 6) hypertension.

Since then there have been many studies elucidating the association of insulin resistance with other clinical and laboratory findings.[11-14] The term Syndrome X has been replaced with the *Insulin Resistance Syndrome* or, most recently, the *Metabolic Syndrome*. This chapter will review the pathogenetic factors of insulin resistance, the abnormalities in the metabolic syndrome, and its association with disease.

MEASUREMENTS OF INSULIN RESISTANCE

There are many ways to assess insulin sensitivity; and they have variable degrees of accuracy and ease of performance.

The euglycemic clamp technique developed by Andres and coworkers is considered the 'gold standard' for assessing insulin resistance.[15] Briefly, the euglycemic clamp is performed by infusing a constant amount of exogenous insulin to achieve a steady-state plasma insulin concentration. A fixed or "clamped" glucose level is then maintained by delivering a variable glucose infusion intravenously. The amount of glucose infused over time to maintain this fixed glucose level is called the M value, or Metabolic Rate. Subjects who are insulin sensitive will require a greater glucose infusion to maintain the fixed glucose level and therefore will have a higher M value than subjects with insulin resistance. Conversely insulin resistance is defined by a low M value. This technique has been adapted to assess many of insulin's actions not only on carbohydrate metabolism, but also on lipid and protein metabolism by using isotopes and variable insulin concentrations. The clamp technique is performed in research centers with trained staff. It is not easily adaptable to assessing insulin resistance in the general clinical setting.

The minimal model developed by Bergman and coworkers is a computer model which uses the glucose and insulin values from a frequently sampled intravenous glucose tolerance test (FSIVGTT) and generates a value, Si, which is a measure of insulin sensitivity.[16] The insulin results can also be used to assess beta cell function by determining the acute insulin release (AIR). In subjects with normal glucose tolerance this test correlates well with the euglycemic clamp for insulin resistance. Since subjects with diabetes have beta cell deficiency, the accuracy of insulin resistance estimates based on insulin values in these subjects is decreased. Usually techniques to increase the insulin response, such as administration of tolbutamide or exogenous insulin, are employed to improve accuracy of this mehod. This technique, though easier to perform than the euglycemic clamp, is still not easily adaptable to assessing insulin resistance in the clinical setting. Moreover, it can only evaluate insulin action on glucose metabolism and cannot assess insulin resistance at the level of the liver or adipose tissue.

Since the oral glucose tolerance test (OGTT) is the most commonly performed test to evaluate glucose tolerance in vivo, attempts have been made to determine if it can also be used to assess insulin sensitivity. Matsuda and DeFronzo developed an index of insulin sensitivity from the OGTT and correlated it to the euglycemic clamp.[17] The equation for insulin sensitivity using the fasting and mean glucose and insulin values during a standard 75 gram 2 hour OGTT is 10,000/square root of [fasting glucose X fasting insulin] X [mean glucose X mean insulin during OGTT].

The Homeostasis Model Assessment (HOMA), developed by Matthews and coworkers, uses computer-aided modeling of fasting glucose and insulin levels to assess insulin resistance.[18] The HOMA equation for insulin sensitivity is defined as fasting insulin multiplied by fasting glucose and divided by 22.5. It is often used in large studies.

The Quick Insulin Sensitivity Check Index (QUICKI) is another method of assessing insulin sensitivity which utilizes fasting insulin and glucose levels. Katz et al demonstrated that the correlation between the QUICKI estimate and the euglycemic clamp was better than the correlation between the clamp and the HOMA or fasting insulin in a combined group of obese, nonobese, and diabetic subjects.[19]

Fasting insulin levels in the presence of normal glucose tolerance have been used to determine degrees of insulin sensitivity.[20] High fasting insulin levels in subjects with normal glucose tolerance typically identify insulin resistance. In the presence of diabetes, however, a fasting insulin level is not reliable since it is confounded by the beta cell defect and insulin deficiency present in people with diabetes. Nevertheless, the fasting insulin levels has been used in several large epidemiological studies in people without diabetes as a way of assessing the relationship between hyperinsulinemia/insulin resistance and a variety of clinical outcomes.[21-23] A recent study suggested that by combining the fasting insulin and triglyceride levels one may further enhance the accuracy. This approach can be used to screen for insulin resistance in the general population.[24] A major drawback of the use of the insulin assay to detect insulin resistance in the clinical setting is the lack of standardization of the insulin assay. The American Diabetes Association (ADA) Task Force on Standardization of the Insulin assay had concluded that the assay is extremely variable between laboratories.[25] Thus, the ADA currently does not recommend screening for insulin resistance using a fasting insulin level.[1]

The euglycemic clamp, minimal model, and OGTT techniques are dynamic interventions, require significant time and effort, and are costly. In contrast the HOMA, QUICKI, and fasting insulin measurements are steady-state assessments of insulin sensitivity and are inexpensive, rapid, and adaptable to assessing insulin sensitivity in a large number of individuals.

PATHOGENESIS OF INSULIN RESISTANCE

Using both in vivo and in vitro techniques, insulin resistance has been identified at the level of the muscle, in which there is impaired insulin-stimulated-glucose uptake, at the level of the liver, in which there is impaired suppression of hepatic glucose production by insulin, and at the level of adipose tissue, in which insulin is ineffective in suppressing lipolysis. In the presence of normal glucose tolerance insulin resistance is associated with compensatory hyperinsulinemia.

Insulin resistance can be due to any one or a combination of the factors listed in Table 1. Though many laboratories have extensively studied this problem, the genetic factors causing insulin resistance are still unclear.[2] A variety of mutations in certain genes have been identified as the cause of insulin resistance in some of the rare and more severe syndromes of insulin resistance (see Chapter VI.6), but no gene has been identified that might be the cause of the majority cases of insulin resistance has been identified.[2]

Table 1. Factors contributing to insulin resistance

Genetic
Fat cell derived signals
    TNFα
    Resistin
    Leptin
Obesity
    Visceral Obesity
Inactivity
Endocrinologic disorders
    Cushing's syndrome
    Acromegaly
    Polycystic ovarian disease
Medications
Hyperglycemia

Numerous studies have a demonstrated a relationship between obesity and insulin resistance.[26-30] Many studies have also shown that weight reduction improves insulin sensitivity.[26-28,30] As early as in the 1950s it was observed that body fat distribution, not just obesity, was important in understanding the diseases associated with obesity.[31] In recent years a number of techniques to assess body composition and adipose tissue distribution have become available. Although waist circumference and waist to hip or waist to thigh ratios are used in large studies to assess visceral adiposity, the most accurate measurements are made using computerized tomography (CT) and magnetic resonance imaging (MRI) often together with dual-energy x-ray absorptiometry scanning.[32-35] These techniques have enabled an examination of the relationship between visceral adiposity and insulin resistance. This relationship may be present independent of the presence of obesity (BMI $\geq$ 30 kg/m^2) and may help explain why individuals who are seemingly of normal weight as assessed by BMI are insulin resistant and may even have the Metabolic Syndrome. In one study of a group of subjects who underwent significant weight loss, improvement in insulin sensitivity correlated with reduction in visceral fat.[36] In studies of African Americans with type 2 diabetes, insulin-sensitive and insulin-resistant variants have been characterized.[37] The insulin-resistant variant had more visceral adiposity and a lipid profile characteristic of the metabolic syndrome as compared to the insulin-sensitive variant.[38-39] Moreover, in subjects with a BMI between 24.5 and 28.5 kg/m,[2] the frequency distribution on insulin action was bimodal with almost equal numbers having normal insulin action and insulin resistance (figure 1).[40]

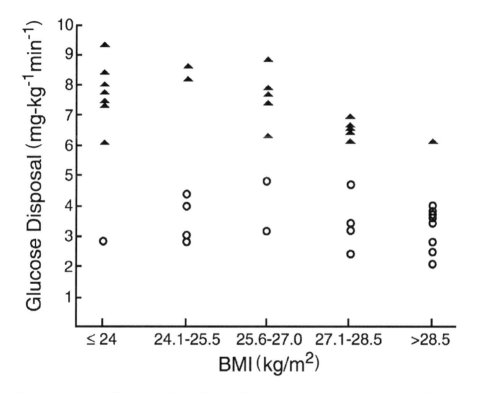

Figure 1. Distribution of insulin-mediated glucose disposal in relation to BMI during a 1mU/kg/min insulin infusion. (▲) and (○) represent insulin-sensitive and insulin-resistant subjects respectively. (From Banerji MA, Lebovitz HL. Insulin action in black Americans with NIDDM. Diabetes Care 15:1295, 1992, with permission.)

In longitudinal studies of Japanese American men, accumulation of visceral adiposity predicts the development of insulin resistance and subsequent diabetes.[41-42] In a small study of 43 mildly obese postmenopausal women, those women who were metabolically normal (that is with normal insulin sensitivity) had less visceral adiposity than the women who were metabolically abnormal (with insulin resistance) despite the fact that the total adiposity was the same for both groups of women.[43] In contrast, studies in Pima Indians, who have the highest reported prevalence of type 2 diabetes in the world, the relationship between insulin resistance and visceral adiposity is less clear.[44] Pima Indians with similar amounts of visceral and subcutaneous adipose tissue as age, gender, and BMI-matched Caucasians were significantly more insulin resistant and secreted more insulin for the same glucose tolerance. Moreover, there was no correlation between the degree of insulin resistance and the amount of visceral fat in the Pima Indians, though this correlation did exist for the Caucasian group.[45]

A number of studies have suggested that free fatty acids, which are elevated in obesity, may play a role in the pathogenesis of insulin resistance by inhibiting insulin—stimulated glucose uptake and increasing hepatic gluconeogenesis.[46-47]

In rat studies tumor necrosis factor alpha (TNFα) has been implicated in contributing to insulin resistance. These findings however have not been corroborated in human studies as of yet.[2] Leptin, the adipocyte-derived hormone identified in 1994, correlates with body fat mass, but its role in causing insulin resistance in humans has not been elucidated.[48] Recently a novel adipocyte-derived protein named resistin has been identified in mice. This protein seems to be increased in genetic and diet-induced obesity. Resistin gene expression is downregulated with the treatment of the thiazolidinedione, rosiglitazone.[49] The role of resistin in insulin resistance in humans has not been elucidated.

Inactivity or lack of physical exercise has been associated with insulin resistance and both acute and chronic physical training have been shown to dramatically improve insulin sensitivity (see chapter VII.4).[50]

INSULIN RESISTANCE AND CLINICAL DISEASE

Insulin resistance is associated with a number of clinical entities. Many studies in many populations have shown that insulin resistance is a powerful predictor of the risk for the development of type 2 diabetes.[51-54] When the beta cell is unable to maintain the compensatory hyperinsulinemia required to maintain normal glucose tolerance, hyperglycemia develops.[55] A number of studies have also shown a relationship between hypertension and insulin resistance in some ethnic groups. Though studies in Caucasians show a relationship, there does not seem to be one in Pima Indians.[56-57] In studies of African Americans who have high rates of hypertension the data are less clear, with some studies showing a relationship and others showing none.[58-59]

Women with polycystic ovary syndrome (PCOS), one of the more common endocrine disorders in women, have been reported to have elevated fasting and post glucose load insulin levels as compared to weight-matched women without PCOS.[60] Moreover women with PCOS are at greater risk for glucose intolerance and elevated LDL.[61-62] Treatment strategies aimed at reducing insulin resistance have been successful in treating this syndrome (see chapter IX.4).[62]

Several endocrinological disorders have also been associated with insulin resistance. These include, among others, hypercortisolism (endogenous or exogenous) and excess growth hormone, as seen in acromegaly.[63-64] In contrast, growth hormone deficiency has also been associated with insulin resistance. Growth hormone deficient individuals, when replaced with growth hormone, improve their insulin sensitivity and decrease their visceral adipose tissue.[65-66]

INSULIN RESISTANCE AND THE METABOLIC SYNDROME

Since the original description of Syndrome X, a number of other clinical and laboratory abnormalities have become associated with the metabolic syndrome (Table 2). In the report from ADA sponsored Consensus Development Conference on Insulin Resistance, a distinction was made between insulin resistance and the Insulin Resistance Syndrome.[1] The latter was described in the report as a constellation of associated clinical and laboratory findings consisting of glucose intolerance, central obesity dyslipidemia (increased triglycerides, decreased HDL, increased small dense LDL), hypertension, increased prothrombotic and antifibrinolytic factors, and an increased risk of atherosclerotic vascular disease.

Table 2. Abnormalities associated with the metabolic syndrome

Insulin Resistance
Central Obesity
Dyslipidemia
    Increased fasting plasma triglycerides
    Decreased HDL-cholesterol
    Small, dense LDL pattern
Hypertension
Pro-coagulant state
    Increased plasma fibrinogen
    Increased PAI-1
Microalbuminuria
Increased Homocysteine
Increased Uric Acid

A number of groups, including World Health Organization (WHO), American Association of Clinical Endocrinologists (AACE), and National Cholesterol Education Program (NECP) have begun to put forth their own list of the criteria that can be used to diagnose the metabolic syndrome (Table 3).[67-69] A summary of the overlapping criteria is presented in Table 3.

Table 3. Summary of criteria for diagnosis of the metabolic syndrome

Insulin Resistance
Glucose intolerance, impaired fasting glucose tolerance or type 2 diabetes
Hypertension
Elevated fasting triglycerides, $\geq$ 150 mg/dl
Low HDL-cholesterol[1]
Central Obesity[2]

1-< 35 mg/dl (WHO, AACE), < 40 mg/dl (NCEP-ATPIII), for men ; < 39 mg/dl (WHO), < 45 mg/dl (AACE), < 50 mg/dl (NECP-ATPIII) for women.

2- Waist:hip ratio > 0.90 (WHO), waist circumference > 102 cm (> 40in) (AACE, NECP-ATPIII) for men; waist :hip ratio > 0.85 (WHO), waist circumference > 88 cm (> 35 in) (AACE, NCEP-ATPIII) for women; or BMI > 30 kg/m2 (WHO).

WHO criteria also include microalbuminuria (urinary albumin excretion rate $\geq$ 20 ug/min or albumin:creatinine ratio $\geq$ 30 mg/G) as part of the syndrome.[67] AACE criteria include hyperuricemia and acanthosis nigricans as major criteria and hypercoagulability, microalbuminuria, vascular endothelial dysfunction, polycystic ovarian syndrome, and coronary heart disease as minor criteria.[69]

RISK FOR THE METABOLIC SYNDROME

A number of factors increase the risk for the development of the metabolic syndrome, particularly weight gain and sedentary lifestyle. Middle-aged men participating in the Kuopio Ischemic Heart Disease Risk Factor Study from Eastern Finland, who gained > 10% of their youthful (age 20 years) weight by middle-age, were more likely to have metabolic abnormalities consistent with the metabolic syndrome (such as hypertension, hyperinsulinemia, and dyslipidemia) as compared to those men whose weight remained stable over time.[70] In the Bruneck Study, a population-based survey on atherosclerosis and its risk factors in Bruneck (a small town in northeastern Italy), insulin resistance was present in 9.6% of the population as assessed by HOMA. Interestingly, 5.1% of the population had normal weight and no metabolic abnormalities, but were insulin resistant. Hypertriglyceridemia and low HDL-cholesterol were as likely to accompany insulin resistance as was type 2 diabetes while there was less of an

730

association between hypertension, hypercholesterolemia, and hyperuricemia and insulin resistance.[71]

Recent reports show that the prevalence of overweight/obesity is increasing in children in the United States and so is the prevalence of type 2 diabetes in children.[72-73] Assessment of insulin resistance and clustering of metabolic abnormalities associated with the metabolic syndrome in African American children aged 5-10 years without diabetes showed a positive correlation with insulin resistance, blood pressure, triglycerides and cholesterol. Girls were more insulin resistant than the boys.[74]

THE METABOLIC SYNDROME AND CARDIOVASCULAR DISEASE

Many studies have looked at the relationship between hyperinsulinemia/ insulin resistance and the development of cardiovascular disease.[21-23] However studies have also shown a relationship between insulin resistance and the clustering of other cardiovascular risk factors of the metabolic syndrome, such as the dyslipidemia and glucose intolerance.[71,75-77] It needs to be determined if the risk for cardiovascular disease associated with insulin resistance and the metabolic syndrome is greater than the contribution of the sum of the individual cardiovascular risk factors.

In the Insulin Resistance Atherosclerosis Study (IRAS), a large epidemiological study evaluating a triethnic cohort (African American, Hispanics and non-Hispanic whites) in four communities in the United States, insulin resistance measured by the FSIVGTT seemed to be associated with intimal medial thickness of the carotid arteries, a surrogate marker for cardiovascular risk, in Hispanic and non-Hispanics whites, but not in African Americans.[78] When factors common to the metabolic syndrome are included in the model, the association between insulin resistance and measures of atherosclerosis diminished. In contrast, the Rancho Bernardo study, a 5-year prospective study of men and women without diabetes, did not show a relationship between hyperinsulinemia and cardiovascular morbidity or mortality.[79] However in a 5-year prospective case controlled study of over 2000 men, the Quebec Heart Study, hyperinsulinemia was an independent predictor of ischemic heart disease.[23] In this study fasting insulin levels were used a marker of insulin resistance. The degree to which insulin resistance alone (independent of the metabolic syndrome) is predictive of atherosclerosis remains unclear. Moreover, since many of the studies linking the metabolic syndrome with cardiovascular disease are in men, its applicability to women needs to be further explored. In studying women, the point at which the woman is in her reproductive cycle will need to be assessed. Menopause is accompanied by an increase in cardiovascular morbidity and mortality and is also associated with an increase in many factors characteristic of the metabolic syndrome, especially increased visceral adiposity with insulin resistance and dyslipidemia.[80]

SUMMARY

In summary, insulin resistance, defined as impaired response to the metabolic and/or mitogenic actions of insulin, is prevalent in increasing numbers of the population. Its presence results in the increased risk for a variety of disease entities, the most common being type 2 diabetes. Coupled with a number of other metabolic abnormalities, including dyslipidemia, a pro-coagulant state, and hypertension, it results in the metabolic syndrome. A growing body of evidence suggests the metabolic syndrome may play a key role in the pathogenesis in atherosclerosis and cardiovascular disease.

REFERENCES

1. American Diabetes Association. Consensus Development Conference on Insulin Resistance. Diabetes Care. 21:310-314, 1998.
2. Mattaei, S, Stumvoll M, Kellerer M, Haring, H. Pathophysiology and pharmacological treatment of insulin resistance. Endocrine Reviews 21:585-618, 2000.
3. Himsowrth HP, Kerr RB. Insulin-sensitive and insulin-insensitive types of diabetes mellitus. Clin Sci 4:119-152, 1939.
4. Cahill GF. Physiology of insulin in man. Diabetes 20:785- 799, 1971.
5. Bagdade JD, Bierman EL, Porte D Jr. The significance of basal insulin levels in the evaluation of the insulin response to glucose and non-diabetic subjects. J Clin Invest 46:1549-1557, 1967.
6. Polonsky KS, Given BD, Hirsch L et al. Quantitative study of insulin secretion and clearance in normal and obese subjects. J Clin Invest 81: 435-441, 1988.
7. Modan M, Halkin H, Fuchs Z, Lusky A, Chetrit A, Segal P, Eshkol A, Almog S, Shefi M. Hyperinsulinemia—a link between glucose intolerance, obesity, hypertension, dyslipoproteinemia, elevated serum uric acid and internal cation imbalance. Diabete et Metabolisme 13:375-80, 1987.
8. Modan M, Halkin H, Lusky A, Segal P, Fuchs Z, Chetrit A. Hyperinsulinemia is characterized by jointly disturbed plasma VLDL, LDL, and HDL levels. A population-based study. Arteriosclerosis 8:227-236, 1988.
9. Modan M, Halkin H. Hyperinsulinemia or increased sympathetic drive as links for obesity and hypertension. Diabetes Care 14:470-487, 1991.
10. Reaven GM. The role of insulin resistance in human disease. Diabetes 37: 1595-1607, 1988.

11. Ferrannini E, Buzzigoli C, Bonadonna R, Giorico M, Oleggini M, Graziadei L, Pedrinelli R, Brandi L, Bevilacqua S. Insulin resistance in essential hypertension. N Engl J Med 317:350-357. 1987.

12. DeFronzo RA, Ferrannini E. Insulin resistance: a multifaceted syndrome responsible for NIDDM, obesity, hypertension, dyslipidemia, and atherosclerotic cardiovascular disease. Diabetes Care 14:173-194, 1991.

13. Yudkin JS, Abnormalities of coagulation and fibrinolysis in insulin resistance. Diabetes Care 22 (Suppl.3): C25-C30, 1999.

14. Brunzell JD, Hokanson JE. Dyslipidemia of central obesity and insulin resistance. Diabetes Care 22 (Suppl. 3): C10-C13, 1999.

15. DeFronzo R, Tobin J, Andres R. Glucose clamp technique: a method for quantifying insulin secretion and insulin resisatnce. Am J Physiol 237:E 214-E223, 1979.

16. Bergman RN, Prager R, Volund A, Olefsky M. Equivalence of the insulin sensitivity index in man derived by the minimal model method and the euglycemic clamp. J Clin Invest 79:790-800, 1987.

17. Matsuda M, DeFronzo R. Insulin sensitivity indices obtained from oral glucose tolerance testing. Diabetes Care 22:1462-1470, 1999.

18. Matthews DR, Hosker JP, Rudenski AS, Naylor BA, Treacher DF, Turner RC. Homeostasis model assessment: insulin resistance and beta-cell function from fasting plasma glucose and insulin concentrations in man. Diabetologia 28:412-419, 1985.

19. Katz A, Nambi SS, Mather K, et al. Quantitative insulin sensitivity check index: a simple, accurate method for assessing insulin sensitivity in humans. J Clin Endocrinol Metab 85:2402-2410.

20. Laakso M. How good a marker is insulin level for insulin resistance? Am J Epidemiol 137:959-965, 1993.

21. Ducimentiere P, Eschwege E, Papz L, Richard JL, Claude JR, Rosselin G. Relationship of plasma insulin to the incidence of myocardial infarction and coronary heart disease. Diabetologia 19:205-210, 1980.

22. Fontbonne A, Charles MA, Thibult N, Rochard JL, Claude JR, Warnet JM, Rosselin GE, Eschwege E. Hyperinsulinemia as a predictor of coronary heart disease mortality in a healthy population: the Paris Prospective Study, 15-year follow-up. Diabetologia, 34:356-361, 1991.

23. Depres J-P, Lamarche B, Mauriege P, Cantin B, Dagenais GR, Moorjani S, Lupien P-J. Hyperinsulinemia as an independent risk factor for ischemic heart disease. N Engl J Med, 334:952-957, 1996.

24. McAuley KS, Williams SM, Mann JI, Walker RJ, Lewis-Barned NJ, Temple LA, Duncan AW. Diagnosing insulin resistance in the general population. Diabetes Care 24:460-464, 2001.

25. American Diabetes Association: Task Force on Standardization of the Insulin Assay (Task Force Report). Diabetes 45:242-256, 1996.

26. Olefsky JM, Kolterman OG, Scarlett JA. Insulin action and resistance in obesity and non-insulin-dependent type 2 diabetes mellitus. Am J Physiol 243:E15-E30, 1982.

27. Su HY, Sheu, WH, Chin HM, Jeng CY, Reaven GM. Effect of weight loss on blood pressure and insulin resistance in normotensive and hypertensive obese individuals. Am J Hypertension 8:1067-1071,1995.

28. Niskanen L, Uusitupa M, Sarlund H, Siitonen O, Paljarvi L, Laasko M. The effects of weight loss on insulin sensitivity, skeletal muscle composition, and capillary density in obese non-diabetic subjects. Int J Obes 20:154-160, 1996.

29. Maggio CA, Pi-Sunyer FX. The prevention and treatment of obesity. Diabetes Care 20:1744-1766, 1997.

30. Muscelli E, Camastra S, Catalano C, Galvan AQ, Ciociaro D, Baldi S, Ferrannini E. Metabolic and cardiovascular assessment in moderate obesity: effect of weight loss. J Clin Endocrinolo Metab 82:2937-2943, 1997.

31. Vague J. The degree of masculine differences of obesities: a factor determining predisposition to diabetes, atherosclerosis, gout, and uric calculous disease. Am J Clin Nutr 4:20-34, 1956.

32. Kvist H, Sjostrom L, Tylen U. Adipose tissue volume determinations in women by computerized tomography: technical considerations. Int J Obesity 10:53-67, 1986.

33. Kvist H, Chowdhury B, Gangard U, Tylen U, Sjostrom L. Total and visceral adipose tissue volume derived from measurements with computerized tomography in adult men and women: predictive equations. Am J Clin Nutr 48:1351-13621, 1988.

34. Abate N, Burns D, Peshock RM, Garg, Grundy SM. Estimation of adipose tissue mass by magnetic resonance imaging: validation against dissection in human cadavers. J Lipid Res 35:1490-1496, 1994.

35. Tataranni PA, Ravussin E. Use of dual X-ray absorptiometry in obese individuals. Am J Clin Nutr 55:730-734, 1995.

36. Goodpaster BH, Kelley DE, Wing RR, Meier A, Thaete FL. Effects of weight loss on regional fat distribution and insulin sensitivity in obesity. Diabetes 48:839-847, 1999.

37. Banerji MA, Lebovitz HE. Insulin-sensitive and insulin-resistant variants in NIDDM. Diabetes 38:784-792, 1989.

38. Banerji MA, Chaiken RL, Gordon D, Kral JG, Lebovitz HE. Does intra-abdominal adipose tissue in black men determine whether NIDDM is insulin resistant or insulin-sensitive? Diabetes 44:141-146, 1995.

39. Banerji MA, Lebowitz J, Chaiken RL, Gordon D, Kral J, Lebovitz HE. Relationships of visceral adipose tissue and glucose disposal is independent of sex in black NIDDM subjects. Am J Physiol. 273:E425-E432., 1997.

40. Banerji MA, Lebovitz HL. Insulin action in black Americans with NIDDM. Diabetes Care 15:1295-1302, 1992.

41. Bergstrom RW, Newell-Morris LL, Leonetti DL. Association of elevated fasting C-peptide level and increased intra-abdominal fat distribution with development of NIDDM in Japanese-American men. Diabetes 39:104-111, 1990.

42. Boyko EJ, Fujimoto WY, Leonetti DL, Newell-Morris L. Visceral adiposity and risk for type 2 diabetes: A prospective study among Japanese-Americans. Diabetes Care 23:465-471, 2000.

43. Brochu, M., Tchernof, A., Isabelle, D., et al. What are the physical characteristics associated with a normal metabolic profile despite a high level of obesity in postmenopausal women? J Clin Endocrinol Metab 86:1020-1025, 2001.

44. Knowler WC, Bennett PH, Hamman RF, Miller M. Diabetes incidence and prevalence in Pima Indians: A 19-fold greater incidence than in Rochester, Minnesota. Am J Epidemiol 108:497-505, 1978.

45. Gautier, J., Milner, M.R., Elam, E., Chen, K., et al. Visceral adipose tissue is not increased in Pima Indians compared with equally obese Caucasians. Diabetologia 42: 28-34, 1999.

46. Saloranta C, Groop L. Interactions between glucose and FFA metabolism in man. Diabetes Metab Rev 12:15-36, 1996.

47. Boden G. Role of fatty acids in the pathogenesis of insulin resistance and NIDDM. Diabetes 46:3-10, 1997.

48. Zhang Y, Proenca R, Maffei M, Barone M, Leopold L, Friedman JM. Positional cloning of the mouse obese gene. Nature 375:425-432, 1994.

49. Steppan CM, Bailey ST, Bhat S, Brown EJ, Banerjee RR, Wright CM, Patel HR, Ahima RS, Lazar MA. The hormone resistin links obesity to diabetes. Nature 409:307-312, 2001.

50. Perseghin G, Price TB, Petersen KF, Roden M, Cline GW, Gerow K, Rothman DL, Shulman GI. Increased glucose transport-phosphorylation and muscle glycogen synthesis after exercise training in insulin-resistant subjects. N Engl J Med 335:1357-1362. 1996.

51. Colditz GA, Willet WC, Stampfer MJ, Manson JE, Hennkens CH, Arky RA, Speizer FE. Weight as a risk factor for clinical diabetes in women. Am J Epidemiol 132:501-513, 1990.

52. Knowler WC, Pettit PJ, Savage PJ, Bennett PH. Diabetes incidence in Pima Indians : contributions of obesity and parental diabetes. Am J Epidemiol 113:144-156, 1981.

53. Modan M, Karasik A, Halkin H, Fuchs Z, Lusky A, Shitrit A, Modan B. Effects of past and concurrent body mass index on prevalence of glucose intolerance and type 2 (non-insulin-dependent) diabetes and on insulin response: the Israel Study of Glucose Intolerance , Obesity, and Hypertension. Diabetologia 29:82-89. 1996.

54. Holbrook TL, Barrett-Connor E, Wingard DL. The association of lifetime weight and weight control patterns with diabetes among men and women in an adult community. Int J Obesity 13:723-729, 1989.

55. Kahn SE. The importance of β-cell failure in the development and progression of type 2 diabetes. J Clin Endocrinol Metab 86:4047-4058, 2001.

56. Ferrannini E, Buzzigoli G, Bonadonna R, Giorico MA, Oleggini M, Graziadei L, Pedrinelli R, Brandi L, Bevilacqua S. Insulin resistance in essential hypertension. N Engl J Med 317:350-357, 1987.

57. Saad MF, Lillioja S, Nyomba BL, Castillo C, Ferraro R, De Gregorio M, Ravussin E, Knowler WC, Bennett PH, Howard BV, Bogardus C. Racial differences in the relation between blood pressure and insulin resistance. N Engl J Med 324:733-739, 1991.

58. Falkner B, Hulman S, Tannenbaum J, Kushner H. Insulin resistance and blood pressure in young black men. Hypertension 16:706-711, 1990.

59. Chaiken RL, Banerji MA, Huey H, Lebovitz HE. Do blacks with NIDDM have an insulin-resistance syndrome? Diabetes 42:444-449, 1993.

60. Burghen GA, Givens JR, Kitabchi AE. Correlation of hyperandrogenism with hyperinsulinism in polycystic ovarian disease. J Clin Endocrinol Metab 50:113-116, 1980.

61. Dunaif A, Graf M, Mandeli J et al. Characterization of groups of hyperandrogenic women with acanthosis nigricans, impaired glucose tolerance, and/or hyperinsulinemia. J Clin Endocrinol Metab 65:499-507, 1987.

62. Dunaif A, Thomas A. Current concepts in the polycystic ovary syndrome. Annu Rev Med 52:401-419, 2001.

63. Rizza RA, Mandarino LJ, Gerich JE. Mechanisms of insulin resistance in man. Assessment using the insulin dose-response curve in conjunction with insulin-receptor binding. Am J Med 70:169-176, 1981.

64. Fineberg SE, Merimee TJ, Rabinowitz D, Edgar PJ. Insulin secretion in acromegaly. J Clin Endocrinol Metab 30:288-292, 1970.

65. Fowelin J, Attvall S, Lager I, Bengtsson BA. Effects of treatment with recombinant human growth hormone on insulin sensitivity and glucose metabolism in adults with growth hormone deficiency. Metabolism 42:1443-1447, 1993.

66. Sesmilo G, Biller BMK, Lievadot J, Hayden D, Hanson G, Rifai N, Klibanski A. Effects of growth hormone administration on inflammatory and other cardiovascular risk markers in men with growth hormone deficiency. Ann Intern Med 133:111-122, 2000.

67. Alberti KGMM, Zimmet PZ for the WHO Consultation: Definition, diagnosis, and classification of diabetes mellitus and its complications. Part 1: Diagnosis and Classification of Diabetes Mellitus. Diabetic Medicine 15:539-553, 1998.

68. AACE: Diagnostic criteria and operational definition developed by American College of Clinical Endocrinologists. www.AACE.com/members/socio/syndormex.php. 2001.

69. Executive Summary of the Third Report of the National Cholesterol Education Program (NCEP) Expert Panel on Detection, Evaluation, and Treatment of High Blood Cholesterol in Adults (Adult Treatment Panel III). JAMA 285:2486-2496, 2001.

70. Everson, S., Lynch JW, Goldberg, D., Kaplan GA, Helmrich, S., Salonen JT, Lakka TA. Weight gain and the risk of developing insulin resistance syndrome. Diabetes Care, 21: 1637-1643, 1998.

71. Bonora, E., Kiechl, S., Willeit, J., Oberhollenzer, F., Egger G, Targher G, Alberiche M, Bonadonna RC, Muggeo M. Prevalence of Insulin resistance in metabolic disorders. The Bruneck Study. Diabetes, 47: 1643-1649, 1998.

72. Flegal KM. The obesity epidemic in children and adults: current evidence and research issues. Med Sci Sports Exer 32 (suppl.11):S509-514, 1999.

73. American Diabetes Association. Type 2 diabetes in children and adolescents (consensus statement) Diabetes Care 23:381-389, 2000.

74. Young-Hyman, D, DeLuca F, Schlundt D, Counts D, Herman L. Evaluation of the Insulin resistance Syndrome in 5- to 10-year-old overweight/obese African-American children. Diabetes Care 24: 1359-1364, 2001.

75. Isomaa, B, Lahti K, Almgren P, Nissen M, Tuomi T, Taskinen MR, Forsen B, Groop L. Cardiovascular morbidity and mortality associated with the metabolic syndrome. Diabetes Care 24: 683-689, 2001.

76. Haffner SM, Mykkanen L, Festa A, Burke JP, Stern MP. Insulin resistant prediabetic subjects have more atherogenic risk factors than insulin-sensitive prediabetic subjects. Circulation 101:975-980, 2000.

77. Greenlund KJ, Rith-Najarian S, Valdez R, Croft JB, Casper ML. Prevalence and correlates of the insulin resistance syndrome among Native Americans. Diabetes Care 22:441-447,1999.

78. Howard G, O'Leary DH, Zaccaro D, Haffner S, Rewers M, Hamman R, Selby JV, Saad MF, Savage P, Bergman R, for the IRAS Investigators. Insulin sensitivity and atherosclerosis. Circulation 93:1809-1817, 1996.

79. Ferrara A, Barrett-Connor EL, Edelstein SL. Hyperinsulinemia does not increase the risk of fatal cardiovascular disease in elderly men or women without diabetes: the Rancho Bernardo Study, 1984-1991. Am J Epidemiol 140:857-869,1994.

80. Rendell M, Hulthen UL, Tornquist C, Groop L, Mattiasson I. Realtionship between abdominal fat compartments and glucose and lipid metabolism in early postmenopausal women. J Clin Endocrinol Metab 86:744-749, 2001.

IX. Diabetes Prevention

Asha Thomas-Geevarghese and Kevan C. Herold

PREVENTION OF TYPE 1 DIABETES MELLITUS

Overview

Studies carried out over the past three decades in animal models and in patients suggest that Type 1 diabetes mellitus is an autoimmune disease. Elsewhere, in Chapter V, this work is reviewed and current concepts of disease pathogenesis are discussed. These studies indicate that the Type 1 diabetes is due to the T cell mediated destruction of the beta cells in the islets of Langerhans. The risk of diabetes in the general population in North America is approximately 12.5/100,000, although this number has been increasing.[1] The risk of Type 1 diabetes is higher among families with another relative with Type 1 diabetes. The genetic locus most highly linked to the disease is the major histocompatibility locus (MHC), and over 90% of Caucasian individuals express either HLA DR3 and/or DR.[2] Prediction of future diabetes, however, is not possible on a genetic basis alone. For example, the concordance rate for identical twins is < 50%, indicating that either environmental or developmental events (such as T cell development) affect the progression of diabetes.

The ability of serologic studies to identify individuals at risk for diabetes in the general population is under investigation. Among relatives of patients with diabetes, serologic markers can identify patients at high risk.[3] This originally was suggested by identification of autoantibodies (islet cell antibodies-ICA) in relatives of patients with Type 1 diabetes years before the diagnosis of disease. In general, the risk of development of Type 1 diabetes in relatives of individuals with the disease is highest in relatives with autoantibodies such as ICA or biochemical markers such as anti-GAD65, anti-ICA512, or anti-insulin autoantibodie.[4] Several studies have evaluated the use of serologic and metabolic markers to predict progression to diabetes in relatives of patients with the disease.[5] Riley et al found that the risk of diabetes among first degree relatives of patients with disease was about 1.7 % over 7 years but was 31.2% among the 3.1% who were ICA+. The risk increased dramatically, however, in subjects younger than 20 years of age and in those from multiplex families or with the highest titers of ICA.[6] Natural history data is consistent with studies in animal models of the disease, suggesting that with progression to disease, there is diversification of the autoimmune response. In DAISY (Diabetes Autoimmunity Study in the Young), the initial marker of autoimmunity, anti-insulin antibodies, could be detected as early as 9 months of age.[7] Of 5 individuals with insulin autoantibodies, before age 1 year, 4 progressed to diabetes. Others have reported that the ability to predict future disease can be considerably enhanced when there is evidence of impaired insulin secretory capacity either in the form of diminished first phase insulin response to intravenous glucose or as impaired response to oral glucose.[8]

The progression to diabetes among high-risk individuals has been well characterized recently in the **Diabetes Prevention Trial-1 (DPT-1)** and other studies (Figure 1).[9] In a cohort of first degree relatives who were ICA+ and had either insulin autoantibodies with diminished first phase insulin responses to intravenous glucose or impaired oral glucose tolerance, 11% of individuals developed diabetes/year.[10] After 5 years of follow-up, 60% of high-risk individuals had developed disease, but even after 5 years, there was no evidence of a plateau of disease risk. The results of this study provide further evidence that clinical presentation occurs after a matured, diversified immune response, because the risk of diabetes was highest among those with 2 or more biochemical autoantibodies compared to those with fewer.

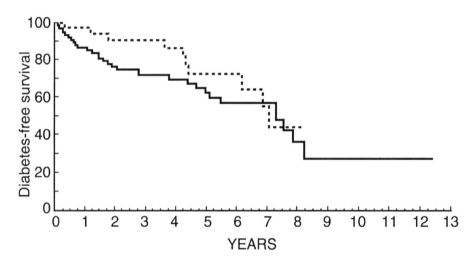

Figure 1. Probability of remaining IDDM-free comparing 103 relatives and 57 schoolchildren aged 5-17 yr who tested positive for ICA. Solid line, relatives; broken line, schoolchildren. (Reprinted with permission from Schatz et al. J Clin Invest 93:2403-2407, 1994.)

Loss of insulin secretory capacity during development of Type 1 diabetes

At the time of the first appearance of markers of autoimmunity, insulin secretory capacity is assumed to be near normal, at least in response to intravenous glucose. With time, insulin responses to intravenous glucose may be impaired, but responses to oral glucose are not. Ultimately, responses to oral glucose deteriorate, and the diagnosis of diabetes may be made. At the time of diagnosis and even 1 year after diagnosis, all patients still can make detectable levels of insulin after stimulation.[10-12] In fact, many individuals in the Diabetes Control and Complications Trial were found to make "clinically meaningful" levels of insulin (defined as a stimulated level > 0.2 pmol/ml) associated with improved glycemic control.[13] By 5 years of disease, however, detectable levels of insulin production are rare. Age appears to be an important modifier of the natural history of disease both in the prediabetic period and following diagnosis. Individuals over the age of 18 showed a much slower progression to diabetes in the DPT-1 trial. The term "latent autoimmune diabetes of adults" (LADA) applies to individuals with diabetes presenting beyond childhood years in whom autoantibodies can be detected. These individuals invariably progress to insulin dependence but do so at a much slower rate than children < 18 years of age.[14]

These clinical studies suggest that: 1) Individuals at risk for development of disease can be identified among first-degree relatives of patients with diabetes; 2) Interventions could be appropriately targeted to high-risk individuals to prevent disease onset. (Unresolved is the certainty of disease prediction balanced with the safety of the proposed intervention before proceeding to intervention trials.); 3) Clinically significant insulin secretion is present before diagnosis and even after the diagnosis of Type 1 diabetes; and 4) Interventions that could prevent ongoing beta cell destruction would be valuable before after the onset of diabetes.

Studies in Animal Models

In animal models of Type 1 diabetes, several approaches have shown to prevent the development of disease. In the NOD mouse, the most studied model of autoimmune diabetes, many manipulations have been reported to prevent development of autoimmune diabetes when administered at an early stage in development.[15] These include both antigen specific approaches (treatment with insulin or a dominant negative GAD transgene expressed in the beta cells) to non-specific approaches such as changes in animal housing, diet, or immunization with Complete Freund's Adjuvant. Some of these studies have suggested clinical approaches that are now in development. For example, in the BB/W rat and the NOD mouse, parenteral administration of insulin prevented onset of the disease.[16, 17] Further studies suggested that the mechanism did not involve a metabolic effect of insulin because insulin B chain, which is not metabolically active, was able to prevent disease. Zhang et al reported that oral insulin would also prevent diabetes and induced a regulatory population that could inhibit the transfer of disease.[18] More recently, Karounas found that an insulin analog will prevent the development of diabetes in the NOD mouse.[19] This altered insulin is thought to function as an "altered peptide ligand" that has been described in which the signal delivered to the TCR by the peptide induces anergy of T cells.[20] Lee et al found that a single chain insulin analog, expressed in hepatocytes as a transgene, would prevent diabetes in the NOD mouse.[21]

Blocking expression of glutamic acid decarboxylase 65 (GAD), a major autoantigen in Type 1 diabetes, in the islets has been found to prevent disease development. When a dominant negative GAD was expressed as a transgene in islet cells, GAD reactive T cells did not develop, and insulitis and diabetes were blocked.[22] Immunization with GAD delayed recurrent diabetes in NOD mice receiving islet transplants.[23] Heat shock protein 60 (HSP 60) has also been implicated as an important autoantigen in the NOD and multi-dose streptozotocin induced mouse models of Type 1 diabetes mellitus. Expression of HSP 60 in the thymic medullary epithelium reduced diabetes and insulitis in the NOD mouse.[24, 25, 26]

Oxidative injury has been thought to be a mechanism leading to beta cell injury and death, possibly through the effects of nitric oxide produced in the islet inflammatory lesions.[27] Hence, nicotinamide has been found to prevent diabetes in the NOD mouse, possibly by blocking the injurious effects of free radicals generated in the inflammatory lesions. Alteration of the phenotype of the autoimmune response to islet antigens is a common finding in several approaches at disease prevention such as oral interferon-alpha administration and others.[28]

Finally, non-FcR binding anti-CD3 specifically anergized previously activated Th1 cells, those thought to mediate beta cell destruction in Type 1 diabetes. Chatenoud et al originally reported that anti-CD3 mAb treatment was able to reverse diabetes when NOD mice were treated at the appearance of hyperglycemia.[29,30] The mechanism of non-FcR binding anti-CD3 is thought to involve anergy of activated Th1 cells. Interestingly, the mAb was most effective in later stages of the disease than if given at the time of first appearance of insulitis, consistent with the finding that activated Th1 cells are those found in the islet at the time of diagnosis, whereas cells of other phenotypes may be present at earlier stages.[31]

Previous Interventions to Stop the Progression of Type 1 Diabetes

With the assumption that strategies to prevent diabetes in high-risk individuals would also prevent deterioration in insulin secretion in new onset disease, potential preventive treatments have first been tested in patients with new onset disease. Over the past 2 decades, a number of interventions have been able to affect the natural history of disease in the short term. Stiller et al first reported that treatment of patients with new onset Type 1 diabetes with cyclosporin A increased the rates of non-insulin requiring remissions.[32] This finding was confirmed by Bougneres et al who found that the rate of complete remission after 9 months of treatment with cyclosporin A was greater in diabetics than in control subjects. Interestingly, insulin reserve, rather than immunologic factors best predicted clinical response to cyclosporin A.[33] Although cyclosporin A was effective in the short term, it was unable to maintain remissions with continued treatment. All cyclosporin treated individuals eventually lost their non-insulin requiring remissions within 4 years.[34] The concern about renal toxicity caused by cyclosporin A as well as the lack of long term efficacy has led most investigators to abandon its use in this setting and there has been little enthusiasm for its use for prevention of diabetes.

Other immunologic interventions have had limited success in patients with new onset disease. Silverstein et al reported that treatment with azathioprine and prednisone increased insulin production in patients with new onset diabetes.[35] Eisenbarth found that anti-thymocyte globulin and prednisone caused clinical remission in patients with recent onset disease, but failed to cause lasting improvement, and the toxicity of this treatment approach led the investigators to abandon its use.[36] More recently, methotrexate failed to induce a meaningful remission when given to patients with recent diagnosis of disease.[37] Shah et al found that individuals treated with an aggressive regimen of insulin at the time of diagnosis of diabetes had improvement in C-peptide responses compared to untreated control subjects one year following the metabolic intervention.[38] Keller et al noted that treatment of individuals at high risk for disease with daily subcutaneous injections of insulin reduced the rate and timing of disease onset.[39] In the DCCT, individuals with recent onset Type 1 diabetes assigned to the "intensive" treatment arm were found to have improved beta cell reserve and less hypoglycemia than those assigned to conventional therapy.[13] In contrast, oral insulin had no effect on residual beta cell function when given at the onset of Type 1 diabetes mellitus.[40]

Other Trials for Treatment of New Onset Disease

Two Phase II trials of non-FcR binding humanized anti-CD3 antibodies for treatment of new onset Type 1 diabetes are ongoing. As discussed above, this approach is different from previous immune suppressive treatments because it induced tolerance to autoimmune diabetes at the time of disease onset, presumably by blocking the diabetogenic Th1 response.

Studies suggesting the importance of insulin as an autoantigen and the ability to induce tolerance to antigen reactive cells with an altered form of the antigen have led to the development of new trials in which altered insulin peptides will be administered to patients with new onset disease. Studies in models of Type 1 diabetes have suggested that cells reactive with a peptide of HSP 60 expressed by inflamed islet cells may destroy insulin producing cells.[41] A trial of immunization with a heat shock protein peptide (DiaPep) is also in phase I/II trials.

In addition, other Phase I/II trials are ongoing involving oral interferon-alpha, anti-IL-2 receptor antibody, with or without mycophenolate mofetil, subcutaneous insulin with adjuvant, and others are in stages of development.

Recent and Ongoing Type 1 Diabetes Prevention Trials

The Schwabing insulin prophylaxis trial showed a delay in onset of Type 1 diabetes in high-risk individuals treated with insulin.[42] This trial involved a relatively small cohort of subjects. In contrast, administration of insulin to individuals in the "high risk" arm of the DPT-1 failed to prevent or delay the onset of Type 1 diabetes. This trial, the largest of its kind, involved screening of over 80,000 relatives of individuals with Type 1 diabetes in order to identify a high-risk cohort of 349 individuals. Despite the preclinical and pilot clinical studies suggesting efficacy of this approach, the incidence curves of the intervention and observation groups were virtually identical over a 5-year period.

Other approaches are either in testing or in development for the treatment of new onset or prophylaxis of disease. For relatives with moderate risk for developing diabetes (defined as less than 50% over 5 years and including individuals who have ICA but who do not have impaired metabolic responses to oral or intravenous glucose), a trial of oral insulin is ongoing part of the DPT-1. This trial will conclude in 2003.[43]

The ENDIT (European Nicotinamide Diabetes Intervention Trial) will test whether treatment with nicotinamide, an anti-oxidant, will prevent onset of the disease in high-risk individuals. This trial is based on animal studies suggesting that islet destruction may be mediated by free radical formation during the inflammatory response, and anti-oxidants can interfere with islet destruction that occurs through this mechanism.[43]

PREVENTION OF TYPE 2 DIABETES

Overview

Type 2 diabetes has become a national and international epidemic involving both adults and children. It is a critical public health priority with a prevalence of 12.3 percent in the United States population. More recently, Type 2 diabetes has been recognized with increasing frequency in pediatric patients, particularly those with a strong family history of the disease, those who are obese, and members of certain ethnic groups.

Overall, the annual rate of progression to diabetes with impaired glucose tolerance is 1 to 10 percent.[44,45] Age, obesity, a family history of diabetes, ethnicity, and the presence of impaired glucose tolerance have been shown to increase the risk of developing diabetes.[46] Both genetic and environmental factors contribute to the disease. As with Type 1 diabetes mellitus, progression to Type 2 diabetes occurs in clinical stages beginning with normal glucose tolerance. Glucose tolerance is then described as "impaired" but there are both quantitative and qualitative defects in insulin secretion. Finally, frank diabetes occurs when insulin secretory capacity cannot meet metabolic demands. Unlike the relatively small risk for having markers of Type 1 diabetes (about 3 percent) in first-degree relatives of patients, the risk of disease is much higher in relatives of patients with Type 2 diabetes. Therefore, there are many more individuals who would be candidates for Type 2 diabetes prevention trials.

The strategies involved in disease prevention involve the 3 mechanisms responsible for disease pathogenesis including impaired insulin production, peripheral resistance to insulin, and hepatic insensitivity to insulin action. In general, one may view disease presentation as a failure of insulin production and insulin action to meet metabolic demands. Therefore, reduction in metabolic demands would be a suitable approach to prevent disease manifestations in the presence of impaired insulin production and/or action. Three specific areas, including exercise, diet and weight loss, and certain pharmacologic interventions have been areas of focus in the prevention of diabetes.

Exercise

Exercise has been shown to prevent development of Type 2 diabetes in high-risk groups. A number of studies have looked at the effect of insulin on delaying the onset of diabetes. In a study of 5990 male alumni from an American university followed over 10 years, 202 pts (3.3 percent) developed Type 2 diabetes mellitus. The relative risk was lower in patients who exercised regularly even when adjusted for obesity, hypertension, and a family history of diabetes. The benefit was greatest in obese patients and not present in thin subjects who were at a lower risk of Type 2 diabetes.[47] Total expenditure of energy during leisure time was protective in middle-aged men. In fact, there was a 6 percent decrease in the incidence for each 500 kcal/week expenditure of energy through exercise. Similar findings were reported in the Malmo Feasibility Study.[48]

More recently, the **Finnish Diabetes Prevention Study** examined the effect of intensive diet and exercise on progression from impaired glucose tolerance to diabetes. In this study although the average weight loss was small (4.2 +/-5.1 kg) the effect on the incidence was substantial with the risk of diabetes 58 percent higher in the control group.[49] However, this study did not look at whether it was diet or exercise, which caused this dramatic change.

The **United States Diabetes Prevention Program (DPP)** was recently completed. The DPP is a randomized clinical trial designed to evaluate the safety and efficacy of interventions that may delay or prevent development of diabetes in people at increased risk for Type 2 diabetes. There were three treatment groups: intensive lifestyle intervention with a goal of weight reduction by 7% through diet and exercise, metformin 850 mg bid or placebo.[50] There were 3,234 individuals with IGT enrolled (mean age- 51, mean BMI-34) with average follow-up of 3 years. Both lifestyle modification and therapy with metformin prevented or delayed the onset of Type 2 diabetes in individuals with IGT. 29% of the placebo group developed diabetes versus 14% of the lifestyle modification group and 22% of the metformin group. Thus, lifestyle modification and metformin groups reduced the risk of Type 2 diabetes by 58% and 31% respectively.

How does exercise impact upon glycemic control? During exercise, the primary beneficial effect on glycemic control on non-diabetic patients is improved tissue sensitivity to insulin and increased peripheral uptake of glucose. To meet the demands of exercise, the metabolic

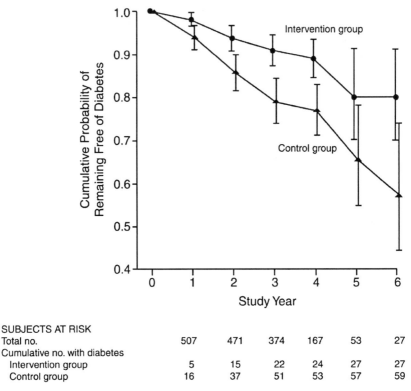

SUBJECTS AT RISK						
Total no.		507	471	374	167	53	27
Cumulative no. with diabetes						
Intervention group		5	15	22	24	27	27
Control group		16	37	51	53	57	59

Figure 2. Proportion of Subjects without Diabetes during the Trial.
The vertical bars show the 95 percent confidence intervals for the cumulative probability of remaining free of diabetes. The relative risk of diabetes for subjects in the intervention group, as compared with those in the control group, was 0.4 (p<0.001 for the comparison between the groups). (Reprinted with permission from Tuomilehto et al. N Engl J Med 344: 1343-50, 2001.)

changes that occur with exercise involve direct uptake of glucose by gluconeogenesis from amino acid and lipid precursors that can provide glucose as muscle stores are depleted. Long-term moderate exercise can lead to more efficient muscle use of energy by increasing mitochondrial enzymes, the number of slow-switch muscle fibers, and the development of new muscle capillaries.[51] In addition, insulin-responsive glucose transporters (GLUT4) which promote glucose uptake, are translocated from intracellular stores to the cell surface[52] ith a resulting increase in insulin sensitivity.[53] In the diabetic patient, these responses are modified and long-term studies of the effects of exercise have not been encouraging primarily due to poor compliance with the exercise regimen.

Weight Loss

Body fat appears to be the most modifiable risk factor in the development of Type 2 diabetes.[54] As 50% of the population of the United States is overweight, this becomes an increasingly important area of public health. The risk of Type 2 diabetes attributable to obesity is up to 75%.[55] More active individuals and those with a lower BMI have a lower incidence of diabetes[47] nd the likelihood of development of diabetes is correlated with weight gain and decreased physical activity.[56] In obesity, IGT is the result of decreased insulin action.[57] Concentrations of free fatty acids are excessive in individuals with abdominal obesity and amplify insulin resistance. Again, both genetics and environment play a role as societies that have changed toward a westernized diet and lifestyle have an increased prevalence of IGT and Type 2 diabetes.

How does weight loss affect the prediabetic state? A number of studies have investigated this question. In one study, 154 overweight nondiabetic patients who had one or both parents with diabetes were randomly assigned to 2 years of decreased caloric and fat intake, exercise with a goal of 1,500 kcal/week of moderate activity or the combination of diet plus exercise or to a no treatment control group. Weight loss from 0 to 2 years reduced the risk of developing Type 2 diabetes.[46] In fact, *even modest losses in weight reduced the risk of developing diabetes.* Though it was expected that the diet plus exercise group would have better maintenance of their weight than diet alone, at 2 years both groups maintained the same degree of weight loss. Other studies have confirmed the reduced progression from IGT to diabetes with weight loss programs including gastric stapling by as much as 30-fold.[58] To assess mechanisms for the improved glycemic control through weight loss, hyperinsulinemic glucose clamps were performed in 20 obese subjects with normal glucose tolerance or mild diabetes before and on the 4th and on the 28th day of reduced energy diets.[59] In both groups, energy restriction reduced fasting plasma glucose and the percent of hepatic glucose output after 4 days. By day 28, insulin sensitivity increased in all subjects with substantial weight loss (6.3 +/- 0.4 kg) more markedly in diabetic patients. A reduction in abdominal fat was associated with a later increase in insulin sensitivity and fall in fasting plasma glucose. The abdominal adipocytes appear to have increased sensitivity to catecholamine-induced lipolysis and higher lipid turnover. The association between increased central obesity and insulin resistance had been noted in a number of cross-sectional studies.[60, 61]

Diet

In addition to weight gain playing a key role in the progression from IGT to Type 2 diabetes, long-term intake of fat and/or saturated fat appears to have an effect independent of weight gain.[62, 63] A reduction in fat intake may be useful in prevention of disease. In a five-year follow-up of a one year randomized study of a reduced fat diet versus a usual diet in patients with

IGT, the reduced fat diet group had increased weight loss at one year and improved glucose tolerance. A lower proportion had impaired glucose tolerance and Type 2 diabetes at one year.[64] One of the potential mechanisms of delaying the onset of diabetes by diet is the reduction of non-esterified fatty acids (NEFA). These fatty acids are a key energy source for most body tissues, particularly during periods of food deprivation. One of its roles is to heighten the responsiveness of the pancreatic beta cell to variety of insulin secretagogues. Recent studies suggest that high levels of NEFA or very-low density lipoprotein (VLDL) might also have a harmful effect in the beta cell as well as muscle. Potential mechanisms of the lipotoxicity include a NEFA induced beta cell dysfunction mediated by overproduction of nitric oxide. Another possibility is that fat-laden islets undergo an accelerated rate of apoptosis and that increased ceramide synthesis, driven by excess availability of NEFA, is a mediator of this process.[65] Insulin secretion is modulated not only by glucose levels, but also by the concentration and nature of the free fatty acids. A very high ratio of saturated to unsaturated NEFA in the blood might promote hypersecretion of insulin and thus contribute to hyperinsulinemia, dyslipidemia, and insulin resistance that accompany the overconsumption of dietary saturated fat.

A dietary fatty acid, conjugated linoleic acid (CLA), has received attention due to its protective properties against cancer and heart disease. It is a naturally occurring fatty acid with anti-carcinogenic and anti-atherogenic properties which activates PPAR alpha in the liver. It shares functional similarities to ligands of PPAR gamma, the thiazolidinediones, which are potent insulin sensitizers. It is found in meats, pasteurized dairy products, and processed cheeses. In a study of prediabetic rats, the CLA was shown to normalize impaired glucose tolerance, improve hyperinsulinemia, and lower circulating free fatty acids.[66] The insulin sensitizing effects appear to be due to activation of PPAR gamma.

Pharmacologic Intervention

Drugs such as biguanides (metformin) and thiazolidinediones (rosiglitazone and pioglitazone) that improve insulin resistance or affect pancreatic beta cell dysfunction have been investigated in the prevention of the onset of Type 2 diabetes mellitus. Metformin is effective only in the presence of insulin and its major effect is to increase insulin action, though the mechanism is not known. Postreceptor effects include suppression of hepatic glucose output, increased insulin-mediated glucose utilization in muscle and lover, and a lipolytic effect that lowers serum free fatty acid concentrations. In the BIGuanides and Prevention of Risks in obesity (BIGPRO1), a one-year prospective study of 324 nondiabetic men who had central obesity and others features of syndrome X including insulin resistance, hypertension, and hyperlipidemia looked at the effect of metformin versus placebo.[67] The men in the treatment group had slightly more weight loss and lower fasting glucose that the placebo group. The

748

results suggest that it may be a useful adjunct to exercise and diet but needs further study. In another study in adolescents with a family history of diabetes, a decrease in glucose, BMI and fasting insulin were noted with metformin treatment for six months. This may suggest a role for intervention at an earlier age.[68] Thiazolidinediones improve glucose utilization by muscle and decrease hepatic glucose production. They also act by increasing insulin secretion in response to glucose in patients with impaired glucose tolerance.[69] These effects have been seen in various animal models of Type 2 diabetes and in humans. In the OLEFT rat (Otsuka Long-Evans Tokushima Fatty) treatment with troglitazone before onset of diabetes reduced fasting glucose, insulin, cholesterol, triglyceride, and free fatty acid levels. The pancreatic wet weight and insulin content were higher in the treated group and they had less islet cell destruction. The troglitazone, in a dose 10-15 times higher than that used in humans, was shown to prevent and reverse the metabolic derangement in genetically determined diabetes.[70] In other animal studies, metformin treated Zucker diabetic fatty rats treated from 6 to 12 weeks of age gained less weight than troglitazone treated rats, but both drugs prevented hyperglycemia by 12 weeks and increased the insulin secretory response of the pancreas.[71]

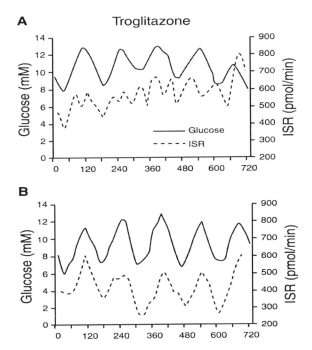

Figure 3. Glucose and ISR profiles during oscillatory glucose infusion. Example of improved entrainment before (A) and after (B) troglitazone. Glucose profiles are shown in solid lines, and ISR profiles are shown in dotted lines. The normalized spectral power increased in this subject from 1.7 to 14.9. (Reprinted with permission from Cavaghan et al. J Clin Invest 100 (3) : 530-537, 1997.)

Troglitazone, since withdrawn from the market in the United States and United Kingdom due to hepatic toxicity, was used in humans comparing fourteen obese patients with IGT receiving 12 weeks of troglitazone and compared to 7 patients receiving placebo.[69] Troglitazone reduced integrated glucose and insulin responses to oral glucose by 10% and 39% respectively, increased the insulin sensitivity index, and increased insulin secretion rates by 52%. The ability of the beta cell to entrain to an exogenous oscillatory glucose infusion was improved by 49%, suggesting that in addition to increasing insulin sensitivity, troglitazone would improve the dysfunctional responses of beta cells characteristic of IGT (Figure 3). This appears to be an important factor in the observed improvement in glucose tolerance.

In clinical studies, troglitazone has been shown to improve peripheral insulin sensitivity in obese subjects with both normal and impaired glucose tolerance by lower plasma insulin levels while maintaining normoglycemia in prospective and placebo controlled studies.[72] Rosiglitazone and pioglitazone may have similar effects in slowing the progression to Type 2 diabetes.[73,74] In vitro experiments have shown troglitazone-induced increases in GLUT1 mRNA and protein in adipocytes, suggesting a potential mechanism for insulin independent glucose disposal.[75] Chronic exposure of pancreatic islets to supraphysiologic levels of glucose may play a secondary pathogenic role in type 2 diabetes (i.e. "glucotoxicity"). It has been postulated that chronic oxidative stress may play a role in glucose toxicity. In a study to evaluate the potential effects of anti-oxidants, N-acetyl-L-cysteine (NAC) or aminoguanidine (AG), both antioxidants, were given to Zucker diabetic fatty rats from 6 to 12 weeks of age. Both drugs prevented a rise in blood oxidative stress markers and partially prevented hyperglycemia, glucose intolerance, defective insulin secretion as well as decrements in B cell insulin content, and insulin gene expression.[76]

An unexpected role for angiotensin converting enzyme (ACE) inhibitors was uncovered in the **HOPE trial (Heart Outcomes Prevention Evaluation)** in pts with underlying cardiovascular disease. Of the 5720 patients who were nondiabetic at study onset, 257 developed diabetes during the 4.5 year follow-up period. There were fewer cases of newly diagnosed diabetes in the ramipril (3.6%) vs. placebo (5.4%), p< 0.001 groups. ACE inhibitors may delay or prevent the onset of Type 2 diabetes.[77] The potential mechanisms are being investigated, but increased insulin sensitivity, decreased hepatic clearance of insulin, an anti-inflammatory effect and pancreatic blood flow have been suggested.[78]

The studies available suggest a role for pharmacologic intervention in certain patients. Many of the studies evaluating the effects of different drug interventions on prediabetic states do not have long enough follow-up to assess if the onset of diabetes is postponed or arrested. In addition, the absence of hyperglycemia does not necessarily prevent abnormalities in insulin secretion. Longer studies are needed to assess the long-term effects of the therapies and the number needed to treat to prevent one case of diabetes.

SUMMARY

Several approaches for the prevention of Type 1 diabetes are now in early stages of development. These approaches are based on animal studies although the precise mechanism for their effects is generally not clear. Screening studies can identify relatives of patients with diabetes who are at high risk for developing the disease within 5 to 7 years. As trials are developed, screening interested families becomes vitally important to identify the needed cohorts for new trials. A new infrastructure termed "TrialNet" has been developed by the National Institutes of Health (NIDDK) to help in carrying out these types of trials of prophylaxis and treatment of new onset disease. This type of organization is needed to conduct trials for prevention of Type 1 diabetes, as evident from the experience from the DPT-1 in which more than 80,000 individuals were screened. TrialNet is expected to be functional by the end of 2001.

Type 2 diabetes is widely prevalent and has a high rate of progression in the United States. Weight loss and exercise have clearly demonstrated benefit in delaying the onset of disease. Application of these findings to the general population and to those at risk for disease is an ongoing task. Pharmacologic therapies are still under investigation. Longer studies will be needed in the event of a successful immediate effect to determine whether these drugs fundamentally alter the deterioration of beta cell capacity. The preliminary data concerning ACE inhibitors are compelling and further study is needed.

REFERENCES

1. LaPorte RB, Chang Y-F. Prevalence and incidence of insulin-dependent diabetes, In "Diabetes in America," 2nd ed. National Diabetes Data Group, National Institutes of Health. Publication No. 95-1468, 1995.
2. Castano L, Eisenbarth GS. Type-I diabetes: a chronic autoimmune disease of human, mouse, and rat. Annu Rev Immunol 8:647-79, 1990.
3. Hagopian WA, Sanjeevi CB, Kockum I, Landin-Olsson M, Karlsen AE, Sundkvist G, Dahlquist G, Palmer J, Lernmark A. Glutamate decarboxylase-, insulin-, and islet cell-antibodies and HLA typing to detect diabetes in a general population-based study of Swedish children. J Clin Invest 95(4):1505-11, 1995.

4. Hagopian WA, Karlsen AE, Gottsater A, Landin-Olsson M, Grubin CE, Sundkvist G, Petersen JS, Boel E, Dyrberg T, and Lernmark A. Quantitative assay using recombinant human islet glutamic acid decarboxylase (GAD65) shows that 64K autoantibody positivity at onset predicts diabetes type. J Clin Invest 91(1):368-74, 1993.

5. Ziegler AG, Hummel M, Schenker M, and Bonifacio E. Autoantibody appearance and risk for development of childhood diabetes in offspring of parents with type 1 diabetes: the 2-year analysis of the German BABYDIAB Study. Diabetes 48(3):460-8, 1999.

6. Riley, WJ, Maclaren NK, Krischer J, Spillar RP, Silverstein JH, Schatz DA, Schwartz S, Malone J, Shah S, Vadheim C et al. A prospective study of the development of diabetes in relatives of patients with insulin-dependent diabetes. N Engl J Med 323(17): 1167-72, 1990.

7. Yu, L, Robles DT, Abiru N, Kaur P, Rewers M, Kelemen K, Eisenbarth GS. Early expression of anti-insulin autoantibodies of humans and the NOD mouse: evidence for early determination of subsequent diabetes. Proc Natl Acad Sci USA 97(4):1701-6, 2000.

8. Eisenbarth GS, Gianani R, Yu L, Pietropaolo M, Verge CF, Chase HP, Redondo MJ, Colman P, Harrison L, and Jackson R. Dual-parameter model for prediction of type I diabetes mellitus. Proc Assoc Am Physicians 110(2): 126-35, 1998.

9. Schatz D, Krischer J, Horne G, Riley W, Spillar R, Silverstein J, Winter W, Muir A, Derovanesian D, Shah S, et al. Islet cell antibodies predict insulin-dependent diabetes in United States school age children as powerfully as in unaffected relatives. J Clin Invest 93(6):2403-7, 1994.

10. Madsbad S, Faber OK, Binder C, McNair P, Christiansen C, Transbol I. Prevalence of residual beta-cell function in insulin-dependent diabetics in relation to age at onset and duration of diabetes. Diabetes 27(Suppl 1):262-4, 1978.

11. Roder ME, Knip M, Hartling SG, Karjalainen J, Akerblom HK, and Binder C. Disproportionately elevated proinsulin levels precede the onset of insulin-dependent diabetes mellitus in siblings with low first phase insulin responses. The Childhood Diabetes in Finland Study Group. J Clin Endocrinol Metab 79(6):1570-5, 1994.

12. O'Meara NM, Sturis J, Herold KC, Ostrega DM, Polonsky KS, Alterations in the patterns of insulin secretion before and after diagnosis of IDDM. Diabetes Care 18(4):568-71, 1995.

13. Effect of intensive therapy on residual beta-cell function in patients with type 1 diabetes in the diabetes control and complications trial. A randomized, controlled trial. The Diabetes Control and Complications Trial Research Group. Ann Intern Med 128(7):517-23, 1998.

14. Carlsson A, Sundkvist G, Groop L, Tuomi T. Insulin and glucagon secretion in patients with slowly progressing autoimmune diabetes (LADA). J Clin Endocrinol Metab 85(1):76-80, 2000.
15. Delovitch TL, Singh B. The nonobese diabetic mouse as a model of autoimmune diabetes: immune dysregulation gets the NOD. Immunity 7(6):727-38, 1997.
16. Bertrand S, De Paepe M, Vigeant C, Yale JF. Prevention of adoptive transfer in BB rats by prophylactic insulin treatment. Diabetes 41(10): 1273-7, 1992.
17. Atkinson, MA, Maclaren NK, Luchetta R. Insulitis and diabetes in NOD mice reduced by prophylactic insulin therapy. Diabetes 39(8): 933-7, 1990.
18. Zhang ZJ, Davidson L, Eisenbarth G, Weiner HL. Suppression of diabetes in nonobese diabetic mice by oral administration of porcine insulin. Proc Natl Acad Sci U S A 88(22):10252-6, 1991.
19. Karounos DG, Bryson JS, Cohen DA. Metabolically inactive insulin analog prevents type I diabetes in prediabetic NOD mice. J Clin Invest 100(6):1344-8, 1997
20. Evavold BD, Sloan-Lancaster J, Allen PM. Tickling the TCR: selective T-cell functions stimulated by altered peptide ligands. Immunol Today 14(12):602-9, 199.
21. Lee HC, Kim SJ, Kim KS, Shin HC, Yoon JW. Remission in models of type 1 diabetes by gene therapy using a single- chain insulin analogue. Nature 408(6811): 483-8, 2000
22. Yoon JW, Yoon CS, Lim HW, Huang QQ, Kang Y, Pyun KH, Hirasawa K, Sherwin RS, Jun HS. Control of autoimmune diabetes in NOD mice by GAD expression or suppression in beta cells. Science 284(5417):1183-7, 199.
23. Tian J, Clare-Salzler M, Herschenfeld A, Middleton B, Newman D, Mueller R, Arita S, Evans C, Atkinson MA, Mullen Y, Sarvetnick N, Tobin AJ, Lehmann PV, Kaufman DL.Modulating autoimmune responses to GAD inhibits disease progression and prolongs islet graft survival in diabetes-prone mice. Nat Med 2(12):1348-53, 1996.
24. Quintana FJ, Rotem A, Carmi P, Cohen IR. Vaccination with empty plasmid DNA or CpG oligonucleotide inhibits diabetes in nonobese diabetic mice: modulation of spontaneous 60-kDa heat shock protein autoimmunity. J Immunol 165(11):6148-55, 2000.
25. Birk OS, Cohen IR. T-cell autoimmunity in type 1 diabetes mellitus. Curr Opin Immunol 5(6):903-9, 1993.
26. Birk OS, Douek DC, Elias D, Takacs K, Dewchand H, Gur SL, Walker MD, Van der Zee R, Cohen IR, Altmann DM. A role of Hsp60 in autoimmune diabetes: analysis in a transgenic model. Proc Natl Acad Sci U S A 93(3):1032-7, 1996.
27. Rothe H, Kolb H. Strategies of protection from nitric oxide toxicity in islet inflammation. J Mol Med 77(1):40-4, 1999.

28. Brod SA, Malone M, Darcan S, Papolla M, Nelson L. Ingested interferon alpha suppresses type I diabetes in non-obese diabetic mice. Diabetologia 41(10):1227-32, 199.

29. Chatenoud L, Thervet E, Primo J, Bach JF. Anti-CD3 antibody induces long-term remission of overt autoimmunity in nonobese diabetic mice. Proc Natl Acad Sci U S A 91(1):123-7, 1994.

30. Chatenoud L, Primo J, Bach JF. CD3 antibody-induced dominant self tolerance in overtly diabetic NOD mice. J Immunol 158(6):2947-54, 1997.

31. Fox CJ, Danska JS. IL-4 expression at the onset of islet inflammation predicts nondestructive insulitis in nonobese diabetic mice. J Immunol 158(5):2414-24, 1997.

32. Stiller CR, Dupre J, Gent M, Jenner MR, Keown PA, Laupacis A, Martell R, Rodger NW, von Graffenried B, WolfeBM. Effects of cyclosporine immunosuppression in insulin-dependent diabetes mellitus of recent onset. Science 223(4643):1362-7, 1984.

33. Bougneres PF, Carel JC, Castano L, Boitard C, Gardin JP, Landais P , Hors J, Mihatsch MJ, Paillard M, Chaussain JL et al. Factors associated with early remission of type I diabetes in children treated with cyclosporine. N Engl J Med 318(11):663-70, 1988.

34. De Filippo G, Carel JC, Boitard C, Bougneres PF. Long-term results of early cyclosporin therapy in juvenile IDDM. Diabetes 45(1):101-4, 1996.

35. Silverstein J, Maclaren N, Riley W, Spillar R, Radjenovic D, Johnson S. Immunosuppression with azathioprine and prednisone in recent-onset insulin-dependent diabetes mellitus. N Engl J Med 319(10):599-604, 1988.

36. Eisenbarth GS, Srikanta S, Jackson R, Rabinowe S, Dolinar R, Aoki T, Morris MA. Anti-thymocyte globulin and prednisone immunotherapy of recent onset type 1 diabetes mellitus. Diabetes Res 2(6):271-6, 1985.

37. Buckingham BA, Sandborg CI. A randomized trial of methotrexate in newly diagnosed patients with type 1 diabetes mellitus. Clin Immunol 96(2):86-90, 2000.

38. Shah SC, Malone JI, Simpson NE. A randomized trial of intensive insulin therapy in newly diagnosed insulin-dependent diabetes mellitus. N Engl J Med 320(9):550-4, 1989.

39. Keller RJ, Eisenbarth GS, Jackson RA. Insulin prophylaxis in individuals at high risk of type I diabetes. Lancet 341(8850):927-8, 1993.

40. Pozzilli P, Pitocco D, Visalli N, Cavallo MG, Buzzetti R, Crino A, Spera S, Suraci C, Multari G, Cervoni M, Manca Bitti ML, Matteoli MC, Marietti G, Ferrazzoli F, Cassone Faldetta MR, Giordano C, Sbriglia M, Sarugeri M, Ghirlanda G. No effect of oral insulin on residual beta-cell function in recent-onset type I diabetes (the IMDIAB VII). IMDIAB Group. Diabetologia 43(8):1000-4, 2000.

41. Elias D, Cohen IR. The hsp60 peptide p277 arrests the autoimmune diabetes induced by the toxin streptozotocin. Diabetes 1996. 45(9):1168-72, 2000.

42. Fuchtenbusch M, Rabl W, Grassl B, Bachmann W, Standl E, Ziegler AG. Delay of type I diabetes in high risk, first degree relatives by parenteral antigen administration: the Schwabing Insulin Prophylaxis Pilot Trial. Diabetologia 41(5):536-41, 1998.

43. Schatz DA, Bingley PJ. Update on major trials for the prevention of type 1 diabetes mellitus: the American Diabetes Prevention Trial (DPT-1) and the European Nicotinamide Diabetes Intervention Trial (ENDIT). J Pediatr Endocrinol Metab 14(Suppl 1): 619-22, 2001.

44. Edelstein SL, Knowler WC, Bain RP, Andres R, Barrett-Connor EL, Dowse GK, Haffner SM, Pettitt DJ, Sorkin JD, Muller DC, Collins VR, Hamman RF. Predictors of progression from impaired glucose tolerance to NIDDM: an analysis of six prospective studies. Diabetes 46(4):701-10, 1997.

45. Sato Y. Diabetes and life-styles: role of physical exercise for primary prevention. Br J Nutr 84 Suppl 2:S187-90, 2000.

46. Wing RR, Venditti E, Jakicic JM, Polley BA, Lang W. Lifestyle intervention in overweight individuals with a family history of diabetes. Diabetes Care 21(3):350-9, 1998.

47. Helmrich SP, Ragland DR, Leung RW, Paffenbarger Jr RS. Physical activity and reduced occurrence of non-insulin-dependent diabetes mellitus. N Engl J Med 325(3):147-52, 1991.

48. Eriksson KF, Lindgarde F. Prevention of type 2 (non-insulin-dependent) diabetes mellitus by diet and physical exercise. The 6-year Malmo feasibility study. Diabetologia 34(12):891-8, 1991.

49. Tuomilehto J, Lindstrom J, Eriksson JG, Valle TT, Hamalainen H, Ilanne-Parikka P, Keinanen-Kiukaanniemi S, Laakso M, Louheranta A, Rastas M, Salminen V, Uusitupa M. Prevention of type 2 diabetes mellitus by changes in lifestyle among subjects with impaired glucose tolerance. N Engl J Med 344(18): 1343-50, 2001.

50. The Diabetes Prevention Program Research Group. Reduction in the incidence of type 2 diabetes with lifestyle intervention or metformin. N Eng J. Med 346:393-403, 2002.

51. Henriksson J. Effects of physical training on the metabolism of skeletal muscle. Diabetes Care 15(11):1701-11, 1992.

52. Rodnick KJ, Holloszy JO, Mondon CE, James DE. Effects of exercise training on insulin-regulatable glucose-transporter protein levels in rat skeletal muscle. Diabetes 39(11):1425-9, 1990.

53. Devlin JT. Effects of exercise on insulin sensitivity in humans. Diabetes Care 15(11):1690-3, 1992.

54. Kuczmarski RJ, Flegal KM, Campbell SM, Johnson CL. Increasing prevalence of overweight among US adults. The National Health and Nutrition Examination Surveys, 1960 to 1991. Jama 272(3):205-11, 1994.

55. Manson JE, Spelsberg A. Primary prevention of non-insulin-dependent diabetes mellitus. Am J Prev Med 10(3):172-84, 1994.

56. Collins VR, Dowse GK, Toelupe PM, Imo TT, Aloaina FL, Spark RA, Zimmet PZ. Increasing prevalence of NIDDM in the Pacific island population of Western Samoa over a 13-year period. Diabetes Care 17(4):288-96, 1994.

57. Lillioja S, Mott DM, Howard BV, Bennett PH, Yki-Jarvinen H, Freymond D, Nyomba BL, Zurlo F, Swinburn B, Bogardus C. Impaired glucose tolerance as a disorder of insulin action. Longitudinal and cross-sectional studies in Pima Indians. N Engl J Med 318(19):1217-25, 1988.

58. Long SD, O'Brien K, MacDonald Jr KG, Leggett-Frazier N, Swanson MS, Pories WJ, Caro JF. Weight loss in severely obese subjects prevents the progression of impaired glucose tolerance to type II diabetes. A longitudinal interventional study. Diabetes Care 17(5):372-5, 1994.

59. Markovic TP, Jenkins AB, Campbell LV, Furler SM, Kraegen EW, Chisholm DJ. The determinants of glycemic responses to diet restriction and weight loss in obesity and NIDDM. Diabetes Care 21(5):687-94, 1998.

60. Kissebah AH, Vydelingum N, Murray R, Evans DJ, Hartz AJ, Kalkhoff RK, Adams PW. Relation of body fat distribution to metabolic complications of obesity. J Clin Endocrinol Metab 54(2):254-60, 1982.

61. Bjorntorp P. Abdominal obesity and the development of noninsulin-dependent diabetes mellitus. Diabetes Metab Rev 4(6):615-22, 1988.

62. Feskens EJ, Virtanen SM, Rasanen L, Tuomilehto J, Stengard J, Pekkanen J, Nissinen A, Kromhout D. Dietary factors determining diabetes and impaired glucose tolerance. A 20-year follow-up of the Finnish and Dutch cohorts of the Seven Countries Study. Diabetes Care 18(8):1104-12, 1995.

63. Marshall JA, Hoag S, Shetterly S, Hamman RF. Dietary fat predicts conversion from impaired glucose tolerance to NIDDM. The San Luis Valley Diabetes Study. Diabetes Care 17(1):50-6, 1994.

64. Swinburn BA, Metcalf PA, Ley SJ. Long-term (5-year) effects of a reduced-fat diet intervention in individuals with glucose intolerance. Diabetes Care 24(4):619-24, 2001.

65. McGarry JD, Dobbins RL. Fatty acids, lipotoxicity and insulin secretion. Diabetologia 42(2):128-38, 1999.

66. Houseknecht KL, Vanden Heuvel JP, Moya-Camarena SY, Portocarrero CP, Peck LW, Nickel KP, Belury MA. Dietary conjugated linoleic acid normalizes impaired glucose tolerance in the Zucker diabetic fatty fa/fa rat. Biochem Biophys Res Commun 1998. 244(3):678-82, 1999.

67. Fontbonne A, Charles MA, Juhan-Vague I, Bard JM, Andre P, Isnard F, Cohen JM, Grandmottet P, Vague P, Safar ME, Eschwege E. The effect of metformin on the metabolic abnormalities associated with upper-body fat distribution. BIGPRO Study Group. Diabetes Care 19(9):920-6, 1996.

68. Freemark M, Bursey D. The effects of metformin on body mass index and glucose tolerance in obese adolescents with fasting hyperinsulinemia and a family history of type 2 diabetes. Pediatrics 107(4):E55, 2001.

69. Cavaghan MK, Ehrmann DA, Byrne MM, Polonsky KS. Treatment with the oral antidiabetic agent troglitazone improves beta cell responses to glucose in subjects with impaired glucose tolerance. J Clin Invest 100(3):530-7, 1997.

70. Jia DM, Tabaru A, Nakamura H, Fukumitsu KI, Akiyama T, Otsuki M. Troglitazone prevents and reverses dyslipidemia, insulin secretory defects, and histologic abnormalities in a rat model of naturally occurring obese diabetes. Metabolism 49(9):1167-75, 2000.

71. Sreenan S, Sturis J, Pugh W, Burant CF, Polonsky KS. Prevention of hyperglycemia in the Zucker diabetic fatty rat by treatment with metformin or troglitazone. Am J Physiol 271(4 Pt 1): E742-7, 1996.

72. Nolan JJ, Ludvik B, Beerdsen P, Joyce M, Olefsky J. Improvement in glucose tolerance and insulin resistance in obese subjects treated with troglitazone. N Engl J Med, 1994. 331(18):1188-93.

73. Antonucci T, Whitcomb R, McLain R, Lockwood D, Norris RM. Impaired glucose tolerance is normalized by treatment with the thiazolidinedione troglitazone. Diabetes Care 20(2):188-93, 1997.

74. Smith SA, Lister CA, Toseland CD, Buckingham RE. Rosiglitazone prevents the onset of hyperglycaemia and proteinuria in the Zucker diabetic fatty rat. Diabetes Obes Metab 2(6):363-72, 2000.

75. Tafuri SR. Troglitazone enhances differentiation, basal glucose uptake, and Glut1 protein levels in 3T3-L1 adipocytes. Endocrinology 137(11):4706-12, 1996.

76. Tanaka Y, Gleason CE, Tran PO, Harmon JS, Robertson RP. Prevention of glucose toxicity in HIT-T15 cells and Zucker diabetic fatty rats by antioxidants. Proc Natl Acad Sci U S A 96(19):10857-62, 1999.

77. Yusuf S, Sleight P, Pogue J, Bosch J, Davies R, Dagenais G. Effects of an angiotensin-converting-enzyme inhibitor, ramipril, on cardiovascular events in high-risk patients. The Heart Outcomes Prevention Evaluation Study Investigators. N Engl J Med 342(3):145-53, 2000.

78. Carlsson PO, Berne C, Jansson L. Angiotensin II and the endocrine pancreas: effects on islet blood flow and insulin secretion in rats. Diabetologia 1998. 41(2):127-33, 2000.

Pertinent Internet Web Sites:
National Institutes of Health: www.nih.gov
National Institute of Diabetes & Digestive & Kidney Diseases: www.niddk.nih.gov
Juvenile Diabetes Research Foundation International: www.jdf.org

X. Resources for Patients with Diabetes

Eileen Reilly, Laura Ronen, and Mary Beyreuther

INTRODUCTION

Providing complete comprehensive care for the patient with diabetes can be challenging for the healthcare professional. It is often necessary to seek additional support from outside the office. The care of the diabetic patient can be supplemented by the input from organizations or agencies that can assist with the many facets of diabetes. The following list includes a number of diabetes resources available both for the general public and for the health professionals.

The Center for Disease Control and Prevention (CDC), the National Institutes of Health (NIH), and the Indian Health Service (IHS) are all agencies within the Department of Health and Human Services. The CDC seeks to promote healthy behaviors by providing accurate health information through its many partnerships. The IHS Diabetes Program concentrates on preventing and controlling diabetes within American Indian and Native Alaskan communities. Two of the institutes within the NIH that deal specifically with diabetes and diabetes-related disease are the National Institute of Diabetes and Digestive and Kidney Diseases (NIDDK) and the National Eye Institute (NEI).

The NIDDK disseminates information on diabetes related topics through its National Diabetes Clearinghouse. One can order copies of fact sheets or booklets on topics as varied as devices for taking insulin, complications of diabetes, Medicare coverage and financial assistance. The NIDDK sponsors research via its Diabetes Research and Training Centers. These centers are involved in diabetes education and community outreach as well.

The NEI was established to protect and prolong the vision of Americans. It conducts its own research and supports research at over 250 medical centers around the country. Laser treatment of diabetic retinopathy was developed in the course of NEI funded research. The NEI also conducts education programs to increase awareness of services and devices that are available for people with vision impairment.

The American Heart Association (AHA), the American Diabetes Association (ADA) and the American Dietetic Association are voluntary organizations dedicated to educating the public and to improving health.

The AHA promotes education and awareness, defines risk factors of heart disease and emphasizes the importance of screening. AHA also publishes research information, statistics and clinical guidelines.

The ADA's mission is to prevent and cure diabetes and to improve the lives of all people affected by the disease.

It does this with advocacy programs, funding research and providing information about type 1 and type 2 diabetes via its magazine, *Diabetes Forecast,* and website. Medications for diabetes are described in detail; new products, such as glucose monitoring devices, are reviewed. Guidelines for laboratory values are provided along with monitoring strategies. The website can link the consumers with free screenings, education programs and support groups in their local area.

The American Dietetic Association works at the state, local and national levels to influence policy on nutrition related issues. Some examples are food labeling, medical nutrition therapy and food programs. The association's website provides dietary advice on multiple topics, such as, for example, how to choose leaner cuts of meat, to decrease fat in recipes, to determine appropriate serving sizes and to improve the health value of holiday eating. One can also obtain a referral to a registered dietitian.

The above websites include strategies for reducing the risk of cardiovascular and cerebrovascular disease and for weight management. Information about recommended books, which can be purchased online, is also offered by these three groups.

The pharmaceutical industry is another strong asset that can be utilized in the care of the patients with diabetes. In addition to manufacturing medications, many companies provide educational pamphlets about their products as well as general diabetes education materials and support services. Pharmaceutical companies often have programs which assist indigent patients in obtaining medications. They also organize continuing education programs for those caring for these patients.

Manufacturers and suppliers of diabetes equipment donate supplies to patients that may not be able to afford these supplies and produce educational products to enhance understanding of the disease. Home blood glucose monitoring devices are often given freely to diabetes centers. This measure not only relieves the patient of the financial burden of purchasing this device, but also enables the diabetes educator to demonstrate the process of measuring blood glucose and to observe the patients' ability to perform this measurement accurately.

Journals offer information, which can supplement the diabetes education provided by the diabetes team, and offer health tips or guidelines for managing diabetes. An issue may be devoted to heart disease, hyperlipidemia, or foot care and may give suggestions on how to handle some difficult scenarios encountered in daily life.

Patients contribute by writing or offering support or advice on a particular topic. Some journals offer a "pen pal" section where patients can correspond with others who have similar interests.

Agencies, such as the American Foundation for the Blind and the National Limb Loss Information Center, can assist patients who developed some of the devastating complications of diabetes. These agencies can provide information about support groups and local resources. There are international associations that also help meet the needs of the diabetic patient.

The list below consists of the most reliable providers of information. Information obtained from these resources can help to augment a patient's understanding of diabetes, but should not be used to replace a comprehensive evaluation by a diabetes team consisting of a physician, a diabetes nurse educator and a registered dietitian.

ASSOCIATIONS:
American Association of Clinical Endocrinologists (AACE)
1000 Riverside Avenue, Suite 205
Jacksonville, FL 32304
Phone: (904) 353-7878
Fax: (904) 353-8185
Internet: http://www.aace.com

American Association of Diabetes Educators
444 North Michigan Avenue, suite 1240
Chicago, Illinois 60611
Phone: (312) 424-2426
Fax: (312) 424-2427
Diabetes Educator Access Line: (800) 832-6874
Internet: http://www.aadenet.org

American Diabetes Association
1660 Duke Street
Alexandria, Virginia 22314
Phone: (888) 342-2387
Fax: (703) 549-6995
http://www.diabetes.org

American Dietetic Association
216 West Jackson Boulevard, Suite 800
Chicago, Illinois 60606-6995
Phone: (312) 899-0040, (800) 342-2383, (800) 366-1655 (consumer nutrition hotline)
Fax: (800) 899-1976
Internet: http://www.eatright.org

American Heart Association
National Center
7272 Greenville Avenue
Dallas, Texas 75231
Phone: (214) 373-6300; check individual states for local chapter phone numbers.
Internet: http://www.americanheart.org

American Podiatric Medical Association (APMA)
9312 Old Georgetown Road
Bethesda, MD 20814-1698
Phone: (800) 366-8227
Fax: (301) 530-2752
Internet: http://www.apma.org

Diabetes Exercise and Sports Association (DESA)
1647 West Bethany Home Road, #B
Phoenix, AZ 85015
Phone: (800) 898-4322
Fax: (602) 433-9331
Internet: http://www.diabetes-exercise.org

Endocrine Society
4350 East West Highway, Suite 500
Bethesda, MD 20814-4410
Phone: (301) 941-0200
Fax: (301) 941-0259
Internet: http://www.endo-society.org

Juvenile Diabetes Research Foundation International (JDRF)
120 Wall Street, 19th floor
New York, NY 10005
Phone: (800) 533-2873, (212) 785-9500
Fax: (212) 785-9595
Internet: http://www.jdrf.org

National Kidney Foundation
30 East 33rd Street, Suite 1100
New York, NY 10016
Phone: (800) 622-9010
Internet: http://www.kidney.org

Pedorthic Footwear Association (PFA)
7150 Columbia Gateway Drive, Suite G
Columbia, MD 21046-1151
Phone: (800) 673-8447
Fax: (410) 381-1167
Internet: http://www.pedorthics.org

ASSOCIATIONS FOR PEOPLE WITH DISABILITIES:
American Foundation for the Blind
15 West 16th Street
NYC, NY 10011
Phone: (800) 232-5463

National Federation of the Blind
1800 Johnson Street
Baltimore, MD 21230
Phone (410) 659-9314
Internet: http://www.nfb.com

National Limb Loss Information Center
900 East Hill Avenue Suite 285
Knoxville, TN 37915-2568
Phone: (888) 267-5669
Internet: http://www.nllicfo@amputee-coaltion.org

INTERNATIONAL ASSOCIATIONS:
British Diabetic Association
10 Queen Anne Street
London W1G9LH
ENGLAND
Phone: 020-7323-1531
Internet: http://www.diabetes.org.uk

Canadian Diabetes Association
15 Toronto Street, Suite 800
Toronto, Ontario M5C2E3
CANADA
Phone: (416) 363-3373
Internet: http://www.diabetes.ca

Diabetes New Zealand
Wilford House
115 Molesworth Street
Thorndon, Wellington
NEW ZEALAND
Phone: 64 4 499 7145
Internet: http://www.diabetes.org.nz

International Diabetes Institute
260 Kooyoong road
Caulfield, Victoria 3162
AUSTRALIA
Phone: (03) 9258-5050
Internet: http://www.idi.org.au

International Diabetic Athletes Association
1647-B West Bethany Home Road
Phoenix, Arizona 85015
Phone: (800) 898-4322; (602) 433-2113

GOVERNMENT AGENCIES:
Centers for Disease Control and Prevention
National Center for Chronic Disease Prevention and Health Promotion
Division of Diabetes Translation
2858 Woodcock Boulevard
Davidson Building
Atlanta, GA 30341-4002
Phone: (877)-232-3422
Internet: http://www.cdc.gov/diabetes

Indian Health Service
Diabetes Program
5300 Homestead Road, N.E.
Albuquerque, New Mexico 87110
Phone: (505) 248-4182
Fax: (505) 248-4188
Internet: http://www.ihs.gov/medicalprograms/diabetes

National Diabetes Education Program
1 Information Way
Bethesda, Maryland 20892-3560
Phone: (800) 438-5383
Internet: http://ndep.nih.gov

National Diabetes Information Clearinghouse (NDIC)
1 Information Way
Bethesda, MD 20892-3560
Phone: (800) 860-8747
Internet: http://www.niddk.nih.gov/health/diabetes/diabetes.htm

National Eye Institute
National Eye Health Education Program
2020 Vision Place
Bethesda Maryland 20892-3633
Phone: (800) 869-2020 (to order materials); (301)-496-5248
Internet: http://www.nei.nih.gov

U.S. Public Health Service
Office of Minority Health Resource Center
P.O. Box 37337
Washington, DC 20013-7337
Phone: (800) 444-6472
Fax: (301) 230-7198
Internet: http://www.niddk-nih.gov/health/diabetes/ndic.htm

OUTREACH PROGRAMS:
Diabetes Assistance & Resources Program (DAR)
Phone: (888)-Diabetes
Internet: http://www.diabetes.org/dar

African American Program
Phone: (888)-Diabetes
Internet: http://www.diabetes.org/africanamerican

Awakening the Spirit
Phone: (888)-Diabetes
Internet: http://www.diabetes.org.awakening

JOURNALS:
Diabetes Self Management
P.O. box 52890
Boulder, CO 80322-2890
Phone: (800) 234-0923
Internet: http://diabetes-self-mgmt.com

Diabetes Forecast
1701 North Beauregard Street
Alexandria, VA 22311
Phone: (800) 806-7801
Internet: http://www.diabetes.org/diabetesforecast

Diabetes Interview
6 School Street, Suite 160
Fairfax, Ca 94930
Phone: (800) 488-8468
Internet: http://www.diabetes interview.com

PHARMACEUTICAL COMPANIES and MEDICAL EQUIPMENT MANUFACTURERS :

Abbott Laboratories Inc.
MediSense Products
4A Crosby Drive
Bedford, MA 01730-1402
Phone: (800) 527-3339
Internet: http://www.abbottdiagnostics.com

Amira
4742 Scotts Valley Drive
Scotts Valley, CA 95066
Phone: (800) 654-0619
Internet: http://www.amira.com

Animas
590 Lancaster Avenue
Frazer, PA 19355
Phone: (877) 937-7867
Internet: http://www.animascorp.com

Aventis Pharmaceuticals
300 Somerset Corporate Boulevard
P.O. Box 6977
Bridgewater, NJ 08807-0977
Phone: (800) 207-8049 Indigent Program (800) 321-0855
Internet: http://www.diabeteswatch.com

Bayer Pharmaceuticals
400 Morgan Lane
West Haven, CT 06516
Phone: (800) 288-8371 Indigent Patient (800) 998-91080
Internet: http://www.pharma.bayer.com

BD Consumer Healthcare
11 Jennifer drive
Holmdel, NJ 07733
Phone: (800) 316-1611
Internet: http://www.bd.com

Bristol-Myers Squibb
602 White Oak Ridge Road
Short Hills, NJ 07078
Phone: (800) 332-2056 Patient Assistance (800) 437-0994
Internet: http://www.bms.com

Can-Am Care
Cimetra Industrial Park Box 98
Chazy, NY 12921
Phone: (800) 461-4414
Internet: http://www.invernessmedical.com

Cell Robotics Inc.
Personal Lasette
2715 Broadbent Parkway, NE
Albuquerque, NM 87107
Phone: (800) 846-0590 ext. 100
Internet: http://www.cellrobotics.com

Disetronic
5151 Program Avenue
St. Paul, MN 55112
Phone: (800) 280-7801
Internet: http://www.disetronic-usa.com

Eli Lilly and Company
82 Plymouth Avenue
Maplewood, NJ 07040
Phone: (800) 545-5979 Lilly Cares (800) 545-6962
Internet: http://www.lilly.com

Glaxo SmithKline Beecham Pharmaceuticals
45 River Drive South
Jersey City, NJ 07310
Phone: (888) 825-5249 Patient Assistance (888) 825-5249
Internet: http://www.gsk.com

Lifescan
1000 Gibraltar Drive
Milpitas, CA 95035-6312
Phone: (800) 227-8862
Internet: http://www.lifescan.com

Medic Alert Foundation
2323 Colorado Avenue
Turlock, CA 95382
Phone: (888) 633-4298
Internet: http://medicalert.org

Minimed
263 Nob Hill Drive
Elmsford, NY 10523
Phone: (800) 646-4633
International Headquarters Phone: (818) 362-5958
Internet: http://www.minimed.com

Novo Nordisk
100 College Road West
Princeton, NJ 08540
Phone: (800) 727-6500 Indigent Program (800) 727-6500
Internet: http://www.novonordisk.com

Paddock Laboratories Inc.
3940 Quebec Avenue North
Minneapolis, MN 55427
Phone: (800) 328-5113
Fax: (763) 546-4842
Internet: http://paddocklabs.com

Pfizer
Pfizer for Living
P.O. Box 29179
Shawnee Mission, KS 66201-9911
Phone: (888) 999-5657 Pfizer Prescription Assistance
Internet: www.pfizer.com

Roche Diagnostics
9115 Hague Road
P.O. Box 50457
Indianapolis, IN 46256
Phone: (317) 845-2000
Internet: http://www.roche.com

Therasense
1360 South Loop Road
Alameda, CA 94502
Phone: (888) 522-5226
Internet: http://www.therasense.com

DIABETES PRODUCT SUPPLY COMPANIES:
American Medical Supplies
P.O. Box 294009
Boca Raton, FL 33429-4009
Phone: (800) 575-2345
Internet: http://www.diabeticmedicare.com

Diabetic Care Center
31122 Vine Street
Cleveland, OH 44095
Phone: (800) 633-7167
Internet: http://www.diabeticare.com

Diabetic Express
31128 Vine Street
Phone: (800) 338-4656
Internet: http://www.diabeticexpress.com

Diabetic Healthcare Services
P.O. Box 309
Hudson, OH 44236
Phone: (800) 353-7318
Internet: no current website available

Diabetic Promotions
P.O. Box 5400
Willowick, OH 44095-0400
Phone: (800) 433-1477
Internet: http://www.info@diabeticpromotions.com

Express Med
6530 West Campus Oval
New Albany, OH 43054-8777
Phone: (800) 651-4902
Internet: http://www.expressmed.com

Liberty Medical Supply Inc.
10045 South Federal Highway
Port St. Lucie, FL 34952
Phone: (800) 633-2001
Internet: http://www.libertymedical.com

INDEX

trans-golgi network 72
treatment of type 1 diabetes mellitus 569
tricylic antidepressants 647
triglycerides 460
troglitazone 713, 749, 750
Troglitazone in Prevention of Diabetes (TRIPOD) Study 604
tumor necrosis factor (TNF) 82, 320, 728
twin studies 126, 180, 657
type 1 diabetes 100, 153
type 1a diabetes 153
type 1b diabetes 153
type 2 diabetes mellitus 64, 101, **179**
type A insulin resistance syndrome 263
type B insulin resistance syndrome 266
tyrosine kinase 79
UKPDS (see United Kingdom Prospective Diabetes Study)
Ultralente insulin 575
uncoupling proteins 659
unequal limb syndrome 399
United Kingdom Prospective Diabetes Study (UKPDS) 29, 294, 319, 331, 344, 357, **498**, 597, 607, **619**
University Group Diabetes Program (UGDP) 621
University of Texas (UT) Risk Classification System 401
vacuum device 430
vagal activation 67
vagotomy 66
vascular endothelial growth factor (VEGF) 320, 335
vascular endothelium 386
vasoactive intestinal polypeptide (VIP) 67, 421, 441
venous beading 333
very low density lipoproteins (VLDL) 462

Veterans Affairs Cooperative Study in Glycemia Control 499, 622
VIPoma 239
Virchow, Rudolph 23
virilization 259
viruses 118, 161
vision loss 339
vitamins 536
vitiligo 483
von Hohenheim (Paracelsus) 20
von Mering, Joseph 22
Wagner A 26
waist circumference
waist to hip or waist to thigh ratios
warning symptoms for hypoglycemia 300
Watanabe CK 26
weight goals 661
weight loss 532, 553, 604, 712, 747
weight regulation 658
Willis, Thomas 21
Wisconsin Epidemiologic Study of Diabetic Retinopathy (WESDR) 330, 495, 623
Wolfram syndrome 123
World Health Organization 222, 729
xanthoderma 481
Yalow RS 27
Zollinger-Ellison (ZE) syndrome 239
Zucker diabetic fatty rat 65, 749
Zuelzer, Georg Ludwig 23